Brain Injury Medicine:
Board Review

Brain Injury Medicine:
Board Review

Brain Injury Medicine: Board Review

First Edition

Blessen C. Eapen, MD

Chief
Physical Medicine and Rehabilitation
VA Greater Los Angeles Health Care System
Los Angeles, California
United States
Associate Clinical Professor
Department of Medicine
Division of Physical Medicine and Rehabilitation
David Geffen School of Medicine at UCLA
Los Angeles, CA, United States

David X. Cifu, MD

Associate Dean for Innovation and Systems Integration
Herman J. Flax Professor
Chairman
Department of Physical Medicine and Rehabilitation
Virginia Commonwealth University School of Medicine
Richmond, Virginia
United States
Senior TBI Specialist
U.S. Department of Veterans Affairs
Principal Investigator
Chronic Effects of NeuroTrauma Consortium (CENC-LIMBIC)

ELSEVIER

Elsevier
1600 John F. Kennedy Blvd.
Ste 1800
Philadelphia, PA 19103-2899

BRAIN INJURY MEDICINE: BOARD REVIEW, FIRST EDITION   ISBN: 978-0-323-65385-5

Library of Congress Control Number: 2020936404

Content Strategist: Humayra R. Khan
Director, Content Development: Ellen Wurm-Cutter
Senior Content Development Specialist: Kathleen Nahm
Publishing Services Manager: Shereen Jameel
Project Manager: Aparna Venkatachalam
Designer: Bridget Hoette

Printed in China

Last digit is the print number: 9 8 7 6 5 4 3 2

Working together
to grow libraries in
developing countries

www.elsevier.com • www.bookaid.org

Blessen C. Eapen, MD

To my devoted parents, Eapen M. Chacko and Aleyamma Eapen,
for your unwavering support, love, prayers, and always believing in me.
To my loving wife, Tracy, and my sons, Elijah and Ayden, for continuing
to inspire me to be a better person, husband, and father.
To my brother, Binay, for being my role model and to all of my family
and friends for your continuous words of encouragement and support.
To my VA Greater Los Angeles family, to my current and past trainees,
and to my mentors for keeping me honest and pushing me to be a better teacher,
researcher, and physician.
To all the busy clinicians who took time out of their busy schedules to author
chapters in this book and for their dedication to caring for brain injury survivors
and advancing the field of brain injury medicine.
Finally, I would like to thank God, without whom none of this would be possible.

David X. Cifu, MD

I would like to dedicate this book to the people in my life who give me joy
and make me a better person—Hilary, Gabriella, and Isabelle—and to the members
of my teams in Richmond and nationally who give me support and make me a better
academician.

Contributors

Ruth E. Alejandro, MD, FAAPMR
Attending Physician
Pediatric Rehabilitation Medicine Department
Blythedale Children's Hospital
TBI Inpatient Unit & Day Hospital
Program Site Director, NYPH/Columbia & Cornell
    PM&R residency program
Program Site Director, NYMC/Metropolitan Hospital
    PM&R residency program
Valhalla, NY
United States
Assistant Clinical Professor
Department of Rehabilitation and Regenerative Medicine
New York Presbyterian Hospital - Columbia University
    College of Physicians & Surgeons
New York, NY
United States

Gemayaret Alvarez, MD
Assistant Professor
Physical Medicine and Rehabilitation
University of Miami
Miami, Florida
United States
Medical Director of Neurorehabilitation
Jackson Memorial Hospital
Miami, Florida
United States

Dixie Aragaki, MD
Professor
Department of Medicine, Division of PM&R
David Geffen School of Medicine at UCLA
Los Angeles, California
United States
Program Director
PM&R Residency
VA Greater Los Angeles Healthcare System
Los Angeles, California
United States

Breton M. Asken, PhD, ATC
Postdoctoral Neuropsychology Fellow
Department of Neurology
Memory and Aging Center
University of California, San Francisco
San Francisco, California
United States

Abana Azariah, MD
Brain Injury Medicine Fellow
Brain Injury, Physical Medicine and Rehabilitation
Moss Rehab/Einstein Healthcare Network
Elkins Park, Pennsylvania
United States

Nazanin Bahraini, PhD
Director of Education
Rocky Mountain MIRECC
Department of Veterans Affairs
Aurora, Colorado
United States
Associate Professor
Psychiatry
University of Colorado School of Medicine
Aurora, Colorado
United States
Associate Professor
Physical Medicine & Rehabilitation
University of Colorado School of Medicine
Aurora, Colorado
United States

K. Chase Bailey, PhD, ABPP-CN
Assistant Professor
Psychiatry
University of Texas Southwestern Medical Center
Dallas, Texas
United States

Jaclyn Barcikowski, DO, MA
Attending Physician
Physical Medicine and Rehabilitation
Moss Rehab
Elkins Park, Pennsylvania
United States

Saurabha Bhatnagar, MD, FAAPMR
Chief Medical Officer
Head of Technology and Performance
United Health Care
Instructor
Harvard Medical School
Boston, Massachusetts
Untied States

Sheital Bavishi, DO
Assistant Professor–Clinical
Physical Medicine and Rehabilitation
The Ohio State University Wexner Medical Center
Columbus, Ohio
United States
Medical Director, Brain Injury Program
Dodd Inpatient Rehabilitation Hospital
The Ohio State University Wexner Medical Center
Columbus, Ohio
United States
Residency Program Director
Department of Physical Medicine and Rehabilitation
The Ohio State University
Columbus, Ohio
United States

James J. Begley, MD, MS
Assistant Professor
Physical Medicine & Rehabilitation
Case Western Reserve University
Cleveland, Ohio
United States
Brain Injury Medicine Fellowship Program Director
Case Western Reserve University/MetroHealth Program
Director, Stroke Rehabilitation
MetroHealth Rehabilitation Institute
Columbus, Ohio
United States

Kimberly Benson, PT, DPT
Polytrauma/TBI Rehabilitation Research Fellow
Physical Medicine and Rehabilitation Service
Veterans Affairs Medical Center
Washington, District of Columbia
United States

Amy O. Bowles, MD
Chief, Brain Injury Rehabilitation Service
Department of Rehabilitation Medicine
Brooke Army Medical Center, JBSA
Ft. Sam Houston, Texas
United States
Associate Professor
Department of Rehabilitation Medicine
Uniformed Services University of the Health Sciences
Bethesda, Maryland
United States
Adjunct Associate Professor
Department of Rehabilitation Medicine
University of Texas Health Science Center at San Antonio
San Antonio, Texas
United States

Juan Cabrera, MD
Assistant Professor
Department of Physical Medicine & Rehabilitation
UT Southwestern Medical Center
Dallas, Texas
United States

David Cancel, MD, JD
Director
Pediatric Rehabilitation Medicine Fellowship
Albert Einstein College of Medicine/Montefiore Medical
    Center
Bronx, New York
United States
Assistant Professor
Physical Medicine and Rehabilitation
Montefiore Medical Center
Bronx, New York
United States

Douglas B. Cooper, PhD
Senior Scientific Director
Defense and Veterans Brain Injury Center
San Antonio VA Polytrauma Rehabilitation Center
San Antonio, Texas
United States
Adjunct Associate Professor
Department of Psychiatry
University of Texas Health Science Center (UT-Health)
San Antonio, Texas
United States

Stephen Correia, PhD, ABPP-CN
Director of Research
Memory & Aging Program
Butler Hospital
Director of Psychology
Butler Hospital
Associate Professor
Department of Psychiatry and Human Behavior
Brown University
Providence, Rhode Island
United States

Kelly M. Crawford, MD
Assistant Professor
Department of Physical Medicine and Rehabilitation
Carolinas Rehabilitation
Charlotte, North Carolina
United States
Medical Director
Brain Injury Program
Carolinas Rehabilitation
Charlotte, North Carolina
United States
Program Director
Brain Injury Medicine Fellowship
Carolinas Rehabilitation
Charlotte, North Carolina
United States

Jovany Cruz Navarro, MD
Assistant Professor
Anesthesiology
Assistant Professor
Neurosurgery
Baylor College of Medicine
Houston, Texas
United States

Laurie Dabaghian, MD
**Director of Consult Services at Hackensack University
  Medical Center**
Department of Physical Medicine & Rehabilitation
JFK Johnson Rehabilitation Institute
Edison, New Jersey
United States

Kevin Dalal, MD
Assistant Professor
Physical Medicine and Rehabilitation
University of Miami
Miami, Florida
United States

Samantha DeDios-Stern, PhD
Clinical Neuropsychology Postdoctoral Fellow
Psychiatry
University of Illinois at Chicago
Chicago, Illinois
United States

Yi Deng, MD
Assistant Professor
Anesthesiology
Baylor College of Medicine
Houston, Texas
United States

Sima A. Desai, MD
Assistant Professor
Physical Medicine and Rehabilitation
Carolinas Rehabilitation
Charlotte, North Carolina
United States

Craig DiTommaso, MD
Medical Director
Physical Medicine and Rehabilitation
Post Acute Medical Rehabilitation of Humble
Humble, Texas
United States

Blessen C. Eapen, MD
Chief
Physical Medicine and Rehabilitation
VA Greater Los Angeles Health Care System
Los Angeles, California
United States
Associate Professor
Department of Medicine
UCLA
Los Angeles, California
United States

Jason Edwards, DO
Brain Injury Medicine Fellow
Physical Medicine & Rehabilitation
Northwestern University Feinberg School of Medicine
Shirley Ryan Ability Lab
Chicago, Illinois
United States

David L. Eng, MD
Resident
Physical Medicine and Rehabilitation
UT Southwestern Medical Center
Dallas, Texas
United States

Dmitry Esterov, DO
Instructor
Physical Medicine and Rehabilitation
Mayo Clinic
Rochester, Minnesota
United States

Christopher M. Falco, MD
Assistant Professor
Physical Medicine and Rehabilitation
McGovern Medical School at the University of Texas
  Health Sciences Center at Houston
Houston, Texas
United States
Medical Director
Neurobehavioral Program
TIRR Memorial Hermann Hospital
Houston, Texas
United States

Samantha Fernandez Hernandez, MD
Research Coordinator
Neurosurgery
Baylor College of Medicine
Houston, Texas
United States

Lauren E. Fulks, MD
Resident Physician
Physical Medicine and Rehabilitation
University of Texas Southwestern
Dallas, Texas
United States

Heidi Fusco, MD
Assistant Professor of Rehabilitation Medicine
Department of Physical Medicine and Rehabilitation
New York University Langone Medical Center
New York, New York
United States

Gary Noel Galang, MD
Director of TBI Services
PMR
UPMC
Pittsburgh, Pennsylvania
United States

Ekua Gilbert-Baffoe, MD
Brain Injury Medicine Fellow
Physical Medicine and Rehabilitation
JFK Johnson Rehabilitation Institute
Edison, New Jersey
United States

Jessica M. Gill, PhD, RN, FAAN
Senior Investigator
Intramural Research Program
Bethesda, Maryland
United States

David Glazer, MD, FABPMR (BIM)
Medical Director
Polytrauma Rehabilitation Center
McGuire VA Medical Center
Richmond, Virginia
United States
Assistant Professor
Department of Physical Medicine and Rehabilitation
Virginia Commonwealth University School of Medicine
Richmond, Virginia
United States

Gary Goldberg, BASc, MD, FABPMR (BIM)
Clinical Adjunct Professor
Physical Medicine and Rehabilitation
Medical College of Virginia
Virginia Commonwealth University Health System
Richmond, Virginia
United States
Director, Electrodiagnostic Center
Physical Medicine and Rehabilitation Service
Hunter Holmes McGuire VA Medical Center
Richmond, Virginia
United States

David Andrés González, PhD, ABPP-CN
Clinical Assistant Professor
Department of Neurology
University of Texas Health Science Center at San Antonio
San Antonio, Texas
United States

Christine Greiss, DO
Director, The Concussion Program
Clinical Assistant Professor
Physical Medicine & Rehabilitation
Hackensack Meridian Health–JFK Johnson Rehabilitation
    Institute
Edison, New Jersey
United States

Zaid Haddadin, MD, PhD
Resident Physician
Radiology
UCLA
Los Angeles, California
United States

Saman Hazany, MD
Neuroradiologist
Greater Los Angeles VA Healthcare System
Los Angeles, California
United States
Associate Professor of Radiology
David Geffen School of Medicine at UCLA
Associate Professor of Radiology
Keck School of Medicine of USC
Los Angeles, California
United States

Kelly M. Heath, MD, FABPMR (BIM)
Assistant Professor
Physical Medicine and Rehabilitation
University of Pennsylvania
Philadelphia, Pennsylvania
United States
Director Polytrauma Rehabilitation
Rehabilitation Medicine
CMC Veterans Health Care System
Philadelphia, Pennsylvania
United States

Justin Sup Hong, MD
Brain Injury Program Director
Penn State Health Rehabilitation Hospital
Hummelstown, Pennsylvania
United States
Brain Injury Medicine Fellowship Director
Assistant Professor
Department of Physical Medicine and Rehabilitation
Penn State College of Medicine
Hershey, Pennsylvania
United States

Peter Horvath, MD
International Research Scholar
Department of Neurosurgery
Virginia Commonwealth University
Richmond, Virginia
United States
PhD Student
Department of Neurosurgery
University of Pecs
Pecs, Baranya
Hungary

Jimmy C. Huang, MD
Radiology
VA Greater Los Angeles Health Care System
Los Angeles, California
United States
Associate Clinical Professor
Department of Radiological Sciences
UCLA
Los Angeles, California
United States

Brian Im, MD
Director of Brain Injury Rehabilitation
Assistant Professor
NYU Department of Physical Medicine and Rehabilitation
NYU Rusk Rehabilitation
New York, New York
United States

Neil Jasey, MD
Director
Brain Injury Services
Kessler Institute for Rehabilitation
West Orange, New Jersey
United States
Director
Brain Injury Medicine Fellowship Program
Rutgers/NJMS
Newark, New Jersey
United States
Clinical Associate Professor
Physical Medicine and Rehabilitation
Rutgers/New Jersey Medical School
Newark, New Jersey
United States

Dara D. Jones, MD
Fellow
Physical Medicine & Rehabilitation
Montefiore Medical Center
Bronx, New York
United States

Cherry Junn, MD
Assistant Professor
Program Director, Brain Injury Medicine Fellowship
Rehabilitation Medicine
University of Washington
Seattle, Washington
United States

Jan Kennedy, PhD
Senior Clinical Research Director
Defense & Veterans Brain Injury Center
General Dynamics Information Technology
Falls Church, Virginia
United States
Neuropsychologist
Neurology Service/DVBIC
Brooke Army Medical Center
Ft. Sam Houston, Texas
United States

Kimbra Kenney, MD
Associate Professor
Neurology
Uniformed Services University of the Health Sciences
Bethesda, Maryland
United States
Service Chief, Research Operations
NICoE
WRNMMC
Bethesda, Maryland
United States

Daniel W. Klyce, PhD, ABPP
Assistant Professor
Board Certified Rehabilitation Psychologist
Department of Physical Medicine and Rehabilitation
Virginia Commonwealth University School of Medicine
Richmond, Virginia
United States

Sunil Kothari, MD
Assistant Professor
H. Ben Taub Department of Physical Medicine and
    Rehabilitation
Baylor College of Medicine
Houston, Texas
United States
Attending Physician
Brain Injury & Stroke Program
TIRR–Memorial Hermann
Houston, Texas
United States

Richard D. Kunz, MD
Assistant Clinical Professor
Physical Medicine and Rehabilitation
VCU Health System
Richmond, Virginia
United States

Kirk Lercher, MD, MBS
Director
Brain Injury Medicine
Department of Rehabilitation and Human Performance
Mount Sinai Medical Center
New York, New York
United States
Director
Brain Injury Medicine Fellowship Program
Icahn School of Medicine at Mount Sinai Hospital
New York, New York
United States
Assistant Professor
Department of Rehabilitation and Human Performance
Icahn School of Medicine at Mount Sinai Hospital
New York, New York
United States

Jaime M. Levine, DO
Medical Director
Brain Injury Rehabilitation, Extended Recovery Unit
Physical Medicine and Rehabilitation
JFK–Johnson Rehabilitation Institute
Edison, New Jersey
United States
Assistant Clinical Professor
Physical Medicine and Rehabilitation
Rutgers–Robert Wood Johnson Medical School
New Brunswick, New Jersey
United States
Assistant Clinical Professor
Physical Medicine and Rehabilitation
Hackensack Meridian School of Medicine at Seton Hall
    University
Jersey City, New Jersey
United States

Katherine Lin, MD
Polytrauma/Traumatic Brain Injury Fellow
Department of Rehabilitation
South Texas Veterans Healthcare System
San Antonio, Texas
United States

Matthew Lin, MD
Assistant Professor
Physical Medicine and Rehabilitation
McGovern Medical School at UTHealth
Houston, TX
United State

Rani Haley Lindberg, MD
Associate Professor
Physical Medicine and Rehabilitation
University of Arkansas for Medical Sciences
Little Rock, Arkansas
United States

Geoffrey S.F. Ling, MD, PhD
Professor
Neurology
Johns Hopkins
Baltimore, Maryland
United States
Interim Vice Chair for Research
Neuroscience and Spine Institute
Inova Fairfax Hospital
Fairfax, Virginia
United States

Susan Loughlin, PharmD, BCPS
Clinical Pharmacist
Pharmacy
TIRR Memorial Hermann Hospital
Houston, Texas
United States

Suzanne McGarity, PhD
Clinical Psychologist
Rocky Mountain MIRECC for Suicide Prevention
Rocky Mountain Regional VA Medical Center
Aurora, Colorado
United States
Department of Physical Medicine and Rehabilitation
University of Colorado School of Medicine
Aurora, Colorado
United States

Meghan J. McHenry, MD
Chief, Physical Medicine and Rehabilitation
Department of Pain Management
Brooke Army Medical Center
San Antonio, Texas
United States

Ondrea McKay, MD
Assistant Professor
Physical Medicine & Rehabilitation
Rutgers New Jersey Medical School
Newark, New Jersey
United States

Stephen T. Mernoff, MD, FAAN
Associate Professor of Neurology, Clinician Educator
Alpert Medical School of Brown University
Providence, Rhode Island
United States
Chief, Neurology Section
Providence VA Medical Center
Providence, Rhode Island
United States

Lindsay Mohney, DO
Assistant Professor
Physical Medicine and Rehabilitation
University of Arkansas for Medical Sciences
Little Rock, Arkansas
United States

Emma Nally, MD
Attending Physician
Physical Medicine and Rehabilitation
MedStar National Rehabilitation Hospital
Washington, District of Columbia
United States

Benjamin N. Nguyen, MD
Professor
PM&R
University of Texas Southwestern Medical Center
Dallas, Texas
United States

Morgan O'Connor, MD
Attending Physician
Interventional Pain Management
Spine & Nerve Diagnostic Center
Roseville, California
United States

Justin B. Otis, MD
Neuropsychiatry Fellow
Behavioral Neurology
Neurology
University of Colorado School of Medicine
Aurora, Colorado
United States

Sanjog Pangarkar, MD
Professor
Department of Medicine, Division of PM&R
David Geffen School of Medicine at UCLA
Los Angeles, CA, United States
Director, Inpatient & Interventional Pain Service
Department of Physical Medicine & Rehabilitation
Department of Veterans Affairs
Los Angeles, California
United States

Komal G. Patel, DO
Brain injury medicine fellow
Physical Medicine and Rehabilitation
Donald and Barbara Zucker School of Medicine at
    Hofstra/Northwell Health
Manhasset, New York
United States

Claudia Robertson, MD
Professor
Department of Neurosurgery
Baylor College of Medicine
Houston, Texas
United States

Rosanna C. Sabini, DO
Associate Professor
Physical Medicine & Rehabilitation
Donald and Barbara Zucker School of Medicine at
    Hofstra/Northwell
Hempstead, New York
United States
Program Director, Brain Injury Medicine Fellowship
Physical Medicine & Rehabilitation
Donald and Barbara Zucker School of Medicine at Hofstra/
    Northwell
Manhasset, New York
United States
Director
Northwell Health Concussion Program
New York
United States
Chair
Physical Medicine & Rehabilitation
Southside Hospital - Northwell Health
Bay Shore, New York
United States

Fabienne Saint-Preux, MD
Resident Physician
Department of Physical Medicine and Rehabilitation
New York University Langone Medical Center
New York, New York
United States

Angelle Sander, PhD, FACRM
Associate Professor
H. Ben Taub Department of Physical Medicine
    & Rehabilitation
Baylor College of Medicine
Houston, Texas
United States
Director
Brain Injury Research Center
TIRR Memorial Hermann
Houston, Texas
United States

Andrea L.C. Schneider, MD, PhD
Neurocritical Care Fellow
Neurology
Johns Hopkins University School of Medicine
Baltimore, Maryland
United States

Joel Dan Scholten, MD
Director
Physical Medicine and Rehabilitation
Veterans Health Administration
Washington, District of Columbia
United States

Billie Schultz, MD
Assistant Professor
Physical Medicine and Rehabilitation
Mayo Clinic
Rochester, Minnesota
United States

Ronald T. Seel, PhD
Executive Director
Professor
CERSE/Department of Physical Medicine and Rehabilitation
Virginia Commonwealth University School of Medicine
Richmond, Virginia
United States

Miriam Segal, MD
Brain Injury Medicine Fellowship Program Director
Department of Physical Medicine and Rehabilitation
Moss Rehab at Elkins Park
Albert Einstein Medical Center
Elkins Park, Pennsylvania
United States

G. Sunny Sharma, MD
Assistant Professor
Physical Medicine and Rehabilitation
University of Texas Southwestern Medical Center
Dallas, Texas
United States

Jason R. Soble, PhD, ABPP-CN
Assistant Professor of Clinical Psychiatry and Neurology
Psychiatry
University of Illinois College of Medicine
Chicago, Illinois
United States

Eric T. Spier, MD
Physician
CNS
Craig
Denver, Colorado
United States

Lillian Flores Stevens, PhD
Research Psychologist
Mental Health Service
Hunter Holmes McGuire VA Medical Center
Richmond, Virginia
United States

Affiliate Assistant Professor
Department of Psychology
Virginia Commonwealth University
Richmond, Virginia
United States
Affiliate Instructor
Department of Physical Medicine and Rehabilitation
Virginia Commonwealth University School of Medicine
Richmond, Virginia
United States

Katharine Stout, PT, DPT, MBA
Clinical Affairs Lead
Defense and Veterans Brain Injury Center
Defense Health Agency/J9
Silver Spring, Maryland
United States

Bruno S. Subbarao, DO
Medical Director,
Polytrauma/TBI Program
Phoenix Veterans Healthcare System
Phoenix, Arizona
United States

Rebecca N. Tapia, MD
Section Chief
Polytrauma Rehabilitation Center
South Texas Veterans Healthcare System
San Antonio, Texas
United States
Associate Professor
Department of Rehabilitation Medicine
UT Health San Antonio
San Antonio, Texas
United States

Alphonsa Thomas, DO
Director of Outpatient Clinical Services
Physical Medicine and Rehabilitation
Hackensack Meridian Health–JFK Shore Rehabilitation
    Institute
Brick, New Jersey
United States

Christopher Ticknor, MD
Adjunct Professor
Psychiatry
UT Health San Antonio
San Antonio, Texas
United States

Alex B. Valadka, MD
Professor and Chair
Department of Neurosurgery
Virginia Commonwealth University
Richmond, Virginia
United States

Monica Verduzco-Gutierrez, MD
Professor and Chair
Department of Rehabilitation Medicine
Joe R. and Teresa Lozano Long School of Medicine
UT Health San Antonio
San Antonio, Texas

Ketan Verma, MD
Housestaff
Department of Neurosurgery
Virginia Commonwealth University
Richmond, Virginia
United States

Nicholas Vlahos, DO
Physical Medicine & Rehabilitation Physician
Memorial Health University Medical Center
Savannah, Georgia
United States
Brain Injury Medicine Fellow
Brain Injury, Physical Medicine and Rehabilitation
South Texas Veterans Health Care System, San Antonio
Texas
United States

Thomas Watanabe, MD
Clinical Director, Drucker Brain Injury Center
Moss Rehab at Elkins Park
Einstein Healthcare Network
Elkins Park, Pennsylvania
United States
Associate Professor
Department of Physical Medicine and Rehabilitation
Temple University School of Medicine
Philadelphia, Pennsylvania
United States

Justin Louis Weppner, DO
Assistant Professor
Director, Neurorehabilitation
Department of Physical Medicine and Rehabilitation
University of Virginia
Charlottesville, Virginia
United States

J. Kent Werner, Jr., MD, PhD
Assistant Professor
Department of Neurology
Uniformed Services University of Health Sciences
Bethesda, Maryland
United States
Adjunct Assistant Professor
Department of Neurology
Johns Hopkins University
Baltimore, Maryland
United States

Victoria C. Whitehair, MD
Director of Brain Injury Rehabilitation
Physical Medicine and Rehabilitation
MetroHealth Rehabilitation Institute
Cleveland, Ohio
United States
Assistant Professor
Physical Medicine and Rehabilitation
Case Western Reserve University
Cleveland, Ohio
United States

Bonny S. Wong, MD
Brain Injury Medicine Fellow
Spaulding Rehabilitation Hospital
Harvard Medical School
Boston, Massachusetts
United States

Jean E. Woo, MD
Brain Injury Medicine Fellow
H. Ben Taub Department of Physical Medicine
    and Rehabilitation
Baylor College of Medicine
Houston, Texas
United States

Hal S. Wortzel, MD
Director, Neuropsychiatric Consultation Services
Rocky Mountain MIRECC
VA Eastern Colorado Health Care System
Aurora, Colorado
United States
Michael K. Cooper Professor of Neurocognitive Disease
Department of Psychiatry
University of Colorado School of Medicine
Aurora, Colorado
United States

Paul Ki Yoo, DO
Brain Injury Medicine Fellow
Physical Medicine and Rehabilitation
Icahn School of Medicine at Mount Sinai
New York, New York
United States

Mauro Zappaterra, MD, PhD
Director of Multidisciplinary Care and Clinical Research
Director of Multidisciplinary Care and Clinical Research
Synovation Medical Group
Pasadena, California
United States
VA Staff Physician
Physical Medicine and Rehabilitation Residency Program
Greater Los Angeles VA Healthcare System
Los Angeles, California
United States

Preface

Traumatic brain injury (TBI) has been a part of the human race since we began traveling upright and had our arms freed up to hurl projectiles and hunt. But the importance of a specialized field of healthcare dedicated specifically to the assessment, management, and long-term care of individuals who have sustained one or more TBIs of a range of severity has only been recognized in the past decade. Similarly, although the challenges of providing care for individuals with TBIs and their families has been a priority of the US military since it was founded in 1776, it has really only been with the most recent conflicts in the Middle East that the true impact of TBIs has been recognized by healthcare systems across the Departments of Defense and Veterans Affairs, academia, and the private sector.

Brain Injury Medicine: Board Review offers a comprehensive and yet concise resource tool for anyone who is studying the field as part of their training or in preparation for certifying examinations and for more experienced practitioners who desire to keep up to date with the most evidence-influenced clinical approaches to assessment and management. More than 130 of the nation's leading experts across the wide range of brain injury medicine elements have been brought together in this book to create more than 60 chapters that offer authoritative yet practical approaches to diagnosis, acute management, and long-term care.

The topics range from mainstream neurosurgical and trauma acute care of TBI to cutting-edge imaging, biomarker and electrophysiologic assessment, and a diverse assortment of rehabilitation topics. The focus of the book is on identifying the clinically relevant core elements of each area so that a clinician or trainee can easily grasp these key components; however, there are also evidence-based recommendations and state-of-the-art research that will allow the reader to take their approach to the individual with acquired brain injury to the next level.

Brain Injury Medicine offers a unique approach that complements existing textbooks in the field by providing well-defined foundational clinical principles that allow the reader to both understand the essential information and integrate this information directly into practice. It is a resource that can be used by entry-level trainees and experienced, advanced practitioners to enhance their understanding and their effectiveness.

Acknowledgements

This *Brain Injury Medicine: Board Review* book represents the combined work of more than 120 authors with a range of healthcare backgrounds from across the United States and with varying interests and experiences in the practice of this specialty. This high number and diversity of experts were necessary to allow this text to reflect the full breadth of all that must be learned and applied to appropriately assess and manage individuals with traumatic brain injury.

Although we have attempted to capture as much of the scientific theory and knowledge related to both brain injury and to brain injury medicine as possible, the true art of healthcare is to take this vast corpus of knowledge and translate and integrate that into everyday practice. Although this evidence-based approach to care takes years of training, mentorship, and experience, the handbook offers a concise, useful, and informative resource that will give everyone from trainees to the seasoned clinicians access to the key elements needed to move to expert status.

We are indebted to all of the authors who worked so diligently to bring together the essential information relevant to the field in this single source. Although it is a handy and convenient reference that may be used for independent study, reviewing for certification exams, or to support practice, we urge all practitioners to rely on multiple sources of information and the oversight and advice of established practitioners. We would also like to acknowledge our academic and clinical institutions: the US Department of Veterans Affairs Physical Medicine and Rehabilitation Program Office and VA Medical Centers in Greater Los Angeles, Richmond, and San Antonio; the University of California in Los Angeles; and the Virginia Commonwealth University.

Contents

Brain Injury Medicine:
Board Review

Brain Injury Medicine:
Board Review

Brain Anatomy and Physiology

1

Neuroanatomy Correlates

JASON R. SOBLE, PHD, ABPP-CN, SAMANTHA DEDIOS-STERN, PHD,
DAVID ANDRÉS GONZÁLEZ, PHD, ABPP-CN, AND K. CHASE BAILEY, PHD, ABPP-CN

OUTLINE

This chapter provides a foundational overview of basic structural and functional neuroanatomy relevant to brain injury. As such, the coverage is not exhaustive, and the reader is referred to authoritative texts[1-3] for more comprehensive detail. Moreover, although descriptive, the summary of each neuroanatomical structure/connection is not prescriptive, in that similar structural lesions can result in strikingly diverse functional neurobehavioral presentations among individual patients.[4-5] Finally, neuroanatomical structures and associated functions are presented as discrete

units here for review, but the human brain is a highly complex, connected, and integrated organ such that lesions rarely produce a singular functional deficit.

Structural Organization of the Brain

The command center of the human CNS, the brain is enclosed in the skull and meninges and structurally divided into the brainstem, cerebellum, and cerebrum. Beneath the cerebral cortex lie several key subcortical structures and connective pathways. The brain is made up of gray matter (cell bodies), which comprises the cortex and some subcortical structures (e.g., basal ganglia), and myelinated white matter, which transmits information to and from connected gray matter for integration/processing. The cortex is folded to allow for greater surface area within the skull, which produces its characteristic grooves (sulci) and folds (gyri). Cardinal directions and key landmarks within the brain are summarized later (Box 1.1; Figs. 1.1 and 1.2).

Skull and Meninges

The brain is encased within bone and surrounded by three membrane layers that provide protection and buoyancy and anchor it within the skull (Box 1.2). Moving from inside the brain laterally to the skull, the mnemonic PADS (**p**ia mater, **a**rachnoid mater, **d**ura mater, **s**kull) identifies the relative positions of the meninges (Figs. 1.3–1.7).[1,3,6-7]

Vasculature

This section presents a brief review of the primary circulations, arteries/branches, and neuroanatomical structures supplied by them (Box 1.3). Broadly, the vascular supply in the brain can be segmented into anterior (fed by paired internal carotid arteries) and posterior circulations (fed by paired vertebral arteries). The three primary arteries are also listed, along with divisions, and underlying neuroanatomical regions/structures are supplied with Fig. 1.8, providing coronal and axial visualization.[1,8]

Watershed areas (i.e., anterior cerebral artery [ACA] and middle cerebral artery [MCA] area and MCA and posterior cerebral artery[PCA] area) refer to cortical neuroanatomical regions fed by the most distal reaches of each artery that are most vulnerable to diminished blood flow.

Cerebrospinal Fluid System

Cerebrospinal fluid (CSF) is produced in the choroid plexus in the lateral ventricles, and its function is to cushion the brain and provide a mechanism for toxin/chemical transmission for cleaning. The relative volume of CSF remains generally stable (150 cc) in adults and is constantly being produced (20 cc/hour). Thus primary/secondary insults to the CNS that affect either production or absorption rates are relevant, as both can result in hydrocephalus (Box 1.4).[1]

- CSF Flow Pathway (see Figs. 1.1–1.9): Lateral ventricles → foramen of Monro to the third ventricle → aqueduct of Sylvius to the fourth ventricle/foramina (medial and lateral) to subarachnoid space → reabsorbed at rate of 4 to 5 times per day in arachnoid granulations

Brainstem

In addition to connecting the spinal cord to the brain via sensory-motor tracts, the brainstem is responsible for consciousness and involuntary, life-sustaining functions (Box 1.5 and Fig. 1.10).[1,3,7,9-11]

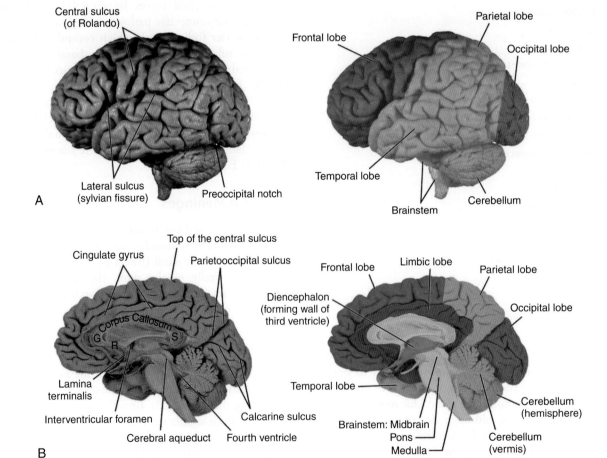

• **Fig. 1.1** Lateral and medial views of the adult brain; G = genu; R = rostrum; S = splenium. (From Gross anatomy and general organization of the CNS. In: Vanderah TW, Gould DJ. *Nolte's the Human Brain: An Introduction to Its Functional Anatomy.* 7th ed. Philadelphia, PA: Elsevier; 2016:58. Fig. 3.2.)

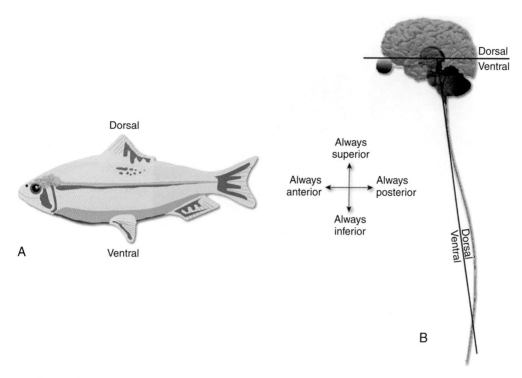

Dorsal

Ventral

Always
superior

Always
anterior ←——→ Always
posterior

Always
inferior

Dorsal
Ventral

A   Ventral

Dorsal
Ventral

B

• **Fig. 1.2** Explanation of directional terms for referring to the CNS. (From Gross anatomy and general organization of the CNS. In: Vanderah TW, Gould DJ. *Nolte's the Human Brain: An Introduction to Its Functional Anatomy.* 7th ed. Philadelphia, PA: Elsevier; 2016:57. Fig. 3.1.)

• BOX 1.2   Summary of the Coverings of the Brain ("PADS")

Meninge	Location/Function	Injury Characteristics
Pia mater	• Thin, innermost layer • Attached to the brain • Contours to the sulci and gyri of the brain • Forms a perivascular space by surrounding initial entry point of blood vessels	• Bleeds below the pia mater, involves hemorrhage in the actual brain parenchyma (e.g., intraparenchymal bleeds, interventricular hemorrhage)
Arachnoid Mater	• Thin layer between the pia and dura • Appears similar to a spider's web • Cerebrospinal fluid (CSF) is present and is reabsorbed in the arachnoid granulations	• Bleeds below the arachnoid are subarachnoid hemorrhages and can result from both traumatic and nontraumatic (e.g., aneurysm rupture) etiologies • Hydrocephalus is common after subarachnoid hemorrhage caused by dense blood product resulting in poor CSF reabsorption
Dura Mater	• Thick and hard outermost layer between the arachnoid and inner skull surface • Contains venous sinuses that drain cerebral blood • Separates the right and left cerebral hemispheres (falx cerebri) and the cerebral hemispheres from the cerebellum (tentorium cerebri)	• Bleeds between the dura and skull are epidural hematomas and result in a rapidly expanding hemorrhage from tearing of meningeal arteries (e.g., middle meningeal artery) • Bleeds between the dura and arachnoid are subdural hematomas and result from tearing of bridging veins; these can be acute or slow, in which symptoms do not become apparent until the bleed has enlarged

Skull	• Hard bone structure that encases the brain
	• Skull base is internally divided by boney ridges that form the cavities in which the ventral aspect of different brain regions rest:
	  • Anterior cranial fossa: frontal lobe
	  • Middle cranial fossa: temporal lobe
	  • Posterior cranial fossa: cerebellum and brainstem
		• Traumatic brain injury can occur from brain tissue striking the boney internal protuberances and cavities within the skull

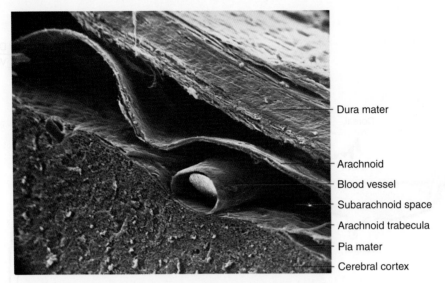

• **Fig. 1.3** Electron micrograph of the meningeal layers of a dog. (From Meningeal coverings of the brain and spinal cord. In: Vanderah TW, Gould DJ. *Nolte's the Human Brain: An Introduction to Its Functional Anatomy.* 7th ed. Philadelphia, PA: Elsevier; 2016:85. Fig. 4.2.)

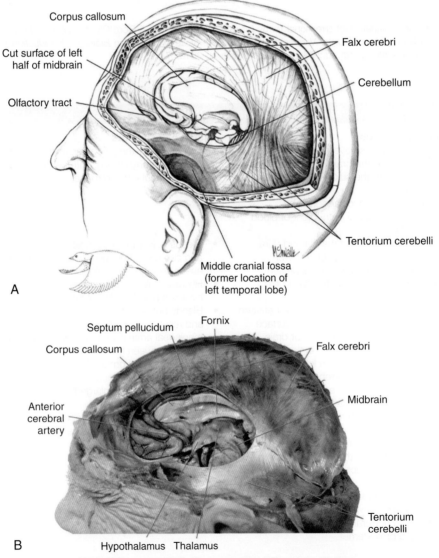

• **Fig. 1.4** Prosections demonstrating the shape and spatial relationships of the dural folds. (From Meningeal coverings of the brain and spinal cord. In: Vanderah TW, Gould DJ. *Nolte's the Human Brain: An Introduction to Its Functional Anatomy.* 7th ed. Philadelphia, PA: Elsevier; 2016:86. Fig. 4.3.)

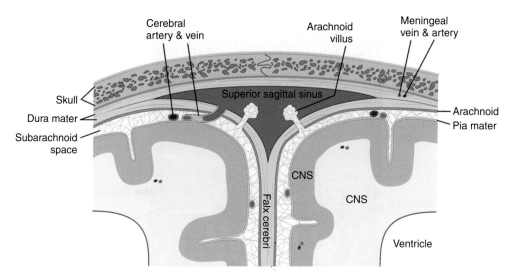

• **Fig. 1.5** Coronal section through the superior sagittal sinus displaying the movement of cerebrospinal fluid (CSF); CNS = central nervous system. (From Meningeal coverings of the brain and spinal cord. In: Vanderah TW, Gould DJ. *Nolte's the Human Brain: An Introduction to Its Functional Anatomy.* 7th ed. Philadelphia, PA: Elsevier; 2016:86. Fig. 4.5.)

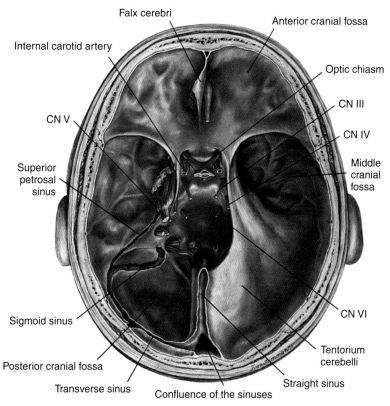

• **Fig. 1.6** View of the base of the skull demonstrating the major sinuses; CN = cranial nerve. *CN,* Cranial nerve. (From Meningeal coverings of the brain and spinal cord. In: Vanderah TW, Gould DJ. *Nolte's the Human Brain: An Introduction to Its Functional Anatomy.* 7th ed. Philadelphia, PA: Elsevier; 2016:88. Fig. 4.6.)

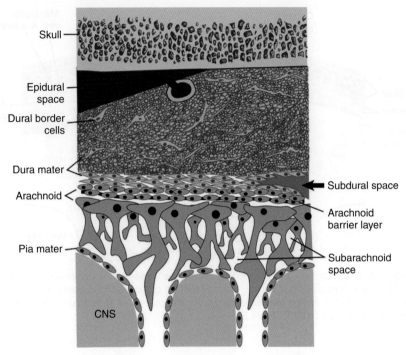

• **Fig. 1.7** View of the meningeal layers. *CNS,* Central nervous system. (From Meningeal coverings of the brain and spinal cord; CNS = central nervous system. In: Vanderah TW, Gould DJ. *Nolte's the Human Brain: An Introduction to Its Functional Anatomy.* 7th ed. Philadelphia, PA: Elsevier; 2016:96. Fig. 4.14.)

• **BOX 1.3** **Summary of Major Cerebral Arteries and Associated Distributions**

Artery	Division	Associated Neuroanatomical Region
Anterior cerebral artery (ACA)	Main	Anterior/medial frontal lobe and aspects of anterior parietal lobe (sensorimotor cortex)
	Deep	Head of the putamen/caudate
	Inferior	Lateral temporal lobe/parietal lobe
Middle cerebral artery (MCA)	Superior (demarcated by Sylvian fissure)	Lateral frontal lobe (dorsolateral region) and peri-Rolandic cortex
	Deep	Medial putamen/caudate
Lenticulostriate	Smallest vessels of MCA	Basal ganglia and internal capsule
Posterior cerebral artery (PCA)	Main	Inferior/medial temporal and occipital lobe
	Deep	Thalamus

Cranial Nerves

The brainstem also contains 10 of the 12 cranial nerve pairs. The cranial nerves are part of the peripheral nervous system and control sensory and motor functions of the head and neck (Box 1.6). In general, cranial nerves innervate ipsilaterally, though one notable exception is the trochlear nerve (IV), which innervates the superior oblique muscles of the contralateral eye (Figs. 1.11 and 1.12).[1,7,12]

Cerebellum

The cerebellum is a large structure in the posterior fossa and is connected to dorsal aspects of the brainstem by the cerebellar peduncles. Its primary function is to smoothly coordinate motor movements and assist with motor planning. Lesions typically result in ipsilateral ataxia. Recent research has also identified contributions of the cerebellum to cognition, including implicit learning, although this is still developing. Neuroanatomically, the cerebellum is made

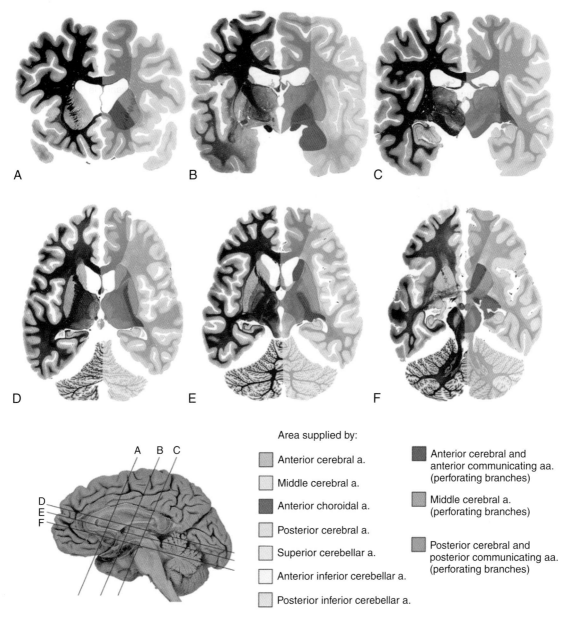

Area supplied by:

- Anterior cerebral a.
- Middle cerebral a.
- Anterior choroidal a.
- Posterior cerebral a.
- Superior cerebellar a.
- Anterior inferior cerebellar a.
- Posterior inferior cerebellar a.
- Anterior cerebral and anterior communicating aa. (perforating branches)
- Middle cerebral a. (perforating branches)
- Posterior cerebral and posterior communicating aa. (perforating branches)

• **Fig. 1.8** Coronal and axial views of the cerebral blood supply; a. = artery; aa. = arteries. *a*, Artery; *aa*, arteries. (From Blood supply of the brain. In: Vanderah TW, Gould DJ. *Nolte's the Human Brain: An Introduction to Its Functional Anatomy.* 7th ed. Philadelphia, PA: Elsevier; 2016:141. Fig. 6.22.)

• BOX 1.4 Overview of Hydrocephalus

Cerebrospinal Fluid (CSF) Dysfunction	Cause(s)	Potential Etiologies
Communicating hydrocephalus	• CSF overproduction • CSF underreabsorption	• Arachnoid granulation dysfunction • Subarachnoid or interventricular hemorrhage • Meningitis
Noncommunicating hydrocephalus	• Obstruction blocking flow at one or more points along the CSF pathway	• Space-occupying lesion or tumor • Edema caused by injury/trauma • Increased intracranial pressure • Obstruction caused by worsening of a congenital defect

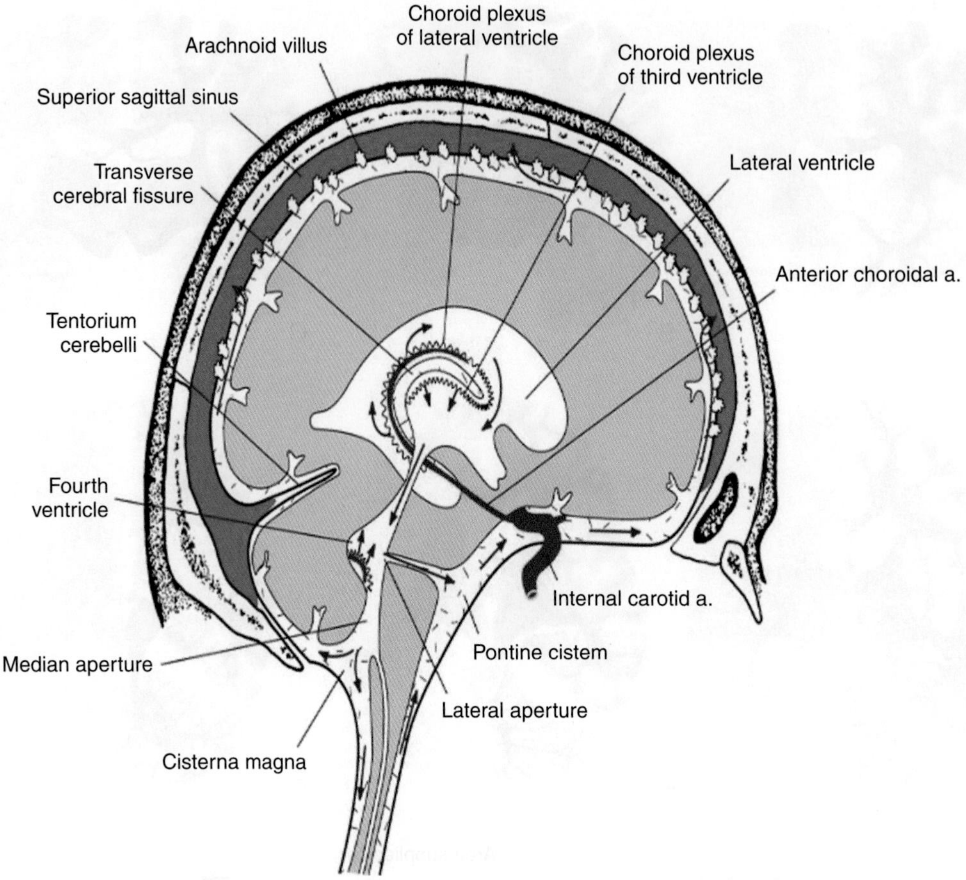

• **Fig. 1.9** View of the path of cerebrospinal fluid flow; a. = artery. *a,* Artery. (From Ventricles and cerebrospinal fluid. In: Vanderah TW, Gould DJ. *Nolte's the Human Brain: An Introduction to Its Functional Anatomy.* 7th ed. Philadelphia, PA: Elsevier; 2016:110. Fig. 5.10.)

• BOX 1.5	Structures of the Brainstem

Brainstem Structure	Function
Medulla	• Regulation of involuntary autonomic functions (e.g., heart rate, breathing, blood pressure) and reflexes (e.g., vomiting, swallowing) • Junction between the spinal cord and brain • Decussation of corticospinal fibers (pyramidal tracts) • Neurotransmitter production (e.g., serotonin in the raphe nuclei)
Pons	• Modulation of arousal, consciousness, and sleep regulation via the reticular formation, which extends into the midbrain • Breathing intensity • "Bridge" connecting the brainstem to the cerebrum and cerebellum • Sensory and motor relay • Neurotransmitter production (e.g., norepinephrine in the locus coeruleus)
Midbrain	• Cerebrospinal fluid flow from third to fourth ventricle (cerebral aqueduct) • Orienting eyes and directing visual attention toward relevant stimuli, notably moving stimuli; visual fixation (superior colliculus) • Main auditory pathway hub; guiding auditory attention; auditory startle response (inferior colliculus) • Motor control and coordination • Connects the forebrain and basal ganglia to the hindbrain • Neurotransmitter production (dopamine in the substantia nigra)

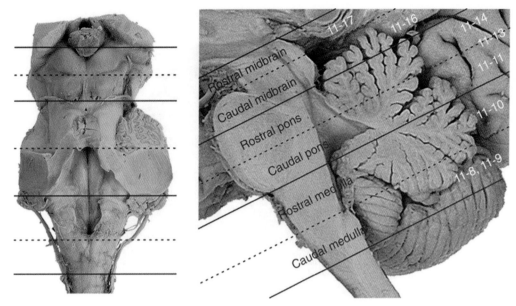

• **Fig. 1.10** Views of the brainstem. (From Organization of the brainstem. In: Vanderah TW, Gould DJ. *Nolte's the Human Brain: An Introduction to Its Functional Anatomy.* 7th ed. Philadelphia, PA: Elsevier; 2016:278. Fig. 11.6.)

•BOX 1.6 Overview of the Cranial Nerves

Nerve	Location	Sensory/Motor	Primary Function(s)
Olfactory (I)	Olfactory bulb	Sensory	Smell
Optic (II)	Retina	Sensory	Vision
Oculomotor (III)	Midbrain	Motor	All eye movements except for downward and lateral gaze Pupillary constriction
Trochlear (IV)	Midbrain	Motor	Eye movements (downward gaze)
Trigeminal (V)	Pons	Both	Facial sensation Muscles of mastication
Abducens (VI)	Pons	Motor	Eye movements (lateral gaze)
Facial (VII)	Pons	Both	Taste (anterior 2/3 of tongue) Lacrimation Salivation Muscles of facial expression
Vestibulocochlear (VIII)	Pons	Sensory	Hearing Equilibrium
Glossopharyngeal (IX)	Medulla	Both	Taste (posterior 1/3 of tongue) Visceral sensory and motor functions Gag reflex Pharyngeal muscles (swallowing)
Vagus (X)	Medulla	Both	Parasympathetic innervation to organs Abdominal visceral sensation Laryngeal muscles (voice) Palate elevation Pharyngeal muscles (swallowing)
Accessory (XI)	Medulla	Motor	Sternomastoid and trapezius muscles (head turning; shoulder elevation)
Hypoglossal (XII)	Medulla	Motor	Tongue movement

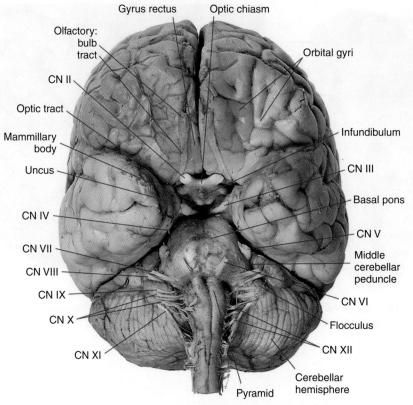

Gyrus rectus
Optic chiasm
Olfactory: bulb tract
Orbital gyri
CN II
Optic tract
Infundibulum
Mammillary body
CN III
Uncus
Basal pons
CN IV
CN V
CN VII
Middle cerebellar peduncle
CN VIII
CN IX
CN VI
CN X
Flocculus
CN XI
CN XII
Cerebellar hemisphere
Pyramid

• **Fig. 1.11** Inferior view of the brain displaying cranial nerves (CNs) II through XII. (From Gross anatomy and general organization of the CNS. In: Vanderah TW, Gould DJ. *Nolte's the Human Brain: An Introduction to Its Functional Anatomy.* 7th ed. Philadelphia, PA: Elsevier; 2016:68. Fig. 3.17.)

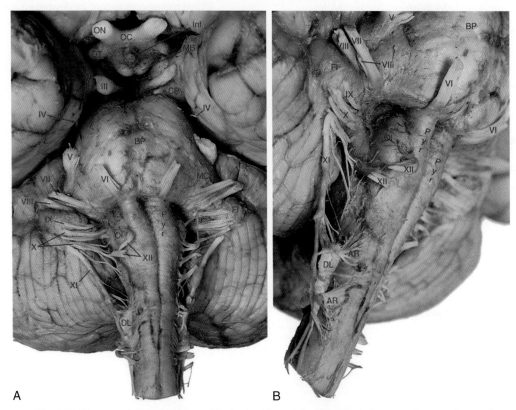

A   B

• **Fig. 1.12** Close-up of the inferior view of the brain with cranial nerves. (From Gross anatomy and general organization of the CNS. In: Vanderah TW, Gould DJ. *Nolte's the Human Brain: An Introduction to Its Functional Anatomy.* 7th ed. Philadelphia, PA: Elsevier; 2016:68. Fig. 3.18.)

• BOX 1.7 Overview of the Cerebellum and Functions by Region

Region	Neuroanatomical Composition	Key Functions
Vestibulocerebellum	• Flocculonodular lobe • Inferior vermis	• Regulates balance and eye movements through connections with the vestibular system
Spinocerebellum	• Vermis • Intermediate portions of the cerebellar hemispheres	• Controls the medial motor systems (proximal trunk muscles) • Maintaining posture, gait, and eye movements
Cerebrocerebellum	• Lateral cerebellar regions	• Controls lateral motor systems (distal appendicular muscles) • Planning and executing movements

up of the vermis and two hemispheres that are divided into intermediate and lateral regions. These have been divided into three distinct areas with specific functions: (1) vestibulocerebellum, (2) spinocerebellum, and (3) cerebrocerebellum (Box 1.7 and Fig. 1.13).[1,13-14]

Cerebrum

The cerebrum comprises four paired lobes (discussed later; Fig. 1.14). In normal/typical functional neuroanatomical organization, the dominant left cerebral hemisphere is responsible for language functions, whereas the nondominant right hemisphere is specialized for visuospatial processing, although intraindividual variability certainly exists. In right-handed individuals, a majority (92%–96%) have left hemisphere language dominance. Among left-handed individuals, the majority (~77%) also have left hemisphere language dominance, but there is a larger percentage with

right hemisphere or bilateral language dominance.[15-16] Box 1.8 provides a summary of common functional neurobehavioral specializations by hemisphere.[8]

Frontal Lobes

The frontal lobes are the largest lobes and account for roughly one-third of human neocortex. Given their location and size, they are particularly vulnerable to damage caused by traumatic brain injury (TBI). The frontal lobes are defined posteriorly by the central sulcus and inferiorly and laterally by the Sylvian fissure. They are commonly divided into three anatomical areas by function: primary motor cortex, premotor and supplementary motor cortex, and prefrontal cortex (Fig. 1.15).
1. The primary motor cortex or motor strip (Box 1.9) is directly anterior to the central sulcus at the precentral gyrus and is organized somatotopically with a motor homunculus (Fig. 1.16).

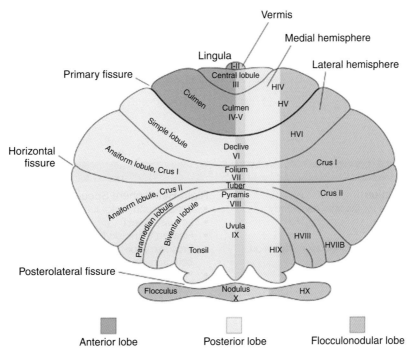

• **Fig. 1.13** Schematic of the cerebellum. (From Cerebellum. In: Vanderah TW, Gould DJ. *Nolte's the Human Brain: An Introduction to Its Functional Anatomy.* 7th ed. Philadelphia, PA: Elsevier; 2016:498. Fig. 20.4.)

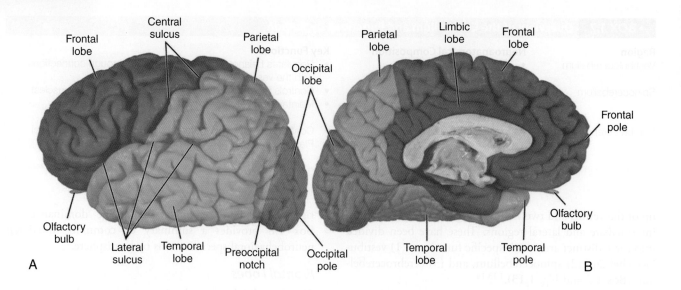

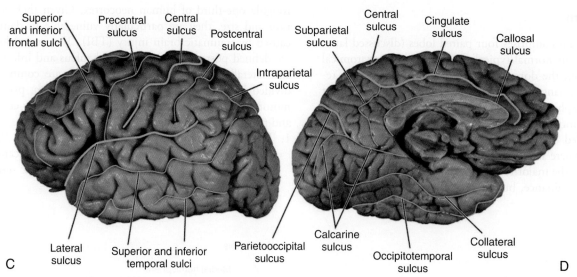

• **Fig. 1.14** Lobes of the cerebral hemisphere with major sulci. (From Gross anatomy and general organization of the CNS. In: Vanderah TW, Gould DJ. *Nolte's the Human Brain: An Introduction to Its Functional Anatomy.* 7th ed. Philadelphia, PA: Elsevier; 2016:61. Fig. 3.8.)

• **BOX 1.8** **Breakdown of Hemispheric Specialization**

Left Hemisphere Specialization
- Sensory and motor functions for the right hemi-body
- Right visual field
- Hearing for speech sounds
- Core language functions (e.g., comprehension, repetition, fluent expression)
- Reading
- Writing
- Mathematical computation
- Memory for verbal/auditory stimuli

Right Hemisphere Specialization
- Sensory and motor functions for the left hemi-body
- Left visual field
- Hearing for music/tones
- Prosodic aspects of speech (e.g., being able to express and comprehend sarcasm)
- Higher order visuospatial processing (e.g., ability to integrate and appreciate whole patterns, mental rotation)
- Spatial orientation/attention
- Memory for visual stimuli (e.g., faces, locations)

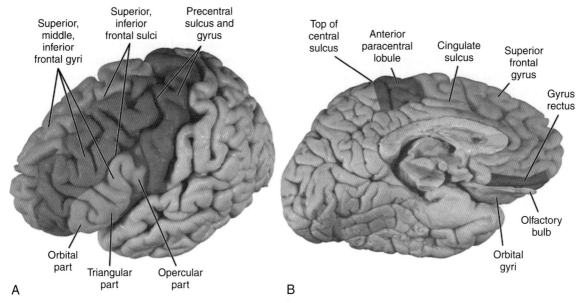

• **Fig. 1.15** Lateral, medial, and inferior surfaces of the frontal lobe. (From Gross anatomy and general organization of the CNS. In: Vanderah TW, Gould DJ. *Nolte's the Human Brain: An Introduction to Its Functional Anatomy.* 7th ed. Philadelphia, PA: Elsevier; 2016:61. Fig. 3.10.)

• BOX 1.9   Overview of the Frontal Lobes: Primary Motor Cortex

Key Functions
- Mediating motor movement for the contralateral side of the body (motor homunculus)
- Control of facial movements

Result of Lesions
- Contralateral hemiplegia or hemiparesis in the corresponding part of the body
- Expressive language deficits caused by oral apraxia (inability to coordinate muscle movements needed for speech)

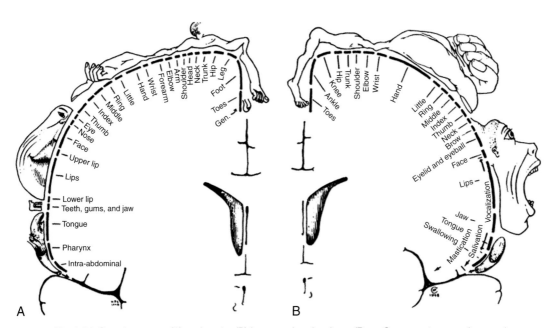

• **Fig. 1.16** Somatosensory (A) and motor (B) homunculus drawings. (From Gross anatomy and general organization of the CNS. In: Vanderah TW, Gould DJ. *Nolte's the Human Brain: An Introduction to Its Functional Anatomy.* 7th ed. Philadelphia, PA: Elsevier; 2016:79. Fig. 3.31.)

2. The premotor and supplementary motor cortices (Box 1.10) are directly anterior to the primary motor cortex and connect directly to the corticospinal and corticobulbar tracts, the basal ganglia, primary motor cortex, thalamus, and parietal and dorsolateral cortices. Broca's area is located in the lateral premotor area of the language-dominant hemisphere (usually left). The frontal eye fields are also part of the premotor cortex.
3. The remainder of the frontal lobe is the prefrontal cortex (Box 1.11), which is responsible for higher level cognitive functions. The prefrontal cortex may be divided into dorsolateral, orbitofrontal/ventromedial, and medial frontal/anterior cingulate regions. Lesions to each area produce distinct frontal syndromes.[17-20]

Temporal Lobes

The temporal lobes are divided from the frontal and parietal lobes by the Sylvian fissure, although they have no sharp posterior demarcation from the occipital lobes when viewed laterally. Their primary functions include audition, language, memory, and aspects of visual processing. Key limbic structures, including the hippocampal formation and amygdala, are embedded deep within the medial temporal lobes and play key roles in memory consolidation and emotional processing/emotion-based learning, respectively. Wernicke's area is located in the superior temporal gyrus of the language-dominant hemisphere (usually left) (Box 1.12 and Fig. 1.17).[1-2]

Parietal Lobes

The parietal lobes are defined anteriorly by the central sulcus and posteriorly by the parietooccipital sulcus when viewed from the brain's lateral surface. Broadly, the functions of the parietal lobes include bodily sensation, visuospatial processing, spatial attention/awareness, and other higher level abilities. The parietal lobe may be divided into

---

• BOX 1.10 Overview of the Frontal Lobes: Premotor and Supplementary Motor Cortex

Key Functions
- Motor sequencing and fine motor movements of nonoverlearned motor skills
- Expressive language (Broca's area)
- Control of frontal eye fields for directing voluntary eye movements

Result of Lesions
- Motor apraxias of the contralateral side and discoordination of movements
- Expressive aphasia (Broca's aphasia) characterized by dysfluent speech and impaired repetition but intact comprehension
- Contralateral voluntary eye movement deficits

• BOX 1.11 Overview of the Frontal Lobes: Prefrontal Cortex

Region	Key Functions	Result of Lesions
Dorsolateral prefrontal cortex	Cognitive executive functions: • Planning • Problem solving • Self-monitoring • Working memory	• Poor problem solving/reasoning • Perseveration • Stimulus-bound behaviors • Decreased working memory and related difficulties with memory retrieval
Orbitofrontal/ventromedial prefrontal cortex	• Inhibition • Social comportment • Judgment	• Disinhibition • Impulsivity • Emotional lability • Decreased social skills
Medial frontal/anterior cingulate prefrontal cortex	• Initiating voluntary action	• Apathy/abulia • Akinetic mutism • Lower extremity weakness (if extending to the precentral gyrus)

• BOX 1.12 Overview of the Temporal Lobes

Key Functions
- Auditory perception and localization of sound (primary auditory cortex/superior temporal/Heschl's gyrus)
- Language comprehension (Wernicke's area)
- Object recognition; perception of form and color (inferior temporal gyrus)
- Emotional processing (medial temporal lobe, temporal pole)
- Memory consolidation (medial temporal)

Result of Lesions
- Cortical deafness
- Receptive aphasia (Wernicke's aphasia) characterized by fluent speech and impaired comprehension and repetition
- Associative agnosia, prosopagnosia
- Emotional deficits
- Amnesia: anterograde (decreased memory for events occurring after the lesion) or retrograde (decreased memory for events for a period immediately before lesion onset, with persevered earlier memories)

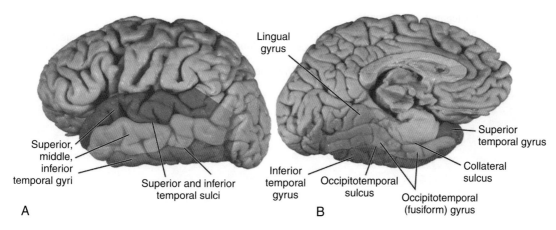

Lingual gyrus

Superior temporal gyrus

Collateral sulcus

Occipitotemporal (fusiform) gyrus

Superior, middle, inferior temporal gyri

Superior and inferior temporal sulci

Inferior temporal gyrus

Occipitotemporal sulcus

A

B

• **Fig. 1.17** Lateral, medial, and inferior surfaces of the temporal lobe. (From Gross anatomy and general organization of the CNS. In: Vanderah TW, Gould DJ. *Nolte's the Human Brain: An Introduction to Its Functional Anatomy.* 7th ed. Philadelphia, PA: Elsevier; 2016:64. Fig. 3.12.)

three sections: postcentral gyrus, superior parietal lobule, and inferior parietal lobule (Box 1.13 and Fig. 1.18).[1-2,21]

Occipital Lobes

The occipital lobes are located posterior to the parietooccipital sulcus, directly posterior to the parietal and temporal lobes. Their main function is visual processing. The primary visual cortex is located along the banks of the calcarine fissure on the medial surface of the brain. The lingual and cuneus represent portions of the medial occipital lobe below and above the calcarine fissure, which are responsible for processing information from the upper and lower visual fields, respectively (Box 1.14 and Fig. 1.19).[1-2]

Subcortical Structures

Thalamus

The thalamus is part of the diencephalon. It is rostral to the midbrain and with the hypothalamus it forms walls of the third ventricle. It is a major relay and processing station for somatosensory information and the termination of the reticular activating system (RAS), such that dysfunction may result in impairments in sensation or arousal/attention. It also has reciprocal connections with widespread cortical and basal ganglia structures, such that it is also involved in motor and cognitive processes. There are multiple nuclei within the thalamus, which are divided by Y-shaped white matter (the thalamic medullary laminae) and coated by the reticular nucleus (Fig. 1.20). This creates five broad groupings with relay and nonspecific association functions (Box 1.15).[1,8]

Hypothalamus and Pituitary Gland

The hypothalamus and pituitary gland lie ventral to the thalamus and are critical parts of the hypothalamic–pituitary–adrenal (HPA) axis (which regulates the autonomic nervous system), the endocrine system, and homeostasis and also have important limbic system connections.[1]

• BOX 1.13 Overview of the Parietal Lobes

Region	Key Functions	Result of Lesions
Postcentral gyrus (primary somatosensory cortex)	• Processing touch sensation for the contralateral side of the body (somatosensory homunculus)	Sensory loss to corresponding area of the body
Superior parietal lobule	• Higher order somatosensory processing • Integrates information with other sensory areas and connects to motor structures • Spatial attention • Body position in space	• Hemispatial neglect • Most commonly seen after right-sided lesions causing a left-side neglect related to the right hemisphere's specialization for spatial attention
Inferior parietal lobule (includes supramarginal gyrus and angular gyrus)	• Integrates information for visuospatial abilities • Mathematical computation • Perception • Language	• Dyscalculia • Agraphia • Finger agnosia • Right–left confusion • Conduction aphasia

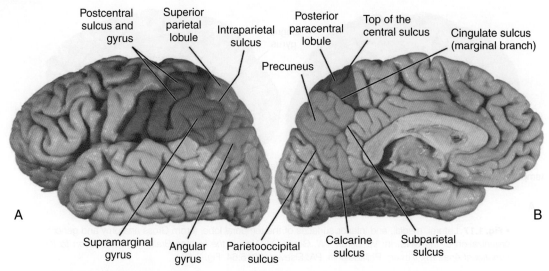

• **Fig. 1.18** Lateral, medial, and inferior surfaces of the parietal lobe. (From Gross anatomy and general organization of the CNS. In: Vanderah TW, Gould DJ. *Nolte's the Human Brain: An Introduction to Its Functional Anatomy.* 7th ed. Philadelphia, PA: Elsevier; 2016:61. Fig. 3.11.)

• BOX 1.14   **Overview of the Occipital Lobes**

Key Functions
- Processing visual information from the opposite visual field (primary visual cortex)

Result of Lesions
- Cortical blindness/visual field cuts dependent on the location of the lesion

---

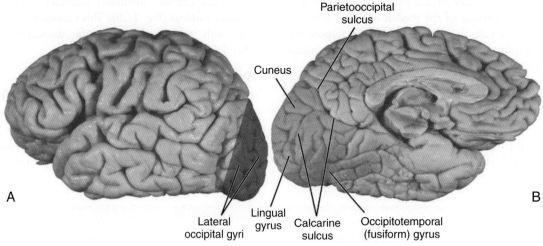

• **Fig. 1.19** Lateral, medial, and inferior surfaces of the occipital lobe. (From Gross anatomy and general organization of the CNS. In: Vanderah TW, Gould DJ. *Nolte's the Human Brain: An Introduction to Its Functional Anatomy.* 7th ed. Philadelphia, PA: Elsevier; 2016:65. Fig. 3.13.)

Epithalamus/Subthalamus

The epithalamus lies dorsal and posterior to the thalamus, with its most prominent structure being the pineal gland. The subthalamus is ventral to the thalamus, and its most prominent structures are the subthalamic nuclei (STN), which are lateral to the hypothalamus. Although sometimes considered part of the diencephalon, the STN are often considered a part of the basal ganglia, because their primary connections are with the basal ganglia and are a part of the indirect frontal–basal ganglia–thalamic loop.[1,8]

Basal Ganglia

The basal ganglia are a collection of gray matter structures involved in processing and modulating frontal and limbic streams, including motor, cognitive, and emotional abilities (see the frontal-subcortical circuitry section). Although

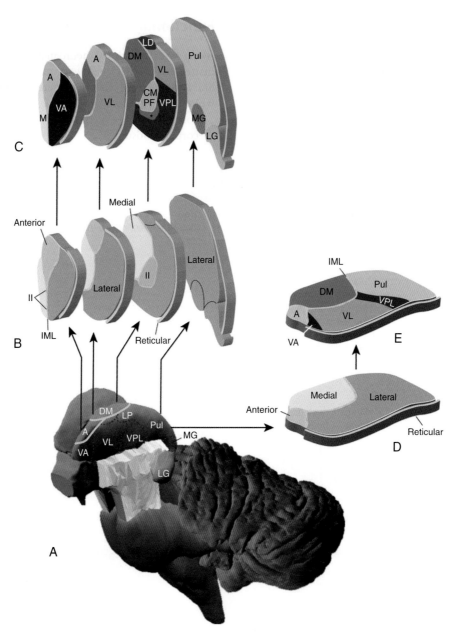

• **Fig. 1.20** Subdivisions of the thalamus. (From The thalamus and internal capsule. In: Vanderah TW, Gould DJ. *Nolte's the Human Brain: An Introduction to Its Functional Anatomy.* 7th ed. Philadelphia, PA: Elsevier; 2016:398. Fig. 16.6.)

• BOX 1.15   Overview of Thalamic Regions and Nuclei

Thalamic Region/Group	Important Nuclei	Function(s)
Lateral	• Ventral posterior lateral nucleus (VPL)	• Somatosensory relay
	• Ventral posteromedial nucleus (VPM)	• Somatosensory relay
	• Lateral geniculate nucleus (LGN)	• Visual relay
	• Medial geniculate nucleus (MGN)	• Auditory relay
	• Ventral lateral nucleus (VL)	• Basal ganglia and cerebellar relay
	• Ventral anterior nucleus (VA)	• Diffuse basal ganglia and cerebellar relay
	• Pulvinar nucleus	• Diffuse connections related to orienting attention
Medial	• Dorsomedial nucleus	• Diffuse limbic and frontal connections, part of lateral limbic circuit
Anterior	• Anterior thalamic nucleus (ATN)	• Part of Papez (medial limbic) circuit
Intralaminar	• Centromedian nucleus	• Diffuse connections as part of alertness and consciousness; some movement regulation
Reticular	• Reticular nucleus	• Connects with and regulates other thalamic nuclei

there is some variation in what structures are believed to make up the basal ganglia, the main structures are lateral and ventral to the lateral ventricles and anterior to the thalamus (Box 1.16 has a review of structures). They are divided by the internal capsule, with the putamen and globus pallidus being lateral to the internal capsule and caudate and thalamic nuclei being medial to the internal capsule (Fig. 1.21).[1,8]

Functional Brain Connectivity/Pathways

Along with individual neuroanatomical structures, white matter connectivity/pathways also are critical for overall brain functioning. In brief, there are three main types of white matter fibers:

1. commissural fibers connect interhemispheric areas (e.g., corpus callosum);

• BOX 1.16 | **Summary of Basal Ganglia Structures and Functions**

Basal Ganglia Structure	Substructure	Function

Striatum	• Caudate
	  • Head
	  • Body
	  • Tail
	• Putamen
	• Nucleus accumbens
		• Different entries for the three direct and indirect functional streams

Globus pallidus	• Internal segment (GPi) • External segment (GPe)	• Common exit for different direct and indirect functional streams
Substantia nigra	• Pars compacta • Pars reticula	• Primary dopamine supplier

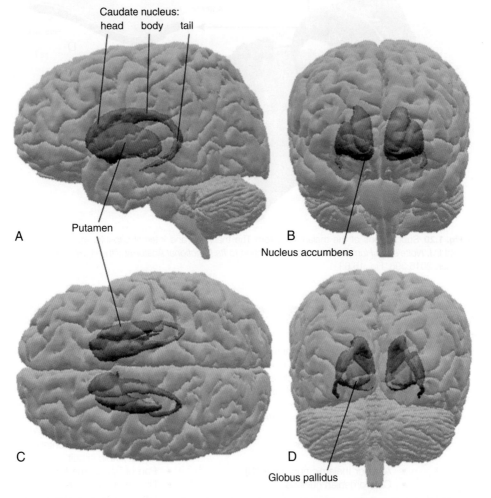

• **Fig. 1.21** View of the basal ganglia. (From Basal nuclei. In: Vanderah TW, Gould DJ. *Nolte's the Human Brain: An Introduction to Its Functional Anatomy*. 7th ed. Philadelphia, PA: Elsevier; 2016:479. Fig. 19.5.)

Summary of Key Sensory-Motor Pathways

Pathway	Function	Level of Decussation
Lateral corticospinal	Motor	Medullary pyramids
Medial lemniscus	Sensory (proprioception, fine touch/two-point discrimination, vibration)	Lower medulla
Spinothalamic	Sensory (pain, temperature, crude touch)	Spinal cord

2. projection fibers connect cortical to subcortical, hindbrain, and spinal cord regions (e.g., sensory-motor tracts); and
3. association fibers connect intrahemispheric cortical areas (e.g., arcuate fasciculus).

Although discussion of all relevant white matter connections is beyond the scope of this chapter, key white matter pathways underlying major neurobehavioral functions are discussed later on.

Sensory-Motor

The primary afferent sensory tracts are divided into dorsal (posterior) column/medial lemniscus and the anterolateral/spinothalamic tracts (Box 1.17). Descending motor information is transmitted to the spinal cord via the lateral corticospinal tract.[1]

Motor information is processed and integrated via complex hierarchical feedback loops. The primary CNS structures implicated in motor functioning are basal ganglia and cerebellum with relay through thalamus and pons to cortex (primary and association areas). Roughly 85% of fibers cross at the medullary pyramid and run contralateral, and 15% continue ipsilaterally in white matter columns to form the anterior corticospinal tract (Fig. 1.22). Lesions to upper and lower motor neurons are associated with diverse dysfunction (Box 1.18).

Lateral corticospinal pathways (see Figs. 1.23 and 1.24)
• Cortex → corona radiata → posterior limb of internal capsule (somatotopic map preserved here, so face and

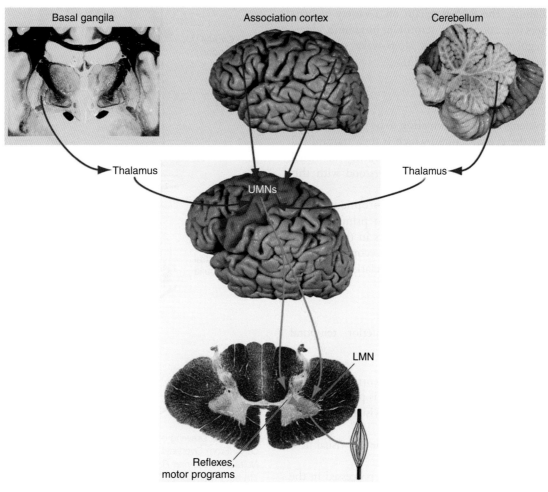

• **Fig. 1.22** View of key structures involved in motor control. (From Overview of motor systems. In: Vanderah TW, Gould DJ. *Nolte's the Human Brain: An Introduction to Its Functional Anatomy.* 7th ed. Philadelphia, PA: Elsevier; 2016:463. Fig. 18.7.)

• **BOX 1.18** | **Upper and Lower Motor Neuron Damage**

Motor Neuron Type	Origin	Dysfunction
Upper motor neurons	• Primary motor cortex • Central brainstem	• Rigidity • Babinski reflex • Hoffman reflex
Lower motor neurons	• Spinal cord anterior horn	• Flaccidity • Decreased tone • Fasciculations

arms medial and legs lateral, but so tightly bundled that lesions typically affect the whole body) → cerebral peduncles → ventral pons → rostral medulla/medullary pyramids and cervicomedullary junction (transition from medulla to spinal cord—85% decussate here) → lateral corticospinal tract → spinal cord gray matter → synapse onto anterior horn cells.[1]

Attention/Arousal[1,22]

The RAS refers to interconnected nuclei in the brainstem, pons, medulla, and hypothalamus to the prefrontal cortex via the thalamus. The RAS is reliant on a variety of neurotransmitters (e.g., dopamine, serotonin, histamine, glutamate) to regulate consciousness, sleep–wake cycle, and simple/sustained attention (Fig. 1.25).

Vision/Visuoperception[1]

The visual system requires information to be perceived most anteriorly by the eye structures, which is then transmitted posteriorly to the occipital lobe. The journey of visual information is complex, but easily understood with this roadmap:
• Information perceived via the retina → optic nerve → lateral geniculate body of thalamus → primary visual cortex. Rudimentary processing occurs in the primary visual cortex then is refined in the secondary visual cortex with integration via association cortices (Fig. 1.26).
• There are two visual streams.
  • "what"
  • travels ventrally through the inferior temporal cortex
  • "where"
  • travels dorsally through the parietal cortex
• The rule of thumb is that information is processed "upside down and backward" from what is visually perceived (Fig. 1.27).
  • The right occipital lobe processes the left visual field and vice versa.
  • The upper half of the visual field is processed in the lingual gyrus of the occipital lobe (divided by calcarine fissure), and the lower half is processed in the cuneus.

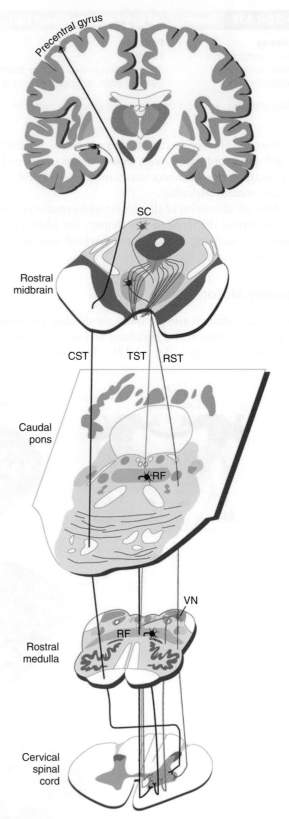

• **Fig. 1.23** Drawing of the motor pathway from the brain to the spinal cord. (From Overview of motor systems. In: Vanderah TW, Gould DJ. *Nolte's the Human Brain: An Introduction to Its Functional Anatomy.* 7th ed. Philadelphia, PA: Elsevier; 2016:465. Fig. 18.8.)

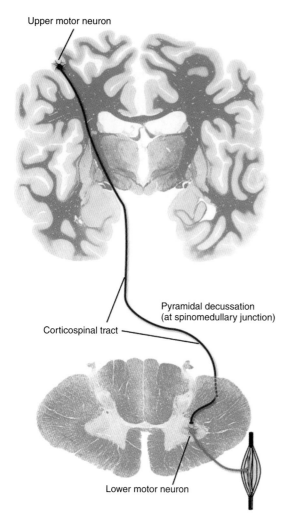

• **Fig. 1.24** Path of the corticospinal tract. (From Gross anatomy and general organization of the CNS. In: Vanderah TW, Gould DJ. *Nolte's the Human Brain: An Introduction to Its Functional Anatomy.* 7th ed. Philadelphia, PA: Elsevier; 2016:81. Fig. 3.33.)

Language/Speech

The language network is subdivided into dorsal and ventral streams (analogous to the visuoperceptual ones) and motor-articulation aspects (Fig. 1.28). The dorsal stream is related to connecting auditory representation to articulatory (motor) representation. The ventral stream is related to connecting auditory perception to semantic representation/meaning. Within the dorsal aspects of the language network, the most classically important pathway has been the arcuate fasciculus, which is considered a part of the superior longitudinal fasciculus.

- Arcuate fasciculus:
  - Connects Wernicke's with Broca's area
  - Lesions result in repetition deficits and phonemic paraphasias and naming problems. See conduction and transcortical aphasias.

The ventral stream of the language network is less understood but may include multiple tracts such as the uncinate fasciculus, extreme capsule, middle longitudinal fasciculus, and inferior longitudinal fasciculus. Of these, the uncinate is the most researched tract.

- Uncinate fasciculus:
  - Connects anterior temporal with frontal
  - Lesions result in semantic knowledge and naming deficits and some frontal syndromes.

Motor abilities also are critical to speech. Language-motor tracts include corticobulbar tracts, frontal-striatal loops, and corticocerebellar loops. Corticobulbar tracts descend from the motor cortex via the internal capsule to relevant cranial nerve nuclei (e.g., V, VII, XII). The motor stream of frontal-subcortical loops is a complex system that generally originates from the motor and premotor cortices, preferentially connects with the putamen, and continues the direct–indirect loops (see later section). Frontocerebellar

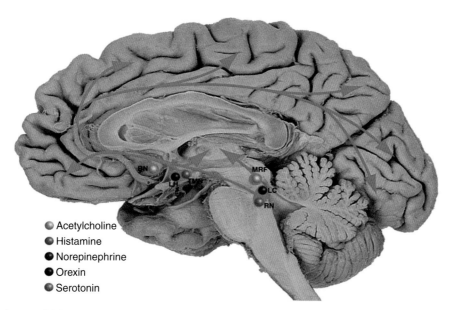

- Acetylcholine
- Histamine
- Norepinephrine
- Orexin
- Serotonin

• **Fig. 1.25** Major components of the reticular activating system (RAS) involved in attention/arousal. (From Cerebral cortex. In: Vanderah TW, Gould DJ. *Nolte's the Human Brain: An Introduction to Its Functional Anatomy.* 7th ed. Philadelphia, PA: Elsevier; 2016:572. Fig. 22.31.)

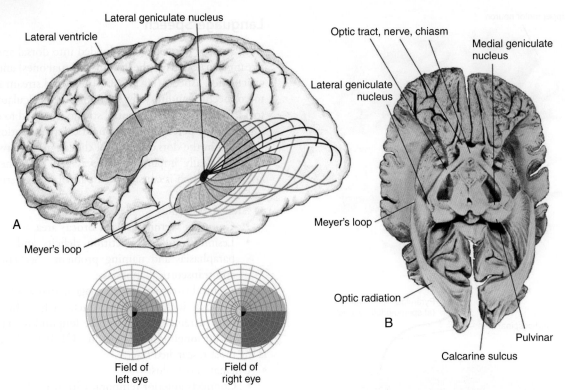

• **Fig. 1.26** View of the major visual system structures and associated pathways. (From The visual system. In: Vanderah TW, Gould DJ. *Nolte's the Human Brain: An Introduction to Its Functional Anatomy.* 7th ed. Philadelphia, PA: Elsevier; 2016:444. Fig. 17.28.)

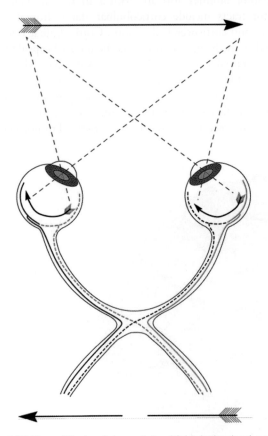

• **Fig. 1.27** View of the breakdown of visual fields in the visual system. (From The visual system. In: Vanderah TW, Gould DJ. *Nolte's the Human Brain: An Introduction to Its Functional Anatomy.* 7th ed. Philadelphia, PA: Elsevier; 2016:442. Fig. 17.26.)

loops communicate via the ventrolateral thalamic nucleus. Lesions to these different motor aspects may result in different types of dysarthria (e.g., ataxic dysarthria) and disruptions in speech initiation or prosody.[1,23-24]

Memory

The most prominent memory circuit is the Papez circuit (also called the medial limbic circuit, or hippocampal–diencephalic–cingulate circuit [Fig. 1.29]). Its primary pathway (where {} denotes white matter) is:

- Hippocampus → {fornix} → mammillary bodies → {mamillothalamic tracts} → anterior thalamic nuclei → cingulate → {cingulum} → parahippocampal gyrus.

Degradation of any node or pathway in the Papez circuit tends to result in impaired declarative memory. Recent research has revealed that there is some redundancy in this circuit, with some connections going to multiple nodes. As such, a dense anterograde amnesia may not result until multiple nodes are damaged (as in Wernicke-Korsakoff syndrome, where damage typically extends to both mammillary bodies and anterior thalamic nuclei).[1,25]

Frontal-Subcortical Circuitry

The frontal lobes are the most highly connected in the brain, containing a dense network of reciprocal connections (Box 1.19 and Fig. 1.30). Most of the major white

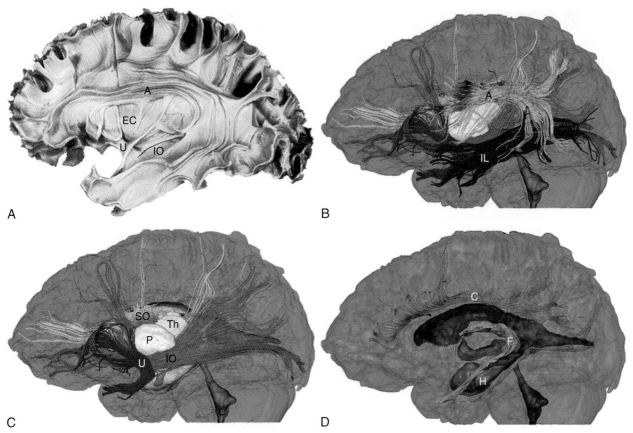

• **Fig. 1.28** View of white matter fibers as seen on dissection (A) and diffusion tensor images (B–D). *A,* Arcuate fasciculus; *C,* cingulum; *EC,* extreme capsule; *F,* fornix; *H,* hippocampus; *IL,* inferior longitudinal fasciculus; *IO,* inferior occipitofrontal fasciculus; *P,* putamen; *SO,* superior occipitofrontal fasciculus; *Th,* thalamus; *U,* uncinated fasciculus. (From Cerebral cortex. In: Vanderah TW, Gould DJ. *Nolte's the Human Brain: an Introduction to Its Functional Anatomy.* 7th ed. Philadelphia, PA: Elsevier; 2016:549. Fig. 22.9.)

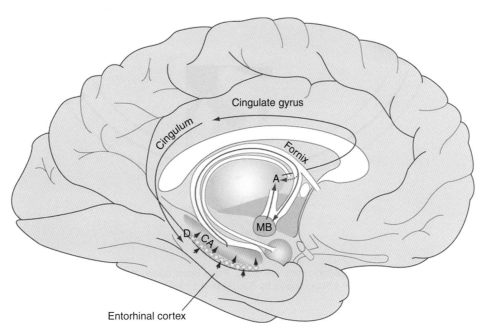

• **Fig. 1.29** Drawing of Papez circuit; A = anterior thalamic nucleus; MB = mammillary bodies; D = dentate gyrus; CA = cornu Ammon. (From Formation, modification, and repair of neuronal connections. In: Vanderah TW, Gould DJ. *Nolte's the Human Brain: an Introduction to Its Functional Anatomy.* 7th ed. Philadelphia, PA: Elsevier; 2016:621. Fig. 24.20.)

Frontal-Subcortical

Pathway	Structures	Function
Direct loop	• Cortex	Excitatory
	• Striatum	
	• Globus pallidus internal segment (GPi) GPi/ substantia nigra	
	• Thalamus	
Indirect loop	• Cortex	Inhibitory
	• Striatum	
	• Globus pallidus external segment (GPe)	
	• Subthalamic nuclei (STN)	
	• GPi/substantia nigra	
	• Thalamus	

matter tracts and networks have nodes with some part of the frontal lobes. Beyond the tracts already discussed, there are prominent frontal–subcortical tracts. In particular, direct and indirect frontal–basal ganglia–thalamic loops may have excitatory, inhibitory, or modulatory effects. These loops appear to have three primary functional streams: motor (oculomotor is sometimes separated), associative (i.e., cognition), and limbic processes. This explains why disorders thought to primarily affect the basal ganglia (e.g., Parkinson's or Huntington's disease) often have motor, cognitive, and psychiatric sequelae. The three functional streams use the same direct and indirect loops but connect to different nuclei within the structures (e.g., limbic channel connects to nucleus accumbens to globus pallidus internal segment (GPi) to dorsomedial and ventral anterior thalamic nuclei).[1,8,19]

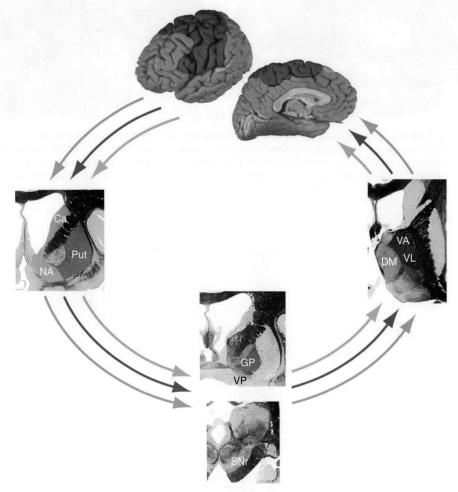

• **Fig. 1.30** View of the frontal-subcortical pathways. (From Basal nuclei. In: Vanderah TW, Gould DJ. *Nolte's the Human Brain: an Introduction to Its Functional Anatomy.* 7th ed. Philadelphia, PA: Elsevier; 2016:481. Fig. 19.8.)

Review Questions

1. Intracranial bleeds from tearing of bridging veins commonly result in a(n) _____, which occurs between the _____ and _____.
   a. epidural hematoma, skull and dura
   b. subdural hematoma, dura and arachnoid
   c. subarachnoid hemorrhage (SAH), arachnoid and pia
   d. intraparenchymal hemorrhage, pia and brain parenchyma

2. A 45-year-old man is being monitored on the neurointensive care unit for an arteriovenous malformation discovered after a moderate traumatic brain injury. You are consulted to assist with diagnosis given that the neuroimaging department is backed up and the patient is becoming increasingly somnolent with periods of confusion/agitation. What condition and associated etiology is highest on your differential given the clinical diagnoses and symptom presentation?
   a. Communicating hydrocephalus secondary to SAH
   b. Noncommunicating hydrocephalus secondary to Chiari malformation
   c. Communicating hydrocephalus secondary to arachnoidal tumor
   d. Extracommunicating hydrocephalus secondary to meningitis

3. A patient presents with an epidural hematoma after a motorcycle accident. On examination, he is observed to have dilated and nonresponsive ("blown") pupils caused by dysfunction of _____, likely caused by herniation compressing the _____.
   a. cranial nerve IV, pons
   b. cranial nerve IV, midbrain
   c. cranial nerve III, midbrain
   d. cranial nerve VI, pons

Answers on page 385.
Access the full list of questions and answers online. Available on ExpertConsult.com

References

1. Blumenfeld H. *Neuroanatomy Through Clinical Cases.* 2nd ed. Sunderland, MA: Sinauer Associates; 2010.
2. Martin JH. *Neuroanatomy Text and Atlas.* 4th ed. New York, NY: McGraw-Hill; 2012.
3. Nolte J. *The Human Brain*: An Introduction to Its Functional Anatomy. 6th ed. Philadelphia, PA: Mosby; 2009.
4. Lezak MD, Howieson DB, Bigler ED, Tranel D. *Neuropsychological Assessment.* 5th ed. New York, NY: Oxford University Press; 2012.
5. Heilman KM, Valenstein E. *Clinical Neuropsychology.* New York, NY: Oxford University Press; 2003.
6. Chen S, Luo J, Reis C, Manaenko A, Zhang J. Hydrocephalus after subarachnoid hemorrhage: pathophysiology, diagnosis, and treatment. *Biomed Res Int.* 2017;2017:8584753.
7. Goldberg S. *Clinical Neuroanatomy Made Ridiculously Simple.* 3rd ed. Miami, FL: MedMaster Inc; 2007.
8. Schoenberg MR, Marsh PJ, Lerner AJ. Neuroanatomy primer: structure and function of the human nervous system. In: Schoenberg MR, Scott JG, eds. *The Little Black Book of Neuropsychology: A Syndrome-Based Approach.* New York, NY: Springer; 2011: 59-126.
9. Casseday JH, Fremouw T, Covey E. The inferior colliculus: a hub for the central auditory system. In: Oertel D, Fay RR, Popper AN, eds. *Integrative Functions in the Mammalian Auditory Pathway.* New York, NY: Springer; 2002:238-318.
10. Gandhi NJ, Katnani HA. Motor functions of the superior colliculus. *Annu Rev Neurosci.* 2011;34:205-231.
11. Ruchalski K, Hathout GM. A medley of midbrain maladies: a brief review of midbrain anatomy and syndromology for radiologists. *Radiol Res Pract.* 2012;2012:258524.
12. Wilson-Pauwels L, Akesson EJ, Stewart PA, et al. *Cranial Nerves in Health and Disease.* 2nd ed. Lewiston, NY: BC Decker; 2002.
13. Kandel ER, Schwartz JH, Jessell TM, Siegelbaum SA, Hudspeth AJ. *Principles of Neural Science.* 5th ed. New York, NY: McGraw-Hill; 2013.
14. Koziol LF, Budding D, Andreasen N, et al. Consensus paper: the cerebellum's role in movement and cognition. *Cerebellum.* 2014;13(1):151-177.
15. Knecht S, Dräger B, Deppe M, et al. Handedness and hemispheric language dominance in healthy humans. *Brain.* 2000;123(Pt 12):2512-2518.
16. Pujol J, Deus J, Losilla JM, Capdevila A. Cerebral lateralization of language in normal left handed people studied by functional MRI. *Neurology.* 1999;52(5):1038-1043.
17. Festa JR, Lazar RM, Marshall RS. Ischemic stroke and aphasic disorders. In: Morgan JE, Ricker JH, eds. *Textbook of Clinical Neuropsychology.* New York, NY: Taylor & Francis; 2008:363-383.
18. Filley CM. *Neurobehavioral Anatomy.* Boulder, CO: University Press of Colorado; 2011.
19. Miller BL, Cummings JL. *The Human Frontal Lobes*: Functions and Disorders. 2nd ed. New York, NY: Guilford Press; 2007.
20. Scott JG, Schoenberg MR. Frontal lobe/executive functioning. In: Schoenberg MR, Scott JG, eds. *The Little Black Book of Neuropsychology: A Syndrome-Based Approach.* New York, NY: Springer; 2011:219-248.
21. Thiebaut de Schotten M, Dell'Acqua F, Forkel S, et al. A lateralized brain network for visuospatial attention. *Nat Neurosci.* 2011;14(10):1245-1246.
22. Scott JG. Arousal: the disoriented, stuporous, agitated or somnolent patient. In: Schoenberg MR, Scott JG, eds. *The Little Black Book of Neuropsychology: A Syndrome-Based Approach.* New York, NY: Springer; 2011:139-147.
23. Dick AS, Tremblay P. Beyond the arcuate fasciculus: consensus and controversy in the connectional anatomy of language. *Brain.* 2012;135(Pt 12):3529-3550.
24. Dick AS, Bernal B, Tremblay P. The language connectome: new pathways, new concepts. *Neuroscientist.* 2014;20(5):453-467.
25. Catani M, Dell'acqua F, Thiebaut de schotten M. A revised limbic system model for memory, emotion and behaviour. *Neurosci Biobehav Rev.* 2013;37(8):1724-1737.

2

Basic Brain Neuroscience and Pathophysiology

GARY GOLDBERG BASC, MD, FABPMR(BIM), AND DAVID GLAZER, MD, FABPMR(BIM)

This chapter serves as a brief overview in outline form of basic brain neuroscience and pathophysiology with specific relevance to the practice of brain injury medicine. This limited review is intended to help establish a very basic neuroscientific foundation for understanding human functionality and pathophysiological processes through which it may be degraded by brain injury. For further details regarding relevant basic brain neuroscience, the reader is referred to reference textbooks in basic and cognitive neuroscience.[1-5] Anatomical details and basic functional anatomy of the central nervous system (CNS) are covered in Chapter 1. In this chapter, the general functional organization of the CNS is discussed followed by a review of basic pathophysiology of traumatic brain injury (TBI). A scheme for the overall organization of various functional brain subsystems is shown in Box 2.1.

General State Controls Over Functional Brain Networks

Systematically ordered groups of cell bodies organized into several systems of nuclei are found in the reticular core of the brainstem and midbrain and project widely throughout the CNS, releasing specific neurotransmitters.

Such neurotransmitters—often called neuromodulators—have a modulatory influence over local synaptic transmission across broad swaths of the CNS, including the cerebral cortex, cerebellum, basal ganglia, limbic system nuclei, and spinal cord.

These nuclear systems have been called components of a reticular activating system (RAS) based in gray matter of the reticular core of the brainstem and midbrain regions.

Conceptualize this general structure as a central multifunctional control system that exerts widespread global state parameter influences over the local dynamics of functional brain networks distributed throughout various subsystems of the CNS.

Each separate nuclear system is associated with a specific neurotransmitter.

Targets to which these cells project may have a range of different receptors all responding to the same neurotransmitter. The effect on the target varies depending on which receptor is activated. Four of these key neuromodulatory systems are characterized in Table 2.1.

Large-scale whole-brain functional neural network dynamics exerting *cognitive control*[6-8]—conceived of as the capacity of neural systems to support cognitive operations such as attention, memory, and executive function—can then be studied in terms of the interaction between these central neuromodulatory parametric controls and the local network dynamics of the functional connectome operating in different brain regions. There are a multitude of functional brain networks identifiable throughout the CNS distributed across multiple spatial scales; here we will focus exclusively on the large-scale functional networks involving the cerebral cortex, called intrinsic connectivity networks (ICNs), because these networks are most directly connected to the dynamics of cognitive control. Traumatic axonal injury (TAI) involving cerebral white matter significantly disrupts the operation of these networks, manifesting

Summary: an Overview of Functional Organization of the Human Brain

Neuroautonomic Visceral Subsystems
Visceral Sensorimotor Subsystems
Visceral Efferent (Motor) Cranial Nerve (CN) Subsystems
General visceral efferent (GVE) (smooth/cardiac muscle and glands)
1. GVE fibers carry parasympathetic autonomic axons. The following CNs carry general visceral efferent fibers:
   A. CN III (Edinger-Westphal nucleus): Preganglionic fibers from the Edinger-Westphal nucleus terminate in the ciliary ganglion and the postganglionic fibers innervate the pupil.
   B. CN VII (superior salivatory nucleus): The preganglionic fibers from the superior salivatory nucleus terminate in the pterygopalatine and submandibular ganglion. The postganglionic fibers innervate the lacrimal gland (from the pterygopalatine ganglion) and the submandibular and sublingual gland (from the submandibular ganglion).
   C. CN IX (inferior salivatory nucleus): The preganglionic fibers from the inferior salivatory nucleus terminate in the otic ganglion, and the postganglionic fibers innervate the parotid gland.
   D. CN X (dorsal motor nucleus): The dorsal motor nucleus innervates the abdominal viscera.
   Special visceral efferent (SVE) (to branchial/pharyngeal musculature)
2. CN V (muscles of mastication, first branchial arch)
3. CN VII (muscles of facial expression, second branchial arch)
4. CN IX (stylopharyngeus muscle, third branchial arch)
5. CN X (muscles of the soft palate and pharynx, fourth branchial arch)
6. CN XI (muscles of the larynx/sternocleidomastoid [SCM]/trapezius, sixth branchial arch)

Visceral Afferent (Sensory) CN Subsystems
General visceral afferent (GVA) (from internal organs, vasculature, glands)
1. CNs IX and X
   Special visceral afferent (SVA) (from olfactory and taste/gustatory receptors)
2. CNs I (olfactory), VII, IX, and X (gustatory)

Spinal Efferent Subsystems
Sympathetic spinal efferent subsystem (SympSE)
1. Intermediolateral nucleus of lateral gray column of spinal cord
2. Extends from T1 down to L2 spinal levels
3. Sympathetic ganglionic chain
   Parasympathetic spinal efferent subsystem (ParasympSE)
4. Pelvic splanchnic efferents to S2–S4 sacral roots

Central Autonomic Network (CAN)
1. Anterior cingulate cortex
2. Ventromedial prefrontal cortex
3. Insular cortex
4. Amygdala

E. Hypothalamus
F. Periaqueductal gray matter
G. Parabrachial nucleus of the pons
H. Locus coeruleus (norepinephrine)
I. Nucleus of the tractus solitarius
J. Ventrolateral reticular formation of the medulla
K. Medullary raphe nuclei (serotonin)

Special Somatic Afferent (Sensory) Subsystems (SSA)
1. Visual
   A. Visual afferent subsystem
   B. Visuomotor/oculomotor subsystem
2. Auditory
3. Vestibular

General Somatic Efferent (Motor) Subsystems (GSE)
1. Primary motor cortex
2. Premotor cortical areas
3. Corticobulbar and corticospinal motor tracts
4. GSE cranial motor nuclei
5. Subcortically originating descending spinal motor tracts
   A. Lateral tracts
      Rubrospinal
   B. Ventromedial tracts
      Tectospinal
      Vestibulospinal
      Pontine (medial) reticulospinal
      Medullary (lateral) reticulospinal
6. Spinal motor neuron nuclei and related segmental subsystem
7. Motor units as basic element of somatomotor function

General Somatic Afferent (Sensory) Subsystems (GSA)
1. Primary, secondary, and supplementary somatosensory cortex
2. Sensory relay nuclei of the thalamus
3. GSA cranial sensory nuclei
4. Dorsal column/medial lemniscal subsystem ("epicritic" modalities)
5. Spinothalamic/anterolateral fasciculus subsystem ("protocritic" modalities)
6. Receptors and DRG neurons as basic somatosensory elements

Neuromodulatory Subsystems of the Reticular Activating System (Table 2.1)

Cerebral Premotor Associative and Attentional Cognitive Functional Networks (Table 2.2)

Cortically Reentrant Motor Efferent Modulatory Support Subsystems
1. Cerebellum
2. Basal ganglia

Greater Limbic Subsystem
1. Hippocampus
2. Amygdala
3. Hypothalamus

in disorders of cognitive control. The brain is a dynamic system transitioning between different momentary mind/brain states in a microgenetic process through which complex behaviors emerge.[9]

Developing concepts in cognitive control based on studies of resting-state functional magnetic resonance imaging (rs-fMRI) indicate cognition emerges through coordinated interaction between multiple anticorrelated ICNs, including those described in Table 2.2.[10,11]

Dynamic transitioning between different cortical networks and associated brain states is facilitated through interactions between ICN dynamics and the neuromodulatory systems sending control signals up out of the reticular core of brainstem and midbrain.[12]

TABLE 2.1 **Four Major Neuromodulatory Systems of the Human Brain** *Neurotransmitters, Receptors, Anatomy, and Functional Characteristics*

Neurotransmitter	Receptor	Source Nuclear System(s)	Projection Sites	Presumed Function	Effect on Cognition	Main Behavioral Effects
Serotonin[51]	$5HT_1$	Raphe nuclear system	Cerebral cortex, Thalamus, Limbic system	Passive coping	Inhibitory	Sleep, Mood, Adaptation
	$5HT_2$			Active coping	Facilitatory	Pain, Memory
	$5HT_{3,4,5,6,7}$			Not well understood	Mixed	Arousal
Dopamine[52]	D_1 family	Substantia nigra, Ventral tegmental area	Dorsal striatum, Limbic areas, Prefrontal cortex	Generate response options	Facilitatory	Movement selection, Attention, Reward
	D_2 family			Selection of responses	Inhibitory	Initiation, Arousal
Norepinephrine[53–54]	Alpha-1	Locus coeruleus, Heteromeric CNS-type, Homomeric CNS-type	Hypothalamus, Amygdala, Hippocampus, Cerebral cortex, Thalamus	Cognition, Memory	Facilitatory	Attention
	Alpha-2				Inhibitory	Sleep
	Beta-1				Facilitatory	Reaction speed, Working memory
	Beta-2				Facilitatory	Plasticity
	Beta-3				Facilitatory	Environmental monitoring, Vigilance
Acetylcholine[55–56]	mAChR M1 group	Basal forebrain (basal nucleus of Meynert)	Prefrontal cortex, Visual, auditory, and somatosensory cortex		Facilitatory	Learning, Memory, Consolidation, Plasticity, Arousal, Goal-directed Attention, Behaviorally relevant stimulus detection
	mAChR M2 group		Amygdala (basal), Hippocampus			
	nAChR				Mixed	

TABLE 2.2 Functional Intrinsic Connectivity Brain Networks Identified with Resting State Functional Magnetic Resonance Imaging				
Network Name	Function	Activation	Deactivation	Functional Hubs
Default mode (DMN) AKA task-negative (TNN)	Internal cognition Thinking about self Thinking about others Remembering Projecting future Endogenous Autobiographical	Self-referential Abstraction Immobile Detachment Not engaged in an external task	Active performance of an external goal-oriented concrete demanding task Externally oriented cognition Anticorrelated with task-positive network	PCC and precuneus vmPFC Angular gyrus
Central executive (CEN) AKA task-positive (TPN) AKA fronto-parietal network (FPN)	Externally directed attention/cognition External awareness Exogenous	Attention-demanding tasks	Anticorrelated with DMN	lPFC PPC Frontal eye fields dmPFC
Salience (SN)	Switch between DMN and "external" engagement Switch from DMN to CEN	Detection of salient features of external environment	Quiescent external circumstances without active salient external event(s)	Anterior insula dACC
Dorsal attention (DAN)	Volitional orienting of attention to a specific task Strategic top-down control	Endogenously directed focused exploratory attentional control	DMN activation	Intraparietal sulcus Frontal eye fields
Ventral attention (VAN)	Stimulus-driven attention Task-relevant reorientation to salient stimulus Bottom-up control	Exogenously directed reactive reorienting attentional control	Volitionally focused goal-driven attention	Temporoparietal junction Ventral frontal cortex

dACC, Dorsal anterior cingulate cortex; *dmPFC*, dorsomedial prefrontal cortex; *lPFC*, lateral prefrontal cortex; *PCC*, posterior cingulate cortex; *PPC*, posterior parietal cortex; *vmPFC*, ventromedial prefrontal cortex.

Basic Neurophysiology of Cognitive Control

There are two different modes of brain activation corresponding to two different philosophical conceptions of cortical function associated with cognitive control:
- The "connectionist theory" of localization of specific functional modules in different specialized cortical regions that become functionally networked and
- The "holistic theory" of functional pluripotentiality, which recognizes significant redundancy and functional overlap allowing for substantial neuroplasticity and flexibility.[13]

In the first activation mode, referred to as the high-modularity mode, activation of cerebral cortex occurs in segregated networks with specialized functions. This corresponds to linking up of functional modules into dynamic subsystems generating the coordinated capacity to meet cognitive demands of a task.

In the second activation mode, referred to as the low-modularity or integrative mode, there is a broad diffuse activation of cortical fields without segregation into distinct focal modules.

Recent studies of time-resolved fMRI (tr-fMRI) have demonstrated that although the brain is organized into dynamic functional networks based on correlational analysis of rs-fMRI,[12] rapid fluctuations occur between segregated states of high modularity and integrated states of low modularity.[14,15] Dynamic switching between these states is associated with outflow from ascending neuromodulatory systems in the brainstem reticular core.[16] Tractography using diffusion tensor imaging to map cerebral white matter tracts demonstrates dynamic functional connectivity is more closely aligned with structural connectivity during low-modularity integrated cognitive brain states.[17] Complex network theory has been applied to understanding how dynamic functional network connectivity enables the brain to flexibly engage in complex activities.[18] Successful cognitive function is associated with the capacity for dynamic reconfiguration of brain network topologies in response to cognitive demands of a task.[19,20] Effects of brain injury can be conceptualized in this context as diminished functional network dynamics.[21,22] Impaired dynamics can be tracked longitudinally following brain injury[23] and used to establish connectomic indicators of severity of injury and project recovery.[24]

Characteristics of functional brain network dynamics such as network modularity have significant implications for recovery process and potential impact of rehabilitation interventions.[25]

Pathophysiology of Brain Injury and Recovery in Space and Time

Brain injury is a highly complex heterogeneous condition involving the most complex organ in the body. Etiologic processes involved in the production of acquired brain injury span every known disease category. We focus here on pathophysiology associated with mechanical trauma and will limit the discussion to a general overview of broad pathophysiological principles without examining details of the pathomechanics or injury classification and assessment (see Chapters 1 and 4). Several review articles cover aspects of brain injury pathophysiology in much further detail than can be addressed here.[26-31] An overview of TBI pathophysiology is provided in Fig. 2.1.[27]

The pathophysiology of brain injury is best understood in the context of normal functioning of the CNS addressed earlier.

The disrupting mechanisms involve both spatial distribution of injury and temporal unfolding of injury-induced pathodynamics.

The spatial classification of injury falls into two categories: focal and diffuse.

Brain functional networks are made up of specialized focal nodes formed from spatially concentrated collections of locally interconnected neurons (i.e., cortical gray matter) and interconnecting axonal pathways (i.e., subcortical white matter tracts) that link up network nodes forming interconnecting "edges" of the network.[30]

Focal injuries primarily manifest as consequences of nodal dysfunction.

Diffuse injuries (e.g., diffuse axonal shearing injury) produce effects related to impaired dynamic communication between network nodes and more generally impaired coordination of contextual dynamic network switching.[23,31] This results in reduced ability to dynamically reconfigure functional brain network connectivity in response to cognitive task demands.

Recovery can be understood as resolution of injury-induced network pathodynamics. For example, dynamic ICN topology reemerges with recovery of consciousness in individuals with disorders of consciousness caused by severe TBI.[32]

In the time domain, the pathogenic process can be parsed into:
- primary mechanical tissue injury at the moment of impact and immediate injury consequences, and
- secondary pathodynamics precipitated by the primary mechanical tissue disruption.

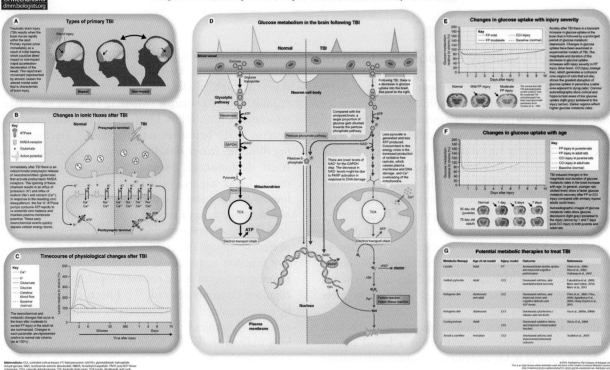

• **Fig. 2.1** Pathophysiology of TBI. (From Prins M, Greco T, Alexander D, Giza CC. The pathophysiology of traumatic brain injury at a glance. *Dis Model Mech.* 2013;6[6]:1307-1315. doi:10.1242/dmm.011585.)

The primary mechanical effects can be differentiated into effects produced by inertially transmitted forces and direct impact forces (see Fig. 2.1A).

Inertial (i.e., acceleration/deceleration) forces result in both translational and rotational movement of the cranial vault and its contents. These forces are transmitted through the neck to the head from rapid back-and-forth and twisting motion of the trunk, thus placing the spinal cord and the soft tissues of the neck also at risk for mechanical injury (see Chapters 22 and 54).

Directly applied impact forces can be divided into:
- deforming force applied perpendicular to the cranial surface and
- tangentially applied torque that induces differential rotation between skull and intracranial structures resulting in a more diffuse distribution and layered absorption of rotational mechanical energy involving shear strain effects on brain tissue.

A classification scheme for TBI subtypes is shown in Fig. 2.2.

Focal Injury

Focal mechanical trauma can result in vascular injury and hemorrhage with resultant bleeding into different extracranial and intracranial spaces, including subgaleal, epidural, subdural, subarachnoid, intraparenchymal, and intraventricular spaces.

The bleeding process and volume of blood extravasated is influenced by various factors, including the type and size of vessel from which the bleeding occurs and the back pressure in the space into which the bleeding occurs. Clotting dysfunction can also precipitate larger accumulations of blood (e.g., patients on anticoagulant medication).

Mechanical trauma can also result in local bruising of brain tissue. Contusional focal injury most commonly involves frontal and temporal lobes caused by close relationship to adjacent sharp edges of internal skull configuration.

Similar focal injuries may result from inertial forces associated with rapid acceleration/deceleration movement of the head inducing movement of the brain relative to sharp edges of internal cranial surfaces:
- "Coup" injury is located directly beneath the site of mechanical impact.
- "Contrecoup" injury localized to the opposite side of the brain as result of translational force effects and rebound motion; often worse than direct coup injury.

Severe head trauma involving both impact and nonimpact inertial forces can produce multiple focal contusions involving both sides of the brain.

Contusions most often involve cortical regions and are often characterized by mechanical tissue deformation and intraparenchymal hemorrhage caused by local vessel injury. This leads to local edema and ischemia, resulting in neuronal necrosis, focal atrophy, and eventual tissue resorption with surrounding reactive gliosis.

There can be continued hemorrhagic progression over the first few postinjury days and "blossoming" of contusion caused by continuing hemorrhage and accumulating reactive cerebral edema. This may lead to progressive elevation of intracranial pressure (ICP). The functional effects of focal injury relate to the location, size, and depth of the affected tissue and the distribution of damaged regions within the cerebral hemispheres and secondary effects of cerebral edema and elevated ICP.

In injuries with rotational strain and resultant tissue shearing, in addition to diffuse axonal shearing in subcortical white matter of the cerebral hemisphere (see later), focal contusions can develop at:
- local sites of shear strain concentration where there is a rapid transition in tissue density (e.g., gray–white matter interfaces);

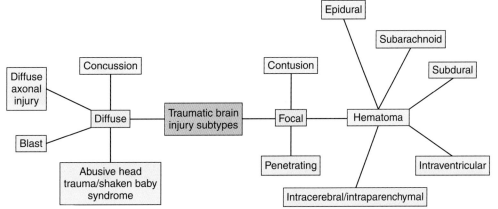

• **Fig. 2.2** Classification scheme for traumatic brain injury (TBI) subtypes. There are several variants of TBI that often coexist and have significant overlap. They can be broadly divided into focal and diffuse injuries. The clinical presentation and prognosis vary depending on the individual nature of the injury and other factors. The inherent variability makes it challenging to establish definitive optimal treatment, and there is recognition of the value of an individualized approach. (From Hill CS, Coleman MP, Menon DK. Traumatic axonal injury: mechanisms and translational opportunities. *Trends Neurosci.* 2016;39[5]:311-324. doi:10.1016/j.tins.2016.03.002 [Fig. 2.1].)

- rapid transitions in segmental moment of inertia caused by differences in the distribution of tissue mass around the axis of rotation associated with changes in shape,
  - midbrain (with transition from brainstem to cerebrum),
  - corpus callosum interface with mesial hemispheric structures; or
- medial temporal lobe (i.e., involving the uncus) and brainstem contusion caused by cerebral edema and elevated ICP associated with subfalcine and transtentorial tissue herniation.

Diffuse Injury

Diffuse injury, particularly involving axons in white matter tracts, with resulting brain network dysfunction is a prominent pathophysiological characteristic of TBI characterized by:

- Multifocal damage with dispersed spread of shearing forces, resulting in widespread mechanical injury to axons and small thin-walled capillary vessels
  - Shearing forces tend to converge in certain regions as noted earlier, so that "diffuse" pattern of injury is really a recognizable pattern of multifocal damage that tends to concentrate in certain vulnerable regions both macroscopically and microscopically.
- Multifocal axonal injury referred to as diffuse axonal injury (DAI) or multifocal TAI
- Diagnosed by histopathology in postmortem brain microscopy (see Fig. 2.3)
  - May vary from minimal distortion of structure to complete tearing

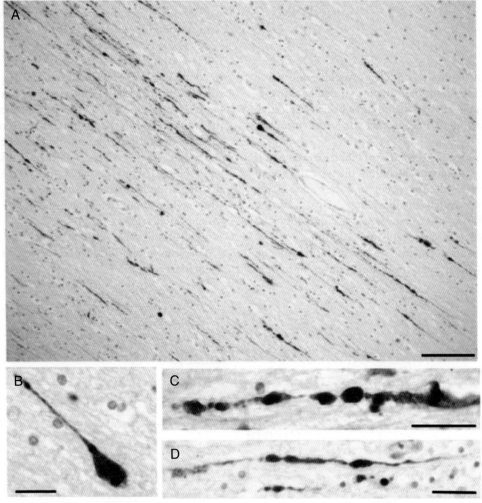

• **Fig. 2.3** Micrograph images of axonal pathology following traumatic brain injury in humans using amyloid precursor protein (APP) immunochemistry. **(A)** Extensive axonal pathology with classic varicosities and axonal bulb formation in a region of the corpus callosum. Scale bar: 100 microns. **(B)** High magnification of a single axon immunoreactive for APP displaying the classical morphology of an axonal bulb. Scale bar: 15 microns. **(C)** and **(D)** High magnification of a single axon with accumulating APP. Axons are morphologically varicose, exhibiting multiple points of transport interruption giving the appearance of beads on a ring. Scale bars: 30 microns. (From Johnson VE, Stewart W, Smith DH. Axonal pathology in traumatic brain injury. *Exp Neurol.* 2013;246:35-43. doi:10.1016/j.expneurol.2012.01.013 [Fig. 2.1].)

- May vary from a limited to extensive multifocal distribution involving cerebral white matter, corpus callosum, and rostral brainstem[33]
- Clinical confirmation of TAI can be difficult because damage is microscopic and scattered and therefore not readily identifiable on conventional neuroimaging.
- MRI is more sensitive in identifying diffuse acute injury compared with computed tomography.

The clinical approach to diagnosis is covered in Chapter 14. Imaging methods for the detection and assessment of TAI after an injury event are covered in Chapter 15.

Interruption of ascending projections from brainstem reticular core can affect ICN dynamics in the cerebral cortex, providing a pathophysiological basis for immediate loss of consciousness or a period of significant alteration of consciousness (e.g., confusion, posttraumatic amnesia, slowed cognition).[34]

Mechanical damage to axonal membrane precipitates calcium ion (Ca^{2+}) influx, initiating calcium-mediated pathological cascade 6p, resulting in:
- Impaired axonal transport
- Focal axonal swelling
- Impaired action potential transmission
- Localized resorption
- Target deafferentation and generalized Wallerian degeneration[35,36]
- Focal degeneration of cytoskeleton with neurofilament compaction in axonal interior without subsequent swelling; axon undergoes process of rapid degradation and resorption[37,38]
- Unmyelinated axons more vulnerable to mechanical trauma than myelinated axons[39]
- Cascade of Ca^{2+}-mediated secondary injury processes affecting axons similar to effects on neurons reviewed in the next section[33-36]

A graphical summary of molecular mechanisms and potential therapeutic targets in TAI is shown in Fig. 2.4.[40]

Secondary Injury Processes Initiated by the Primary Injury

Initial stages after injury involve secondary alterations in:
- Regional cerebral blood flow (rCBF)
  - Regional neural activity, cerebral metabolic rate (CMR), and rCBF are normally closely matched through a fine-grained regionally precise autoregulatory process that links the blood supply to the metabolic requirement of the active neural tissue.
  - With respect to rCBF, one immediate effect of injury is a loss of rCBF autoregulation; cerebral perfusion becomes totally dependent on systemic blood pressure rather than on the metabolic requirements of the tissues.
  - Regional or global hypoperfusion can result in cerebral ischemia, particularly in the context of multiple trauma and hypotension caused by hemorrhagic shock.

- Vascular Trauma:
- Brain injury can be secondarily worsened by direct damage to major intracerebral vascular structures and a lack of naturally occurring vasodilating substances.
- Cerebrovascular factors that can exacerbate the primary trauma include:
  - Potentiation of prostaglandin-induced vasoconstriction with resulting vasospasm.
  - Prolonged posttraumatic vasospasm associated with diffuse ischemia and poor prognosis.
  - Arterioles and arteries, although appearing intact, can show persisting impaired vascular reactivity to normal endothelial-dependent pathways along with impaired smooth muscle responsivity.
  - May render brain especially susceptible to posttraumatic secondary insults threatening cerebrovascular blood supply such as hypotension or hypoxia.
  - Can be a brief period of cerebral hyperperfusion in the early stages of injury (see Fig. 2.1C) either in reaction to initial phase of hypoperfusion or as result of systemic hypertension, precipitating increased intracranial blood volume, and elevated ICP.
  - Altered perfusion states may reflect postinjury changes in regional cerebral metabolism, with relative pathophysiological ischemia or hyperemia reflecting a mismatch between rCBF and CMR rather than adaptive changes to postinjury cerebral metabolic activity.
- CMR
  - CMR as reflected by cerebral oxygen and glucose consumption may be persistently reduced in the acute postinjury state. Degree of metabolic failure relates to severity of primary insult, with outcome being worse in patients with persistently and significantly lowered CMR. This has been related to injury-induced mitochondrial dysfunction with impaired adenosine triphosphate (ATP) production and mitochondrial Ca^{2+} influx and overload (see Fig. 1D). More typically, acute elevation of CMR and glucose consumption initially is observed related to rapid, transient release of excitotoxic neurotransmitters such as glutamate occurring soon after injury driving the brain into a transient hypermetabolic state. Magnitude of excitotoxin elevation and its duration correlate with injury severity. Widespread neural excitation caused by overactivation of excitatory glutamate receptors (particularly the N-methyl-D-aspartate[NMDA receptors]) then produces massive efflux of K^+ leading to a rise in extracellular K^+ along with a cellular influx of Na^+ and Ca^{2+} secondary to excitotoxin-induced repetitive neuronal firing. Observed acute elevation of CMR in response to altered transmembrane ionic gradients leading to metabolic crisis precipitated by requirement for acute increase in available intracellular energy substrate and upregulation of ATP production to restore transmembrane ionic balance and resting membrane potential through ATP-dependent

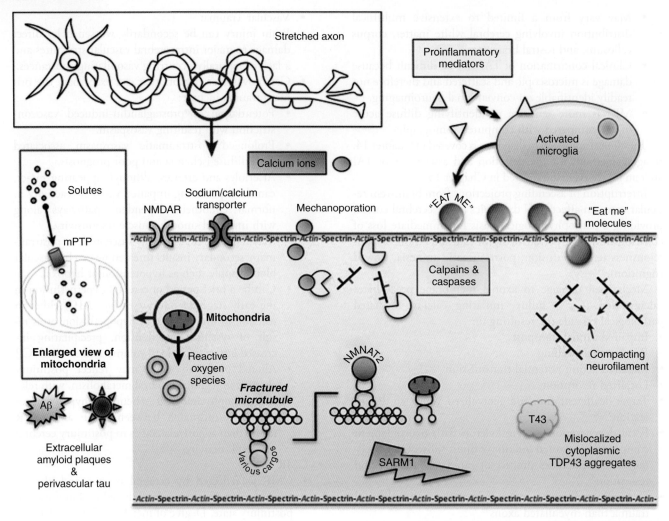

• **Fig. 2.4** Summary of molecular mechanisms and therapeutic targets in traumatic axonal injury. Mechanical stretch of the axon leads to undulation and activation of various injury pathways illustrated here. Direct membrane mechanoporation and opening of exchange channels lead to calcium influx. This activates calpains, which degrade structural proteins. Proinflammatory cytokines have broad effects, including initiation of caspase-mediated proteolysis and microglia recruitment. Calcium influx also triggers generation of the mPTP, with subsequent solute influx and mitochondrial dysfunction/death. Reactive oxygen species are generated and result in oxidative damage. Neurofilaments compact and aberrant protein including TDP43 and amyloid fibrils accumulate. Microtubules are fractured; this leads to impairment of axon transport with failure to deliver nicotinamide mononucleotide adenylyltransferase 2 (NMNAT2) and subsequent Wallerian degeneration. Although NMDA channels are shown on the axon for simplicity, most are localized on dendrites and dendritic spines of neurons. *mPTP,* Mitochondrial permeability pore—when induced in mitochondria by tissue injury, this allows solute influx, leading to mitochondrial swelling and death; *NMDAR,* a glutamate receptor/ion channel that is a channel for calcium ion influx; *SARM1,* Sterile alpha and HEAT/Armadillo motif containing 1; *TDP43,* transactive response DNA-binding protein 43 kDA—a nuclear-pore transport protein, the cytoplasmic mislocalization and aggregation of which are associated with chronic traumatic encephalopathy, frontotemporal dementia, and amyotrophic lateral sclerosis. (From Hill CS, Coleman MP, Menon DK. Traumatic axonal injury: mechanisms and translational opportunities. *Trends Neurosci.* 2016;39[5]:311-324. doi:10.1016/j.tins.2016.03.002 [Fig. 2.3].)

membrane ionic exchange pump. Hypermetabolic response to excitation-induced ionic flows can be associated with an elevation in brain lactate with shift to anaerobic glycolysis. Lactate tends to normalize within a few days in TBI survivors but continues to climb and remain elevated at 5 to 10 times baseline brain lactate level in fatal TBI. These acute injury-induced alterations in neurotransmitter action lead to

significant imbalance between excitatory and inhibitory influences in brain activity required for normal cognition.

Increasing intracellular Ca^{2+} also is commonly observed after TBI. Additional Ca^{2+} released from intracellular stores flows into the cell through voltage-gated Ca^{2+} channels and through membrane "mechanoporation" (i.e., mechanical disruption of the cellular membrane leading to increased ionic permeability). Accumulation of intracellular Ca^{2+} activates mitochondrial Ca^{2+} uptake, leading to intramitochondrial Ca^{2+} overloading, resulting in oxidative stress and impaired ATP production under conditions during which, as noted earlier, increased ATP supply is critically essential to restore disrupted transmembrane ionic gradients.

Increased intracellular Ca^{2+} induces cell damage through multiple pathways:
- activation of Ca^{2+} dependent proteases,
- generation of reactive oxygen and nitrogen species(ROS/RNS), and
- mitochondrial dysfunction caused by Ca^{2+} overload

In summary, TBI precipitates early excitotoxin-induced transmembrane ionic fluxes and neurotransmitter disturbances initiating disruption in normal cellular function affecting rCBF, CMR, glucose metabolism, free radical production, and mitochondrial energy production failure.

Subacute Cerebral Metabolic Rate Depression

The acute period of elevated CMR is typically followed by prolonged period of CMR depression associated with persisting global reduction in brain glycolysis.[41] Magnitude of CMR reduction and time required to return to baseline reflects both the severity and extent of injury and age of the injured person. Associated polytrauma and hypoxia/anoxia can have a deleterious impact. Clinical course typically parallels gradual return to normal CMR. Explanation for persisting post-TBI relative energy production failure not known. One possibility is reduced CBF with reduced supply of glucose to the brain. Another explanation could be reduced glucose transport across blood-brain barrier into brain tissue. Finally, there may be issues with intracellular glycolysis and an impaired ability to generate ATP efficiently through intramitochondrial oxidative metabolism. Increased intracellular production of free radicals—ROS and RNS—caused by excitotoxicity and overwhelming of limited endogenous antioxidant system. Excessive production of ROS after TBI can induce peroxidation of cellular and vascular structures, protein oxidation, DNA damage, and inhibition of the mitochondrial electron transport chain contributing to metabolic failure. These mechanisms can all contribute to immediate cell death and necrosis. As noted later, inflammatory processes and apoptosis can be induced by oxidative stress via effects of elevated intracellular Ca^{2+} and accumulation of ROS (Fig. 2.5).

Neuroinflammation

- TBI associated with full-blown activation of an immunological/inflammatory tissue response including release of proinflammatory cellular mediators: cytokines, prostaglandins, and complement plus release of growth factors.
- Injured and adjacent tissue eliminated through microglial phagocytosis after which astrocytes produce precursors leading to reactive gliosis and synthesis of fibrous scar tissue.
- Cytotoxic edema can also accompany this process.

- Upregulation of various proinflammatory enzymes such as tumor necrosis factor, interleukin-1-beta, and interleukin-6 occurs within hours after significant brain injury along with release of vasoconstrictors (leukotrienes and prostaglandins).
- Neuroinflammatory reaction can lead to multiple punctures through cell membranes (i.e., "mechanoporation") and enhanced Ca^{2+} influx furthering the calcium-facilitated tissue breakdown outlined earlier.
- All of these factors can lead to an aggravation of secondary brain damage caused by ischemia associated with reduced tissue perfusion:
  - Local vasoconstriction
  - Adhesion of leukocytes and platelets to inner walls in microvasculature
  - Blood-brain barrier disruption
  - Local edema formation
- Postinjury inflammatory response with phagocytosis and clearing of cellular debris may also serve beneficial neuroprotective role in process of recovering tissue homeostasis and facilitating regeneration and neuroplasticity after injury.[42]

Cell Death After Injury: Necrosis Versus Apoptosis

Cell death after TBI may occur through necrosis and/or apoptosis (i.e., "programmed'" cell death). Necrosis occurs in response to mechanical or hypoxic/ischemic effects leading to metabolic failure. Dead cells are broken down, and residual cellular detritus is removed by inflammatory processes with scar tissue then laid down.

With apoptosis, neurons are initially morphologically intact and maintained through adequate energy metabolism but later undergo a delayed process of organized dissolution hours or days after the injury event. Apoptosis involves an energy-consuming process with discrete but progressive disintegration of membrane, lysis of internal nuclear membranes, chromatin condensation, and spontaneous fragmentation of the DNA (see Figure 1D).

There is the possibility of antiapoptotic therapy given within a reasonable window of opportunity to block programmed cell death.

An overall summary of various cellular and molecular processes involved in secondary brain injury is shown in Fig. 2.6.

Summary

- Improving knowledge of pathophysiology of TBI can lead to improved interventions to limit brain damage and cognitive dysfunction after mechanical trauma.
- See Chapter 60 for more on pathophysiological mechanisms for development of chronic traumatic encephalopathy and risk of late neurodegeneration associated with recurrent injury exposures not discussed here.[43]

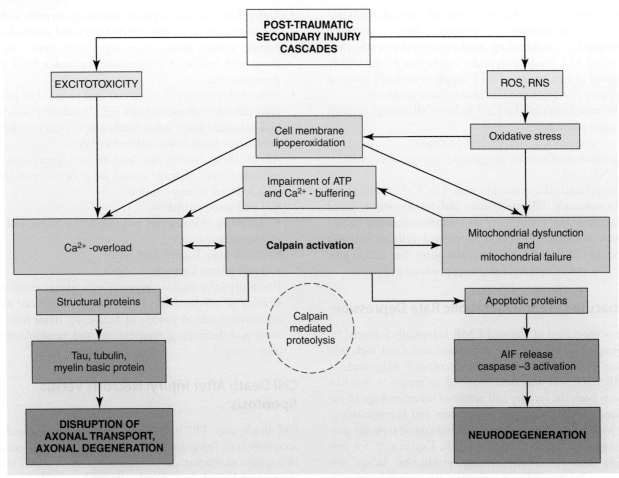

• **Fig. 2.5** Hypothetical relationship between traumatic brain injury (TBI)–induced oxidative damage, axonal degeneration, and neurodegeneration. Secondary injury cascade in TBI induces oxidative stress related to increase of free radicals, reactive oxygen and nitrogen species (ROS/RNS), and increase calcium entry both from intracellular stores and injury-induced increases in glutamate (excitotoxicity). Oxidative stress induces cell membrane lipoperoxidation and calcium release, which activates calpain. ROS and RNS induce oxidative damage in neuronal mitochondria and compromise Ca^{2+} homeostasis. Activated calpain mediates further Ca^{2+} entry, forming a positive feedback loop and induces mitochondrial membrane permeability and releases the apoptosis inducing factor (AIF) from mitochondria. Caspase-3 is also activated by Calpain-1. The released AIF and activated caspase-3 together induce neurodegeneration. Activated calpain proteolyzes large groups of cellular proteins varying from structural proteins and soluble proteins (e.g., apoptotic proteins). Changing either or both the structure or activity of the protein substrates can have important effects such as axonal deterioration and neuronal death. *AIF,* Apoptosis inducing factor; *ATP,* adenosine triphosphate. (From Frati A, Cerretani D, Fiaschi AI, et al. Diffuse axonal injury and oxidative stress: A comprehensive review. *Int J Mol Sci.* 2017;18:2600. doi: 10.3390/ijms18122600.)

• Animal models of brain trauma have contributed significantly to advances in understanding of underlying mechanisms, but verification is needed that similar mechanisms are demonstrable in human TBI using neuroimaging techniques and special technologies such as cerebral microdialysis.

• Individual biological factors, such as genetically determined predisposing factors, may create differential vulnerability to the effects of a given mechanical trauma.

• Comorbid conditions and demographic factors such as the age and sex of the injured person can have significant influence on pathophysiological process and the eventual outcome (see Chapters 48 and 51).

• Multiple psychological and socioeconomic factors including history of psychiatric disorder, substance abuse, and socioeconomic status have a negative impact on outcome (see Chapter 8).[44,45]

• The ultimate clinical goal, as elusive as it can be given the complexity of pathophysiology and the rigor of executing multicenter randomized controlled trials to achieve adequate numbers of subjects, is to:
  • Discover interventions that rescue and preserve brain tissue before irreversible damage has occurred or
  • Interfere with secondary late processes, such as oxidative stress,[46] neuroinflammation,[47-49] and neuronal apoptosis[50] with the goal of reducing their delayed deleterious effects.

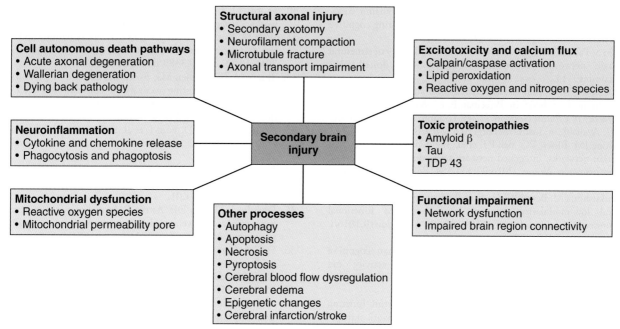

• **Fig. 2.6** Cellular and molecular activities resulting in secondary brain injury. Following a traumatic insult to the brain, an extensive series of various cellular processes is initiated that leads to further neuronal dysfunction and death. The contributes to the complexity of traumatic brain injury but also provides a variety of potential therapeutic targets. *TDP43,* Transactive response DNA-binding protein 43 kDA. (From Hill CS, Coleman MP, Menon DK. Traumatic axonal injury: mechanisms and translational opportunities. *Trends Neurosci.* 2016;39[5]:311-324. doi:10.1016/j.tins.2016.03.002 [Fig. 2.2].)

Review Questions

1. Which of these is not considered a direct result of primary brain injury?
   a. Intracranial hemorrhage
   b. Diffuse axonal injury
   c. Apoptosis
   d. Focal cortical contusion
   e. Contrecoup injury
2. Which cation starts the cascade leading to the breakdown of the axon cytoskeleton, oxidative stress, and mitochondrial failure after brain injury?
   a. Sodium
   b. Calcium
   c. Potassium
   d. Hydrogen
   e. Magnesium
3. Large-scale intrinsic connectivity networks that have been recognized through functional brain imaging include all of the following except:
   a. Default mode network
   b. Salience network
   c. Central executive network
   d. Error detection network
   e. Dorsal attentional network

Answers on page 385.

Access the full list of questions and answers online.

Available on ExpertConsult.com

References

1. Kandel ER, Schwartz JM, Jessel TM, et al., eds. *Principles of Neural Science.* 5th ed. New York, NY: McGraw-Hill Medical; 2013.
2. Nieuwenhuys R, Voogd J, van Huijzen C. *The Human Central Nervous System.* 4th ed. Berlin, Germany: Springer-Verlag; 2008.
3. Bear MF, Connors BW, Paradiso MA. *Neuroscience. Exploring the Brain.* 4th ed. Wolters-Kluwer; 2016.
4. Banich MT, Compton R. *Cognitive Neuroscience.* 4th ed. Cambridge, UK: Cambridge University Press; 2018.
5. Gazzaniga MS, Ivry RB, Mangun GR. *Cognitive Neuroscience. The Biology of Mind.* 5th ed. New York, NY: WW Norton and Company; 2013.
6. Botvinick MM, Cohen JD. The computational and neural basis of cognitive control: charted territory and new frontiers. *Cogn Sci.* 2014;38:1249-1285.
7. Power JD, Schlaggar BL, Lessov-Schlaggar CN, Petersen SE. Evidence for hubs in human functional brain networks. *Neuron.* 2013;79:798-813.
8. Corbetta M, Schulman GL. Control of goal-directed and stimulus-driven attention in the brain. *Nat Rev Neurosci.* 2002;3: 201-205.
9. Brown JW. Theoretical note on the nature of the present. *Process Stud.* 2018;47:163-171.
10. Fox MD, Snyder AZ, Vincent JL, Corbetta M, Van Essen DC, Raichle ME. The human brain is intrinsically organized into dynamic, anticorrelated functional networks. *Proc Natl Acad Sci U S A.* 2005;102:9673-9678. doi:10.1073/pnas.0504136102.

11. Cocchi L, Zalesky A, Fornito A, Mattingley JB. Dynamic cooperation and competition between brain systems during cognitive control. *Trends Cogn Sci*. 2013;17:493-501.

12. Gu S, Pasqualetti F, Cieslak M, et al. Controllability of structural brain networks. *Nat Commun*. 2015;6:8414. doi:10.1038/ncomms9414.

13. Deacon TW. Holism and associationism in neuropsychology. An anatomical synthesis. In: Perecman E, ed. *Integrating Theory and Practice in Clinical Neuropsychology*. London: Routledge; 1989:1-47. Available at: https://doi.org/10.4324/9780429489464.

14. Shine JM, Bissett PG, Bell PT, et al. The dynamics of functional brain networks: integrated network states during cognitive task performance. *Neuron*. 2016;92:544-554. doi:10.1016/j.neuron.2016.09.018.

15. Fukushima M, Betzel RF, He Y, et al. Fluctuations between high- and low-modularity topology in time-resolved functional connectivity. *NeuroImage*. 2018;180:406-416. doi:10.1016/j.neuroimage.2017.08.044.

16. Shine JM, Breakspear M, Bell PT, et al. Human cognition involves the dynamic integration of neural activity and neuromodulatory systems. *Nat Neurosci*. 2019;22(2):289-296. doi:10.1038/s41593-018-0312-0.

17. Fukushima M, Betzel RF, He Y, et al. Structure-function relationships during segregated and integrated network states of human brain functional connectivity. *Brain Struct Funct*. 2018;223:1091-1106. doi:10.1007/s00429-017-1539-3.

18. Papo D, Zanin M, Pineda-Pardo JA, et al. Functional brain networks: great expectations, hard times and the big leap forward. *Philos Trans R Soc Lond B Biol Sci*. 2013;369:20130525. doi:10.1098/rstb.2013.0525.

19. Cohen JR, D'Esposito M. The segregation and integration of discrete brain networks and their relationship to cognition. *J Neurosci*. 2016;36:12083-12094. doi:10.1523/JNEUROSCI.2965-15.2016.

20. Hearne LJ, Cocchi L, Zalesky A, Mattingley JB. Reconfiguration of brain network architectures between resting-state and complexity-dependent cognitive reasoning. *J Neurosci*. 2017;37:8399-8411. doi:10.1523/JNEUROSCI.0485-17.2017.

21. Gilbert N, Bernier RA, Calhoun VD, et al. Diminished neural network dynamics after moderate and severe traumatic brain injury. *PLoS One*. 2018;13:e0197419. doi:10.1371/journal.pone.0197419.

22. Sharp DJ, Scott G, Leech R. Network dysfunction after traumatic brain injury. *Nat Rev Neurol*. 2014;10:156-166. doi:10.1038/nrneurol.2014.15.

23. Meier TB, Bellgowan PSF, Mayer AR. Longitudinal assessment of local and global functional connectivity following sports-related concussion. *Brain Imaging Behav*. 2017;11:129-140. doi:10.1007/s11682-016-9520-y.

24. Churchill NW, Hutchinson MG, Graham SJ, Schweizer TA. Connectomic markers of symptom severity in sports-related concussion: whole-brain analysis of resting-state fMRI. *Neuroimage Clin*. 2018;18:518-526. doi:10.1016/j.nicl.2018.02.011.

25. Arnemann KL, Chen AJW, Novakovic-Agopian T, et al. Functional brain network modularity predicts response to cognitive training after brain injury. *Neurology*. 2015;84:1568-1574. doi:10.1212/WNL.0000000000001476.

26. Werner C, Engelhard K. Pathophysiology of traumatic brain injury. *Br J Anaesth*. 2007;99:4-9. doi:10.1093/bja/aem131.

27. Prins M, Greco T, Alexander D, Giza CC. The pathophysiology of traumatic brain injury at a glance. *Dis Model Mech*. 2013;6:1307-1315. doi:10.1242/dmm.011585.

28. McGinn MJ, Povlishock JT. Pathophysiology of traumatic brain injury. *Neurosurg Clin North Am*. 2016;27:397-407. doi:10.1016/j.nec.2016.06.002.

29. Kaur P, Sharma S. Recent advances in pathophysiology of traumatic brain injury. *Curr Neuropharmacol*. 2018;16:1224-1238. doi:10.2174/1570159X15666170613083606.

30. Sporns O. Graph theory methods: applications in brain networks. *Dialogues Clin Neurosci*. 2018;20:111-121.

31. Wolf JA, Koch PF. Disruption of network synchrony and cognitive dysfunction after traumatic brain injury. *Front Syst Neurosci*. 2016;10:43. doi:10.3389/fnsys.2016.00043.

32. Threlkeld ZD, Bodien YG, Rosenthal ES, et al. Functional networks reemerge during recovery of consciousness after acute severe traumatic brain injury. *Cortex*. 2018;106:299-308. doi:10.1016/j.cortex.2018.05.004.

33. Adams JH, Doyle D, Ford I, et al. Diffuse axonal injury in head injury: definition, diagnosis and grading. *Histopathology*. 1989;15:49-59.

34. Johnson VE, Stewart W, Smith DH. Axonal pathology in traumatic brain injury. *Exp Neurol*. 2013;246:35-43. doi:10.1016/j.expneurol.2012.01.01.

35. Povlishock JT, Erb DE, Astruc J. Axonal response to traumatic brain injury: reactive axonal change, deafferentation, and neuroplasticity. *J Neurotrauma*. 1992;9(suppl 1):S189-S200.

36. Frati A, Cerretani D, Fiaschi AI, et al. Diffuse axonal injury and oxidative stress: a comprehensive review. *Int J Mol Sci*. 2017;18:E2600. doi:10.3390/ijms18122600.

37. Marmarou CR, Walker SA, Davis CL, et al. Quantitative analysis of the relationship between intra-axonal neurofilament compaction and impaired axonal transport following diffuse traumatic brain injury. *J Neurotrauma*. 2005;22:1066-1080. doi:10.1089/neu.2005.22.1066.

38. Siedler DG, Chuah MI, Kirkcaldie MT, Vickers JC, King AE. Diffuse axonal injury in brain trauma: insights from alterations in neurofilaments. *Front Cell Neurosci*. 2014;8:429. doi:10.3389/fncel.2014.00429.

39. Reeves TM, Phillips LL, Povlishock JT. Myelinated and unmyelinated axons of the corpus callosum differ in vulnerability and functional recovery following traumatic brain injury. *Exp Neurol*. 2005;196:126-137.

40. Hill CS, Coleman MP, Menon DK. Traumatic axonal injury: Mechanisms and translational opportunities. *Trends Neurosci*. 2016;39:311-324. doi:10.1016/j.tins.2016.03.002.

41. O'Connell MT, Seal A, Nortje J, et al. Glucose metabolism in traumatic brain injury: a combined microdialysis and [18F]-2-fluoro-2-deoxy-D-glucose-positron emission tomography (FDG-PET) study. *Acta Neurochir Suppl*. 2005;95:165-168.

42. Morganti-Kossmann MC, Rancan M, Stahel PF, et al. Inflammatory response in acute traumatic brain injury: a double-edged sword. *Curr Opin Crit Care*. 2002;8:101-105.

43. Bramlett HM, Dietrich WD. Long-term consequences of traumatic brain injury: Current status of potential mechanisms of injury and neurological outcomes. *J Neurotrauma*. 2015;32:1834-1848. doi:10.1089/neu.2014.3352.

44. Lingsma HF, Yue J, Maas AI, et al. TRACK-TBI Investigators. Outcome prediction after mild traumatic brain injury: external validation of existing models and identification of new predictors using the TRACK-TBI pilot study. *J Neurotrauma*. 2015;32:83-94. doi:10.1089/neu.2014.3384.

45. van der Naalt J, Timmerman ME, de Koning ME, et al. Early predictors of outcome after mild traumatic brain injury (UPFRONT): an observational cohort study. *Lancet Neurol*. 2017;16:532-540. doi:10.1016/S1474-4422(17)30117-5.

46. Hall ED, Wang JA, Miller DM, et al. Newer pharmacological approaches for antioxidant neuroprotection in traumatic brain injury. *Neuropharmacology*. 2019;145(Pt B):247-258. doi:10.1016/j.neuropharm.2018.08.005.

47. Kumar A, Loane DJ. Neuroinflammation after traumatic brain injury: opportunities for therapeutic intervention. *Brain Behav Immun*. 2012;26:1191-1201. doi:10.1016/j.bbi.2012.06.008.

48. Chiu CC, Liao YE, Yang LY, et al. Neuroinflammation in animal models of traumatic brain injury. *J Neurosci Methods*. 2016;272:38-49. doi:10.1016/j.jneumeth.2016.06.018.

49. Xiong Y, Mahmood A, Chopp M. Current understanding of neuroinflammation after traumatic brain injury and cell-based therapeutic opportunities. *Chin J Traumatol.* 2018; 21:137-151. doi:10.1016/j.cjtee.2018.02.003.

50. Raghupathi R, Graham DI, McIntosh TK. Apoptosis after traumatic brain injury. *J Neurotrauma.* 2009;17:927-938. doi:10.1089/neu.2000.17.927.

51. Hannon J, Hoyer D: Molecular biology of 5-HT receptors. *Behavioural Brain Research.* 2008;195(1):198–213.

52. Romanelli RJ, Williams JT, Neve KA: Dopamine receptor signalling: intracellular pathways to behavior, in Neve KA (ed.). The Dopamine Receptors. *Springer.* 2009, pp. 137–74.

53. Musacchio JM: Enzymes involved in the biosynthesis and degradation of catecholamines, in Iverson L (ed.). Biochemistry of Biogenic Amines. *Springer.* 203, pp. 1–35.

54. Rang HP, Ritter JM, Flower R, Henderson G: Noradrenergic transmission, in Rang & Dale's Pharmacology. *Elsevier Health Sciences.* 2014, pp. 177–196.

55. Itier V, Bertrand D: Neuronal nicotinic receptors: from protein structure to function. *FEBS Letters* 2001;504(3):118–25.

56. Ishii M, Kurachi Y: Muscarinic acetylcholine receptors. *Current Pharmaceutical Design* 2006;12(28):3573–81

Traumatic Brain Injury Severity and Patterns

SECTION 2

Traumatic Brain Injury Severity and Patterns

3

Mild, Moderate, and Severe Traumatic Brain Injury

JUAN CABRERA, MD

OUTLINE

Traumatic brain injury (TBI) is defined by the Centers for Disease Control and Prevention as a disruption of normal brain function that can be caused by an external force, such as a bump, blow, or jolt to the head, or a penetrating head injury.[1] Although different medical specialties or organizations will use different language, the defining characteristics for a TBI are:

- Acquired external force (nondegenerative, noncongenital, not related to birth trauma)
- Resulting in alteration in physiological brain function (temporary or permanent)

One of the most critical aspects in the evaluation and treatment of TBI is the assignment of injury severity. Unfortunately, however, no single classification system of TBI exists that encompasses all the clinical, pathological, and cellular/molecular features of this complex process.[2] In this chapter, we review the most commonly used definitions and classification schema for TBI.

Definitions

Mild Traumatic Brain Injury

The American Congress of Rehabilitation Medicine (ACRM) provided the first diagnostic criteria for mild TBI in 1993. This foundational definition is "a traumatically induced physiological disruption of brain function" with the criteria in the list that follows but excluding any Glasgow Coma Scale (GCS) score less than 13 after 30 minutes. The subsequent diagnostic criteria for moderate and severe TBI have been rooted in this original definition.

- Any loss of consciousness (LOC) (not to exceed 30 minutes)
- Any loss of memory immediately before or after injury event (not to exceed 24 hours)
- Any alteration of metal status (dazed, disoriented, confused, etc.)
- Any focal neurological deficits that may or may not be transient[3]

Complicated Mild Traumatic Brain Injury

Inconsistencies with inclusion criteria for studies concerning mild traumatic brain injuries resulted in the introduction of the term *complicated* mild TBI (mTBI) in 1990. At the time of publication, a complicated mTBI was defined as a closed head injury with GCS 13 to 15 but differentiated from an "uncomplicated" mTBI by the presence of a depressed skull fracture and/or any injury-related intracranial abnormalities (e.g. hemorrhage, contusion, edema). Over time, the term has been simplified to include any mTBI with radiographic intracranial abnormalities. This term has largely been used for outcome-related research studies.[4,5]

TABLE 3.1	Severity of Traumatic Brain Injury		
	Mild	Moderate	Severe
GCS	13–15	9–12	3–8
Structural Imaging	Normal	Normal or abnormal	Normal or abnormal
LOC	0–30 min	>30 min, <24 h	>24 h
AOC	Up to 24 h	>24 h	>24 h
PTA	0–1 day	>1 day, <7 days	>7 days

AOC, Alteration of consciousness/mental state; *GCS*, Glasgow Coma Scale; *LOC*, loss of consciousness; *PTA*, posttraumatic amnesia.

Common Classification Systems

Glasgow Coma Scale

The most common classification system for assigning TBI severity remains the GCS, first published by Jennet and Teasdale[6] in 1974 (Table 3.1). High-yield information with regard to GCS, however, includes:
- Use best available score within first 24 hours to diagnose severity
- With LOC, GCS is serially measured until consciousness is regained.
- Best motor response provides the greatest prognostic factor for recovery.[7]

Loss of Consciousness

Duration for LOC after TBI has also been used to measure severity of TBI. According to Greenwald et al., mild TBI is defined as alteration or LOC less than 30 minutes, moderate TBI is defined as greater than 30 but less than 6 hours, with severe TBI including LOC greater than 6 hours.[8] In contrast, Department of Defense (DoD) and Department of Veterans Affairs (VA) Clinical Practice Guidelines (CPG) uses 24 hours of LOC to differentiate between moderate and severe TBI[9] (see Table 3.1).

Posttraumatic Amnesia

The time between injury event and ability to demonstrated continuous memory has been well documented as early as 1932 and has been labeled as posttraumatic amnesia (PTA).[10] Duration of PTA has been largely used for outcome studies but can also be used to assign TBI severity when accurately measured.[11]

Department of Defense/Department of Veterans Affairs Clinical Practice Guidelines

The DoD, VA, and Defense and Veterans Brain Injury Center (DVBIC) have collaborated with other federal and civilian medical professionals to develop the most up-to-date evidence-based clinical guidelines and definitions. The VA/DoD CPG is intended for use not only by the VA and Armed Forces but also by the general public. The VA/DoD CPG publication provides a classification table for diagnosis of TBI severity using the variables discussed earlier[9] (see Table 3.1).

Less Common Classification Systems

Abbreviated Injury Scale

The Association for the Advancement of Automotive Medicine developed an anatomical-based coding system called the Abbreviated Injury Scale (AIS) in 1969 with the goal of describing and classifying severity of traumatic injuries.[12] With regards to TBI, the AIS has been used in epidemiological studies but has not gained widespread use for clinical purposes:[13]
- Mild TBI: AIS 1 to 2
- Moderate TBI: AIS 3 to 4
- Severe TBI: AIS greater than 5

Simplified Motor Score

Despite the widespread use of the GCS, it has been widely criticized for poor interrater reliability and complexity. The three-point Simplified Motor Score (SMS) was created to simplify the diagnosis for severity of TBI. Retrospective studies comparing SMS to GCS reveal that the SMS performs as well as the GCS for classifying severity and predicting outcome. The SMS has largely been used for outcomes-based research and has not gained clinical popularity as a classification system.[14,15]

Review Questions

1. A 34-year-old male presents to your outpatient clinic with a self-reported history of recent head trauma from a fall while inebriated. The event was unwitnessed, and the details are unclear. The patient reports persistent cognitive symptoms, headaches, and balance deficits. Which of these options has the best diagnostic value?
   a. Thorough physical examination including Montreal Cognitive Assessment.[12]
   b. Neuropsychological testing
   c. Computed tomography (CT) of brain
   d. Magnetic resonance imaging (MRI) of brain

2. A patient with a history of mild TBI (mTBI) 4 days ago presents to the emergency room (ER) with seizure activity. Electroencephalogram (EEG) demonstrates a seizure locus in the left frontotemporal lobe and head CT demonstrates subdural hematoma (SDH). What is the most likely assumption about the initial diagnosis?
   a. The patient is suffering a late onset seizure
   b. The patient likely has a history of undiagnosed epilepsy
   c. The initial assessment incorrectly identified the severity of injury
   d. The patient was not properly medicated for seizure prophylaxis after a concussion

3. A 67-year-old male patient is brought into the ER after involvement in a motorcycle accident. The patient's initial Glasgow Coma Scale (GCS) score was 8 and has improved to an 11 in the ER. Which of these is the best predictor of outcome?
   a. Best motor response of 5
   b. Verbal response of 4
   c. Eye opening and verbal response score total greater than 8
   d. None of the above

Answers on page 385.
Access the full list of questions and answers online.
Available on ExpertConsult.com

References

1. Centers for Disease Control and Prevention. *Traumatic Brain Injury & Concussion.* Available at: https://www.cdc.gov/traumaticbraininjury/index.html Access date: March 23, 2020.
2. Silver J, McAllister T, Yudofsky S. *Textbook of Traumatic Brain Injury.* 2nd ed. Arlington, VA: American Psychiatric Publishing, Inc.; 2014.
3. Mild Traumatic Brain Injury Committee of the Head Injury Interdisciplinary Special Interest Group of the American Congress of Rehabilitation Medicine. Definition of mild traumatic brain injury. *J Head Trauma Rehabil.* 1993;8(3):86-87.
4. Williams DH, Levin HS, Eisenberg HM. Mild head injury classification. *Neurosurgery* 1990;27(3):422-428.
5. Iverson GL, Lange RT, Wäljas M, et al. Outcome from complicated versus uncomplicated mild traumatic brain injury. *Rehabil Res Pract.* 2012;2012:415740.
6. Teasdale G, Jennett B. Assessment of coma and impaired consciousness. *Lancet.* 1974;2:81-84.
7. Jennett B. Defining brain damage after head injury. *J R Coll Physicians Lond.* 1979;13(4):197-200.
8. Greenwald BD, Burnett DM, Miller MA. Congenital and acquired brain injury. 1. Brain injury: epidemiology and pathophysiology. *Arch Phys Med Rehabil.* 2003;84(3 suppl 1):S3-S7.
9. Department of Veterans Affairs, Department of Defense: *VA/DoD Clinical Practice Guideline for Management of Concussion/Mild Traumatic Brain Injury (mTBI), Version 2.0.* 2016. Available at: https://www.healthquality.va.gov/guidelines/Rehab/mtbi/mTBICPGFullCPG50821816.pdf. Access date March 23, 2020.
10. Russell WR. Cerebral involvement in head injury. *Brain.* 1932;55:549-603.
11. Zafonte RD, Mann NR, Millis SR, Black KL, Wood DL, Hammond F. Posttraumatic amnesia: its relation to functional outcome. *Arch Phys Med Rehabil.* 1997;78(10):1103-1106.
12. Association for the Advancement of Automotive Medicine. *Abbreviated Injury Score.* Available at: https://www.aaam.org/abbreviated-injury-scale-ais/. Access date: March 23, 2020.
13. Savitsky B, Givon A, Rozenfeld M, Radomislensky I, Peleg K. Traumatic brain injury: it is all about definition. *Brain Inj.* 2016;30(10):1194-1200.
14. Caterino JM, Raubenolt A. The prehospital simplified motor score is as accurate as the prehospital Glasgow coma scale: analysis of a statewide trauma registry. *Emerg Med J.* 2012;29:492-496.
15. Thompson DO, Hurtado TR, Liao MM, Byyny RL, Gravitz C, Haukoos JS. Validation of the Simplified Motor Score in the out-of-hospital setting for the prediction of outcomes after traumatic brain injury. *Ann Emerg Med.* 2011;58(5):417-425.

4

TBI by Pattern: Penetrating, Nonpenetrating, and Blast Injury

NICHOLAS C. VLAHOS, DO, AND REBECCA N. TAPIA, MD

Traumatic brain injuries (TBIs) are sustained through a variety of mechanisms. The three broad classifications are discussed in Table 4.1.

Understanding the underlying mechanism of injury can help guide prognosis and treatment. Please note that most established guidelines relate specifically to closed or non-penetrating head injuries, and this injury pattern is covered more extensively in other chapters. In this chapter we will review the unique features and key differences of both penetrating and blast injury.

Penetrating Brain Injury

Epidemiology

- Penetrating brain injury (PBI) is the deadliest form of TBI.
  - It is estimated that 70% to 90% of victims will die before arrival to the hospital, and approximately 50% more will die during resuscitation attempts in the emergency department.[7]
- The prognosis for PBI is worse than that of closed brain injury, but it is far less prevalent.[8]

- Based on data from the Department of Defense (DoD), PBI was responsible for only 1.4% of all TBIs sustained by the military between the years 2000 to 2018.[2]
- Gunshot wounds are the leading cause of PBI overall and account for 12% of all TBIs.
- In the United Sates it is estimated that 32,000 to 35,000 civilians die each year from PBI.[7]
- The incidence of PBI is on the rise and is attributed to an increase in gun violence and suicide.[8]
- In 2016" the Centers for Disease Control and Prevention (CDC) reported a 6.3% increase in firearm mortality rate from 2015 to 2016, with suicide and homicide accounting for 59.3% and 37.3% of the total firearm deaths, respectively.[9]

Mechanism of Injury

- PBI is most commonly caused from a firearm projectile; see Table 4.2 for various types of penetrating injuries and Fig. 4.1 for illustration of common patterns of PBI.
- Kinetic energy is transferred through the projectile into the human skull and brain parenchyma.
- The equation for kinetic energy is $E_k = 1/2 \ mv^2$, where m = mass and v = speed.[10]
  - Based on this formula, it is clear that the speed of an object has a greater impact on kinetic energy than its overall mass.
  - This explains why small high-speed projectiles from a firearm often produce greater damage than slow-speed projectiles like knives, which are greater in mass.
- Other important factors that contribute to gunshot wound severity include the shape of the projectile, tumbling, and the firing distance.[10]
  - Shorter firing distances result in less kinetic energy loss before the time of impact and therefore maximize energy transfer to skull and brain.

TABLE 4.1   Mechanisms of Traumatic Brain Injury

Penetrating Brain Injury

A head injury that results from a projectile or object that penetrates through the skull and dura mater. The most common cause is gunshot wounds, but low-velocity objects such as knives and skull fragments are also capable of causing penetrating injury.[1,2]

Nonpenetrating or Closed/Blunt Injury

A head injury that results from direct impact to the skull. This produces linear and rotational forces that are exerted through the brain, resulting in damage to both neuronal and vascular structures. Falls and motor vehicle accidents are the two leading causes of closed injury.[3,4]

Manifestations include:

- Focal/contusions: Localized deformation of brain tissue secondary to blunt forces or vascular disruption (e.g., expanding subdural or epidural hematomas)
- Diffuse axonal injury: Widespread distribution of axonal injury favoring areas of corpus callosum, fornix, and subcortical white matter[5]
- Brainstem lesions: Associated with poorer prognosis (particularly if bilateral) and decerebrate posturing

Blast Injury

A head injury that results from a blast wave created by an explosion. The blast wave causes rapid changes in intracranial pressure, which results in axonal, capillary, and brain tissue damage. Air−fluid interfaces are most susceptible to damage. Improvised explosive devices are the most common cause of blast injury.[6]

TABLE 4.2   Penetrating Brain Injury Wound Patterns

Does not penetrate brain parenchyma	Tangential	• Projectile that strikes the skull at an angle, resulting in superficial scalp damage without penetrating through bone • Can cause skull fracture and cerebral contusion • Wound pattern associated with best prognosis
	Careening	• Projectile penetrates the skull but travels along the periphery of the cortex without penetrating the brain parenchyma • Rare wound pattern
Penetrates brain parenchyma	Penetrating	• Projectile penetrates the skull and brain parenchyma but does not exit
	Perforating	• Projectile enters the skull and brain parenchyma and then exits at a distal site • Most lethal form of penetrating brain injury • Typically caused by close range or high-velocity projectile
	Ricochet	• Projectile enters brain parenchyma and then bounces off the inner aspect of the skull forming new wound tract

From Vakil MT, Singh AK. A review of penetrating brain trauma: epidemiology, pathophysiology, imaging assessment, complications, and treatment. *Emerg Radiol.* 2017;24(3):301-309.

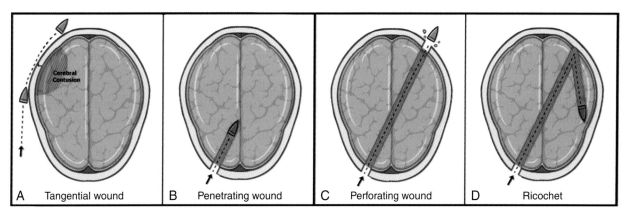

• **Fig. 4.1** Common patterns of penetrating brain injury. (From Vakil MT, Singh AK. A review of penetrating brain trauma: epidemiology, pathophysiology, imaging assessment, complications, and treatment. *Emerg Radiol.* 2017;24[3]:301-309. Illustration by Nicholas Vlahos, DO.)

TABLE 4.3	Mortality Risk Factors	
Demographic Factors	**Epidemiological Factors**	
• Advanced age • Male gender[11] • Low socioeconomic status[4]	• Suicide[1] • Perforating brain injury[11]	
Admission Evaluation Findings	**CT Findings**	
• Abnormal pupillary light reflex • Low admission GCS score[12] • Elevated intracranial pressure • Hypotension • Coagulopathy[11]	• Bihemispheric involvement • Ventricular involvement • Multilobar involvement[4] • Interventricular or subarachnoid hemorrhage. • Mass lesions[11]	

CT, Computed tomography; *GCS,* Glasgow Coma Scale.

TABLE 4.4	Blast Injury Risk Factors	
Increased Risk	**Decreased Risk**
Water medium	Air medium
Close proximity to epicenter	Remote distance to epicenter
Enclosed space	Open space
High-order explosives	Low-order explosives
No body armor	Body armor

From Wolf SJ, Bebarta VS, Bonnett CJ, et al. Blast injuries. *Lancet.* 2009;374:405-415. From Rosenfeld JV, Mcfarlane AC, Bragge P, et al. Blast-related traumatic brain injury. *Lancet Neurol.* 2013;12(9):882-893.

• Suicide-related PBI typically occur at close range and carries a high mortality rate of approximately 95%.[1]

Pathophysiology

• PBI is the result of immediate neuronal and vascular destruction from a traversing projectile through the brain parenchyma.
• This causes permanent cavitation and is followed by high-pressure waves that cause hemorrhage and neuronal membrane disruption at sites distant to the projectile's primary trajectory.[7]
• Cerebral edema rapidly develops and intracranial pressure increases resulting in cerebral ischemia.[3]
• Multiple factors contribute to, the mortality rate of PBI; see Table 4.3 for a brief review.

Blast Brain Injury

Epidemiology

• Blast injury is the most common form of TBI in the military setting.
• Its prevalence has earned it the title of the "signature injury" of both Operation Iraqi Freedom and Operation Enduring Freedom.[6]
• Improvised explosive devices (IEDs) are the leading cause of blast injury overall.
    • Galarneau and colleagues examined registry data of 115 servicemen and found that IEDs accounted for 52% of all TBI. Previous descriptive studies estimate the rate to be approximately 60%.[13]
• The overwhelming majority of blast injuries result in mild TBI.
    • Based on data collected by the DoD from 2000 to 2018, a total of 383,947 service members sustained a TBI, 82.3% of which were classified as mild brain injury.[2]

Mechanism of Injury

Blast-related brain injury comprises four distinct categories:
1. Primary injury: Injury that occurs directly from the transmission of pressure waves through bodily tissue• Primary injury results from an explosion that produces a series of emanating pressure waves.
    • The leading pressure wave, known as the *blast wave,* is characterized by an abrupt increase in atmospheric pressure followed by a period of negative pressure.
    • Rapid change in pressure results in barotrauma, which preferentially affects air-filled organs and air–fluid interfaces.[14]
    • Organs that are most vulnerable to primary injury include the tympanic membranes, lungs, and colon.[15]
2. Secondary injury: Penetrating injury caused by high-velocity projectiles[6]
    • As the blast wave expands, it displaces the surrounding air. This generates high-velocity winds up to several hundred kilometers per hour and is referred to as the *blast winds.*[16]
    • Metallic fragments and foreign bodies are carried by the blast wind and can cause penetrating injury, including PBI.[15]
3. Tertiary injury: Injury that occurs when an individual is thrown into a nearby structure or surface by blast winds[6]
    • Injury is the result of acceleration–declaration forces caused by blunt trauma.
4. Quaternary injury: Explosion-related injuries, illnesses, and diseases not caused by the other listed reasons (miscellaneous injuries)[16]
    • Common injures include thermal and chemical burns, toxin inhalation, radiation exposure, and asphyxiation.[15]

Multiple factors may increase or decrease risk of injury during a blast; see Table 4.4 for a brief review.

Review

As discussed earlier, there are multiple important differences between blast and penetrating head injuries. Please see Table 4.5 for a review of these differences.

TABLE 4.5 Key Points	Blast Injury	Penetrating Injury
Most common cause of injury	Improvised explosive devices	Gunshot wounds
Most common severity	Mild	Severe
Prevalence	Leading cause of military traumatic blast injury (TBI) from 2000–2018[c]	Rare cause of military TBI from 2000–2018[c] (1.4%)
Mechanism of injury	• Primary injury caused by blast wave[b] • Secondary/tertiary injury caused by blast wind • Quaternary injury caused by thermal, chemical, or toxin exposure	• High pressure at the leading edge of projectile results in direct crush injury (<u>missile tract</u>)[a] • Surrounding tissue is also injured trough shearing and compressive forces resulting in <u>cavitation</u>, which is larger than the initial tract
Unique mortality risk factors	Explosion physics[b] • Close proximity to epicenter • Enclosed space • High-order explosive • Water medium	Missile tract[a] • Bihemispheric involvement • Multilobar involvement • Ventricular penetration • Perforating wound pattern

[a]Vakil MT, Singh AK. A review of penetrating brain trauma: epidemiology, pathophysiology, imaging assessment, complications, and treatment. *Emerg Radiol.* 2017;24(3):301-309.
[b]Wolf SJ, Bebarta VS, Bonnett CJ, et al. Blast injuries. *Lancet.* 2009;374:405-415.
[c]Defense and Veterans Brain Injury Center. *DOD Numbers for Traumatic Brain Injury Worldwide: Totals 2000-2018 (Q1).* https://dvbic.dcoe.mil/dod-worldwide-numbers-tbi. Accessed December, 15, 2018.

Review Questions

1. What is the leading cause of penetrating brain injury?
   a. Knife wounds
   b. Gunshot wounds
   c. Shrapnel wounds
   d. Sports related injury
2. In penetrating brain injury, which wound pattern carries the most severe prognosis?
   a. Penetrating
   b. Careening
   c. Perforating
   d. Tangential

3. What component of a blast injury is caused by the blast wave?
   a. Secondary injury
   b. Primary injury
   c. Quaternary injury
   d. Tertiaryinjury

Answers on page 385.
Access the full list of questions and answers online.
Available on ExpertConsult.com

References

1. Vakil MT, Singh AK. A review of penetrating brain trauma: epidemiology, pathophysiology, imaging assessment, complications, and treatment. *Emerg Radiol.* 2017;24(3):301-309.
2. Defense and Veterans Brain Injury Center. *DOD Numbers for Traumatic Brain Injury Worldwide: Totals 2000-2018 (Q1).* Available at: https://dvbic.dcoe.mil/dod-worldwide-numbers-tbi. Accessed December 15, 2018.
3. Bauer D, Tung LM, Tsao WJ. Mechanisms of traumatic brain injury. *Semin Neurol.* 2015;35(1):e14-e22.
4. Antiago LA, Oh BC, Dash PK, Holcomb JB, Wade CE. A clinical comparison of penetrating and blunt traumatic brain injuries. *Brain Inj.* 2012;26:107-125.
5. McGinn M, Povlischock J. Pathophysiology of traumatic brain injury. *Neurosurg Clin N orth Am.* 2016;27(4):397-407.
6. Rosenfeld JV, Mcfarlane AC, Bragge P, Armonda RA, Grimes JB, Ling GS. Blast-related traumatic brain injury. *Lancet Neurol.* 2013;12(9):882-893.
7. Van Wyck DW, Grant GA, Lasowitz DT. Penetrating brain injury: a review of current evaluation and management concepts. *J Neurol Neurophysiol.* 2015;6(6):1-7.
8. Skarupa DJ, Khan M, Hsu A, et al. Trends in civilian penetrating brain injury: a review of 26,871 patients. *Am J Surg.* 2019;218(2):255-260.
9. Xu J, Murphy S, Kochanek K, Bastian B, Arias E. Deaths: final data for 2016. *Natl Vital Stat Rep.* 2018;67(5):1-75.

10. Kazim SF, Shamim MS, Tahir MZ, Enam SA, Waheed S. Management of penetrating brain injury. *J Emerg Trauma Shock.* 2011;4(3):395-402.

11. Part II: Prognosis in penetrating brain injury. *J Trauma.* 2001; 51(suppl 2):S44-S86.

12. Kaufman HH, Makela ME, Lee KF, Haid Jr RW, Gildenberg PL. Gunshot wounds to the head: a perspective. *Neurosurgery.* 1986;18:689-695.

13. Galarneau MR, Woodruff SI, Dye JL, Mohrle CR, Wade AL. Traumatic brain injury during Operation Iraqi Freedom: findings from the United States Navy-Marine Corps Combat Trauma Registry. *J Neurosurg.* 2008;108(5):950-957.

14. Nakagawa A, Manley GT, Gean AD, et al. Mechanisms of primary blast-induced traumatic brain injury: insights from shock-wave research. *J Neurotrauma.* 2011;28(6):1101-1119.

15. DePalma RG, Burris DG, Champion HR, Hodgson MJ. Blast injuries. *N Engl J Med.* 2005;352:1335-1342.

16. Wolf SJ, Bebarta VS, Bonnett CJ, Pons PT, Cantrill SV. Blast injuries. *Lancet.* 2009;374:405-415.

17. Coello AF, Canals AG, Gonzalez JM, Martín JJ. Cranial nerve injury after minor head trauma. *J Neurosurg.* 2010;113(3): 547-555.

5

Brain Death Criteria

CHERRY JUNN, MD

With the advancement of positive-pressure ventilation in the 1950s, patients who sustained a catastrophic brain injury could be supported in hospitals after cessation of brain function. In 1968, an ad hoc committee at Harvard Medical School defined a new criterion for death, wherein the brainstem and higher cortical functions are absent despite preserved cardiac function.[1]

Criteria for Determining Brain Death

Since the release of the Harvard report, criteria for brain death continue to be refined.[2] The American Academy of Neurology (AAN) released a clinician guideline for determining brain death in 2010 (Table 5.1).[3] However, each hospital has its own specific criteria. The information provided here is based on the AAN guideline.

Prerequisites

Two prerequisites must always be met before proceeding with clinical examination:
1. An irreversible coma from a known cause—an untreatable catastrophic neurologic structural injury without known effective intervention
2. Exclusion and treatment of all possible confounding factors, such as hypothermia; hypotension; drug intoxication; poisoning; effects of paralytic, sedative, analgesic, and/or neuromuscular blockers; major metabolic abnormalities (electrolytes, acid base, or endocrine)[4];

and other mimicking condition such as severe Guillain-Barré syndrome

Clinical Examination

Once the prerequisites are met, complete a clinical examination in a stepwise fashion.
1. Absent motor response to noxious stimuli in all limbs (Fig. 5.1 A)
   A. Spinal responses such as a brief, slow movement or flexion in upper limbs or flexion in the fingers that extinguish with repeated stimulation[5] are consistent with brain death.
2. Absent brainstem reflexes (Fig. 5.1 B)
   A. No corneal reflex: No blinking after water or swab touches cornea. Similar to spinal responses, facial myokymia from possible denervation of the facial nucleus is compatible.
   B. Immobile eyes and no reaction to light: eyes can be skewed in position but should not deviate. Nystagmus or other spontaneous movement is not compatible with brain death.
   C. Absent oculocephalic reflex: When the head is turned quickly, the eyes should remain fixed without any movement.
   D. Absent oculovestibular reflex: No eye movement with ice water caloric testing. If the brainstem is intact, then the eyes slowly deviate toward the cold caloric stimulus.
   E. Absent facial movement to noxious stimuli to supraorbital nerve or bilateral condyles of the temporomandibular joint. Jaw reflex is also absent.
   F. Absent cough and gag reflexes

Apnea Test

1. Prerequisites:
   A. Hemodynamically stable with systolic blood pressure ≥ 100 mm Hg
   B. Ventilator set to provide normocarbia (partial pressure of carbon dioxide [$Paco_2$] 35–45 mm Hg)

TABLE 5.1	Checklist for Determination of Brain Death

Prerequisites (all must be checked)
1. Coma, irreversible and cause known
2. Neuroimaging explains coma
3. CNS depressant drug effect absent (if indicated toxicology screen; if barbiturates given, serum level <10 µg/mL)
4. No evidence of residual paralytics (electrical stimulation if paralytics used)
5. Absence of severe acid-base, electrolyte, or endocrine abnormality
6. Normothermia or mild hypothermia (core temperature >36°C)
7. Systolic blood pressure ≥100 mm Hg
8. No spontaneous respiration

Examination (all must be checked)
1. Pupils nonreactive to bright light
2. Corneal reflex absent
3. Oculocephalic reflex absent (tested only if C-spine integrity ensured)
4. Oculovestibular reflex absent
5. No facial movement to noxious stimuli at supraorbital nerve, temporomandibular joint
6. Gag reflex absent
7. Cough reflex absent to tracheal suctioning
8. Absence of motor response to noxious stimuli in all four limbs (spinally mediated reflexes are permissible)

Apnea testing (all must be checked)
1. Patient is hemodynamically stable
2. Ventilator adjusted to provide normocarbia (partial pressure of carbon dioxide [$PaCO_2$] 35–45 mm Hg)
3. Patient preoxygenated with 100% FiO_2 for >10 min to partial pressure of oxygen (PaO_2) >200 mm Hg
4. Patient well oxygenated with a positive end-expiratory pressure (PEEP) of 5 cm of water
5. Provide oxygen via a suction catheter to the level of the carina at 6 L/min or attach T-piece with continuous positive airway pressure (CPAP) at 10 cm H_2O
6. Disconnect ventilator
7. Spontaneous respirations absent
8. Arterial blood gas drawn at 8–10 min patient reconnected to ventilator
9. $PaCO_2$ ≥60 mm Hg or 20 mm Hg rise from normal baseline value

OR:

Apnea test aborted

Ancillary testing (only one needs to be performed; to be ordered only if clinical examination cannot be fully performed because of patient factors, or if apnea testing inconclusive or aborted)
1. Cerebral angiogram
2. HMPAO SPECT
3. EEG
4. TCD

Time of death (date/month/year): _____

Name of physician and signature: _____

CNS, Central nervous system; *EEG*, electroencephalogram; *HMPAO*, hexamethylpropyleneamine-oxime; *SPECT*, single photon emission computed tomography; *TCD*, transcranial Doppler ultrasonography.
From Wijdicks EFM, Varelas PN, Gronseth GS, Greer DM. Evidence-based guideline update: determining brain death in adults-report of the Quality Standards Subcommittee of the American Academy of Neurology. *Neurology.* 2010;74:1911.

C. Preoxygenate with 100% FiO_2 for >10 minutes to achieve partial pressure of oxygen (PaO_2) >200 mm Hg
D. Well oxygenated with a positive end-expiratory pressure (PEEP) of 5 cm of water
2. Steps: (Fig. 5.2)
A. Disconnect from the ventilator.
B. Insert oxygen insufflation catheter to the level of the carina at 6 L/min or attach T-piece with continuous positive airway pressure (CPAP) at 10 cm H_2O.
C. Check for any respiratory movements. Abort if there's movement, refractory hypotension (systolic blood pressure [SBP] <90 mm Hg), or worsening hypoxemia (pulse oximetry <85%).[6]
D. If no respiratory movements for about 8 minutes, obtain arterial blood gas.
E. Apnea is established if blood gas should demonstrate $PaCO_2$ ≥60 mm Hg or 20 mm Hg rise from normal baseline value.

Ancillary Testing

Ancillary test is not mandatory and generally unnecessary. Use if reliability of the neurologic examination is uncertain or if the apnea test cannot be performed. For possible pitfalls, see Table 5.2.

Cerebral Angiography

There are no specific criteria to define cerebral angiograph (CTA) findings consistent with brain injury.[7] Nonetheless, no intracerebral filling in distal middle cerebral arteries[3,6] is compatible with brain death.

Electroencephalography

A complete lack of electrocerebral activity, defined as the absence of electroencephalography (EEG) activity exceeding 2µV in amplitude.[8]

Transcranial Doppler Ultrasonography

Findings consistent with brain death include absence of blood flow. However, presence of small systolic peaks in early systole in setting of elevated ICP or a reverberating flow pattern with forward flow in systole and retrograde flow in diastole (Fig. 5.3) does not preclude brain death.[3,6,8,9]

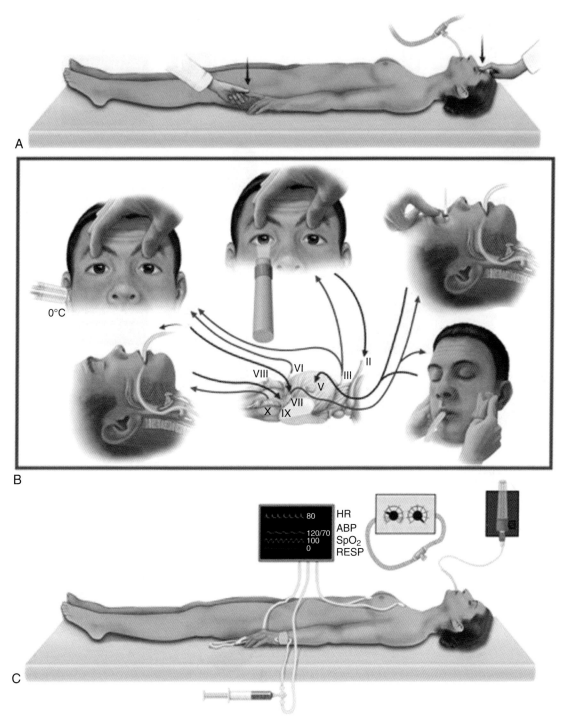

• **Fig. 5.1** Clinical determination of brain death requirement: **(A)** absent motor response or grimacing to noxious stimulation; **(B)** absent brainstem reflexes; and **(C)** no respiratory effort despite adequate CO_2 challenge during formal apnea testing (From Fugate JE. *Bradley's Neurology in Clinical Practice.* 7th ed. Philadelphia, PA: Elsevier; 2016.)

Cerebral Scintigraphy (Technetium Tc 99m Hexametazime)

Compatible with brain death if no brain perfusion: no radionuclide location in the middle cerebral artery, anterior cerebral artery, or basilar artery territories of the cerebral hemispheres.[3,6,7]

Somatosensory-Evoked Potentials

Although not mentioned in the AAN guideline, bilateral loss of the median somatosensory-evoked potentials (SSEPs) is indicative of impending brain death.[10,11] SSEPs can also be used for prognosis; an asymmetrical median SSEP is associated with severe residual deficit.[10]

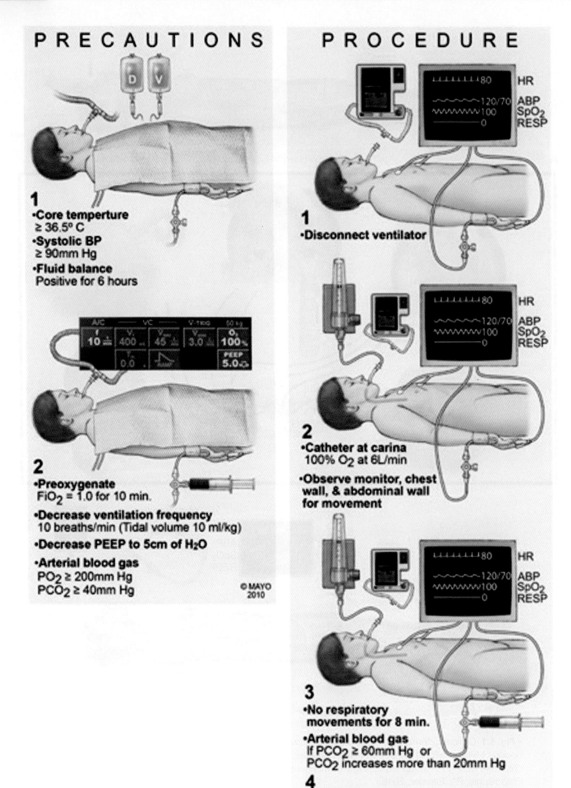

PRECAUTIONS

1
- Core temperture
  ≥ 36.5° C
- Systolic BP
  ≥ 90mm Hg
- Fluid balance
  Positive for 6 hours

2
- Preoxygenate
  FiO_2 = 1.0 for 10 min.
- Decrease ventilation frequency
  10 breaths/min (Tidal volume 10 ml/kg)
- Decrease PEEP to 5cm of H_2O
- Arterial blood gas
  PO_2 ≥ 200mm Hg
  PCO_2 ≥ 40mm Hg

© MAYO
2010

PROCEDURE

1
- Disconnect ventilator

2
- Catheter at carina
  100% O_2 at 6L/min
- Observe monitor, chest
  wall, & abdominal wall
  for movement

3
- No respiratory
  movements for 8 min.
- Arterial blood gas
  If PCO_2 ≥ 60mm Hg or
  PCO_2 increases more than 20mm Hg

4
- Reconnect ventilator 10 breaths/min.

DOCUMENT BRAIN DEATH

• **Fig. 5.2** Apnea test. (From Wijdicks EF. Brain death guidelines explained. *Semin Neurol.* 2015;35(2): 105-115.)

TABLE 5.2 Pitfalls of Ancillary Tests

Cerebral angiogram	Image variability with injection of arch or selective arteries Image variability with injection and/or push technique No guidelines or interpretation
Transcranial Doppler ultrasonographic scan	Technical difficulties and skill dependent Normal in anoxic-ischemic injury
EEG	Artifacts in intensive care settings Vulnerable to confounders; information limited assessment of subcortical structures
Somatosensory evoked potentials	Absent in comatose patients without brain death
CT angiogram	Interpretation difficulties Retained blood flow in 20% of cases Possibility to miss slow flow states because of rapid acquisition of images
Nuclear brain scan	Areas of perfusion in thalamus in patients with anoxic injury or skull defect
SSEPs	High sensitivity but poor specificity

CT, Computed tomography; *EEG,* electroencephalogram; *SSEPs,* somatosensory-evoked potentials.
From Kramer AH. Ancillary testing in brain death. *Semin Neurol.* 2015;35(2):125-138.
From Wijdicks EF. The case against confirmatory tests for determining brain death in adults. *Neurology.* 2010;75(1):77-83.

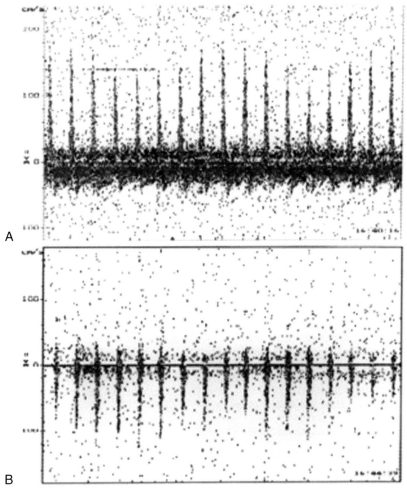

• **Fig. 5.3** Transcranial Doppler ultrasonography (TCD). **(A)** Reverberating flow pattern and **(B)** small systolic spikes. (From Adamczyk P. *Bradley's Neurology in Clinical Practice.* 7th ed. Philadelphia, PA: Elsevier; 2016.)

Ethical and Legal Concerns

In the United States, a model definition of death has been outlined by the Uniform Determination of Death Act (UDDA)[13]: "an individual who has sustained either (a) irreversible cessation of circulatory or respiratory functions, or (b) irreversible cessation of all function of the entire brain, including brainstem, is dead."

Although all 50 states adopted a version of the UDDA, significant variations are present,[14] leading to policy deficiencies that can result in error.[3] Policy variability also exists internationally.[15] For this difficult diagnosis with controversies, evaluation must be standardized and systematic to obtain zero error rate.

Review Questions

1. Which of these findings is not compatible with brain death?
   a. Asymmetrical median somatosensory-evoked potentials (SSEPs)
   b. Reverberating arterial flow on transcranial Doppler ultrasonography (TCD)
   c. No brain perfusion with nuclear medicine scan
   d. Small peaks in early systole on TCD
2. Which of these is a possible major confounding factor that should be excluded before a diagnosis of brain death?
   a. Bladder temperature of 36°C
   b. Hyperglycemia (180 mg/dL)
   c. Propofol infusion, stopped 5 hours before the examination
   d. Partial pressure of oxygen (Pao_2) of 100 mg Hg

3. Which of these does NOT necessitate a termination of an apnea test?
   a. Worsening hypoxemia with pulse oximetry <85%
   b. Systolic blood pressure <85 mm Hg
   c. No respiratory movement 5 minutes after starting the test
   d. Evidence of respiratory movement 5 minutes after starting the test

Answers on page 386.
Access the full list of questions and answers online.
Available on ExpertConsult.com

References

1. Wijdicks EFM. *Brain Death*. 3rd ed. New York, NY: Oxford University Press; 2017.
2. Beecher HK. A definition of irreversible coma: Report of the Ad Hoc Committee of the Harvard Medical School to Examine the Definition of Brain Death. *JAMA*. 1968;205:337-340.
3. Wijdicks EF. Determining brain death. *Continuum (Minneap Minn)*. 2015;21(5):1411-1424.
4. Wijdicks EFM, Varelas PN, Gronseth GS, Greer DM. Evidence-based guideline update: determining brain death in adults: Report of the Quality Standards Subcommittee of the American Academy of Neurology. *Neurology*. 2010;74(23):1911-1918.
5. Wijdicks EF. Brain death guidelines explained. *Semin Neurol*. 2015;35(2):105-115.
6. Wijdicks EFM. The case against confirmatory tests for determining brain death in adults. *Neurology*. 2010;75(1):77-83.
7. Rabinstein AA. Coma and brain death. *Continuum (Minneap Minn)*. 2018;24(6):1708-1731.
8. Kramer AH. Ancillary testing in brain death. *Semin Neurol*. 2015;35(2):125-138.
9. Adamczyk P, Liebeskind DS. Chapter 40. Vascular imaging. In: *Bradley's Neurology in Clinical Practice e-book*. 7th ed. Philadelphia, PA: Elsevier; 2016:459-485.e4.
10. Cant BR, Hume AL, Judson JA, Shaw NA. The assessment of severe head injury by short-latency somatosensory and brainstem auditory evoked potentials. *Electroencephalogr Clin Neurophysiol*. 1986;65(3):188-195.
11. Wagner AK, Arenth PM, Kwasnica C, McCullough EH. Chapter 43 Traumatic brain injury. In: *Braddom's Physical Medicine and Rehabilitation E-book*. 5th ed. Philadelphia, PA: Elsevier; 2016:961-998.e13.
12. Keely GC, Gorsuch AM, McCabe JM, Wood WH, Deacon JC, Hill MK, Pierce WJ, Langrock PF. Uniform determination of death act. InNational Conference of Commissioners on Uniform State Laws 1980.
13. Greer DM, Wang HH, Robinson JD, Varelas PN, Henderson G V, Wijdicks EFM. Variability of brain death policies in the United States. *JAMA Neurol*. 2016;73(2):213-218.
14. Wahlster S, Wijdicks EF, Patel PV, et al. Brain death declaration: practices and perceptions worldwide. *Neurology*. 2015;84(18):1870-1879.
15. Fugate JE, Wijdicks EFM. Chapter 4. Brain death, vegetative state and minimally conscious states. In: *Bradley's Neurology in Clinical Practice e-book*. 7th ed. Philadelphia, PA: Elsevier; 2015:51-56.

Epidemiology and Risk Factors

6

Epidemiology and Public Health and Prevention

KELLY M. HEALTH, MD, FABPMR (BIM) AND JACLYN BARCIKOWSKI, DO, MA

Epidemiology and Public Health

Definition of Traumatic Brain Injury

The Centers for Disease Control and Prevention (CDC) defines a traumatic brain injury (TBI) as an "injury to the head from blunt or penetrating trauma or from acceleration–deceleration forces resulting in one or more of the following: period of decreased or loss of consciousness, any amnesia before or after the injury, objective neurological deficits, any altered consciousness (i.e. confusion, disorientation, slowed thinking)."[1] Forces from explosive blasts, particularly among US service members, can also cause TBI.[2]

Traumatic Brain Injury Classification

TBIs occur across a spectrum of severity and are classified based on specific factors (Table 6.1), with the majority of TBIs (75%–90%) categorized as being mild TBI. The majority of patients who sustain a mild TBI experience symptom resolution with no lasting clinical sequelae. However, approximately 10% of these patients experience persistent symptoms.[3,4]

Statistics on TBI are limited and likely an underestimation largely because of the variability of definitions and classification of TBI across studies and databases. Epidemiological studies are usually based on hospital admission or discharge records, emergency department (ED) records, or death certificates[5] and do not account for persons who did not seek medical attention, had outpatient evaluation, or those who received care at a federal facility (i.e., US military personnel or those seeking care at a Veterans Affairs hospital).[6]

Incidence and Trends of Traumatic Brain Injury

Data from the CDC in 2014 estimated that approximately 2.87 million TBI-related ED visits, hospitalizations, and deaths occurred in the United States.

Of the 2.87 million cases reported[7,8]:

- Approximately 288,000 were hospitalized and discharged
- 56,800 had TBI-related deaths, making up one-third of all injury-related deaths

Total combined rates for TBI-related ED visits from 2006 to 2014 have increased by 53%, while hospitalizations have decreased by about 8%, and deaths have decreased by 6% from 2006 to 2014.[7] The number of ED visits was highest for children 0 to 4 years of age and for persons 75 years of age and older.[7,8]

Causes of Traumatic Brain Injury

Overall leading causes of TBI in 2014 based on CDC reports:[7,8]

- Falls were the overall leading cause of TBI, accounting for almost half (48%) of all TBI-related ED visits.

TABLE 6.1	Criteria Used to Classify Traumatic Brain Injury Severity			
Criteria	Mild	Moderate	Severe
LOC	0–30 min	>30 min and <24 h	>24 h
PTA	<24 h	>24 h and <7 days	>7 days
Glasgow Coma Scale score	13–15	9–12	<9
Structural Imaging	Normal	Normal or abnormal	Normal or abnormal

LOC, Loss of consciousness; *PTA,* posttraumatic amnesia.

- Falls disproportionately affect children and adults ages 75 and older.
  - Falls caused 49% of all TBI-related ED visits among children ages 0 to 17 years and 81% of all TBI-related ED visits among adults ages 75 and older
- Being struck by or against an object was the second leading cause of TBI-related ED visits.[7,8]
- Falls were the leading cause of TBI-related hospitalizations (52%), and motor vehicle accidents (MVA) were the second leading cause of TBI-related hospitalizations (20%).[7,8]

Traumatic Brain Injury–Related Death

During 2014, surveillance data from the CDC showed that there were approximately 56,800 TBI-related deaths each year. The first overall leading cause of all TBI-related deaths in 2014 was intentional self-harm. Falls and MVA were the second and third most common causes of overall TBI-related deaths respectively. Further data on overall rates of TBI-related deaths by mechanism of injury can be found in Fig. 6.1 from the CDC.

TBI-related deaths varied by age group[7]:
- Homicide was the leading cause of death for children ages 0 to 4 years.
- MVAs were the leading cause of death for persons 15 to 24, 25 to 34, and adults ages 75 years or older.
- Intentional self-harm was the leading cause of death for persons 45 to 64 years of age.
- Falls were the leading cause of death for persons 65 years of age or older.

Risk Factors and Characteristics

- TBI morbidity and mortality more common in males than females across all age groups.[1,9]
- Children ages 0 to 4 years, older adolescents ages 15 to 19 years, and adults ages 65 years and older are most likely to sustain a TBI.[4]
  - Different anatomical characteristics increase their risk of a TBI in the pediatric population. Children have larger and heavier heads relative to their bodies

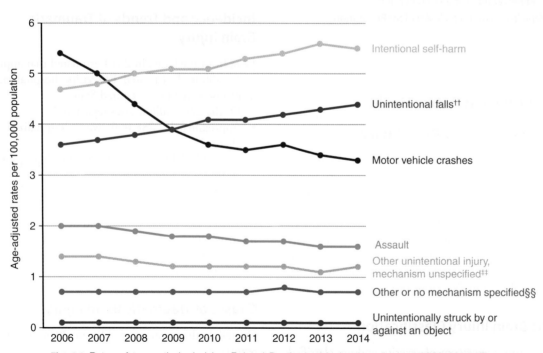

• **Fig. 6.1** Rates of traumatic brain injury-Related Deaths by Mechanism of Injury, 2006–2014. (From Centers for Disease Control and Prevention. National Vital Statistics System. Traumatic Brain Injury and Concussion. Available from https://www.cdc.gov/traumaticbraininjury/data/tbi-deaths.html.)

compared with adults. Additionally, their neck musculature and ligaments are weaker, making them more susceptible to injury. The disproportionate head weight in a child affects the movement of the head during a fall or external blow.[11,12]

- Adults over the age of 75 years have the highest rates of TBI-related hospitalization and mortality.[4,7]
- 25% to 50% of all patients with acute TBI were intoxicated at the time of injury.[13]

Sports and Recreational Injury

The majority of TBIs resulting from recreational and sporting activities are classified as concussions.[9] According to data from the National Electronic Injury Surveillance System (NEISS), from 2001 to 2012, the rate of ED visits for sports and recreation-related injuries that included a diagnosis of concussion or TBI more than doubled among children aged 19 years and younger.[14]

Sports with the highest incidence of concussion, in decreasing order, are American football, hockey, rugby, soccer, and basketball.[9,15] In sports with similar playing rules, the reported incidence of concussion is higher in female versus male athletes.[15]

In American football, the most common mechanism of injury was player-to-player contact. Studies of professional players show that quarterbacks, wide receivers, running backs, and defensive backs have a three times greater risk of concussion versus linemen. Among high school football players, linemen and running backs were more likely to incur concussions.[15,16]

Military Personnel

- TBI is the signature injury from the Iraq and Afghanistan wars.[17]
- From 2000 to the first quarter of 2010, a total of 202,281 US service members were diagnosed with TBIs, and the number of TBIs diagnosed steadily increased during that decade.[18]
- Majority of cases are mild TBI.[2,18]

Economic Cost

A CDC report estimated the economic burden of TBI in the United States to be about $56 billion, with mild TBI making up $16.7 billion of that amount.[1]

Disability

- Data from two states estimate that 3.2 million to 5.3 million persons in the United States are living with a TBI-related disability.[19-21]
- Outcomes at 5 years postinjury based on data from TBI Model Systems[13,22,23]:
  - 57% are moderately or severely disabled.
  - 55% do not have a job (but were employed at the time of their injury).

- 50% return to a hospital at least once.
- 33% rely on others for help with everyday activities.
- 29% are not satisfied with life.
- 29% use illicit drugs or misuse alcohol.
- 12% reside in nursing homes or other institutions.

Injury Prevention

From 2006 to 2014, approximately one-third of all injury-related deaths were associated with TBI.[7] Data from 2006 to 2014 demonstrate that rates for TBI-related ED visits have increased. These increasing rates may reflect growing public awareness of the signs and symptoms of TBI and the importance of medical evaluation and management. Despite increased awareness, morbidity and mortality associated with TBI place a need for comprehensive preventive measures on the public healthcare system.[24]

Fall Prevention

More than one-half of TBIs result from falls and are most common in children ages 0 to 17 and in patients ages 75 years or older.

Preventive measures aimed at various contributing factors based on patient age include:[(24)]

- Safety devices aimed at preventing falls from windows in pediatric population
- Use of protective surfaces and safe borders of soft material (e.g., wood chips, sand, or rubber) in playgrounds
- Balance therapy for postural control and fall prevention in older patients
- Reduction of polypharmacy in elderly patients
- Home modifications for elderly patients (e.g., brighter lighting, removal or repair of tripping hazards, grab bar installation).

Sports and Recreational Injury Prevention

- Bike helmets have been estimated to reduce head, brain, and severe brain injury in all age groups by nearly 70%.[25]
- Prevention measures for American football include helmet design upgrades, limiting the number of players on the field, and eliminating the three-point stance, and the National Football League (NFL) has passed rules limiting head-to-head contact.[24]

Motor Vehicle and Motorcycle Accident Prevention

The National Highway Traffic Safety Administration (NHTSA) reports seat belt use reduces the risk of death by 45% and serious injury by 50% for drivers and front seat passengers in all causes of MVAs. The correct use of car seats, booster seats, and seat belts reduces the risk of serious and fatal injuries in children and adults.[10,12,26,27]

- Car seat use reduces the risk for injury in a crash by 71% to 82% for children compared with seat belt use alone.[12,27]
- Booster seat use reduces the risk for serious injury by 45% for children ages 4 to 8 years compared with seat belt use alone.[12,27]
- Seat belt use reduces the risk for death and serious injury by approximately half and by about 83% when used in

combination with front-impact air bag protection compared with unrestrained drivers.[24,26]

Motorcycle crash deaths are preventable. The single most effective way to reduce mortality is helmet use.[28-31]

- In 2016, helmets saved an estimated 1859 lives.
- In 2016, helmets could have prevented 802 deaths.
- Helmets reduce the risk of death by 37%.
- Helmets reduce the risk of head injury by 69%.

Review Questions

1. What is the leading overall cause of traumatic brain injury (TBI)?
   a. Assault
   b. Motor vehicle accidents
   c. Falls
   d. Struck by or against objects
2. What is the leading cause of TBI-related death in 19-year-olds?
   a. Assault
   b. Motor vehicle accidents
   c. Falls
   d. Struck by or against objects

3. Of the TBIs diagnosed, what is the approximate percentage that are found to be classified as mild?
   a. 50%
   b. 60%
   c. 70%
   d. 80%

Answers on page 386.
Access the full list of questions and answers online.
Available on ExpertConsult.com

References

1. Centers for Disease Control and Prevention. *Report to Congress on Traumatic Brain Injury in the United States: Epidemiology and Rehabilitation*. Atlanta, GA: National Center for Injury Prevention and Control; Division of Unintentional Injury Prevention; 2015.
2. Management of Concussion/mTBI Working Group. VA/DoD clinical practice guideline for management of concussion/ mild traumatic brain injury. *J Rehabil Res Dev*. 2009;46(6): CP1-CP68.
3. Cassidy JD, Carroll LJ, Peloso PM, et al. Incidence, risk factors and prevention of mild traumatic brain injury: results of the WHO Collaborating Centre Task Force on Mild Traumatic Brain Injury. *J Rehabil Med*. 2004;(suppl 43):28-60.
4. *The Report to Congress on Mild Traumatic Brain Injury in the United States: Steps to Prevent a Serious Public Health problem*. Atlanta, GA: National Center for Injury Prevention and Control; 2003. Available at: https://www.cdc.gov/traumaticbraininjury/ pdf/mtbireport-a.pdf. Accessed January 15, 2019.
5. Andelic N. The epidemiology of traumatic brain injury. *Neurol*. 2013;12(1):28-29.
6. Faul M, Xu L, Wald MM, Coronado VG. *Traumatic Brain Injury in the United States: Emergency Department Visits, Hospitalizations and Deaths 2002–2006*. Atlanta, GA: Centers for Disease Control and Prevention, National Center for Injury Prevention and Control; 2010.
7. Centers for Disease Control and Prevention. *Surveillance Report of Traumatic Brain Injury-related Emergency Department Visits, Hospitalizations, and Deaths—United States, 2014*. Atlanta, GA: Centers for Disease Control and Prevention, U.S. Department of Health and Human Services; 2019. Available at: https://www. cdc.gov/traumaticbraininjury/pdf/TBI-Surveillance-Report-FI- NAL_508.pdf

8. Taylor CA, Bell JM, Breiding MJ, Xu L. Traumatic brain injury– related emergency department visits, hospitalizations, and deaths — United States, 2007 and 2013. *MMWR Surveill Summ*. 2017;66(9):1-16.
9. Coronado VG, McGuire LC, Faul M, Sugerman DE, Pearson WS. Traumatic brain injury epidemiology and public health issues. In: Zasler ND, Katz DI, Zafonte RD, eds. *Brain Injury Medicine: Principles and Practice*. New York, NY: Demos Medical Publishing; 2007.
10. Coronado VG, Xu L, Basavaraju SV, et al. Surveillance for traumatic brain injury-related deaths: United States, 1997-2007. *MMWR Surveill Summ*. 2011;60(5):1-32.
11. Figaji AA. Anatomical and physiological differences between children and adults relevant to traumatic brain injury and the implications for clinical assessment and care. *Front Neurol*. 2017;8:685.
12. Arbogast KB, Durbin DR, Cornejo RA, Kallan MJ, Winston FK. An evaluation of the effectiveness of forward-facing child restraint systems. *Accid Anal Prev*. 2004:36(4):585-589.
13. Shandro JR, Rivara FP, Wang J, Jurkovich GJ, Nathens AB, Mac Kenzie EJ. Alcohol and risk of mortality in patients with TBI. *J Trauma*. 2009;66(6):1584-1590.
14. Coronado VG, Haileyesus T, Cheng TA, et al. Trends in sports- and recreation-related traumatic brain injuries treated in US emergency departments: The National Electronic Injury Surveillance System-All Injury Program (NEISS-AIP) 2001-2012. *J Head Trauma Rehabil*. 2015;30(3):185-197.
15. Harmon KG, Drezner JA, Gammons M, et al. American Medical Society for Sports Medicine position statement: concussion in sport. *Br J Sports Med*. 2013;47:15-26.
16. Marar M, McIlvain N, Fields S, Comstock RD. Epidemiology of concussions among united states high school athletes in 20 sports. *Am J Sports Med*. 2012;40(4):747-755.
17. Armed Forces Health Surveillance Center. Causes of medical evacuations from Operations Iraqi Freedom (OIF), New Dawn (OND), and Enduring Freedom (OEF), active and reserve

components, U.S. Armed Forces, October 2001-September 2010. *MSMR.* 2011;18(2):2-7.

18. Defense and Veterans Brain Injury Center. *DoD Worldwide Numbers for Traumatic Brain Injury.* Available at: http://www.dvbic.org/TBI-Numbers.aspx. Accessed January 3, 2019.

19. Selassie AW, Zaloshnja E, Langolis JA, Miller T, Jones P, Steiner C. Incidence of long-term disability following traumatic brain injury hospitalization, United States, 2003. *J Head Trauma Rehabil.* 2008;23(2):123-131.

20. Thurman DJ, Alverson C, Dunn KA, Guerrero J, Sniezek JE. Traumatic brain injury in the United States: a public health perspective. *J Head Trauma Rehabil.* 1999;14(6):602-615.

21. Zaloshnja E, Miller T, Langlois JA, Selassie AW. Prevalence of long-term disability from traumatic brain injury in the civilian population of the United States, 2005. *J Head Trauma Rehabil.* 2008;23(6):394-400.

22. Corrigan JD, Cuthbert JP, Harrison-Felix C, et al. US population estimates of health and social outcomes 5 years after rehabilitation for traumatic brain injury. *J Head Trauma Rehabil.* 2014;29(6):E1-E9.

23. *Traumatic brain Injury Model Systems National Database Syllabus.* Traumatic Brain Injury Model Systems National Data and Statistical Center, 2009.

24. Kneer LM, Elovic E. Primary prevention of traumatic brain injury. In: Zasler ND, Katz DI, Zafonte RD, eds. *Brain Injury Medicine: Principles and Practice.* New York, NY: Demos Medical Publishing; 2007.

25. Thompson DC, Rivara FP, Thompson R. Helmets for preventing head and facial injuries in bicyclists. *Cochrane Database Syst Rev.* 2000;(2):CD001855.

26. National Highway Traffic Safety Administration. *Traffic Safety Facts: Occupant Protection.* U.S. Department of Transportation. Washington, DC: 2009. Available at: https://crashstats.nhtsa.dot.gov/Api/Public/ViewPublication/811160. Accessed January 3, 2019.

27. Arbogast KB, Jermakian JS, Kallan MJ, Durbin DR. Effectiveness of belt positioning booster seats: an updated assessment. *Pediatrics.* 2009;124;1281-1286.

28. National Highway Traffic Safety Administration. *Motorcycles (Traffic Safety Facts Research Note. Report No. DOT HS 812 492).* Washington, DC: U.S. Department of Transportation; 2017. Available at: https://crashstats.nhtsa.dot.gov/Api/Public/ViewPublication/812492. Accessed January 15, 2019

29. National Highway Traffic Safety Administration. *Estimating Lives and Costs Saved by Motorcycle Helmets with Updated Economic Cost Information* (Traffic Safety Facts Research Note. Report No. DOT HS 812 206). Washington, DC: U.S. Department of Transportation; 2015. Available at https://crashstats.nhtsa.dot.gov/Api/Public/ViewPublication/812388. Accessed January 15, 2019.

30. Derrick AJ, Faucher LD. Motorcycle helmets and rider safety: a legislative crisis. *J Public Health Policy.* 2009;30(2):226-242.

31. Liu BC, Ivers R, Norton R, et al. Helmets for preventing injury in motorcycle riders. *Cochrane Database Syst Rev.* 2008;(1):CD004333. doi:10.1002/14651858.CD004333.pub3.

7

Proteomic, Genetic, and Epigenetic Biomarkers in Traumatic Brain Injury

KIMBRA KENNEY, MD, J. KENT WERNER, JR., MD, PhD, AND JESSICA M. GILL, PhD, RN, FAAN

OUTLINE

Biomarker Definition

Biomarkers are critical to understand disease pathophysiology, improve diagnostics, and select therapies.[1-3] Biomarkers are used to determine the presence or absence of a disease, measure response to therapy, or predict likely outcomes. Biomarkers may be useful for patient stratification and to determine target engagement in drug development. Key features of a biomarker include sensitivity (ability to detect true positives), specificity (ability to detect true negatives), and predictive ability (measured by areas under receiver-operating characteristic curves), along with precision, accuracy, stability, and reproducibility.[4] The US Food and Drug Administration (FDA) describes a biomarker as "a defined characteristic that is measured as an indicator of normal biological processes, pathogenic processes, or responses to an exposure or intervention, including therapeutic interventions."[2,5] The FDA delineates four primary biomarker categories: diagnostic, prognostic, predictive, and pharmacodynamic (Fig. 7.1).

Ideal biomarkers are safe, easily accessed, and inexpensive. Although frequently associated with blood measures, they are not limited to biofluids and can include a wide variety of traumatic brain injury (TBI) diagnostics, including imaging (e.g., computed tomography [CT], magnetic resonance imaging [MRI]), neurophysiology (e.g., electroencephalography [EEG], magnetoencephalography [MEG]), cerebrospinal fluid (CSF), saliva, urine, blood, and blood components (e.g., DNA, microRNA [miRNA], exosomal cargo). TBI biomarkers remain largely in the research domain because of the inherent complexities of heterogeneous TBI mechanisms (e.g., blunt, shear, blast) affecting the various central nervous system (CNS) components (e.g., neurons, axons, vascular, astroglial cells) and the protean physiological responses to the acute (primary and secondary cascades) injury, making single biomarker tests at a single time point unlikely. Until recently, no TBI biomarker had been approved by the FDA.[6] This chapter focuses on proteomic, genetic, and epigenetic TBI biomarkers.

Proteomics in Acute Traumatic Brain Injury

The majority of TBI biomarker research has focused on proteomics (initially in CSF, then in blood) as diagnostic biomarkers of acute TBI within the first 24 hours after injury. For peripheral detection, either the blood-brain barrier (BBB) has to be compromised with egress of CNS proteins from the breached CNS space or active transport (e.g., cargo proteins within exosomes) by lipophilic components readily exit from the CNS. Candidate acute TBI biomarkers include markers of BBB integrity,[7-9] neuroinflammation,[10] axonal,[11,12] neuronal,[13] astroglial,[7,11,14] and vascular injury.[15]

The first combination TBI biomarkers to receive FDA approval in acute TBI are plasma glial fibrillary acidic protein (GFAP) and ubiquitin C-terminal hydrolase-L1 (UCH-L1), with the Banyon Brain Trauma Indicator (BTI).[6,16,17]

Diagnostic: Disease characteristics that categorize individuals by the presence of absence of a specific disease
Prognostic: Baseline measurements that categorize individuals by degree of risk for disease progression and inform about the natural history of the disorder
Predictive: Baseline characteristics that categorize individuals by their likelihood of response to a particular treatment
Pharmacodynamic: Dynamic measurements that show if a biological response has occurred in a patient after a therapeutic intervention

• **Fig. 7.1** US Food & Drug Administration biomarker classification. (Adapted from Bogoslovsky T, Gill J, Jeromin A, et al. Fluid biomarkers of traumatic brain injury and intended context of use. *Diagnostics.* 2016;6(4):37. doi.org/10.3390/diagnostics6040037.)

GFAP is an astroglial structural protein that is released with injury; in acute TBI, serum GFAP levels peak 20 hours after injury.[6] UCH-L1, making up 2% of total soluble brain proteins,[18] is a neuron-specific enzyme involved in ubiquitin turnover.[19] It is detectable as early as 1 hour after TBI and peaks earlier than GFAP at 8 hours and then declines slowly over 48 hours after injury.[6]

In the ALERT-TBI trial with 2081 mild and moderate TBI subjects, GFAP and UCH-L1 levels together reliably differentiated TBI with and without CT-detectable intracranial lesions (sensitivity of 97.5% and specificity of 99.6%), and it is currently FDA approved for point-of-care (POC) testing in serum collected within 12 hours of a TBI.[17,20] The test is not approved for the diagnosis of TBI; rather its indication is to identify TBI patients who may have an intracranial lesion that could require surgical intervention. S100B, an abundant astroglial protein, also has a high sensitivity for TBI, with higher levels associated with greater TBI severity and poorer outcomes.[21] Despite widespread use in Europe as a TBI biomarker, its lower specificity in patients with polytrauma caused by extracranial sources and varying levels in young children limits its potential as an acute POC biomarker.[22]

Neurofilament proteins are the major intermediate structural proteins of neuronal axons. Individual intermediate filaments are made up of two of three isoforms—neurofilament light (NF-L), medium (NF-M), and heavy (NF-H) chains—and are associated with large-caliber myelinated axons.[23] Likewise tau is an axonal skeletal protein but is associated with thin, unmyelinated axons.[7] Both (CSF[11,24] and blood[25]) are associated with acute axonal injury, with tau demonstrating less CNS specificity than NF-L in polytrauma cases, likely because of peripheral sources of tau. To date, most studies of NF-L and tau have focused on CSF sources as a diagnostic marker of acute TBI, with CSF NF-L levels the most sensitive of acute axonal injury, including in mild TBI (mTBI) among boxers.[11] Recent studies of plasma tau in acute sports concussion collected within the first 6 hours after injury suggest that higher levels may be prognostic biomarkers of prolonged recovery.[26] Amyloid species—including amyloid precursor protein (APP), amyloid beta 40 ($A\beta_{40}$), and amyloid beta 42 ($A\beta_{42}$)—are associated with neuronal axons and accumulate as early as 2 to 3 hours after TBI with axonal injury.[27] CSF levels of both $A\beta_{40}$ and $A\beta_{42}$ are increased in acute, severe TBI but not acute mTBI,

making it less useful as a diagnostic biomarker of axonal injury.[11]

Biomarkers of BBB disruption, neuroinflammation, and vascular injury are candidate biomarkers that may aid our understanding of TBI pathophysiology. Studies in acute severe TBI have shown BBB disruption with increased CSF to serum albumin ratios and neuroinflammatory responses (interleukin [IL]-1β, IL-6, IL-8, IL-10, TNF alpha)[28] but no similar changes in studies of boxers with mTBI or military personnel with blast exposures, suggesting these are less sensitive as diagnostic TBI biomarkers.[11] Candidate vascular biomarkers include vascular endothelial growth factor, von Willebrand factor, and angiopoietin-1. TBI biomarker discovery projects hypothesize that candidate biomarker analyses from large TBI longitudinal studies that encompass multiple mechanisms and time since injury, partnered with robust data sets and statistical modeling, will advance the field to actuate TBI diagnostic biomarker panels from POC to chronic TBI outcomes.

Proteomics in Chronic Traumatic Brain Injury

Chronic TBI biomarker research focuses on advancing our understanding of the mechanisms responsible for ongoing symptoms and deficits. Clinically, one cannot identify the 10% to 15% of mTBI patients who will remain symptomatic 1 year postinjury or optimal timing for a safe return to play after sports concussions. Candidate prognostic biomarkers of TBI early outcomes include S100B, tau and phosphorylated tau (p-tau), NF-L, αII-spectrin breakdown product (SNTF), and neuroinflammatory markers (IL-6, IL-8, IL-10 and TNF-α). The most promising and sensitive to date are plasma measures of tau, NF-L, and GFAP.[29]

There are few studies of TBI biomarkers in the chronic stage, 6 months after injury. The first studied active duty service members who sustained deployment TBIs and were tested 12 or more months later. They had elevated levels of plasma tau in those with repetitive (≥3) TBI, and tau elevations correlated with increased postconcussive symptoms.[29,30] Rubenstein reported elevated plasma tau, p-tau, and p-tau:tau ratio in a small cohort of severe TBI patients 6 to 8 months after injury.[31] Exosomes, extracellular vesicles thought to be important in cell-to-cell signaling, have a lipid membrane that easily crosses the BBB and are abundant in the peripheral circulation. Their cargo reflects cytoplasmic metabolic status from the cell of origin and is enriched with peptides, enzymes, and RNA (including miRNA). Recent prognostic biomarker studies of chronic TBI have focused on exosomal proteins of central origin. Several studies have reported elevated levels of exosomal tau, p-tau, NF-L, GFAP, and IL-6 years to decades after TBI, with biomarker levels corresponding to postconcussive and affective symptoms and cognitive impairment.[32,33]

Genetics of Traumatic Brain Injury

Evidence is mounting that genetic variation may modulate response to TBI, including TBI recovery and outcomes.[34] The polymorphism with the most support is the ε4 allele of the apolipoprotein E (*APOE*) gene, which encodes for lipoproteins that transport cholesterol in the peripheral circulation. A metaanalysis suggests that the ε4 allele is associated with poorer outcomes after TBI,[35] including a 10-fold risk of dementia and greater cognitive decline 30 years after TBI.[36] Further, boxers with the ε4 allele who had participated in many bouts were more likely to develop chronic traumatic encephalopathy (CTE) than those who had only boxed a few fights.[37] Several other common genetic variants have been associated with chronic effects of neurotrauma (e.g., *DRD2, COMT, BDNF, DAT1, MAO-A*), but their association with neurodegenerative disorders after TBI remains inconclusive.

Recent advances in large-scale genome-wide association studies have helped characterize genetic vulnerability as prognostic biomarkers for a wide range of chronic neurological disorders.[38] Polygenic risk scores (PRS) derived from TBI-related outcomes (e.g., dementia, CTE, posttraumatic headache) could pave the way for a more robust understanding of how genes moderate TBI recovery and may in the future be useful to help predict treatment response.

Epigenetics of Traumatic Brain Injury

Epigenetics refers to factors both inheritable and noninheritable that modify gene activity by a variety of mechanisms that include DNA hyper- and hypomethylation, histone modification (e.g., acetylation), and miRNA regulation of protein translation.[39,40] DNA methylation modulates gene expression through the inhibition or reduction of transcriptional proteins binding to DNA. In TBI, DNA methylation has the potential to affect variability in injury susceptibility, intensity of the acute pathophysiological response to injury, rate and extent of recovery, and the emergence of posttraumatic neurodegeneration. Recent studies have investigated its potential to influence outcomes of chronic psychological and related neurologic disorders, including dementia, TBI, and posttraumatic stress disorder.[41-43] This is a rapidly advancing field in biomarker research, particularly in chronic TBI outcomes.

miRNAs are short lengths of single-stranded RNA (17–25 nucleotides) and are thought to be important in regulating posttranscriptional gene expression[44]. They can be found in several peripheral sources, such as blood, saliva, and urine, with the majority contained within exosomes. There is intense interest in the potential of miRNA expression as a possible acute, chronic, and/or remote TBI diagnostic and prognostic biomarker. There are increasing reports of miRNAs as novel biomarkers for the diagnosis and prognosis of sports concussion[44-46] and mild[44,45] and severe TBI.[45,46] Both blood and salivary miRNAs are easily measured, physiologically relevant, and candidate diagnostic and prognostic TBI biomarkers, but these remain a research endeavor at this time.

Review Questions

1. Current evidence suggests an acute traumatic brain injury (TBI) diagnostic biomarker panel could include which of the following trios:
   a. Apolipoprotein E (APOE) genotyping, diffuse tensor imaging (DTI) sequence on magnetic resonance imaging (MRI), plasma tau
   b. Computed tomography (CT) scan findings, salivary microRNA (miRNA) expression, urinary catecholamine levels
   c. Cerebrospinal fluid (CSF) neurofilament light (N-FL) level, serum cholesterol level, plasma ubiquitin C-terminal hydrolase-L1 (UCHL-1) level
   d. Plasma glial fibrillary acidic protein (GFAP) level, exosomal interleukin (IL)-6 level, susceptibility weighted imaging (SWI) sequence on MRI

2. Recently, a, the US Food and Drug Administration (FDA) approved a TBI serum test for GFAP and ubiquitin C-terminal hydrolase-L1 with a sensitivity of 97.5% for detecting a patient with evidence of TBI on head CT. Given this information, which of the following is true?
   a. A positive test means the patient has a 97.5% chance having evidence of injury on head CT.
   b. A negative test result means that the patient has a 2.5% chance of having no evidence of injury on head CT.
   c. A TBI patient with evidence of injury on head CT has a 2.5% chance of testing negative.
   d. A TBI patient with no evidence of injury on head CT has a 2.5% chance of testing positive.

3. GFAP may be a superior biomarker for TBI than S100B because of which of the following?
   a. S100B is less stable than GFAP.
   b. S100B has lower specificity than GFAP.
   c. S100B does not cross the blood-brain barrier after TBI.
   d. S100B is not expressed in younger children.

Answers on page 386.
Access the full list of questions and answers online.
Available on ExpertConsult.com

References

1. Lesko LJ, Atkinson AJ. Use of biomarkers and surrogate endpoints in drug development and regulatory decision making: criteria, validation, strategies. *Annu Rev Pharmacol Toxicol.* 2001;41:347-366.
2. Robb MA, McInnes PM, Califf RM. Biomarkers and surrogate endpoints: developing common terminology and definitions. *JAMA.* 2016;315:1107-1108.
3. Packard RR, Libby P. Inflammation in atherosclerosis: from vascular biology to biomarker discovery and risk prediction. *Clin Chem.* 2008;54:24-38.
4. Bossuyt PM, Reitsma JB, Bruns DE, et al. The STARD statement for reporting studies of diagnostic accuracy: explanation and elaboration. *Clin Chem.* 2003;49:7.
5. Strimbu K, Tavel J. What are biomarkers? *Curr Opin HIV AIDS.* 2010;5:463-466.
6. Papa L, Brophy GM, Welch RD, et al. Time course and diagnostic accuracy of glial and neuronal blood biomarkers GFAP and UCH0L1 in a large cohort of trauma patients with and without mild traumatic brain injury. *JAMA Neurol.* 2016;73:551-560.
7. Zetterberg H, Hietala M, Jonsson M, et al. Neurochemical aftermath of amateur boxing. *Arch Neurol.* 2006;63:1277-1280.
8. Mondello S, Muller U, Jeromin A, et al. Blood-based diagnostics of traumatic brain injuries. *Expert Rev Mol Diagn.* 2011;11:65-78.
9. Metting Z, Wilczak N, Rodiger LA, Schaaf JM, van der Nalt J. GFAP and S100B in the acute phase of mild traumatic brain injury. *Neurology.* 2012;78:1428-1433.
10. Bell MJ, Kochanek PM, Doughty LA, et al. Interleukin-6 and Interleukin-10 in cerebrospinal fluid after severe traumatic brain injury in children. *J Neurotrauma.* 1997;14:451-457.
11. Neselius S, Brisby H, Theodorsson A, Blennow K, Zetterberg H, Marcusson J. CSF-biomarkers in Olympic boxing: diagnosis and effects of repetitive head trauma. *PLoS One.* 2012;7:e33606.
12. Zurek J, Fedora M. Serum neuron-specific enolase, S100B, NSE, GFAP NF-H secretagogin and Hsp70 as a predictive biomarker of outcome in children with traumatic brain injury. *Acta Neurochir (Wien).* 2012;154(1):93-103.
13. Berger RP, Dulani T, Adelson PD, Leventhal JM, Richichi R, Kochanek PM. Identification of inflicted traumatic brain injury in well-appearing infants using serum and cerebrospinal markers: a possible screening tool. *Pediatrics.* 2006;117:325-332.
14. Kövesdi E, Lückl J, Bukovics P, et al. Update on protein biomarkers in traumatic brain injury with emphasis on clinical use in adults and pediatrics. *Acta Neurochir (Wien).* 2010;152:1-17.
15. Salehi A, Zhang JH, Obenaus A. Response of the cerebral vasculature following traumatic brain injury. *J Cereb Blood Flow Metab.* 2016;37(7):2320-2339.
16. Posti JP, Takala RS, Runtti H, et al. The levels of glial fibrillary acidic protein and ubiquitin C-terminal hydrolase-L1 during the first week after a traumatic brain injury: correlations with clinical and imaging findings. *Neurosurgery.* 2016;79:456-464.
17. *FDA Decision Memorandum, Evaluation of Automatic Class III Designation for Banyon Brain Trauma Indicator.* 13 FEB 2018. https://www.accessdata.fda.gov/cdrh_docs/reviews/DEN170045.pdf..
18. Wilkinson KD, Lee KM, Deshpande S, Duerksen-Hughes P, Boss JM, Pohl J. The neuron-specific protein PGP 9.5 is a ubiquitin carboxyl-terminal hydrolase. *Science.* 1989;246(4930):670-673.
19. Gong B, Cao Z, Zheng P, et al. Ubiquitin hydrolase Uch-L1 rescues beta-amyloid-induced decreases in synaptic function and contextual memory. *Cell.* 2006;126(4):775-788.
20. Vos PI, Jacobs B, Andriessen TM, et al. GFAP and S100B are biomarkers of traumatic brain injury: an observational cohort study. *Neurology.* 2010;75:1786-1793.
21. Thelin EP, Nelson DW, Bellander BM. A review of the clinical utility of serum S100B protein levels in the assessment of traumatic brain injury. *Acta Neurochir (Wien).* 2017;159(2):209-225.
22. Perrot R, Berges R, Bocquet A, Eyer J. Review of the multiple aspects of neurofilament functions, and their possible contribution to neurodegeneration. *Mol Neurobiol.* 2008;38:27-65.
23. Anderson JM, Hampton DW, Patani R, et al. Abnormally phosphorylated tau is associated with neuronal and axonal loss in experimental autoimmune encephalomyelitis and multiple sclerosis. *Brain.* 2008;131:1736-1748.
24. Gatson JW, Barillas J, Hynan LS, Diaz-Arrastia R, Wolf SE, Minei JP. Detection of neurofilament-H in serum as a diagnostic tool to predict injury severity in patients who have suffered mild traumatic brain injury. *J Neurosurg.* 2014;121:1232-1238.
25. Gill J, Merchant-Borna K, Jeromin A, Livingston A, Livingston W, Bazarian J. Acute plasma tau relates to prolonged return to play after concussion. *Neurology.* 2017;88:595-602.
26. Blumbergs PC, Scott G, Manavis J, Wainwright H, Simpson DA, McLean AJ. Staining of amyloid precursor protein to study axonal damage in mild head injury. *Lancet.* 1994;344:1055-1056.
27. Smith DH, Chen XH, Iwata A, Graham DI. Amyloid β accumulation in axons after traumatic brain injury in humans. *J Neurosurg.* 2003;98:1072-1077.
28. Blennow K, Jonsson M, Andreasen N, et al. No neurochemical evidence of brain injury after blast overpressure by repeated explosions or firing heavy weapons. *Acta Neurol Scand.* 2011;123:245-251.
29. Olivera A, Lejbman N, Jeromin A, et al. Peripheral total tau in military personnel who sustain traujatic brain injuries during deployment. *JAMA Neurol.* 2015;72(10);1109-1116.
30. Gill J, Mustapic M, Diaz-Arrastia R, et al. Higher exosomal tau, amyloid-beta 42 and IL-10 are associated with mild TBIs and chronic symptoms in military personnel. *Brain Inj.* 2018;32(10):1277-1284.
31. Rubenstein R, Chang B, Yue JK, et al. Comparing plasma phospho tau, total tau, and phospho tau-total tau ratio as acute and chronic traumatic brain injury biomarkers. *JAMA Neurol.* 2017;74(9):1063-1072.
32. Kenney K, Bu BX, Lai C, et al. Higher exosomal phosphorylated tau and total tau among veterans with combat-related repetitive chronic mild traumatic brain injury. *Brain Inj.* 2018;32(10):1276-1284.
33. Stern RA, Tripodis Y, Baugh CM, et al. Preliminary study of plasma exosomal tau as a potential biomarker for chronic traumatic encephalopathy. *J Alzheimers Dis.* 2016;51(4):1099-1109.
34. Williams DB, Annegers JF, Kokmen E, O'Brien PC, Kurland LT. Brain injury and neurologic sequelae: a cohort study of dementia, parkinsonism, and amyotrophic lateral sclerosis. *Neurology.* 1991;41:1554-1557.
35. Haan M, Aiello A, West N, Jagust W. C-reactive protein and rate of dementia in carriers and non-carriers of Apolipoprotein APOE4 genotype. *Neurobiol Aging.* 2008;29:1774-1782.
36. Isoniemi H, Tenovuo O, Portin R, Himanen L, Kairisto V. Outcome of traumatic brain injury after three decades-relationship to ApoE genotype. *J Neurotrauma.* 2006;23:1600-1608.
37. Jordan BD, Relkin NR, Ravdin LD, Jacobs AR, Bennett A, Gandy S. Apolipoprotein E epsilon4 associated with chronic traumatic brain injury in boxing. *JAMA.* 1997;278:136-140.
38. Chen J, Yu JT, Wojta K, et al. Genome-wide association study identifies MAPT locus influencing human plasma tau levels. *Neurology.* 2017;88:669-676.
39. Mulligan CJ. Insights from epigenetic studies on human health and evolution. *Curr Opin Genet Dev.* 2018;53:36-42.
40. Yokoyama AS, Rutledge JC, Medici V. DNA methylation alterations in Alzheimer's disease. *Environ Epigenet.* 2017;3(2):dvx008. doi:10.1093/eep/dvx008.

41. Nagalakshmi B, Sagarkar S, Sakharkar AJ. Epigenetic mechanisms of traumatic brain injuries. *Prog Mol Biol Transl Sci.* 2018;157:263-298.

42. Nielsen DA, Spellicy CJ, Harding MJ, Graham DP. Apolipoprotein E DNA methylation and posttraumatic stress disorder are associated with plasma ApoE level: a preliminary study. *Behav Brain Res.* 2019;356:415-422.

43. Van Rooij E. The art of microRNA research. *Circ Res.* 2011;108:219-234.

44. Di Pietro V, Ragusa M, Davies D, et al. MicroRNAs as novel biomarkers for the diagnosis and prognosis of mild and severe traumatic brain injury. *J Neurotrauma.* 2017;34(11): 1948-1956.

45. Papa L, Slobounov SM, Breiter HC, et al. Elevations in MicroRNA biomarkers in serum are associated with measures of concussion, neurocognitive, function, and subconcussive trauma over a single national collegiate athletic association division 1 season in collegiate football players. *J Neurotrauma.* 2018;35:1-9.

46. Hicks SD, Johnson J, Carney MC, Bramley H, Olympia RP, Loeffert AC. Overlapping microRNA expression in saliva and cerebrospinal fluid accurately identifies pediatric traumatic brain injury. *J Neurotrauma.* 2018; 35(1):64-72.

8

Prognosis and Recovery Patterns

KOMAL G. PATEL, DO, AND ROSANNA C. SABINI, DO

The Centers for Disease Control and Prevention (CDC) reports that about 150 individuals die of a traumatic brain injury (TBI) daily in the United States. Advancements in medical and surgical care seemingly allow for a higher prevalence of individuals living with a disability related to a TBI—now believed to be between 3.2 and 5.3 million.[1,2] Long-standing disability secondary to a TBI and the difficulty predicting the extent of recovery continue to challenge patients, families, caretakers, and medical practitioners. Clinical aspects of a TBI can aid in determining prognosis of a patient's recovery. With such knowledge, families may be better equipped for weighing medical and surgical decisions and managing their expectations in the setting of the resultant TBI.

Prognostic Factors

To date, there are limited prognostic factors that assist in predicting recovery after a TBI. Researched variables help determine threshold levels of predicting potential outcome. Much of the prognostication that takes place is based on clinical experience, which can lead to selection bias. A survey revealed that only 37% of brain injury physicians agreed that they were assessing prognosis accurately.[3] Furthermore, patients' families generally question functional recovery, which may be difficult to determine based on certain variables. The sections that follow discuss the most commonly researched prognosticating factors.

Age

Poor outcome after a TBI is more commonly experienced in those who are under 4 or over 65 years old.[4] The centripetal model of brain injury severity claims that the stronger the forces the brain is subjected to, the more severe and the deeper the brain lesions will be.[5] A developing brain may be subjected to greater forces given the increased head to neck ratio, whereas elderly adults, whose brains have fully developed, do not have the resiliency of recovery compared with their younger counterparts.[6] As one ages into adulthood, individuals are more likely to have a worsened recovery after a TBI, especially after the age of 40 and an even significantly worsened outcome after the age of 65.[5,7,8] There is also a progressive increase in adverse outcomes in those ages 35 years and older, whereas patients under the age of 18 have significantly better outcomes.[9]

Glasgow Coma Scale

The Glasgow Coma Scale (GCS) not only determines severity of TBI but also assesses and monitors a patient's level of consciousness (Table 8.1).[5,10] A mild TBI is considered a total GCS score of 13 to 15, a moderate TBI is considered a total GCS score of 9 to 12, and a severe injury is considered a total GCS score of 3 to 8.[5] Studies have shown that initial GCS scores are associated with outcomes, and a lower GCS score is associated with a worse outcome.[7] Even so, all outcomes on the Glasgow Outcome Scale (GOS) were still possible in initial GCS scores between 3 and 8.[5] The GCS does not yield a definitive prognosis by itself. An association between lower GCS scores has also been noted with a longer duration of coma and posttraumatic amnesia (PTA).[5] When the GCS is used in prognosticating a patient's recovery, the best total GCS and best motor scores within 24 hours have been shown to correlate with a better

TABLE 8.1	Glasgow Coma Scale	
	Response	Score
Eye opening	Spontaneously	4
	To speech	3
	To pain	2
	None	1
Verbal response	Orientated	5
	Confused	4
	Inappropriate	3
	Incomprehensible	2
	None	1
Motor response	Obeys commands	6
	Localizes to pain	5
	Withdraws from pain	4
	Flexion to pain (decorticate posturing)	3
	Extension to pain (decerebrate posturing)	2
	None	1

recovery.[5,11] Although an objective measurement, the GCS can be confounded by interrater differences, use of paralytics for agitation or intubation, or intoxication with alcohol and/or drugs.

Length of Coma, Vegetative State, and Minimally Conscious State

Consciousness describes an individual's level of arousal, with coma representing the lowest state of arousal. Using level of consciousness in determining a patient's prognosis requires determination of timeframe (e.g., coma 2 weeks, vegetative state 16 weeks). The most basic methodology of measuring coma is the length of time it takes to follows commands. Longer periods of poor arousal are associated with worse prognosis for functional recovery.[5] A good recovery is unlikely when the coma lasts longer than 4 weeks, and severe disability is unlikely when the coma lasts less than 2 weeks.[5]

In general, the longer a patient with a TBI remains in VS or MCS, the longer they will continue to need significant assistance for mobility and self-care. Details regarding how the length of VS and MCS correlate with prognosis are inconsistent because of frequent misclassification of these two states. A clinician needs to be judicious in their clinical assessment of a patient's arousal state because the classification connotates different prognoses and can potentially mislead long-term management plans for family.

Posttraumatic Amnesia

Thought to be one of the most powerful prognostic factors available, PTA is defined as the inability to retain memory after a TBI, such as day-to-day information or ongoing events. It is often evaluated using the Galveston Orientation and Amnesia Test (GOAT) or the Orientation Log (O-Log). The GOAT is a series of questions in reference to orientation and recall of recent events. The O-Log was later developed as an alternative to the GOAT and appears to be a better predictor of outcome. The end of PTA is indicated when the patient has achieved a score of 76 or higher on the GOAT or 25 or higher on the O-Log for two consecutive days.[5] A longer duration of PTA is associated with worsened outcomes.[5] A good recovery, as defined by the GOS, is unlikely when PTA lasts longer than 3 months, and severe disability is unlikely when PTA lasts less than 2 months.[5]

Brainstem Reflexes

Injury to the brainstem involving the midbrain, pons, and medulla oblongata generally has a poor outcome. The presence of decerebrate posturing may indicate a brainstem injury and is associated with a worsened functional recovery compared with decorticate posturing, which indicates a cortical injury.[10]

In addition, absence of a pupillary response, an oculovestibular reflex, and/or an oculocephalic reflex can also indicate an unfavorable outcome.[10]

Presence of Extracranial Injuries

Concomitant extracranial injuries, such as a fracture or visceral damage, may occur in addition to the TBI and imply a greater severity of the trauma. Furthermore, the risk of complications related to the concomitant extracranial injuries may lead to a worsened outcome, such as bleeding or infections.[5] Some studies have noted that there may an associated increased mortality in those who sustain extracranial injuries with moderate brain injuries but not in those who suffered a severe brain injury.

Imaging Findings

Findings on brain neuroimaging can provide insight into a TBI patient's prognosis.[12] The number and extent of findings correlate with recovery, and certain findings—such as traumatic subarachnoid hemorrhage, midline shifts, cisternal compression or obliteration, subdural hematomas, and epidural hematomas—are correlated with worse outcomes.[5] Cistern obliteration and midline shifts are the strongest mortality predictors within 14 days of TBI, whereas a nonevacuated hematoma is the strongest predictor of unfavorable outcome at 6 months.[7] Furthermore, bilateral compared with unilateral findings indicates an increased cerebral involvement and may lead to a worsened outcome.[5] As mentioned earlier, individuals with brainstem involvement, especially captured within the first 8 weeks of neuroimaging, are more strongly associated with worse prognosis than those who have cortical injuries.[5]

Other Factors

Patient clinical factors can also provide relative recovery outcomes. In general, those with a lower Functional Independence Measure (FIM) score, which is a tool used to assess functional ability and need for caregiver support, have poorer outcomes than those with higher FIM scores.[5] Notably, bowel or bladder incontinence can predict a worsened outcome.[5]

Presence of spasticity or flaccidity, which may limit a patient's functional ability, denotes an individual requiring more caregiver assistance.

Somatosensory evoked potentials can also provide insight into recovery. The absence of the N20 response, which is a negative peak at 20 milliseconds, has been correlated with a poor outcome after a TBI.[12]

Relative impact of gender, ethnicity, and educational levels has been researched, but their use in predicting outcome and recovery after a TBI is still debated.

Genetics

There is growing evidence that prognosis and recovery after a TBI may be linked to an individual's genetic predisposition. It has been demonstrated that a patient with the APO-ϵ4 allele who sustains a TBI has a twofold increase a worsened outcome.[5] It is believed that the APO-ϵ4 allele predisposes patients to having larger hematomas, remaining in a comatose state for a longer period, and an increased risk of posttraumatic seizures.[5] Many genes in addition to the APO-ϵ4 allele are currently being investigated for their relationship to recovery after a TBI.

Future Direction

Given the heterogenicity of TBIs and those who sustain them, it has been challenging to predict long-term outcomes early on. More often than not, the passing of time is usually what allows understanding of outcomes, but this is not useful to caregivers who are in need of vital information to assist in management decision making. Advancements in medical management, especially related to secondary injury that occurs after a TBI, may assist with improving recovery, thereby easing prognosis predictions. Furthermore, additional research is needed on the relationship between these predictive variables and how they help in a combined fashion to predict outcomes after a TBI.

Recovery Patterns

Improvements in regulating the secondary neuroinflammatory responses that occurs subsequent to a TBI have not been as successful as the improvements in managing primary injury sustained after a TBI, such as increased intracranial pressures or an expanding bleed.[10] Recovery after the resultant metabolic cascade also has been poorly understood, and much of what is known has been deduced from stroke research. The majority of motor and cognitive recovery after a TBI occurs within 6 months after the injury, with less significant functional recovery afterward.

Neuroplasticity, the brain's inherent recovery mechanism to intrinsic and extrinsic factors, gained momentum after studies demonstrated newly developed neural connections after a neurologic injury. Prior to this conceptualization, recovery after a TBI was believed to be solely compensatory, in which neurologic growth was limited to developing central nervous systems. Neuroplasticity, which is believed to be the brain's primary method of recovery, refers to brain reorganization and functions that can be mediated by structural alterations in brain maps. It may function to improve already existing neural connections, alter long-term potentiation and depression, create axonal and dendritic sprouting, and/or stimulate synaptogenesis/angiogenesis.[5] Neuroplasticity can occur in several ways:

- Vicariation: A specific brain function is taken over by an alternative brain area that was not originally responsible for that function.[5]
- Equipotentiality: The capacity of an anatomically distinct brain area to mediate a rather wide variety of functions.[5]
- Diaschisis: Decrease in function of an area of the brain that is interconnected with the area of damaged brain. Functional recovery is related to a gradual reduction in diaschisis as cerebral blood flow improves.[5]
- Synkinesis: Aberrant axonal regeneration leading to reinnervation of inappropriate muscles.[5]
- Compensation: Alternative strategies used to restore lost function.[5]

Neuroplasticity occurs sequentially in three different time phases. Immediately after the injury, there is a decrease in cortical inhibitory pathways along with cell death, which is thought to recruit and reveal secondary neural connections.[13] Free-radical production induces neural degeneration and death, potentially preventing neuronal regeneration. Cortical pathways may eventually shift from inhibitory to excitatory, allowing for neuronal proliferation and synaptogenesis.[13] Cells are recruited to replace damaged cells and revascularize areas of damaged brain. Days to weeks after the TBI, new axonal sprouting and synaptic connections are upregulated, promoting remodeling and cortical recovery.[13] Chronic changes have also been researched, but no consensus has been established on these alterations.

Studies have shown that environmental stimulation is critical in enhancing neurogenesis.[6,13,14]

Understanding these concepts and the maladaptive neural changes that may occur with neurorecovery can assist with determining a patient's prognosis.

TABLE 8.2	Rancho Los Amigos Cognitive Functioning Scale
Rancho Level	Clinical Correlate
I	No response
II	Generalized response
III	Localized response
IV	Confused, agitated response
V	Confused, inappropriate response
VI	Confused, appropriate response
VII	Automatic, appropriate response
VIII	Purposeful, appropriate response

Measurement Tools

Functional recovery can be measured via a variety of objective tools. Currently, the Disability Rating Scale (DRS) is more commonly used as a measure of general functional change over the course of recovery. It is a 30-point scale that scores impairment, disability, and handicap. The total GCS score measures impairment, whereas disability is measured by how much assistance is needed for feeding, toileting, and grooming (complete, partial, or none).[15] Handicap, on the other hand, measures the level of functioning (ranges from total assist to independent) and employability (ranges from needing no restrictions to not employable).[15]

The Ranchos Los Amigos scale (Table 8.2) can also provide generalized progression of recovery and descriptions of behaviors in TBI patients.[16] As patients progress to the higher stages, their outcomes generally improve. Level IV is the most common stage in which patients begin their acute inpatient rehabilitation program.

Last, the Glasgow Outcome Scale-Extended (GOS-E) is a brief and broad descriptor of clinical outcome (Table 8.3).[17]

TABLE 8.3	Glasgow Outcome Scale (GOS) and Glasgow Outcome Scale-Extended (GOS-E)	
Clinical State (GOS)	Clinical State (GOS-E)	Clinical Function
1 = Dead	1 = Dead	–
2 = Vegetative state	2 = Vegetative state	Unable to interact with environment; unresponsive
3 = Severely disabled	3 = Lower severe disability	Able to follow commands; unable to live independently
	4 = Upper severe disability	Needs full assistance in ADLs
		Needs partial assistance in ADLs
4 = Moderately disabled	5 = Lower moderate disability	Able to live independently
	6 = Upper moderate disability	Unable to return to work or school
		Can partially resume work or previous schoolwork
5 = Good recovery	7 = Lower good recovery	Able to return to work or school
	8 = Upper good recovery	Minor deficits affecting daily life
		Full recovery or minor symptoms not affecting daily life

ADLs, Activities of daily living.

Review Questions

1. Which component of the Glasgow Coma Scale (GCS) has the most predictive value for a better recovery?
   a. Eye opening
   b. Verbal response
   c. Motor response
   d. Following commands
2. Which age groups are more likely to have a poorer prognosis after a traumatic brain injury (TBI)?
   a. ≤4 and >65 years
   b. ≤13 and >50 years
   c. ≤8 and >65 years
   d. ≤4 and >50 years
3. What are the clinical features of a coma patient?
   a. No eye opening, no sleep–wake cycle, no spontaneous/purposeful movements
   b. Intermittent eye opening, no sleep–wake cycle, no spontaneous/purposeful movements
   c. Inconsistent eye opening, presence of sleep–wake cycle, no spontaneous/purposeful movements
   d. No eye opening, presence of sleep–wake cycle, no spontaneous/purposeful movements

Answers on page 386.
Access the full list of questions and answers online. Available on ExpertConsult.com

References

1. Selassie AW, Zaloshnja E, Langlois JA, Miller T, Jones P, Steiner C. Incidence of long-term disability following traumatic brain injury hospitalization, United States, 2003. *J Head Trauma Rehabil.* 2008;23(2):123-131.
2. Zaloshnja E, Miller T, Langlois JA, Selassie AW. Prevalence of long-term disability from traumatic brain injury in the civilian population of the United States, 2005. *J Head Trauma Rehabil.* 2008;23(6):394-400.
3. Perel P, Wasserberg J, Ravi RR, Shakur H, Edwards P, Roberts I. Prognosis following head injury: a survey of doctors from developing and developed countries. *J Eval Clin Pract.* 2007;13(3):464-465.
4. Luerssen TG, Klauber MR, Marshall LF. Outcome from head injury related to patient's age. A longitudinal prospective study of adult and pediatric head injury. *J Neurosurg.* 1988;68(3):409-416.
5. Zasler ND, Katz DI, Zafonte RD. *Brain Injury Medicine: Principles and Practice.* 2nd ed. New York, NY: Demos Medical Pub.; 2013.
6. Kolb B, Harker A, Gibb R. Principles of plasticity in the developing brain. *Dev Med Child Neurol.* 2017;59(12):1218-1223.
7. Collaborators MCT, Perel P, Arango M, et al. Predicting outcome after traumatic brain injury: practical prognostic models based on large cohort of international patients. *BMJ.* 2008;336(7641):425-429.
8. Katz DI, Alexander MP. Traumatic brain injury. Predicting course of recovery and outcome for patients admitted to rehabilitation. *Arch Neurol.* 1994;51(7):661-670.
9. Gomez PA, Lobato RD, Boto GR, De la Lama A, Gonzalez PJ, de la Cruz J. Age and outcome after severe head injury. *Acta Neurochir (Wien).* 2000;142(4):373-380; discussion 380-371.
10. Davis RA, Cunningham PS. Prognostic factors in severe head injury. *Surg Gynecol Obstet.* 1984;159(6):597-604.
11. Marmarou A, Lu J, Butcher I, et al. Prognostic value of the Glasgow Coma Scale and pupil reactivity in traumatic brain injury assessed pre-hospital and on enrollment: an IMPACT analysis. *J Neurotrauma.* 2007;24(2):270-280.
12. Stevens RD, Sutter R. Prognosis in severe brain injury. *Crit Care Med.* 2013;41(4):1104-1123.
13. Sophie Su YR, Veeravagu A, Grant G. Neuroplasticity after traumatic brain injury. In: Laskowitz D, Grant G, eds. *Translational Research in Traumatic Brain Injury.* Boca Raton, FL: CRC Press; 2016.
14. Kolb B, Gibb R. Searching for the principles of brain plasticity and behavior. *Cortex.* 2014;58:251-260.
15. Deepika A, Devi BI, Shukla D. Predictive validity of disability rating scale in determining functional outcome in patients with severe traumatic brain injury. *Neurol India.* 2017;65(1):83-86.
16. Lin K, Wroten M. Ranchos Los Amigos. In: *StatPearls.* Treasure Island, FL: StatPearls Publishing; 2018.
17. Tsyben A, Guilfoyle M, Timofeev I, et al. Spectrum of outcomes following traumatic brain injury-relationship between functional impairment and health-related quality of life. *Acta Neurochir (Wien).* 2018;160(1):107-115.

Emergency Room and Intensive Care Management

9

Prehospital Care of Traumatic Brain Injury

ANDREA L.C. SCHNEIDER, MD, PhD, AND GEOFFREY S.F. LING, MD, PhD

Traumatic brain injury (TBI) is a major cause of disability and death worldwide. Public awareness of the importance of TBI and its sequelae has been increasing because of both the focus on head injuries observed among members of the military in the wars in Iraq and Afghanistan and head injuries seen among professional football players. This has led to new laws and policy changes regarding concussion screening and return-to-play rules in sports and an increase in the number of individuals seeking medical care and evaluation.[1]

In the United States, there were more than 2.8 million TBI-related emergency department visits, hospitalizations, and deaths in 2014; this reflects a 54% increase in the number of emergency department visits between the years of 2006 and 2014.[1] There has also been increased recognition of the importance of prehospital TBI care because nearly half of individuals who die of TBI die within the first 2 hours of injury.[2] In this chapter we review the prehospital evaluation and management of patients with TBI.

Initial Prehospital Assessment and Management

The most critical step in managing TBI is first recognizing that a TBI may have occurred. The inciting event may be subtle, such as elderly victim bumping a car door frame or seemingly insignificant fall during a sporting event when the patient's head briefly hits the ground. If there is any suspicion that a TBI might have happened, the victim must be removed from further risk and assessed for TBI risk immediately. Ideally, assessment will be done using a TBI risk assessment tool and/or a neurologic examination by an advanced medical provider.

Initial management of TBI is focused on the ABCs of airway, breathing and circulation. This is followed by stabilizing the patient, determining severity of injury, and deciding what level of care is needed.

Mild Traumatic Brain Injury/Concussion

Concussion is mild TBI. There has been increased awareness of the seriousness of sports-related concussions. This in turn has resulted in implementation of policy and legal measures to reduce risk of further injury and safe return to play or work. The Centers for Disease Control and Prevention (CDC) reports that between 2001 and 2012, the number of children ages 19 years or younger who received treatment in an emergency room for sports-related head injury doubled, with an estimated 329,290 children treated for sports-related head injuries in 2012.[3]

In the past, especially in youth sports, decisions regarding return to play were made on the sidelines in the prehospital setting, typically by a coach or parent. Fortunately, this is no longer the case. The CDC has helped increase public awareness of the importance of recognizing and properly managing sports-related concussions with the CDC's Heads Up program, introduced in 2003.[4] The Heads Up program provides educational material on prevention, recognition, and response to concussion to five target audiences: healthcare professionals, high school coaches, youth sports coaches, school professionals, and parents.[4]

Recognition and identification of concussion at the time of injury is key to preventing further injury. To this end, the Sport Concussion Assessment Tool (SCAT) was first developed in 2004 and is now in its fifth iteration (SCAT5).[5] The SCAT provides a brief objective and standardized assessment of concussion, including screening of neurocognitive and neurologic functions in addition to symptom assessment.[5]

There are now laws governing the prehospital management of concussion. The first legislation addressing concussion education and victim management was ratified in 2009 when Washington state passed the Zackery Lystedt Law.[6,12] Mr. Lystedt was a high school football player who died after sustaining a number of concussions. By 2014, all 50 states and the District of Columbia passed similar laws governing return-to-play rules for athletes ages 18 years and younger. These laws all share three similar key elements:

- Mandatory education of athletes, coaches, and parents/guardians about concussion
- Removal of youth athlete from practice or play at the time of suspected concussion/head injury
- Return to practice or play only with the written permission of a licensed healthcare provider trained in the evaluation and management of concussion[6]

These laws are intended to raise awareness about the seriousness of sports-related head injuries and on preventing second-impact syndrome (SIS). SIS is rapidly developing diffuse cerebral edema that primarily affects younger victims. SIS is a devastating condition with close to 50% mortality rate. The risk is greatest when a second concussion occurs before symptoms from the first concussion have resolved.[7] More research is needed to clarify risk factors and outcomes after first and repeat injuries to better guide future recommendations for return-to-play rules for athletes.

An important aspect of prehospital management of presumed mild TBI involves identification of those individuals at risk of more serious TBI because they will need urgent evaluation at a medical facility. Clinical clues include multiple vomiting episodes, posttraumatic seizures, focal neurological deficits, and decrease in level of consciousness after an initial lucid interval.

Signs suspicious of skull fracture are raccoon eyes or clear watery nasal discharge concerning for cerebrospinal fluid (CSF) leak.[8]

The SCAT5 should be administered as soon possible after the injury. If positive, the player must not return to play until he or she is evaluated by and receives written clearance for return to play from an advanced medical provider. This is both prudent and the law.

The need for neuroimaging depends on the level of clinical suspicion of intracranial pathology. According to CDC and American College of Emergency Physicians (ACEP) guidelines,[9] the Canadian CT Head Rule,[10] and the New Orleans Criteria for CT scanning in patients with minor head injury,[11] noncontrast head computed tomography (CT) is indicated in head trauma patients with loss of consciousness or posttraumatic amnesia if one or more of these is present:

- Headache
- Vomiting
- Age >60 years, drug/alcohol intoxication
- Posttraumatic seizure
- Glasgow Coma Scale (GCS) score <15
- Focal neurologic deficit
- Coagulopathy
- Evidence of trauma above the clavicle
- Deficits in short-term memory[15]

It is important to note that fewer than 10% of patients with mild TBI have abnormalities detected on noncontrast head CT, and only approximately 1% of these patients need neurosurgery.[18]

Moderate to Severe Traumatic Brain Injury

All moderate to severe TBI patients should be considered as having a potential life-threatening injury. Thus 9-1-1 must be called because these patients invariably will require airway and ventilation management. After emergency medical services (EMS) stabilization in the field, these patients will be taken to a level 1 trauma center where neurointensive care and neurosurgical services can be rendered by a multidisciplinary team of neuro specialty nurses, neurointensivists, neurosurgeons, and trauma specialists. If the patient survives, long-term care will be by neurorehabilitation specialists.

Clinical practice guidelines (CPGs) for moderate to severe TBI have been developed, and the Brain Trauma Foundation has published updated evidence-based guidelines.[13] In the prehospital setting, all severities of TBI victims undergo an initial assessment based on the CPGs of Advanced Trauma Life Support (ATLS) primary survey guidelines.[14] The primary survey is defined using the ABCDE mnemonic: **a**irway and cervical spine stabilization, **b**reathing and ventilation, **c**irculation, **d**isability/neurologic status, and **e**xposure/environment.

First responders need to verify a patent airway to ensure adequate oxygenation and ventilation, paying close attention for signs of airway obstruction including stridor, gurgling, hoarseness, and altered mental status. The cervical spine should be immobilized using a hard collar. Assessment of breathing and ventilation includes inspection, palpation, and auscultation. Circulation is assessed by blood pressure, heart rate, mental status, and inspection for signs of hemorrhage. Disability/neurologic status is assessed by examining pupils, GCS, and assessing for spinal cord injury. After the initial survey is completed, patients should be covered in warm blankets and administered warm intravenous fluids to avoid hypothermia from environmental exposure and transported to trauma medical center. After the primary trauma survey is performed and the patient is stabilized, first responders can proceed to perform a secondary survey, which includes gathering information on the patient's medical history, medications, and allergies, and performing a complete physical examination.

Airway, Ventilation, Oxygenation, and Blood Pressure

The Brain Trauma Foundation guidelines recommend that patients with suspected severe TBI be monitored in the prehospital setting for signs of hypoxemia (<90% oxygen saturation) and hypotension (<90 mm Hg systolic blood pressure [SBP]).[2] Hypoxemia and hypotension have been shown to be strong predictors of poor outcome among patients with severe TBI.[4]

Avoiding hypoxemia (<90% oxygen saturation) in the prehospital setting is recommended because hypoxemia has been shown to be a strong predictor of poor outcome after TBI.[4] Supplemental oxygen can be used in patients who are protecting their airways, whereas patients who are unable to protect their airways (often indicated by GCS score ≤8) or patients with persistent hypoxemia despite supplemental oxygen should be endotracheally intubated using rapid-sequence intubation protocols. During intubation, blood pressure, oxygenation, and end-tidal carbon dioxide ($ETCO_2$) should be measured, and endotracheal tube placement should be confirmed using lung auscultation and $ETCO_2$ measurement. Normocapnia is recommended ($ETCO_2$ 35–40 mm Hg), and hyperventilation ($ETCO_2$ <35 mm Hg) should be avoided unless the patient shows signs of cerebral herniation.[2]

Circulation and Fluid Resuscitation

Fluid resuscitation should be used to treat TBI patients with hypotension (SBP <90 mm Hg) because hypotension has been associated with poor outcomes.[4] Isotonic or hypertonic fluids should be used for resuscitation, and hypotonic fluids should be avoided because of the risk for increased intracranial pressure and cerebral herniation.[2]

Neurological Examination

Pupillary Reflex

The pupillary examination is an important part of the post-TBI prehospital neurological examination and consists of examination of the size, symmetry, and reaction to light of each pupil.[2] The pupillary light reflex is dependent on the function of cranial nerve III (oculomotor nerve). Asymmetry (defined as >1 mm difference in pupil diameter) or fixed, dilated pupils (defined as <1 mm response to bright light) may suggest a herniation syndrome or brainstem ischemia, indicating a need for emergent treatment of increased intracranial pressure.[2]

TABLE 9.1	Glasgow Coma Scale	
Eye Opening		
Opens eyes spontaneously		4
Opens eyes in response to voice		3
Opens eyes in response to pain		2
Does not open eyes		1
Verbal Response		
Oriented		5
Confused		4
Inappropriate words		3
Incomprehensible sounds		2
No verbalization		1
Motor Response		
Obeys command		6
Localizes to painful stimuli		5
Flexion withdrawal to painful stimuli		4
Flexor posturing to painful stimuli		3
Extensor posturing to painful stimuli		2
No movements		1

Glasgow Coma Scale

Prehospital measurement of the GCS score is a reliable measure of the severity of TBI.[2,16] The GCS is a measurement of the severity of neurological impairment based on assessment of eye opening, verbal responses, and motor responses (score range 3–15) (Table 9.1). Categories of TBI severity using the GCS are defined as 13 to 15 for mild injuries, 9 to 12 for moderate injuries, and 3 to 8 for severe injuries.[16] It is important to routinely reassess the GCS of the patient to monitor for neurological changes. The GCS is limited by provider subjectivity, obscuration of level of consciousness in the acute setting by confounders such as medical sedation or intoxication, and the loss of the verbal response component after intubation.

The most valuable aspect of the GCS is that it is a simple-to-obtain, straightforward, well-recognized way of conveying to other providers a patient's neurological state at a given time. A worsening GCS over time is an alarming sign and mandates reassessment and potential intervention.

Cerebral Herniation

Cerebral herniation is a result of increased intracranial pressure and results in parts of the brain shifting across structures. There are multiple different types of cerebral herniation that depend on where the mass effect is located. Uncal herniation is one type of cerebral herniation that occurs when the temporal lobe/uncus puts pressure on the midbrain, compressing the oculomotor nerve and corticospinal tracts causing pupil dilatation and hemiplegia. Clinical signs of cerebral herniation include dilated and unreactive pupils, asymmetrical pupils, hemiplegia, and progressive neurological deterioration (defined as a decrease in GCS by 2 or more points). Vital sign changes may also be seen in cerebral herniation and are characterized by the Cushing reflex triad of hypertension, bradycardia, and irregular breathing.

Treatment of cerebral herniation is based on the Monroe–Kellie doctrine, which states that the sum of the volume of the brain, CSF, and intracranial blood is constant within the fixed volume of the skull and that if there is an increase in any one component, one or both of the other components must decrease or intracranial pressure will increase.[17] In the acute setting, the patient's head should be raised to encourage venous drainage from the brain. Hyperventilation with goal $ETCO_2$ 30 to 35 mm Hg will lead to cerebral vasoconstriction and lowered cerebral blood flow/volume. Osmotherapy using mannitol or hypertonic saline can also help treat cerebral herniation by promoting the osmotic shift of fluid from the intracellular to the interstitial and intravascular space. Finally, sedation including propofol and barbiturates can decrease the cerebral metabolic rate and cerebral blood flow to help reduce intracranial pressure.[18,19] Upon patient arrival at a trauma medical center, neurosurgical evaluation can be performed to determine whether surgical treatments for increased intracranial pressure are warranted.

Summary

TBI is a common condition. Concussion is mild TBI. Anyone suspected of having sustained a concussion must be evaluated and appropriately managed. This is the law throughout the United States. Moderate to severe TBI is associated with significant morbidity and mortality. Given that nearly half of individuals who die of TBI die within the first 2 hours of injury,[2] early recognition of possible TBI events and prehospital evaluation and management of patients with TBI are integral to outcome. CPGs are focused on optimizing general physiology to support the brain recovery. CPGs provide guidance for proper prehospital care and include avoiding hypoxemia and hypotension and identification and treatment of cerebral herniation/increased intracranial pressure.

Presently, this is no cure for TBI. There is no TBI-specific pharmacologic agent that will protect neurons or enhance neuronal recovery. For this, additional research is needed.

Review Questions

1. All of these are treatments for cerebral herniation except
   a. hyperventilation.
   b. hypotonic fluids.
   c. elevation of head of bed.
   d. mannitol.
   e. propofol sedation.
2. Initial evaluation (primary survey) of patients with suspected traumatic brain injury (TBI) includes all of these except:
   a. airway.
   b. circulation.
   c. disability/neurological status.
   d. breathing and ventilation.
   e. past medical history.
3. Using the Glasgow Coma Scale (GCS), a mild TBI is defined as a score of:
   a. 9–12.
   b. 0–3.
   c. 3–8.
   d. 13–15.

Answers on page 387.
Access the full list of questions and answers online.
Available on ExpertConsult.com

References

1. Centers for Disease Control. *Rates of TBI-related Emergency Department Visits, Hospitalizations, and Deaths—United States, 2001–2010.* 2016. Available at: https://www.cdc.gov/traumaticbraininjury/data/rates.html. Access Date: June 1, 2019
2. Badjatia N, Carney N, Crocco TJ, et al. Guidelines for prehospital management of traumatic brain injury 2nd edition. *Prehosp Emerg Care.* 2008;12(suppl 1):S1-52.
3. Kortbeek JB, Al Turki SA, Ali J, et al. Advanced trauma life support, 8th edition, the evidence for change. *J Trauma.* 2008;64(6): 1638-1650.
4. Maas AI, Stocchetti N, Bullock R. Moderate and severe traumatic brain injury in adults. *Lancet Neurol.* 2008;7(8):728-741.
5. Teasdale G, Jennett B. Assessment of coma and impaired consciousness. A practical scale. *Lancet.* 1974;2(7872):81-84.
6. Wilson MH. Monro-Kellie 2.0: The dynamic vascular and venous pathophysiological components of intracranial pressure. *J Cereb Blood Flow Metab.* 2016;36(8):1338-1350.
7. Goldberg SA, Rojanasarntikul D, Jagoda A. The prehospital management of traumatic brain injury. *Handb Clin Neurol.* 2015;127:367-378.
8. Stevens RD, Huff JS, Duckworth J, Papangelou A, Weingart SD, Smith WS. Emergency neurological life support: intracranial hypertension and herniation. *Neurocrit Care.* 2012;17(suppl 1): S60-S65.
9. Coronado VG, Haileyesus T, Cheng TA, et al. Trends in sports- and recreation-related traumatic brain injuries treated in US emergency departments: The National Electronic Injury Surveillance System-All Injury Program (NEISS-AIP) 2001-2012. *J Head Trauma Rehabil.* 2015;30(3):185-197.
10. Sarmiento K, Hoffman R, Dmitrovsky Z, Lee R. A 10-year review of the Centers for Disease Control and Prevention's Heads Up initiatives: bringing concussion awareness to the forefront. *J Safety Res.* 2014;50:143-147.
11. Yengo-Kahn AM, Hale AT, Zalneraitis BH, Zuckerman SL, Sills AK, Solomon GS. The Sport Concussion Assessment Tool: a systematic review. *Neurosurg Focus.* 2016;40(4):E6.

12. Bompadre V, Jinguji TM, Yanez ND, et al. Washington State's Lystedt law in concussion documentation in Seattle public high schools. *J Athl Train*. 2014;49(4):486-492.

13. McLendon LA, Kralik SF, Grayson PA, Golomb MR. The controversial second impact syndrome: a review of the literature. *Pediatr Neurol*. 2016;62:9-17.

14. Levin HS, Diaz-Arrastia RR. Diagnosis, prognosis, and clinical management of mild traumatic brain injury. *Lancet Neurol*. 2015;14(5):506-517.

15. Jagoda AS, Bazarian JJ, Bruns Jr JJ, et al. Clinical policy: neuroimaging and decision making in adult mild traumatic brain injury in the acute setting. *Ann Emerg Med*. 2008;52(6):714-748.

16. Stiell IG, Wells GA, Vandemheen K, et al. The Canadian CT Head Rule for patients with minor head injury. *Lancet*. 2001;357(9266):1391-1396.

17. Haydel MJ, Preston CA, Mills TJ, Luber S, Blaudeau E, DeBlieux PM. Indications for computed tomography in patients with minor head injury. *N Engl J Med*. 2000;343(2):100-105.

18. Smits M, Dippel DW, de Haan GG, et al. External validation of the Canadian CT Head Rule and the New Orleans Criteria for CT scanning in patients with minor head injury. *JAMA*. 2005;294(12):1519-1525.

19. Carney N, Totten AM, O'Reilly C, et al. Guidelines for the management of severe traumatic brain injury, fourth edition. *Neurosurgery*. 2017;80(1):6-15.

20. Beck B, Gantner D, Cameron PA, et al. Temporal trends in functional outcomes after severe traumatic brain injury: 2006-2015. *J Neurotrauma*. 2018;35(8):1021-1029.

10

Acute Emergency Management of Traumatic Brain Injury

PETER HORVATH, MD, KETAN VERMA, MD, AND ALEX B. VALADKA, MD

OUTLINE

General Principles

Acute Management of Traumatic Brain Injury Is Based on Preventing Secondary Insults

- *Primary insult* refers to the initial injury itself.[1]
- Secondary insult is a subsequent deviation from normal physiological conditions that can worsen the effects of the primary insult.

- Common examples: hypotension, hypoxia, elevated intracranial pressure (ICP).
- A recently injured brain is highly vulnerable even to mild physiological derangements that would be well tolerated by an uninjured brain.

Prophylactic Versus Reactive Treatment

- Dozens of clinical trials have failed to identify any effective therapy for traumatic brain injury (TBI).[2,3] There are many possible reasons for these failures, including:
  - Lack of appreciation of the heterogeneity of TBI
  - Failure to use appropriately sophisticated statistical techniques
  - Poor adherence to complex study protocols
  - Lack of sensitivity of outcome instruments
- Current treatment is limited to careful monitoring and prompt intervention when secondary insults occur.
- So far, all attempts at aggressive initiation of therapies to prevent secondary insults have not only failed to improve outcomes but also have usually led to worse outcomes.[1]
  - Examples of failed prophylactic interventions: induced hypertension, neuromuscular paralysis, barbiturate coma, hypothermia, decompressive craniectomy (DC), and many others.
- Even though various treatments may lower ICP, none of these treatments has been shown to improve outcomes in TBI patients.
- Because we have been largely unable to prevent secondary insults, the best we can do is to promptly recognize and treat them when they do occur.

Initial Management Priorities

As in every medical emergency, management priorities begin with the ABCs (airway, breathing, circulation).

Airway

- If endotracheal intubation has not been performed in the prehospital setting, it should be performed immediately on a patient's arrival in the emergency department (ED).

- Cervical spine immobilization must be maintained.
- Nasotracheal intubation or other instrumentation is generally discouraged in patients with head trauma because of the risk of passage of the inserted object through a basilar skull fracture and into the cranial vault.
- Rarely, extensive injury and bleeding from the oropharynx may make it impossible to perform orotracheal intubation, in which case emergency tracheostomy may be required.

Breathing

- After the airway has been secured, the patient should be placed on a mechanical ventilator.
- Ventilation by bag–valve–mask is discouraged because of the tendency of those who are doing the bagging to use excessive tidal volumes and respiratory rates. The reduction in partial pressure of carbon dioxide ($Paco_2$) and subsequent increase in arterial pH lead to constriction of the cerebral arteries, resulting in a decrease in cerebral blood flow (CBF) that may be so severe that the metabolically impaired injured brain may progress to infarction.[1]
- The goal of ventilation is to keep $Paco_2$ in the normal range of 35 to 45 mm Hg.
- Although often used in the past, continuous hyperventilation is no longer recommended because of its adverse effect on outcome, presumably from reduction of CBF.
- If hyperventilation is prolonged, it must be remembered that cerebral arterioles progressively dilate and return to baseline diameter within 24 hours even when $Paco_2$ is maintained at low levels.[4] Thus, nothing has been gained by continuous hyperventilation, and the reduction in bicarbonate ions that might have served to buffer regions of cerebral acidosis could potentially cause harm.
- However, as a short-term intervention during emergencies that may be caused by expansion of a mass lesion, such as sudden neurological deterioration in a patient who develops a dilated pupil and asymmetrical motor examination, hyperventilation may be used to transiently lower ICP while emergency computed tomography (CT) scanning is performed to assess for the presence of a large hematoma that requires immediate surgery. If evaluation reveals that no such hematoma is present, hyperventilation should not be maintained, as discussed earlier.
- As with $Paco_2$, normal levels are also the goal for partial pressure of oxygen (PaO_2). In general, maintaining oxygen saturation above 90% is adequate, but because hypoxia is such a common and potentially devastating secondary insult, many clinicians aim for slightly higher levels, such as 92% to 94%, to create a bit of a buffer.

- Driving PaO_2 to supranormal levels confers no benefit.

Circulation

- Hypotension is among the most frequent and most harmful of secondary insults in TBI patients, and one-third of severe TBI patients suffer cerebral ischemia during the initial hours after injury.[5,6]
- Traditionally, the recommended minimum systolic blood pressure for severe TBI patients was 90 mm Hg or higher. More recent evidence suggests that a goal of 100 mm Hg may be a more appropriate starting point, with some patients—such as those at the younger and older ends of the adult age spectrum—benefiting from a target of 110 mm Hg.[7]
- Another commonly measured parameter is cerebral perfusion pressure (CPP), defined as mean arterial pressure minus ICP. The recommended target range for CPP is 60 to 70 mm Hg.[7]
- Blood pressure management aims to ensure sufficient blood flow to meet the brain's metabolic needs and avoid ischemia.
- In uninjured individuals, the cerebral arteries dilate and constrict as needed to maintain CBF constant even if systemic blood pressure fluctuates widely. This process is known as *autoregulation*.
- The impairment of autoregulation in many TBI patients causes CBF to become "pressure passive," that is, CBF passively rises and falls in response to corresponding changes in blood pressure. As a result, some practitioners in years past routinely used pressors to artificially raise blood pressure in TBI patients because of a belief that this practice had little downside and would avoid cerebral hypoperfusion
- Subsequent work, however, demonstrated that this practice actually worsens outcome, largely because of the pulmonary complications caused by the amount of fluid and pressors needed to maintain artificial elevation of blood pressure and CPP.[8]

Emergency Neurological Assessment

The rapid tempo of resuscitation and stabilization of trauma patients in the ED may make it impossible to obtain a detailed neurological examination. Nevertheless, certain minimum information is crucial for adequate neurological assessment and planning.

The Glasgow Coma Scale Assesses Eye Opening, Verbal Response, and Motor Response

- The best score is used when an examination fluctuates or when the two sides are asymmetrical.[9]
- Each component should be recorded separately, but a single sum score is often used to summarize a patient's neurological status.

- Any right–left asymmetry should be noted.
- Generally, a score of 3 to 8 is described as a severe injury, 9 to 12 is moderate, and 13 to 15 is mild.
- Accurate assessment may be compromised by the presence of alcohol, other drugs, hypothermia, hypotension, and many other factors.

Pupillary Size and Reactivity Convey Critical Information That Is Not Captured in the Glasgow Coma Score

- A dilated pupil may indicate the presence of a large mass lesion that is exerting pressure on the third cranial nerve. The pupilloconstrictor fibers on the periphery of the nerve are vulnerable to compression by large hematomas or edematous brain.
- Bilaterally dilated pupils may indicate the presence of diffuse cerebral edema and high ICP. This is an ominous finding.
- It must be remembered that, in a sizeable minority of cases, a dilated pupil is caused by local ocular trauma and does not indicate an intracranial emergency. However, the burden is on the treating physician to obtain an emergency CT scan to verify that an expanding intracranial hematoma is not present.

Initial Interventions

After the ABCs have been addressed, a series of steps is usually performed, generally simultaneously, by different members of the team.

Laboratory Studies

- Complete Blood Count, Basic Chemistries, Coagulation Studies, Alcohol Level and Toxicology Screens, Blood Type and Crossmatch, Pregnancy Level as Appropriate, Urinalysis, Additional Studies as Appropriate

Relevant Medical History if Available

- Significant comorbidities
- Medications, especially anticoagulants and/or antiplatelet agents

Detailed Systemic Evaluation

- Severe TBI rarely occurs in isolation. Significant associated systemic injuries are the rule rather than the exception.

Imaging

- Chest x-ray in resuscitation bay
- Head CT scan
- Cervical spine CT scan, and other studies as needed

Anticonvulsant Prophylaxis

- Most severe TBI patients receive anticonvulsant prophylaxis.
- The highest-quality studies find that phenytoin prophylaxis prevented seizures during the first 8 days after injury but not later.[10]
- Many clinicians have substituted levetiracetam for a 7-day course of prophylaxis because it is not necessary to check serum levels and because of a perceived lower rate of adverse events.
- Of note: The decrease in seizures during the first week has not been shown to improve long-term outcomes.

Steroids

- Steroids were often administered to TBI patients in the past.
- The rationale was that steroids were known to reduce edema associated with brain tumors, and it was assumed the same would be true for trauma.
- However, large clinical trials have demonstrated that steroids increase the mortality rate after TBI.[11]
- Steroids are no longer given to TBI patients unless a patient has been on steroids for another reason.
- The only level 1 recommendation in the Brain Trauma Foundation's *Guidelines for the Management of Severe Traumatic Brain Injury* is that use of steroids is not recommended for improving outcome or reducing ICP in TBI patients.[7]

Blood Transfusions

- For many years, TBI patients were given red blood cells whenever their hemoglobin dropped below 10 g/dL.
- That level represents the theoretical point at which blood oxygen–carrying capacity (which increases at a higher hemoglobin concentration) and blood viscosity (which decreases at a lower hemoglobin concentration) come into optimal balance.
- However, a large body of literature demonstrated the many adverse effects of blood transfusions, and a hemoglobin transfusion threshold of 7 g/dL was widely adopted for most nonneurologically injured patients.
- It remained unclear whether TBI patients could safely tolerate a hemoglobin transfusion of 7 g/dL until a prospective clinical trial demonstrated lack of benefit and an increase in thromboembolic events by keeping TBI patients at a hemoglobin concentration of 10 g/dL.[12]

Surgical Decision Making

Detailed evidence-based guidelines for surgical decision making have been published. However, the resulting recommendations are based on the lowest level of evidence because it is impossible to conduct randomized studies to obtain class I evidence. For example, a teenager who is known to have a large temporal epidural hematoma and who becomes difficult to arouse would be taken immediately for a craniotomy. Obviously, it would be unethical to enroll him into a clinical trial in which he could potentially be randomized to a control (nonsurgical) group.

Guidelines that are strictly based on available evidence can make only those recommendations that are supported by the evidence. In the example given earlier, a guidelines document could not make a high-level recommendation for surgical evacuation of the hematoma because no randomized, prospective, blinded, controlled trial has been performed to investigate the role of surgery, which is the obviously indicated intervention. For this reason, most recommendations regarding indications for surgery are based on experience and common sense, with support from only class III evidence.

Common Indications for Evacuation of Traumatic Intracranial Hematomas and Contusions

- Midline shift >5 mm in patients with GCS score ≤8
- Significant enlargement of a mass lesion or surrounding edema on repeat CT scanning
- Inability to control ICP in patients with moderate-sized mass lesions who are being managed nonoperatively
- Decrease in GCS score of 2 or more points in patients with moderate-sized mass lesions who are being managed nonoperatively

Situations in Which Surgery May Not Be Necessary

- Bilateral subfrontal (anterior inferior frontal lobe) contusions: Many patients can tolerate very large contusions in this area surprisingly well.
- Cerebral atrophy: Elderly patients and others with significant atrophy have a relatively large amount of intracranial volume that can accommodate sizeable acute mass lesions that might require immediate surgery in younger or nonatrophied patients.
  o Acute subdural hematoma in elderly patients: In asymptomatic patients with significant atrophy, even large acute subdural hematomas can be managed without surgery while they gradually evolve from a solid hematoma to a liquid subacute hematoma, which will resolve spontaneously or drain easily through a bur hole.
- Diffuse brain injury: In the past, some neurosurgeons performed DC in severe TBI patients whose CT scans showed only diffuse injury. The rationale was that removal of a large portion of the skull would permit the brain to swell without the harmful elevation of ICP that would occur if the brain were confined within the rigid skull. The randomized, prospective DEcompressive CRAniectomy (DECRA) trial demonstrated that such a practice actually worsened outcomes in the patients who had surgery.[13] Although the results generated some controversy, it is clear that the operated patients did not experience any benefit from surgery but were still exposed to the many complications of this procedure.

Goals

Acute emergency management of TBI patients has two main goals. The first is to prevent secondary insults, which begins with the ABCs, and continues during resuscitation, evaluation, initial interventions, and possible surgery.

The second goal is to get the patient to the neurosurgical ICU as soon as possible. The ICU environment permits detailed monitoring and rapid intervention when needed, which may be difficult in other settings, especially when a patient is being transported from the ED to the CT scanner to the operating room to various other parts of the hospital.

Review Questions

1. In healthy patients, cerebral blood flow (CBF) remains essentially unchanged even if systemic blood pressure decreases or increases significantly. What word or phrase is used to describe this physiological maintenance of constant CBF?
   a. Autoregulation
   b. Linkage
   c. Metabolic coupling
   d. Optimization
2. A 25-year-old man sustains a severe traumatic brain injury (TBI) in an automobile accident. Shortly after arrival in the emergency department (ED), he becomes hypotensive and is found to have intraabdominal bleeding. His blood pressure is restored after transfusion of several units of packed red blood cells, but after restoration of his blood pressure, his neurological examination is noticeably worse than it had been when he arrived. Which of these best describes this period of hypotension?
   a. Iatrogenic injury
   b. Natural history of disease
   c. Unavoidable complication
   d. Secondary cerebral insult
3. Several large prospective trials have examined the effect of prophylactic hypothermia in severe TBI patients, with the goal of achieving hypothermia as soon as possible after injury. Which of these is the expected result of those trials?
   a. Hypothermia did not improve outcomes.
   b. Most patients did not achieve the target temperature.
   c. Normothermic patients had a higher incidence of hemorrhagic complications.
   d. Pneumonia occurred less frequently in hypothermia patients.

Answers on page 387.
Access the full list of questions and answers online. Available on ExpertConsult.com

References

1. Whitaker-Lea WA, Valadka AB. Acute management of moderate-severe traumatic brain injury. *Phys Med Rehabil Clin N orth Am.* 2017;28(2):227-243.

2. Stein DG. Embracing failure: What the phase III progesterone studies can teach about TBI clinical trials. *Brain Inj.* 2015;29(11):1259-1272.

3. Maas AI, Roozenbeek B, Manley GT. Clinical trials in traumatic brain injury: past experience and current developments. *NeuroRx.* 2010;7(1):115-126.

4. Muizelaar JP, van der Poel HG, Li Z, Kontos HA, Levasseur JE. Pial arteriolar vessel diameter and CO2 reactivity during prolonged hyperventilation in the rabbit. *J Neurosurg.* 1988;69(6):923-927.

5. Bouma GJ, Muizelaar JP, Choi SC, Newlon PG, Young HF. Cerebral circulation and metabolism after severe traumatic brain injury: the elusive role of ischemia. *J Neurosurg.* 1991;75(5):685-693.

6. Bouma GJ, Muizelaar JP, Stringer WA. Ultra-early evaluation of regional cerebral blood flow in severely head-injured patients using xenon-enhanced computerized tomography. *J Neurosurg.* 1992;77(3):360-368.

7. Carney N, Totten AM, O'Reilly C, et al. *Guidelines for the Management Of Severe Traumatic Brain Injury.* Brain Trauma Foundation; 2016. Available at: https://braintrauma.org/uploads/03/12/Guidelines_for_Management_of_Severe_TBI_4th_Edition.pdf. Accessed February 12, 2019.

8. Robertson CS, Valadka AB, Hannay HJ, et al. Prevention of secondary ischemic insults after severe head injury. *Crit Care Med.* 1999;27(10):2086-2095.

9. Teasdale G, Jennett B. Assessment of coma and impaired consciousness. A practical scale. *Lancet.* 1974;2(7872):81-84.

10. Temkin NR, Dikmen S, Wilensky A, Keihm J, Chabal S, Winn HR. A randomized, double-blind study of phenytoin for the prevention of post-traumatic seizures. *N Engl J Med.* 1990;323(8):497-502.

11. Edwards P, Arango M, Balica L, et al. Final results of MRC CRASH, a randomised placebo-controlled trial of intravenous corticosteroid in adults with head injury—outcomes at 6 months. *Lancet.* 2005;365(9475):1957-1959.

12. Robertson CS, Hannay HJ, Yamal JM, et al. Effect of erythropoietin and transfusion threshold on neurological recovery after traumatic brain injury: a randomized clinical trial. *JAMA.* 2014;312(1):36-47.

13. Cooper DJ, Rosenfeld JV, Murray L, et al. Decompressive craniectomy in diffuse traumatic brain injury. *N Engl J Med.* 2011;364(16):1493-1502.

11

Critical Care Management in Traumatic Brain Injury

JOVANY CRUZ NAVARRO, MD, YI DENG, MD, AND
CLAUDIA ROBERTSON, MD

The Centers for Disease Control and Prevention (CDC) reports that about 150 individuals die of a traumatic brain injury (TBI) daily in the United States. Advancements in medical and surgical care seemingly allow for a higher prevalence of individuals living with a disability related to a TBI—now believed to be between 3.2 and 5.3 million.[1,2] Long-standing disability secondary to a TBI and the difficulty predicting the extent of recovery continue to challenge patients, families, caretakers, and medical practitioners. Clinical aspects of a TBI can aid in determining prognosis of a patient's recovery. With such knowledge, families may be better equipped for weighing medical and surgical decisions and managing their expectations in the setting of the resultant TBI.

Because TBI is an extremely heterogeneous condition, it poses a unique set of challenges for the critical care provider. During resuscitation efforts and critical care interventions, the intensivist must consider the brain and systemic organs as a whole to prevent or minimize further brain injury resulting from secondary insults such as hypotension, hypoxia, and metabolic abnormalities. Major efforts have been put toward the development of standardized approaches that follow the recommendations from national and international societies dedicated to the management of TBI. In this chapter we briefly cover the most commonly employed strategies for the critical care management of patients with severe TBI.

Prehospital Management

Currently, there is no therapy to reverse the primary injury associated with TBI. Therefore the main goals of prehospital evaluation and management are to prevent, identify, and treat secondary insults that will result in further brain injury. The two most commonly recognized secondary insults are hypotension and hypoxia, which are particularly deleterious during the first 24 hours after the initial insult.[3-5] In 2007, McHugh et al. reported in a metaanalysis of clinical trials and population-based studies that hypoxia (partial pressure of oxygen [PaO_2] <60 mm Hg) and systolic blood pressure (SBP) less than 90 mm Hg is associated with a higher likelihood of poor outcomes.[4] Some authors have reported that prehospital care aimed to achieve early intubation[6] and normalize blood pressure (BP) may be associated with improved outcomes,[7,8] whereas others have found increased mortality from prehospital intubation.[9]

Endotracheal intubation is recommended for patients with a Glasgow Coma Scale (GCS) of 8 or less or an inability to protect their airway regardless of GCS and/or oxygen saturation below 90%.[10] Although some authors recommend prehospital intubation in patients with severe TBI, its benefit is uncertain, with several studies reporting conflicting results[11] or no benefit,[12] and in some cases, it was associated with decreased survival in moderate to severe TBI patients.[13]

Initial Resuscitation and Management

Before arriving to the neurointensive care unit (NeuroICU), patients are usually resuscitated and stabilized in the emergency department (ED) or operating room (OR). This first contact is crucial for both treatment and prognostication. Initial approach should follow the Advanced Trauma Life Support (ATLS) guidelines, including airway, breathing, circulation, disability (including GCS), and exposure (Table 11.1). *Particular attention should be paid to avoiding hypoxia and hypotension.* A neurological evaluation should be completed as soon as possible to determine the severity of the TBI. If intracranial hypertension is suspected, evaluation and management should be initiated in the ED/OR. If clinical signs of cerebral herniation are imminent, immediate life-saving measures should be instituted. After initial assessment and management, computed tomography (CT) scan of the head should be performed as soon as possible to detect any condition that requires immediate neurosurgical intervention.

If not yet secured, an endotracheal airway should quickly be placed on arrival to the ED. The primary goal during airway instrumentation is to avoid extremes of BP and hypoxia. Induction agents such as propofol should be titrated carefully to prevent excessive vasodilation and subsequent hypotension. Etomidate can be a more suitable option during rapid

TABLE 11.1 **Glasgow Coma Scale (GCS)**

Glasgow Coma Scale (GCS)	Score
Motor Response	
Obeys commands	6
Localizes to pain	5
Withdrawal response to pain	4
Flexion to pain	3
Extension to pain	2
None	1
Verbal Response	
Oriented	5
Confused	4
Inappropriate words	3
Incomprehensible sounds	2
None	1
Eye Opening	
Spontaneously	4
To verbal commands	3
To stimulation	2
None	1

sequence induction because it maintains better hemodynamics. Although some evidence suggests that ketamine does not increase intracranial pressure (ICP),[14] the authors refrain from its use when the suspicion is high for intracranial hypertension. Ventilation and oxygenation should be optimized to prevent hypoxia and extreme hypo- or hypercarbia.

Intensive Care Management

The main goal of critical care management in TBI patients is to limit the development of secondary brain injury, which entails maintenance of cerebral perfusion, optimization of oxygenation/ventilation and BP, and prevention of hyperthermia, seizures, glucose derangements, and other metabolic abnormalities.

Hemodynamic Management

Blood Pressure and Cerebral Perfusion Pressure

The Avoidance of Hypotension Remains a Priority in Traumatic Brain Injury. SBP below 90 mm Hg is an independent predictor of poor outcomes[15] and has been associated with increased mortality.[5] Although hypotension is easily prevented and treated, it has been shown that close to 75% of patients present with at least one episode of hypotension during their intensive care unit (ICU) stay.[16]

Neurogenic and hypovolemic shock account for the most common etiologies of hypotension after severe TBI. Unless significant blood loss associated with scalp laceration or spinal cord injury exists, it is uncommon for isolated head trauma to present with severe hypotension. Consequently, other sources of hypotension should be sought, such as intrathoracic or abdominopelvic trauma or long bone fractures. Occasionally, hypotension can be masked by the Cushing response to intracranial hypertension.

Current recommendation is to maintain SBP 100 mm Hg or higher for patients 50 to 69 years old or at 110 mm Hg or higher for patients 15 to 49 or 70 years or older to decrease mortality and improve outcomes.[17] Optimal cerebral perfusion pressure (CPP) is discussed in the Intracranial Hypertension Management section. One must be aware that the location of the arterial transducer (heart or brain) can have significant effects on CPP determination. In 2013, Kosty et al. surveyed practices at different NeuroICUs across the United States regarding arterial transducer location to determine CPP, and a wide variation in practice was found.[18] The authors recommend placing an arterial transducer at the level of the tragus to estimate the CPP accurately.

Adequate intravenous access should be obtained, including at least two large-bore peripheral intravenous catheters (14–16 gauge) and a central venous catheter as soon as possible. Subclavian venous access is preferable in patients with TBI to minimize the risk of cerebral venous obstruction and vein thrombosis associated with internal jugular vein catheters. Additionally, internal jugular vein cannulation carries a higher likelihood for infection. Ultrasound-guided cannulation is recommended to increase success rate and decrease risk of arterial puncture, pneumothorax, and catheter malposition.[19]

Radial or femoral arterial cannulation should be achieved to actively guide fluid resuscitation with dynamic tests of fluid responsiveness such as pulse pressure variation and stroke volume variation. These variables can be calculated from commercially available minimally invasive devices such as EV1000 and FloTrac/Vigileo. There is good evidence that static measures of volume status such as central venous pressure should no longer be used when guiding fluid resuscitation.[20,21] Pulmonary artery catheter might incur undue risk and is no longer recommended as a first-line intervention.

Resuscitation Fluids

Normal (0.9%) saline is the resuscitation fluid of choice in neurotrauma. Albumin was associated with increased mortality rate in a subset of TBI patients enrolled in the SAFE trial and is typically avoided.[22] Hypotonic solutions (e.g., 5% dextrose, 0.45% saline) should be avoided in the acute setting because they can decrease plasma osmolarity and worsen cerebral edema.[23] Although hypertonic saline can quickly restore BP and improve intracranial hypertension, no survival benefit has been identified, and its routine use is not recommended for resuscitation purposes.[24] Although balanced crystalloid solutions (i.e., Ringer's lactate, PlasmaLyte) are associated with less risk of acute kidney injury in critically ill patients, no benefit was seen among the TBI patients enrolled in the SMART ICU trial.[23] Overall, providers in the NeuroICU should become familiar with the most commonly used resuscitation fluids because the fluid of choice is often based on the individual's hemodynamic and clinical profile (Table 11.2).

Ventilation and Oxygenation

Endotracheal intubation after severe TBI provides airway protection to reduce the risk of aspiration and subsequent development of pneumonia. In addition, it helps to control partial pressure of carbon dioxide ($Paco_2$) and minimize changes to cerebral blood flow (CBF) and ICP. $Paco_2$ and/or end-tidal CO_2 monitoring throughout the acute care phase is recommended with an initial target of normocarbia (35–45 mm Hg). In addition, hypoxia should be avoided and plateau pressure maintained less than 30 mm Hg.

Although therapeutic hyperventilation can be employed to decrease ICP, current guidelines recommend its use only as a temporizing measure, and it should be avoided during the first 24 hours after the initial injury when CBF is critically reduced.[17] Hyperventilation decreases $Paco_2$, leading to cerebral vasoconstriction that may cause secondary ischemia and increased levels of extracellular glutamate and lactate.[25] If hyperventilation is used, multimodal neuromonitoring with jugular venous oxygen saturation ($SjvO_2$) and/or partial brain tissue oxygenation ($PbtO_2$) measurement is recommended to monitor oxygen delivery.[17] Although hyperoxia can be employed in select patients to improve brain tissue oxygenation, its routine use is not recommended because of risk for oxygen toxicity.[26]

TBI is frequently complicated by acute respiratory distress syndrome (ARDS), which requires specific ventilatory therapy, including high levels of positive end-expiratory pressure (PEEP). Historically, elevated intrathoracic pressure resultant from high PEEP has been associated with impaired venous return from the brain and worsened ICP. Recent studies of applied PEEP up to 20 cm H_2O have not revealed significant effect on ICP,[27] and most important, high PEEP in TBI patients who develop ARDS seems to improve brain tissue oxygenation. In conclusion, high PEEP use is reasonable when clinically indicated for management of ARDS *in conjunction* with invasive ICP monitoring.

TABLE 11.2   Composition of Commonly Used Fluids in the Neurointensive Care Unit (NeuroICU)

| Fluid | Osm | mEq/L | | | | g/L | |
		Na	Cl	K	Ca	Lactate	Dextrose
Normal saline 0.9%	308	154	154				
Lactated Ringer's solution	275	130	109	4	3	28	
D5W	278						50
0.45% NaCl	154	77	77				
3% NaCl	1026	513	513				
5% NaCl	1710	855	855				
23.4% NaCl	8008	4004					
5% Dextrose LR	525	130	109	4	3		50
5% Dextrose 0.9% NaCl	561	154	154				50
5% Dextrose 0.45% NaCl	405	77	77				50

Osm: osmolarity, Na – Sodium, K – Potassium, Cl – Chloride, Ca – Calcium, mEq/L – miliequivalents per liter, g/L – grams per liter. D5W – Dextrose 5% in water, LR – Lactated Ringers, NaCl – Sodium chloride.

Seizure Prophylaxis

Convulsive and nonconvulsive seizures may worsen neurological examination and raise ICP, especially when associated with status epilepticus. Additionally, seizures increase metabolic demand on damaged brain tissue, which could lead to secondary injury. The incidence of posttraumatic seizures (PTSs) may be as high as 30% after severe TBI,[28] and up to 20% to 25% of patients may experience some variation of subclinical nonconvulsive seizures.[29] Thus antiseizure medications are recommended to prevent the onset of early PTS after severe TBI.[17] Although the clinical significance of electrographic silent seizures is unclear, continuous electroencephalogram (EEG) monitoring is a reasonable intervention when the neurological examination is disproportionate to the extent of the injury seen on imaging.

Current guidelines recommend prophylactic phenytoin for 7 days after injury.[17] Levetiracetam is another alternative that has shown improved functional outcomes at 6 months after injury and fewer adverse events compared with phenytoin.[30,31] Antiseizure drugs should be continued indefinitely if the patient presents with clinical or electrographic seizures during the acute phase of treatment.

Status epilepticus is a condition that results either from failure of the mechanisms responsible for seizure termination or from the initiation of mechanisms that lead to prolonged seizures.[32] It is defined as more than 5 minutes of continuous clinical or 10 minutes of subclinical or electrographic seizures and/or recurrent clinical seizures without recovery to baseline in between episodes. The main goal is to terminate the seizure activity as soon as possible while concurrently initiating long-term antiseizure therapy. Benzodiazepines such as lorazepam and midazolam represent first-line therapy, whereas CBF-decreasing drugs such as propofol or pentobarbital are reserved for refractory status epilepticus.

Venous Thromboembolism Prophylaxis

Severe TBI patients commonly develop hypercoagulable state and are at higher risk for venous thromboembolism (VTE). The risk of VTE in TBI patients without any prophylaxis has been reported as high as 53%[33] and decreases to around 10% when sequential compression stockings are employed.[34] Certainly, pharmacological VTE prophylaxis can further reduce VTE risk,[35] but it has to be weighed against the risk for hemorrhage expansion, which is greatest within the first 24 to 48 hours.[36,37]

Studies are conflicting regarding VTE prophylaxis and hemorrhage expansion.[38-40] A metaanalysis reported that VTE prophylaxis is safe when initiated within 24 to 48 hours of TBI with bleeding stability demonstrated on imaging.[41] The risk of hemorrhage expansion can be stratified using the modified Berne-Norwood Guide recommended by the American College of Surgeons (Table 11.3).[42] Although currently there is insufficient evidence to support recommendations regarding specific agent, dosing, or timing of chemical VTE prophylaxis, unfractionated heparin or enoxaparin plus compression stockings can be used in most patients, and the benefit is considered to outweigh the risks of hemorrhage expansion.[17] If VTE is identified in patients for whom anticoagulation is contraindicated, an inferior vena cava (IVC) filter should be placed.

Nutrition

Similar to most critical care patients, patients with TBI experience hypermetabolic and hypercatabolic states lasting from 1 week to several months after initial injury. Consequently, initiation of nutrition to meet basal caloric needs by postinjury day 7 is recommended to decrease mortality.[17] Enteral nutrition is superior to parenteral nutrition. If parenteral nutrition is required, strict blood glucose

TABLE 11.3	Modified Berne-Norwood Guide	
Low Risk	**Moderate Risk**	**High Risk**
No moderate or high risk	1. Small subdural/epidural/contusion Or 2. IVH Or 3. SAH with abnormal CT angiogram Or 4. Evidence of progression at 24hrs	1. ICP monitor Or 2. Craniotomy Or 3. Evidence of progression at 72 h
Treatment		
Start pharmacological VTE prophylaxis if CT stable at 24 h	Initiate pharmacological prophylaxis if CT stable at 72 h	Consider inferior vena cava filter placement

CT, computed tomography; *ICP*, intracranial pressure; *IVH*, intraventricular hemorrhage; *SAH*, subarachnoid hemorrhage; *VTE*, venous thromboembolism.

monitoring is necessary to avoid extremes. Whenever possible, postpyloric feeding should be employed to decrease the risk of aspiration pneumonia.[43]

Ulcer Prophylaxis

Gastric ulcers are a frequent source of morbidity in TBI patients. Both proton pump inhibitors and histamine-2 receptor antagonists have been shown to decrease the incidence of gastrointestinal bleeding in NeuroICU patients.[44] However, both have been associated with increased rates of pneumonia, *Clostridium difficile* infection, and drug interactions, calling into a question the role of these agents in critical care.[45]

Coagulopathy

TBI is one of the most common causes of coagulopathy after trauma,[46] and it is associated with an increased risk of hemorrhage enlargement, poor neurological outcomes, and mortality.[47,48] A baseline coagulation profile should be obtained immediately on arrival to the ED, and efforts to correct coagulopathy should be promptly initiated. The international normalization ratio (INR) should be kept at or below 1.4 and platelets at least at 75,000/μL.

Red blood cell (RBC) transfusion thresholds in TBI remain a controversial area. In a single-center randomized clinical trial, transfusion to maintain hemoglobin levels above 10 g/dL failed to improve outcomes and was associated with increased adverse effects compared with 7 g/dL.[49] Overall, RBC transfusion in TBI should be based on the patient's hemodynamics and cerebral oxygenation.

Tracheostomy

Severe TBI patients often require mechanical ventilation as an initial intervention. If the level of consciousness remains depressed after resolution of the acute treatment phase, patients should undergo tracheostomy to ensure patent airway and facilitate liberation from mechanical ventilation. Relative contraindications include elevated ICP, hemodynamic instability, and severe respiratory failure with high oxygen and PEEP requirements. Early tracheostomy ($\leq$8 days) in patients with isolated TBI has been associated with shorter mechanical ventilation, ICU, and hospital days. Therefore TBI patients deemed unlikely to reverse their initial condition should be considered for early tracheostomy ($\leq$8 days).[50]

Glucose Management

Following TBI, both hyperglycemia and hypoglycemia can further exacerbate injury and induce secondary neuronal toxicity and cerebral edema.[51] Strict glucose control (80–110 mg/dL) has not shown to decrease mortality in these patients whereas the risk of hypoglycemia is significantly

increased.[52-54] Thus, it is reasonable to target glucose between 140 and 180 mg/dL, and avoid glucose-containing hypo-osmolar resuscitation fluid.

Temperature Management

Although there is evidence that hyperthermia worsens preexisting injury and neurological outcomes, prophylactic hypothermia has not demonstrated definitive benefits.[55,56] There was significant heterogeneity in study designs in terms of time of initiation, nadir of hypothermia, duration, and rewarming protocol.[57-59] To date the largest randomized trial (Eurotherm3235) was terminated prematurely because of worsened Glasgow Outcome Scale (GOS) scores at 6 months compared with controls, and early (<2.5 hours), short-term (48 hours) prophylactic hypothermia is not recommended based on current guidelines (Evidence IIB).[17,60]

Antibiotics and Infection Prophylaxis

Patients with TBI are at higher risk for infections caused by invasive monitoring and mechanical ventilation, with incidence of external ventricular drain (EVD) infection up to 27% and ventilator-associated pneumonia (VAP) up to 40%.[61,62] Currently, as consistent with general ICU guidelines, TBI patients should not be initiated on prophylactic antibiotics or povidone–iodine oral care to decrease VAP.[17] Early tracheostomy does not affect VAP incidence. Antimicrobial-impregnated catheters received a level III recommendation for EVD management, but focus has been more toward aseptic techniques in placement and daily care of catheters rather than routine antibiotic use.[17,63,64]

Steroids

Steroids currently have no role in severe TBI patients. The CRASH (Corticosteroid Randomisation After Significant Head Injury) study randomized 4000 patients to high-dose methylprednisolone and found worsened mortality at 2 weeks and 6 months.[65] It remains to be seen if low-dose steroids may play a role in TBI management in the future.

Paroxysmal Sympathetic Hyperactivity

Paroxysmal sympathetic hyperactivity (PSH)—formerly known as *sympathetic storming*—is characterized by sudden and labile episodes of tachycardia, hypertension, diaphoresis, tachypnea, fever, increased tone, and posturing.[66] PSH is seen in approximately 10% of TBI patients. Mainstay treatment consists of pain control (enteral or intravenous opioids), sedation (e.g., midazolam, propofol), and sympathetic blockade. Sympathetic blockade can be achieved with nonselective beta blockers such as propranolol and/or α-2 receptor agonists (e.g., clonidine, dexmedetomidine). If control is inadequate, the addition of second-line agents such as gabapentin, bromocriptine, or dantrolene should be considered.[67]

Neuromonitoring

Intracranial hypertension frequently occurs after a traumatic insult to the brain and causes secondary insult to the brain, leading to ischemia, herniation, and death. Although changes in clinical examination and GCS score are helpful, in a comatose or sedated patient, dynamic evolution of injury could be occurring with little to no reliable clinical differentiation. As such, additional monitoring is necessary for early prognosis and intervention.

In the United States, ICP monitoring with EVD is considered the gold standard currently. The Brain Trauma Foundation (BTF) in its third edition guidelines recommended that either (1) all patients with severe TBI, GCS 3 to 8 and an abnormal CT scan or (2) patients over the age of 40, evidence of motor posturing, systolic BP less 90 mm Hg, and normal CT scan receive ICP monitoring.[68] This recommendation was not carried forward strongly in the fourth edition because of perceived low quality of evidence, which simply recommends monitoring ICP in severe TBI patients to reduce in-hospital and 2-week mortality.[17] Normal ICP is 10 to 15 mm Hg and if greater than 22 mm Hg, a stepwise treatment algorithm should be initiated.[17] CPP should be calculated and optimized per patient (covered later).

In addition to ICP monitoring, other adjunct modalities are often used concomitantly in the ICU. The two most common are $PbtO_2$ and cerebral microdialysis, which uses an additional intraparenchymal catheter placed through a secondary burr hole. Measuring local tissue oxygen tension in areas of the brain at risk for further injury (penumbra) allows for more focal intervention that may not be reflected through global ICP measurement. Normal $PbtO_2$ is greater than 40 mm Hg, whereas less 15 mm Hg portends poor outcome and should be intervened through further ICP reduction, CPP optimization, and/or oxygenation carrying capacity augmentation.[69,70]

Similarly, cerebral microdialysis provides a targeted analysis of brain milieu in the at-risk regions. A high lactate/pyruvate ratio above 25 reflects anaerobic metabolism and is independently associated with worsened mortality rate.[71] Regional glutamate levels, glucose fluctuation, and newer biomarkers such as interleukin-6 and matrix-metalloproteinase-9 have all been linked to inflammation, delayed ischemia, and poor outcomes.[72-74] Disadvantages of these techniques include elevated risk of infection and bleeding related to the invasive nature of devices and additional labor cost. Others have argued that the regional snapshot of the brain is irreflective of the global environment. However, Bouzat et al. examined 27 severe TBI patients and demonstrated excellent correlation between cerebral microdialysis and global perfusion and concluded the addition of $PbtO_2$ and microdialysis monitoring was significantly more accurate at

predicting low regional blood flow versus ICP monitoring alone.[75]

Another technique for measuring brain oxygenation is the $SjvO_2$, which entails inserting a special catheter retrograde up the internal jugular vein past the jugular bulb. Continuous measurement of global cerebral venous saturation can then be obtained. Normal $SjvO_2$ is 55% to 75%, with low values indicating an imbalance of oxygen demand versus supply. High values, conversely, can indicate hyperemia or dysfunction in oxygen usage.[76] More recently, near-infrared spectroscopy (NIRS) has been evaluated in TBI patients. It uses a noninvasive optical probe placed on the scalp to measure tissue oxygenation.[77] Although logistical challenges in this population can confound results (e.g., scalp hematoma, skull thickness, extracranial injuries), if NIRS is validated it can offer the potential to supplant invasive techniques as a surrogate measure of cerebral perfusion.

Intracranial Hypertension Management

Elevated ICP after TBI is common and must be promptly treated to avoid devastating neurological outcomes. The overarching goals of ICP management are to optimize cerebral perfusion, prevent ischemia, reduce edema, and support metabolic demand. If the patient has a new, focal space-occupying lesion such as subdural hematoma, surgical evacuation is first-line therapy. Once corrected, global elevation of ICP can then be tackled in a tiered approach (Fig. 11.1).[17,78] Regardless of the patient, certain measures should be instituted if not contraindicated, such as head-of-bed elevation at 30 degrees with neutral neck position to minimize venous outflow obstruction, prevent hyperthermia and shivering, achieve euvolemia, avoid hypoxia, and maintain normocapnia. Aggressive hyperventilation has fallen out of favor because it has been shown to worsen ischemia and death in several studies and should only be instituted in patients with impending herniation.[79-81]

An in-situ EVD allows for CSF removal either in a continuous or intermittent manner and is the primary treatment for TBI-induced hydrocephalus. ICP measured from the EVD allows one to derive CPP, as CPP = MAP – ICP (where MAP is mean arterial pressure. CPP is a major determinant of cerebral perfusion and is linearly correlated with CBF in a TBI patient with dysfunctional autoregulation mechanisms. As such, optimizing CPP at certain thresholds can ameliorate unintended low-CBF consequences. Optimal CPP is controversial. The BTF fourth edition guidelines recommend 60 to 70 mm Hg while avoiding aggressively targeting above 70 mm Hg with vasopressors or fluids.[17] High CPP can reflect cerebral hyperemia and has been linked to increased acute respiratory distress syndrome, presumably from pressor use. There are some who argue for the benefits of individualized CPP management using pressure reactivity index, which essentially identifies BP ranges at which CPP/autoregulation is preserved. This optimal CPP (CPPopt) is then targeted for that patient. The studies

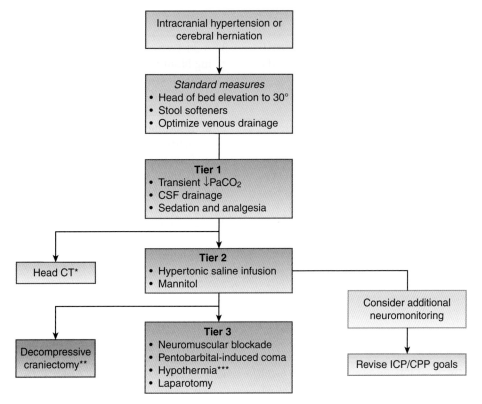

Intracranial hypertension or
cerebral herniation

↓

Standard measures
- Head of bed elevation to 30°
- Stool softeners
- Optimize venous drainage

↓

Tier 1
- Transient ↓PaCO₂
- CSF drainage
- Sedation and analgesia

Head CT*

Tier 2
- Hypertonic saline infusion
- Mannitol

Consider additional
neuromonitoring

↓

Revise ICP/CPP goals

Decompressive
craniectomy**

Tier 3
- Neuromuscular blockade
- Pentobarbital-induced coma
- Hypothermia***
- Laparotomy

* If the brain has not yet been imaged, a noncontrast head CT scan should be performed when the patient can be safely transported.
** Decompressive craniectomy can be performed at any point during this algorithm if indicated
*** Hypothermia should be reserved as a "rescue" therapy when all tier 3 interventions have failed.

• **Fig. 11.1** Tiered algorithm for intracranial pressure management. *CSF,* Cerebrospinal fluid; *CPP,* cerebral perfusion pressure; *CT,* computed tomography; *ICP,* intracranial pressure.

are conflicted; some show improving GOS scores and mortality rates a, whereas others conclude lack of benefit.[82-85] As such, it currently receives a weak recommendation from the Neurocritical Care Society.[86]

Osmotherapy with mannitol has been a mainstay therapy in treating intracranial hypertension for decades. Mannitol decreases ICP by a combination of blood viscosity reduction and osmotic diuresis. More recently, hypertonic saline has achieved potentially even greater ICP reduction than mannitol.[87,88] Nevertheless, current recommendations do not favor one agent over the other, and caution must be exercised in specific situations, such as mannitol in hypovolemic patients and hypertonic saline in grossly hyponatremic patients.

As a third-tier medical therapy, barbiturates such as pentobarbital can be used to control refractory ICP elevation. Barbiturates decrease cerebral metabolism and oxygen consumption, thus reducing CBF and ICP. It is titrated to burst suppression on the EEG but frequently will induce hypotension, necessitating vasopressors. Propofol can also be used for ICP control but has not been shown to benefit mortality or neurological outcomes.

Decompressive craniectomy (DC), whereby a section of the skull is surgically removed to allow for swelling, has been used as an option of last resort. Previously, several

low-level, retrospective, or observational trials were equivocal in their findings.[89-91] Higher level evidence includes two randomized trials: DEcompressive CRAniectomy (DECRA) and Randomised Evaluation of Surgery with Craniectomy for Uncontrollable Elevation of Intracranial Pressure (RESCUEicp).

DECRA found that bilateral craniectomies exhibited no mortality benefit compared with medical management but had better ICP control with shorter ICU stay at the cost of more unfavorable outcomes at 6 months.[92] RESCUEicp had similar study design and found lower mortality but higher rates of severe neurological disability among survivors at 6 months. Taken together, the debate on the utility of DC in medically refractory patients is still ongoing. BTF does recommend that if a surgical option is sought, a large frontotemporoparietal DC is superior over small DC in terms of neurological outcomes.[17]

Summary

The critical care management of patients with severe TBI should be focused on the prevention of secondary injury. Patients should be optimally managed in a specialized neurotrauma center with neurosurgical and neurocritical care providers and the use of standardized guideline-based protocols.

Review Questions

1. In patients with traumatic brain injury (TBI), what is the most reasonable target for glucose control in the intensive care unit?
   a. 50–80 mg/dL
   b. 80–110 mg/dL
   c. 140–180 mg/dL
   d. 180–210 mg/dL
2. Based on the current available evidence, which of these cerebral perfusion pressures (CPP) should be targeted to achieve the best outcome after TBI?
   a. 30 mm Hg
   b. 50 mm Hg
   c. 70 mm Hg
   d. 90 mm Hg

3. A 34-year-old man is admitted to the ICU after sustaining blunt trauma to the head. He is currently intubated, nonresponsive to commands, with a Glasgow Coma Score (GCS) of 4. Which of these interventions should be instituted for the patient at this time?
   a. Inserting external ventricular drain
   b. Starting prophylactic antibiotics
   c. Inducing hypertension
   d. B and C
   e. All of the above

Answers on page 387.
Access the full list of questions and answers online.
Available on ExpertConsult.com

References

1. Schiller JS, Lucas JW, Ward BW, Peregoy JA. Summary health statistics for U.S. adults: National Health Interview Survey, 2010. *Vital Health Stat 10.* 2012;(252):1-207.
2. Taylor CA, Bell JM, Breiding MJ, Xu L. Traumatic brain injury–related emergency department visits, hospitalizations, and deaths — United States, 2007 and 2013. *MMWR Surveill Summ.* 2017;66(9):1-16. doi:10.15585/mmwr.ss6609a1.
3. Brain Trauma Foundation, American Association of Neurological Surgeons, Congress of Neurological Surgeons, et al. Guidelines for the management of severe traumatic brain injury. I. Blood pressure and oxygenation. *J Neurotrauma.* 2007;24(suppl 1):S7-S13. doi:10.1089/neu.2007.9995
4. McHugh GS, Engel DC, Butcher I, et al. Prognostic value of secondary insults in traumatic brain injury: results from the IMPACT study. *J Neurotrauma.* 2007;24(2):287-293. doi:10.1089/neu.2006.0031.
5. Chesnut RM, Marshall LF, Klauber MR, et al. The role of secondary brain injury in determining outcome from severe head injury. *J Trauma.* 1993;34(2):216-222.
6. Denninghoff KR, Nuño T, Pauls Q, et al. Prehospital Intubation is Associated with Favorable Outcomes and Lower Mortality in ProTECT III. *Prehosp Emerg Care.* 21(5):539-544. doi:10.1080/10903127.2017.1315201.
7. Davis DP, Peay J, Sise MJ, et al. Prehospital airway and ventilation management: a trauma score and injury severity score-based analysis. *J Trauma.* 2010;69(2):294-301. doi:10.1097/TA.0b013e3181dc6c7f.
8. Rudehill A, Bellander BM, Weitzberg E, Bredbacka S, Backheden M, Gordon E. Outcome of traumatic brain injuries in 1,508 patients: impact of prehospital care. *J Neurotrauma.* 2002;19(7):855-868. doi:10.1089/08977150260190447.
9. Bukur M, Kurtovic S, Berry C, et al. Pre-hospital intubation is associated with increased mortality after traumatic brain injury. *J Surg Res.* 2011;170(1):e117-e121. doi:10.1016/j.jss.2011.04.005.
10. Badjatia N, Carney N, Crocco TJ, et al. Guidelines for prehospital management of traumatic brain injury 2nd edition. *Prehosp Emerg Care.* 2008;12(suppl 1):S1-S52. doi:10.1080/10903120701732052.
11. Gaither JB, Spaite DW, Bobrow BJ, et al. Balancing the potential risks and benefits of out-of-hospital intubation in traumatic brain injury: the intubation/hyperventilation effect. *Ann Emerg Med.* 2012;60(6):732-736. doi:10.1016/j.annemergmed.2012.06.017.
12. von Elm E, Schoettker P, Henzi I, Osterwalder J, Walder B. Pre-hospital tracheal intubation in patients with traumatic brain injury: systematic review of current evidence. *Br J Anaesth.* 2009;103(3):371-386. doi:10.1093/bja/aep202.
13. Davis DP, Peay J, Sise MJ, et al. The impact of prehospital endotracheal intubation on outcome in moderate to severe traumatic brain injury. *J Trauma.* 2005;58(5):933-939.
14. Zeiler FA, Teitelbaum J, West M, Gillman LM. The ketamine effect on ICP in traumatic brain injury. *Neurocrit Care.* 2014;21(1):163-173. doi:10.1007/s12028-013-9950-y.
15. Manley G, Knudson MM, Morabito D, Damron S, Erickson V, Pitts L. Hypotension, hypoxia, and head injury: frequency, duration, and consequences. *Arch Surg.* 2001;136(10):1118-1123.
16. Chesnut RM, Marshall SB, Piek J, Blunt BA, Klauber MR, Marshall LF. Early and late systemic hypotension as a frequent and fundamental source of cerebral ischemia following severe brain injury in the Traumatic Coma Data Bank. *Acta Neurochir Suppl (Wien).* 1993;59:121-125.
17. Carney N, Totten AM, O'Reilly C, et al. Guidelines for the Management of Severe Traumatic Brain Injury, Fourth Edition. *Neurosurgery.* 2017;80(1):6-15. doi:10.1227/NEU.0000000000001432
18. Kosty JA, Leroux PD, Levine J, et al. Brief report: a comparison of clinical and research practices in measuring cerebral perfusion pressure: a literature review and practitioner survey. *Anesth Analg.* 2013;117(3):694-698. doi:10.1213/ANE.0b013e31829cc765.
19. Lalu MM, Fayad A, Ahmed O, et al. Ultrasound-guided subclavian vein catheterization: a systematic review and meta-analysis. *Crit Care Med.* 2015;43(7):1498-1507. doi:10.1097/CCM.0000000000000973.
20. Bentzer P, Griesdale DE, Boyd J, MacLean K, Sirounis D, Ayas NT. Will this hemodynamically unstable patient respond to a bolus of intravenous fluids? *JAMA.* 2016;316(12):1298-1309. doi:10.1001/jama.2016.12310.
21. Marik PE, Cavallazzi R. Does the central venous pressure predict fluid responsiveness? An updated meta-analysis and a plea for some common sense. *Crit Care Med.* 2013;41(7):1774-1781. doi:10.1097/CCM.0b013e31828a25fd.
22. Van Aken HK, Kampmeier TG, Ertmer C, Westphal M. Fluid resuscitation in patients with traumatic brain injury: what is a

SAFE approach? *Curr Opin Anaesthesiol.* 2012;25(5):563-565. doi:10.1097/ACO.0b013e3283572274.

23. Semler MW, Self WH, Wanderer JP, et al. Balanced crystalloids versus saline in critically ill adults. *N Engl J Med.* 2018;378(9):829-839. doi:10.1056/NEJMoa1711584.

24. Strandvik GF. Hypertonic saline in critical care: a review of the literature and guidelines for use in hypotensive states and raised intracranial pressure. *Anaesthesia.* 2009;64(9):990-1003. doi:10.1111/j.1365-2044.2009.05986.x.

25. Marion DW, Puccio A, Wisniewski SR, et al. Effect of hyperventilation on extracellular concentrations of glutamate, lactate, pyruvate, and local cerebral blood flow in patients with severe traumatic brain injury. *Crit Care Med.* 2002;30(12):2619-2625. doi:10.1097/01.CCM.0000038877.40844.0F.

26. Diringer MN. Hyperoxia: good or bad for the injured brain? *Curr Opin Crit Care.* 2008;14(2):167-171. doi:10.1097/MCC.0b013e3282f57552.

27. Boone MD, Jinadasa SP, Mueller A, et al. The effect of positive end-expiratory pressure on intracranial pressure and cerebral hemodynamics. *Neurocrit Care.* 2017;26(2):174-181. doi:10.1007/s12028-016-0328-9.

28. Temkin NR. Risk factors for posttraumatic seizures in adults. *Epilepsia.* 2003;44(s10):18-20.

29. Zimmermann LL, Diaz-Arrastia R, Vespa PM. Seizures and the role of anticonvulsants after traumatic brain injury. *Neurosurg Clin N Am.* 2016;27(4):499-508. doi:10.1016/j.nec.2016.06.001.

30. Xu JC, Shen J, Shao WZ, et al. The safety and efficacy of levetiracetam versus phenytoin for seizure prophylaxis after traumatic brain injury: a systematic review and meta-analysis. *Brain Inj.* 2016;30(9):1054-1061. doi:10.3109/02699052.2016.1170882.

31. Szaflarski JP, Sangha KS, Lindsell CJ, Shutter LA. Prospective, randomized, single-blinded comparative trial of intravenous levetiracetam versus phenytoin for seizure prophylaxis. *Neurocrit Care.* 2010;12(2):165-172. doi:10.1007/s12028-009-9304-y.

32. Trinka E, Cock H, Hesdorffer D, et al. A definition and classification of status epilepticus-Report of the ILAE Task Force on Classification of Status Epilepticus. *Epilepsia.* 2015;56(10):1515-1523. doi:10.1111/epi.13121.

33. Geerts WH, Code KI, Jay RM, Chen E, Szalai JP. A prospective study of venous thromboembolism after major trauma. *N Engl J Med.* 1994;331(24):1601-1606. doi:10.1056/NEJM199412153312401.

34. Sachdeva A, Dalton M, Lees T. Graduated compression stockings for prevention of deep vein thrombosis. *Cochrane database Syst Rev.* 2018;11:CD001484. doi:10.1002/14651858.CD001484.pub4.

35. Agnelli G, Piovella F, Buoncristiani P, et al. Enoxaparin plus compression stockings compared with compression stockings alone in the prevention of venous thromboembolism after elective neurosurgery. *N Engl J Med.* 1998;339(2):80-85. doi:10.1056/NEJM199807093390204.

36. Norwood SH, Berne JD, Rowe SA, Villarreal DH, Ledlie JT. Early venous thromboembolism prophylaxis with enoxaparin in patients with blunt traumatic brain injury. *J Trauma.* 2008;65(5):1021-1026; discussion 1026-1027. doi:10.1097/TA.0b013e31818a0e74.

37. Salottolo K, Offner P, Levy AS, Mains CW, Slone DS, Bar-Or D. Interrupted pharmacologic thromboprophylaxis increases venous thromboembolism in traumatic brain injury. *J Trauma.* 2011;70(1):19-24; discussion 25-26. doi:10.1097/TA.0b013e318207c54d.

38. Saadeh Y, Gohil K, Bill C, et al. Chemical venous thromboembolic prophylaxis is safe and effective for patients with traumatic brain injury when started 24 hours after the absence of hemorrhage progression on head CT. *J Trauma Acute Care Surg.* 2012;73(2):426-430. doi:10.1097/TA.0b013e31825a758b.

39. Scudday T, Brasel K, Webb T, et al. Safety and efficacy of prophylactic anticoagulation in patients with traumatic brain injury. *J Am Coll Surg.* 2011;213(1):148-153; discussion 153-154. doi:10.1016/j.jamcollsurg.2011.02.027.

40. Kwiatt ME, Patel MS, Ross SE, et al. Is low-molecular-weight heparin safe for venous thromboembolism prophylaxis in patients with traumatic brain injury? A Western Trauma Association multicenter study. *J Trauma Acute Care Surg.* 2012;73(3):625-628. doi:10.1097/TA.0b013e318265cab9.

41. Margolick J, Dandurand C, Duncan K, et al. A systematic review of the risks and benefits of venous thromboembolism prophylaxis in traumatic brain injury. *Can J Neurol Sci.* 2018;45(4):432-444. doi:10.1017/cjn.2017.275.

42. ACS. *ACS TQIP Best Practices in the Management of Traumatic Brain Injury.* Available at: https://www.facs.org/-/media/files/quality-programs/trauma/tqip/tbi_guidelines.ashx

43. Acosta-Escribano J, Fernández-Vivas M, Grau Carmona T, et al. Gastric versus transpyloric feeding in severe traumatic brain injury: a prospective, randomized trial. *Intensive Care Med.* 2010;36(9):1532-1539. doi:10.1007/s00134-010-1908-3.

44. Schirmer CM, Kornbluth J, Heilman CB, Bhardwaj A. Gastrointestinal prophylaxis in neurocritical care. *Neurocrit Care.* 2012;16(1):184-193. doi:10.1007/s12028-011-9580-1.

45. MacLaren R, Reynolds PM, Allen RR. Histamine-2 receptor antagonists vs proton pump inhibitors on gastrointestinal tract hemorrhage and infectious complications in the intensive care unit. *JAMA Intern Med.* 2014;174(4):564-574. doi:10.1001/jamainternmed.2013.14673.

46. Lippi G, Cervellin G. Disseminated intravascular coagulation in trauma injuries. *Semin Thromb Hemost.* 2010;36(4):378-387. doi:10.1055/s-0030-1254047.

47. de Oliveira Manoel AL, Neto AC, Veigas PV, Rizoli S. Traumatic brain injury associated coagulopathy. *Neurocrit Care.* 2015;22(1):34-44. doi:10.1007/s12028-014-0026-4.

48. Zehtabchi S, Soghoian S, Liu Y, et al. The association of coagulopathy and traumatic brain injury in patients with isolated head injury. *Resuscitation.* 2008;76(1):52-56. doi:10.1016/j.resuscitation.2007.06.024.

49. Robertson CS, Hannay HJ, Yamal JM, et al. Effect of erythropoietin and transfusion threshold on neurological recovery after traumatic brain injury: a randomized clinical trial. *JAMA.* 2014;312(1):36-47. doi:10.1001/jama.2014.6490.

50. Alali AS, Scales DC, Fowler RA, et al. Tracheostomy timing in traumatic brain injury: a propensity-matched cohort study. *J Trauma Acute Care Surg.* 2014;76(1):70-76; discussion 76-78. doi:10.1097/TA.0b013e3182a8fd6a.

51. Lam AM, Winn HR, Cullen BF, Sundling N. Hyperglycemia and neurological outcome in patients with head injury. *J Neurosurg.* 1991;75(4):545-551. doi:10.3171/jns.1991.75.4.0545.

52. Bilotta F, Caramia R, Cernak I, et al. Intensive insulin therapy after severe traumatic brain injury: a randomized clinical trial. *Neurocrit Care.* 2008;9(2):159-166. doi:10.1007/s12028-008-9084-9.

53. Yang M, Guo Q, Zhang X, et al. Intensive insulin therapy on infection rate, days in NICU, in-hospital mortality and neurological outcome in severe traumatic brain injury patients: a randomized controlled trial. *Int J Nurs Stud.* 2009;46(6):753-758. doi:10.1016/j.ijnurstu.2009.01.004.

54. Coester A, Neumann CR, Schmidt MI. Intensive insulin therapy in severe traumatic brain injury: a randomized trial. *J Trauma.* 2010;68(4):904-911. doi:10.1097/TA.0b013e3181c9afc2.

55. Thompson HJ, Tkacs NC, Saatman KE, Raghupathi R, McIntosh TK. Hyperthermia following traumatic brain injury: a critical evaluation. *Neurobiol Dis.* 2003;12(3):163-173.

56. Sadaka F, Veremakis C. Therapeutic hypothermia for the management of intracranial hypertension in severe traumatic brain injury: a systematic review. *Brain Inj.* 2012;26(7-8):899-908. doi:10.3109/02699052.2012.661120.

57. Clifton GL, Valadka A, Zygun D, et al. Very early hypothermia induction in patients with severe brain injury (the National Acute Brain Injury Study: Hypothermia II): a randomised trial.

Lancet Neurol. 2011;10(2):131-139. doi:10.1016/S1474-4422(10)70300-8.

58. Clifton GL, Miller ER, Choi SC, et al. Lack of effect of induction of hypothermia after acute brain injury. *N Engl J Med.* 2001;344(8):556-563. doi:10.1056/NEJM200102223440803.

59. Qiu WS, Liu WG, Shen H, et al. Therapeutic effect of mild hypothermia on severe traumatic head injury. *Chin J Traumatol.* 2005;8(1):27-32.

60. Andrews PJD, Sinclair HL, Rodriguez A, et al. Hypothermia for intracranial hypertension after traumatic brain injury. *N Engl J Med.* 2015;373(25):2403-2412. doi:10.1056/NEJMoa1507581.

61. Rebuck JA, Murry KR, Rhoney DH, Michael DB, Coplin WM. Infection related to intracranial pressure monitors in adults: analysis of risk factors and antibiotic prophylaxis. *J Neurol Neurosurg Psychiatry.* 2000;69(3):381-384.

62. Hui X, Haider AH, Hashmi ZG, et al. Increased risk of pneumonia among ventilated patients with traumatic brain injury: every day counts! *J Surg Res.* 2013;184(1):438-443. doi:10.1016/j.jss.2013.05.072.

63. Wang X, Dong Y, Qi XQ, Li YM, Huang CG, Hou LJ. Clinical review: efficacy of antimicrobial-impregnated catheters in external ventricular drainage - a systematic review and meta-analysis. *Crit Care.* 2013;17(4):234. doi:10.1186/cc12608.

64. Ratilal BO, Costa J, Sampaio C, Pappamikail L. Antibiotic prophylaxis for preventing meningitis in patients with basilar skull fractures. *Cochrane database Syst Rev.* 2011;(8):CD004884. doi:10.1002/14651858.CD004884.pub3.

65. Edwards P, Arango M, Balica L, et al. Final results of MRC CRASH, a randomised placebo-controlled trial of intravenous corticosteroid in adults with head injury-outcomes at 6 months. *Lancet.* 365(9475):1957-1959. doi:10.1016/S0140-6736(05)66552-X.

66. Baguley IJ, Perkes IE, Fernandez-Ortega JF, et al. Paroxysmal sympathetic hyperactivity after acquired brain injury: consensus on conceptual definition, nomenclature, and diagnostic criteria. *J Neurotrauma.* 2014;31(17):1515-1520. doi:10.1089/neu.2013.3301.

67. Hendricks HT, Heeren AH, Vos PE. Dysautonomia after severe traumatic brain injury. *Eur J Neurol.* 2010;17(9):1172-1177. doi:10.1111/j.1468-1331.2010.02989.x.

68. Brain Trauma Foundation, American Association of Neurological Surgeons, Congress of Neurological Surgeons, et al. Guidelines for the management of severe traumatic brain injury. VIII. Intracranial pressure thresholds. *J Neurotrauma.* 2007;24(suppl 1):S55-S58. doi:10.1089/neu.2007.9988.

69. Kurtz P, Helbok R, Claassen J, et al. The effect of packed red blood cell transfusion on cerebral oxygenation and metabolism after subarachnoid hemorrhage. *Neurocrit Care.* 2016;24(1):118-121. doi:10.1007/s12028-015-0180-3.

70. Narotam PK, Morrison JF, Nathoo N. Brain tissue oxygen monitoring in traumatic brain injury and major trauma: outcome analysis of a brain tissue oxygen-directed therapy. *J Neurosurg.* 2009;111(4):672-682. doi:10.3171/2009.4.JNS081150.

71. Timofeev I, Carpenter KLH, Nortje J, et al. Cerebral extracellular chemistry and outcome following traumatic brain injury: a microdialysis study of 223 patients. *Brain.* 2011;134(Pt 2):484-494. doi:10.1093/brain/awq353.

72. Kurtz P, Claassen J, Helbok R, et al. Systemic glucose variability predicts cerebral metabolic distress and mortality after subarachnoid hemorrhage: a retrospective observational study. *Crit Care.* 2014;18(3):R89. doi:10.1186/cc13857.

73. Hinzman JM, Wilson JA, Mazzeo AT, Bullock MR, Hartings JA. Excitotoxicity and metabolic crisis are associated with spreading depolarizations in severe traumatic brain injury patients. *J Neurotrauma.* 2016;33(19):1775-1783. doi:10.1089/neu.2015.4226.

74. Helbok R, Schiefecker AJ, Beer R, et al. Early brain injury after aneurysmal subarachnoid hemorrhage: a multimodal neuromonitoring study. *Crit Care.* 2015;19:75. doi:10.1186/s13054-015-0809-9.

75. Bouzat P, Marques-Vidal P, Zerlauth JB, et al. Accuracy of brain multimodal monitoring to detect cerebral hypoperfusion after traumatic brain injury. *Crit Care Med.* 2015;43(2):445-452. doi:10.1097/CCM.0000000000000720.

76. Dash HH, Chavali S. Management of traumatic brain injury patients. *Korean J Anesthesiol.* 2018;71(1):12-21. doi:10.4097/kjae.2018.71.1.12.

77. Davies DJ, Su Z, Clancy MT, et al. Near-infrared spectroscopy in the monitoring of adult traumatic brain injury: a review. *J Neurotrauma.* 2015;32(13):933-941. doi:10.1089/neu.2014.3748.

78. Nathens AB, Cryer HG, Fildes J. The American College of Surgeons Trauma Quality Improvement Program. *Surg Clin North Am.* 2012;92(2):441-54, x-xi. doi:10.1016/j.suc.2012.01.003.

79. Stein NR, McArthur DL, Etchepare M, Vespa PM. Early cerebral metabolic crisis after TBI influences outcome despite adequate hemodynamic resuscitation. *Neurocrit Care.* 2012;17(1):49-57. doi:10.1007/s12028-012-9708-y.

80. Liu S, Wan X, Wang S, et al. Posttraumatic cerebral infarction in severe traumatic brain injury: characteristics, risk factors and potential mechanisms. *Acta Neurochir (Wien).* 2015;157(10):1697-1704. doi:10.1007/s00701-015-2559-5.

81. Spaite DW, Bobrow BJ, Stolz U, et al. Evaluation of the impact of implementing the emergency medical services traumatic brain injury guidelines in Arizona: the Excellence in Prehospital Injury Care (EPIC) study methodology. *Acad Emerg Med.* 2014;21(7):818-830. doi:10.1111/acem.12411.

82. Dias C, Silva MJ, Pereira E, et al. Optimal cerebral perfusion pressure management at bedside: a single-center pilot study. *Neurocrit Care.* 2015;23(1):92-102. doi:10.1007/s12028-014-0103-8.

83. Aries MJ, Czosnyka M, Budohoski KP, et al. Continuous determination of optimal cerebral perfusion pressure in traumatic brain injury. *Crit Care Med.* 2012;40(8):2456-2463. doi:10.1097/CCM.0b013e3182514eb6.

84. Sugimoto K, Shirao S, Koizumi H, et al. Continuous monitoring of spreading depolarization and cerebrovascular autoregulation after aneurysmal subarachnoid hemorrhage. *J Stroke Cerebrovasc Dis.* 2016;25(10):e171-e177. doi:10.1016/j.jstrokecerebrovasdis.2016.07.007.

85. Johnson U, Engquist H, Howells T, et al. Bedside xenon-CT shows lower CBF in SAH patients with impaired CBF pressure autoregulation as defined by Pressure Reactivity Index (PRx). *Neurocrit Care.* 2016;25(1):47-55. doi:10.1007/s12028-016-0240-3

86. Le Roux P, Menon DK, Citerio G, et al. Consensus summary statement of the International Multidisciplinary Consensus Conference on Multimodality Monitoring in Neurocritical Care: a statement for healthcare professionals from the Neurocritical Care Society and the European Society of Intensive C. *Neurocrit Care.* 2014;21(suppl 2):S1-S26. doi:10.1007/s12028-014-0041-5.

87. Cottenceau V, Masson F, Mahamid E, et al. Comparison of effects of equiosmolar doses of mannitol and hypertonic saline on cerebral blood flow and metabolism in traumatic brain injury. *J Neurotrauma.* 2011;28(10):2003-2012. doi:10.1089/neu.2011.1929.

88. Vialet R, Albanèse J, Thomachot L, et al. Isovolume hypertonic solutes (sodium chloride or mannitol) in the treatment of refractory posttraumatic intracranial hypertension: 2 mL/kg 7.5% saline is more effective than 2 mL/kg 20% mannitol. *Crit Care*

Med. 2003;31(6):1683-1687. doi:10.1097/01.CCM.0000063268.91710.DF.

89. Wen L, Wang H, Wang F, et al. A prospective study of early versus late craniectomy after traumatic brain injury. Brain Inj. 2011;25(13-14):1318-1324. doi:10.3109/02699052.2011.608214.

90. Olivecrona M, Rodling-Wahlström M, Naredi S, Koskinen LO. Effective ICP reduction by decompressive craniectomy in patients with severe traumatic brain injury treated by an ICP-targeted therapy. J Neurotrauma. 2007;24(6):927-935. doi:10.1089/neu.2005.356E.

91. Soustiel JF, Sviri GE, Mahamid E, Shik V, Abeshaus S, Zaaroor M. Cerebral blood flow and metabolism following decompressive craniectomy for control of increased intracranial pressure. Neurosurgery. 2010;67(1):65-72; discussion 72. doi:10.1227/01.NEU.0000370604.30037.F5.

92. Cooper DJ, Rosenfeld JV, Murray L, et al. Decompressive craniectomy in diffuse traumatic brain injury. N Engl J Med. 2011;364(16):1493-1502. doi:10.1056/NEJMoa1102077.

12

Complications of Traumatic Brain Injury

SAMANTHA FERNANDEZ HERNANDEZ, MD, JOVANY CRUZ NAVARRO, MD, AND CLAUDIA ROBERTSON, MD

OUTLINE

Traumatic brain injury (TBI) can be a catastrophic event, with a mortality rate up to 40% in severe cases[1] and potential lifelong sequelae in a large number of patients. It is estimated that 1.1% of the US population has long-term disabilities after a TBI, not accounting for those who do not seek treatment, which may increase this number substantially.[2] This chapter focuses on immediate and delayed complications of TBI and their impact on life expectancy in the TBI survivor.

Herniation Syndromes

One of the most important, time-critical, and potentially fatal complications of brain injury with increased intracranial pressure (ICP) is brain herniation, which, if untreated in a timely manner, can quickly lead to irreversible brain injury and death. Brain herniation is defined as the displacement of brain matter from its normal anatomical compartment into a different one and sequential compression of adjacent structures.[3-5] The underlying mechanism of this phenomenon can be explained by the Monro-Kellie doctrine, which states that the sum of volumes of brain parenchyma, blood, and cerebrospinal fluid (CSF) is constant, and an increase in one of these components should be counterbalanced by a decrease in one or both of the remaining volumes.[4] Brain herniation in TBI occurs when there is an occupying lesion (e.g., intracranial hematoma) causing an increase in ICP, presence of cerebral edema, and subsequent displacement and compression of the brain parenchyma.

Herniation syndromes are classified based on their location as either supratentorial or infratentorial (Figs. 12.1 and 12.2).[3-6]

Supratentorial herniation syndromes include uncal, subfalcine, central transtentorial, and transcalvarial herniation. Infratentorial herniation syndromes include tonsillar and reverse transtentorial herniation.

This chapter will discuss the four main types of herniation associated with TBI: uncal, central transtentorial, subfalcine, and tonsillar herniation.

Uncal Herniation

Uncal herniation is the most common type of cerebral herniation and develops when the medial portion of the temporal lobe (uncus) protrudes downward through the tentorial notch, compressing the midbrain[3,4,6] (Figs. 12.1 and 12.3). At early stages the clinical presentation is mainly ophthalmic, with paralysis of the third cranial nerve (oculomotor nerve) first causing an ipsilateral fixed and dilated pupil that will later progress to complete ptosis and a characteristic "down and out" gaze.[3-5] As herniation continues, the ipsilateral superior cerebral peduncle and posterior cerebral artery become affected, leading to contralateral hemiparesis followed by decerebrate posturing and visual cortex infarction

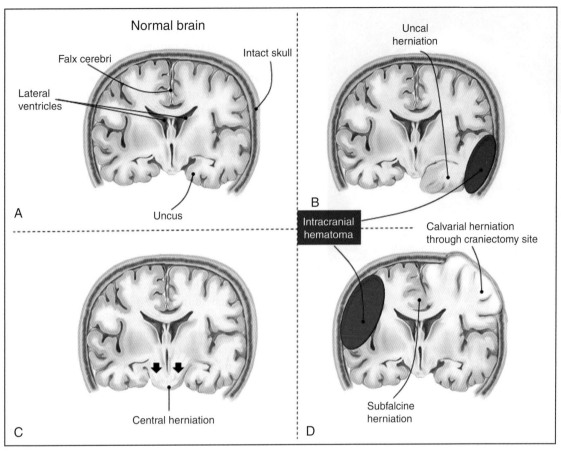

• **Fig. 12.1** **(A)** Schematic representation depicting normal cerebral structures in a coronal plane. **(B)** Left-sided uncal herniation resultant from epidural hematoma. **(C)** Central herniation represented by downward displacement of the diencephalon. **(D)** Subfalcine herniation represented by cingulate gyrus displacement under the falx cerebri and associated transcalvarial herniation through a skull defect.

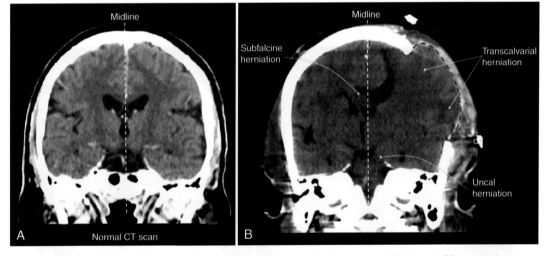

• **Fig. 12.2** **(A)** Coronal computed tomography (CT) image of a normal brain. **(B)** Coronal CT image of a patient who suffered from extensive intracranial bleed and cerebral edema requiring decompressive craniectomy with resultant subfalcine, uncal, and transcalvarial herniations.

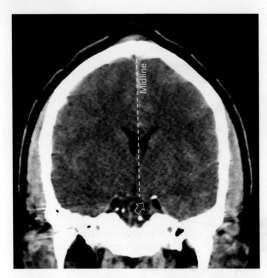

• **Fig. 12.3** Coronal computed tomography image demonstrating left-to-right uncal displacement *(red arrow).*

with subsequent cortical blindness.[4,6] The ascending reticular activating system (ARAS) can also be compromised, and alteration of consciousness will ensue.[5,6]

Central Transtentorial Herniation

When the diencephalon is pushed through the tentorial notch into the foramen magnum, central transtentorial herniation occurs[4] (see Fig. 12.1). This herniation syndrome can concurrently appear with uncal herniation, explaining why some of the early and late clinical signs of both syndromes are fairly similar.[6] In the early stages, central transtentorial herniation (CTH) will present with alteration of consciousness and small reactive pupils.[3,4,6] In

the process of the brainstem being downwardly displaced, the perforating arteries that branch off the basilar artery will stretch and tear, causing the so called *Duret's hemorrhages,*[3,4] seen as linear hyperdensities in the brainstem on computed tomography (CT) scans.[3] Cheyne-Stokes respirations will develop, decorticate posturing will appear, and coma will ensue. If herniation is not reversed, the patient will inevitably progress to the late stage, characterized by decerebrate posturing, fixed and dilated pupils, and respiratory and cardiovascular failure.[3,4]

Subfalcine Herniation

The cingulate gyrus can herniate under the free edge of the falx cerebri when an occupying lesion in one of the cerebral hemispheres begins expanding, giving rise to what is known as *subfalcine herniation*[4] (Figs. 12.1 and 12.4). Ropper et al. have established a direct correlation between the degree of horizontal shift of the pineal gland and the level of consciousness.[7] When there is a pineal gland shift of 6 to 9 cm, stupor appears, and when the shift is greater than 9 mm, it is associated with coma.[7] Progression of the herniation may result in compression of the pericallosal and callosal marginal arteries, medial temporal lobe infarction, and obstructive hydrocephalus caused by compression of the foramen of Monro.[3-5]

Tonsillar Herniation

Tonsillar herniation occurs when the cerebellar tonsils protrude downward through the foramen magnum and can lead to coma, flaccid paralysis, and cardiorespiratory failure caused by compression of the lower medulla[3,4] (Fig. 12.5). This type of herniation carries a high mortality rate.[4,5] The mainstay of treatment for herniation syndromes post-TBI is

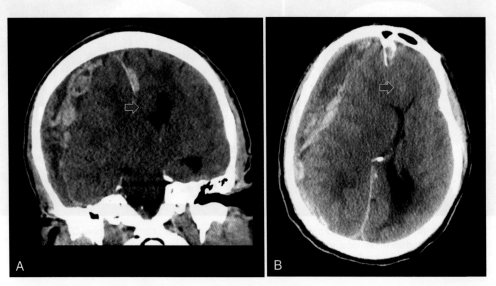

• **Fig. 12.4 (A)** Coronal and **(B)** axial computed tomography image of a patient with a large subdural hematoma with associated subfalcine herniation *(red arrows).*

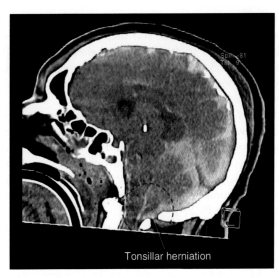

• Fig. 12.5 Sagittal computed tomography image of a patient with cerebellar tonsillar herniation *(red circle)*.

immediate surgical decompression.[6] If clinical signs are rapidly recognized, the chances of a favorable outcome with the appropriate treatment are significantly improved. Herniation secondary to head injury tends to have the worst outcome, and the prognosis depends not solely on the timing of surgery but also on other intracranial and extracranial injuries.[6]

Second-Impact Syndrome

Second-impact syndrome (SIS) is defined as a specific form of cerebral swelling resulting from a second brain injury (usually mild) occurring before symptoms associated with the initial insult have fully resolved.[8-10] The classic scenario is an athlete who sustains a concussion, returns to play before postconcussion symptoms have resolved, sustains a second hit (whether a concussion or a simple tackle that applies acceleration–deceleration forces to the brain), and within 2 to 5 minutes drops to the ground, develops respiratory failure, brain herniation, and catastrophic brainstem compression.[10-12] Possibly one of the most controversial and poorly understood complications of brain injury, SIS can be fatal, resulting in rapid brain herniation within minutes of the second hit and death,[11] making it of vital importance to understand its underlying mechanisms and possible forms of prevention.

This syndrome, mostly seen in athletes and caused by repeated concussions and early return to play (RTP), is hypothesized to be the result of two different mechanisms:

1. Altered metabolism and neuronal cell damage: After a first hit, cerebral protein synthesis is decreased, free radical formation develops, lactic acid starts to build up in the neuronal cells, and extracellular potassium massively increases, subsequently leading to cerebral edema.[9,13,14] At this point the brain has entered a state of hypermetabolism that can last up to 10 days.[9,13] These metabolic changes make the brain more susceptible to a

fatal outcome as a result of subsequent injuries, regardless of their severity.[9,13]
2. Vascular congestion: The brain's vasculature ability to autoregulate after a first TBI is impaired, leading to increased cerebral blood flow, consecutive vascular engorgement, and resultant edema.[8] When a person receives a second hit before symptoms of the first concussion have completely resolved, the brain is still in a state of autoregulatory impairment, and the existing vascular congestion worsens and is further enhanced by trigeminal system dysfunction.[9,11,15] The reason behind the belief that a trigeminal system failure exacerbates cerebral vascular congestion is that when a head trauma occurs, the trigeminal system becomes stimulated, releasing vasoactive peptides such as substance P, neurokinin A, and calcitonin gene-related peptide, which in turn produce vasodilation and increased vascular permeability.[16] The results of these vascular and neurogenic disturbances are increased ICP, uncal and/or tonsillar herniation, and rapidly ensuing brainstem failure.[11]

An important factor affecting the development of SIS is the time elapsed between the first TBI and the second hit. Some authors argue that the second impact must occur within 10 days of the first one, given that the disruption of neuronal metabolism caused by the first concussion is thought to last this long.[13] Other authors believe that the second hit can happen beyond 10 days after the first concussion and still lead to SIS, which is why RTP is recommended until postconcussion symptoms have fully resolved.[10]

The most effective prevention strategy of SIS is delaying RTP until symptoms of the first concussion have fully resolved, despite the time elapsed from onset. Given the findings in animal studies that vascular congestion as a result of mild TBI (mTBI) is often extremely difficult to control, those who sustain the controversial SIS usually have a catastrophic result.

Postconcussion Syndrome

After sustaining a TBI, patients usually report an array of symptoms—some immediate and some late onset—known as *postconcussion symptoms*. These include somatic, cognitive, and/or emotional symptoms, such as headache, dizziness, nausea, memory impairment, fatigue, sleep disturbances, difficulty concentrating, anxiety, irritability, sensitivity to noise and/or light, depression, and cognitive deficits.[17,18] These postconcussion symptoms are usually more prominent in the acute and subacute phases of the TBI and fully resolve within a few weeks to 3 months postinjury.[19] When at least three of those symptoms have not resolved by 3 months, are the result of a TBI, create attention or memory deficits on neuropsychological testing, and result in significant social or occupational functioning impairment, they become part of the persistent postconcussion syndrome (PCS) or postconcussion disorder (PCD), according to the *Diagnostic and Statistical Manual of Mental*

Disorders 4th edition (DSM-IV) criteria.[19,20] Another criterion widely used to diagnose PCS is the one imposed by the *International Classification of Diseases* 10th edition (ICD-10), which requires the syndrome to follow a TBI with at least three of these symptoms: headache; memory impairment; difficulty concentrating; insomnia; intolerance to stress, emotion, or alcohol; fatigue; dizziness; and irritability.[19] A consensus of which criteria to use has yet to be reached, making incidence of PCS difficult to accurately estimate.

Postconcussion symptoms are divided into four domains: somatic, cognitive, sleep, and emotional.[21]

Somatic Symptoms

Headache and dizziness are undoubtedly the most commonly reported somatic symptoms after an mTBI, with headache being reported in up to 85% of patients who have sustained a TBI.[19-21] These symptoms are usually present in the acute phase of the TBI and resolve in the subacute stage, but if PCS develops, their duration may be prolonged.[22]

Posttraumatic headache (PTH) has a peculiar inverse correlation with the severity of brain injury. It has been found that PTH is reported with more frequency after mTBI than in individuals with more severe forms of the injury.[19,23] Tension headache and migraine are also the most common type of headaches reported, with migraine being more common in military blast–associated injuries and tension type in the general population.[19,20,24] Other reported somatic problems are fatigue, sensitivity to noise or light, vertigo, and autonomic nervous system dysfunction.[20]

Cognitive Symptoms

The most common neurocognitive symptoms reported post-TBI are difficulty in executive function, attention deficits, and impairment in memory and information processing speed.[18,19,21] These symptoms are usually resolved by 3 months, and previous studies have found that neuropsychological testing does not accurately correlate with symptom self-report.[19,20]

Emotional Symptoms

The most commonly reported emotional symptoms in PCS are depression, anxiety, irritability, and mood swings.[19,20] Anxiety and irritability usually appear in the acute phase post-TBI, whereas depression tends to appear at later stages.[20] These symptoms usually resolve by 3 months, but some studies have found that around 11% to 17% of TBI survivors meet criteria for a psychiatric disorder[19,20]

Sleep–Wake Disorders

Sleep disturbances have been reported in approximately 30% to 70% of TBI survivors, with insomnia and pleiosomnia being the main complaints followed by circadian rhythm disturbances, parasomnias, and sleep-related breathing disturbances.[25] Some studies have found sleep–wake disorders to persist up to 3 years after a TBI, making this an important late-phase complication of a brain injury that can severely affect the recovery of post-TBI individuals.[25]

There is an ongoing debate surrounding the etiology of PCS and whether it is a result of neuropathologic processes derived from the TBI, preinjury and postinjury physiological and psychogenic factors, or a mix of both.[17,19,26] Female gender, older age, and preinjury psychological problems have been found to be predisposing factors to developing and prolonging PCS.[17,20]

As previously mentioned, most symptoms after a brain injury resolve within 3 months postinjury; therefore, it is of great importance to recognize and diagnose PCS early to start the appropriate management in a prompt manner and prevent further difficulties in the TBI survivor's road to recovery.

Treatment

In general, treatment of PCS is individualized based on the patient's symptoms. Reassurance is often the only intervention needed, because most patients will improve after weeks or a few months. Treatment is usually symptomatic; patients should avoid activities that lead to a possible second concussion while they haven't fully recovered from the initial insult.

Amitriptyline has been used for posttraumatic tensional headache, fatigue, depression, irritability, and insomnia. A trial of propranolol along with amitriptyline may provide relief of refractory PTH.[27] Indomethacin has been reported to be effective as management of paroxysmal posttraumatic hemicrania.[28] Occipital nerve blocks with local anesthetic alone or in combination with steroids are a useful resource for greater occipital neuralgia.[29]

Behavioral treatments are available for sleep–wake disorders. Treatment is aimed toward the dominant symptom or specific sleep disorder and relevant comorbidities. Potential benefits of successful treatment of sleep–wake disorders include improvement in functional outcomes and quality of life.

Current evidence is insufficient to recommend therapies for cognitive and psychological complaints. Donepezil has had promising results in patients with severe TBI, but its effectiveness in PCS remains unclear.[30] When psychological symptoms are particularly prominent, supportive psychotherapy and the use of antidepressant and anxiolytic medications may be helpful.[31] Citalopram and carbamazepine have shown symptomatic improvement in TBI patients with depression.[32]

An extremely important role for the physician is education of the patient and family members, other physicians, and healthcare providers. Many patients are reassured to discover that their symptoms are not unique or unusual but are instead part of a well-known syndrome.

Posttraumatic Epilepsy

Posttraumatic epilepsy (PTE) continues to be one of the most common and disabling complications of TBI, with the particular feature that there is no current effective prophylaxis, and once it develops, seizures tend to be refractory to treatment.[33-36] Seizures after a TBI are fairly common[34] regardless of the severity and have been classified as immediate (happening <24 hours postinjury), early (happening >24 hours but <1 week postinjury), or late (>1 week after injury).[37,38] PTE is defined as the occurrence of at least two unprovoked late-onset seizures associated with TBI.[33] Although antiepileptic drugs (AEDs) are routinely administered post-TBI to prevent posttraumatic seizures (PTS) in the immediate and early stages, there are no data that support the use of prophylactic AED to prevent the development of PTE.[33,35,38]

Studies have shown that the severity of the brain injury directly correlates with the risk of developing PTE,[33] with intracranial hematoma, skull fracture, penetrating brain injury, and loss of consciousness or posttraumatic amnesia lasting greater than 24 hours being the major determinants.[33,38] Age has also been associated with the appearance of late-onset seizures, with younger patients being at higher risk.[34,37]

The mechanism behind posttraumatic seizures is thought to be a combination of persistent neuroinflammation, which has been linked to the development of PTE, and increased neuronal excitability, believed to be the cause of early onset seizures caused by increased hippocampal glutamate excitotoxicity.[33,35]

It is of critical importance to continue developing research methods that will better elucidate the epileptogenic process post-TBI. As with many other complications of brain injury, PTE remains poorly understood, with several promising preclinical model studies aiming to develop the preventive therapy that this brain injury complication so desperately needs.

Chronic Traumatic Encephalopathy

Multiple TBIs have been associated with the development of a neurodegenerative disease called *chronic traumatic encephalopathy* (CTE). CTE is characterized by an array of symptoms encompassing four domains—cognitive, behavioral, memory, and executive function—and specific neuropathologic findings that include the presence of perivascular hyperphosphorylated tau neurofibrillary tangles in neurons and astrocytes in the cortical sulci (pathognomonic postmortem finding), beta-amyloid plaques, and white matter degeneration.[39,40]

CTE has been seen in boxers, soccer players, and military personnel who have been exposed to repetitive brain injuries. The age of onset can vary, ranging from 19 to greater than 65 years, and clinical symptoms usually show approximately 15 years after the exposure to repetitive TBI.[39] Symptoms of this TBI complication are extremely similar to those of PCS, making the clinical recognition of CTE even more challenging.

Stern and colleagues have proposed two different clinical presentations of CTE[41]:

1. Younger age onset (mean age of 35 years): Behavioral symptoms appear first, and cognitive deficits have a late presentation.
2. Older age onset (mean age of 60 years): Cognitive impairment is the first symptom to appear, with behavioral disturbances appearing later in the disease.

This late-phase complication of repetitive TBI, unfortunately, can only be diagnosed by postmortem neuropathology, and there is currently an increased need for the development of a diagnostic tool to aid in its recognition.

Summary

The spectrum of complications of TBI is overwhelmingly broad—ranging from some that are immediate, rapidly fatal, and require an early recognition of clinical signs—to others that can appear late in the course of recovery and disable the patient for the rest of his or her life. There is a need for more research in this subfield of trauma to successfully develop tools that will aid in prevention of such complications and provide the patient with a better opportunity of having a successful recovery.

Review Questions

1. A 46-year-old man presents to the emergency department (ED) after aggravated assault, sustaining multiple blows to the head with a baseball bat and positive loss of consciousness (LOC) of approximately 15 minutes. On examination, his right pupil is 6 mm and nonreactive to light, whereas the left is 3 mm and reactive. He appears obtunded and doesn't follow commands, for which he is intubated emergently for airway protection. On imaging, he is found to have a left frontotemporal–parietal epidural hematoma with midline shift and uncal herniation. Which of these therapies would most likely treat this complication?
   a. Elevate head of bed 30 degrees
   b. Intravenous mannitol
   c. STAT operating room (OR) decompressive craniectomy
   d. Hyperventilation to 25 to 30 mm Hg
2. A 21-year-old unrestrained male driver presents to the ED after a motor vehicle accident in which he was ejected from the car. Computed tomography (CT) scan

of the head shows a large right temporal epidural hematoma, and he undergoes an emergent decompressive hemicraniectomy. An external ventriculostomy device is placed for intracranial pressure monitoring, and he is transported to the neurointensive care unit (NeuroICU) for further management. He remained intubated and sedated on propofol. Three hours later, the patient shows a decerebrate posturing, and on examination, his pupils are fixed and dilated. Repeat CT head scan is performed. What will the scan most likely show?

a. Subfalcine herniation
b. Tonsillar herniation
c. New ischemic areas
d. Central transtentorial herniation and new multiple hemorrhagic areas

3. A 23-year-old college football player sustains a blow to the head during a game and experiences brief LOC of approximately 30 seconds. His coach clears him to go back to the game, and within 3 minutes, the player falls to the ground and becomes unresponsive. On arrival to the ED, the patient is not able to breathe, and pupils are fixed and dilated on examination. He is intubated emergently for airway protection and taken for a CT head scan STAT. The scan shows a large frontotemporal hyperdensity and central transtentorial herniation. Within minutes, the patient as a cardiac arrest, resuscitation efforts are unsuccessful, and he subsequently dies. What relevant medical history will this patient most likely have?

a. Previous recent concussion with persistent postconcussive symptoms
b. Polycystic kidney disease with multiple Berry aneurysms
c. Transient ischemic attack
d. Meningioma

Answers on page 388.
Access the full list of questions and answers online. Available on ExpertConsult.com

References

1. Stocchetti N, Zanier ER. Chronic impact of traumatic brain injury on outcome and quality of life: a narrative review. *Crit Care.* 2016;20(1):1-10.
2. Wilson L, Stewart W, Dams-O'Connor K, et al. The chronic and evolving neurological consequences of traumatic brain injury. *Lancet Neurol.* 2017;16(10):813-825.
3. Kan PKY, Chu MHM, Koo EGY, Chan MTV. Brain herniation. *Complicat Neuroanesthesia.* 2016;3–13.
4. Benson C, Young GB. Herniation syndromes. *Encycl Neurol Sci.* 2014;2:554-556.
5. Young GB. Impaired consciousness and herniation syndromes. *Neurol Clin.* 2011;29(4):765-772.
6. Ponce FA. Brain herniation; surgical management. *Encycl Neurol Sci.* 2014;484-485.
7. Ropper AH. Herniation. *Handb Clin Neurol.* 2008;90:79-98.
8. McCrory PR, Berkovic SF. Second impact syndrome. *Neurology.* 1998;50(3):677-683. doi:10.1212/WNL.50.3.677.
9. McLendon LA, Kralik SF, Grayson PA, Golomb MR. The controversial second impact syndrome: a review of the literature. *Pediatr Neurol.* 2016;62:9-17.
10. Cantu RC. Dysautoregulation/second-impact syndrome with recurrent athletic head injury. *World Neurosurg.* 2016;95:601-602.
11. Cantu RC. Second impact syndrome. *Clin Sports Med.* 1998;17(1):37–44.
12. Cantu RC, Gean AD. Second-impact syndrome and a small subdural hematoma: an uncommon catastrophic result of repetitive head injury with a characteristic imaging appearance. *J Neurotrauma.* 2010;27(9):1557-1564.
13. Bey T, Ostick B. Second impact syndrome. *West J Emerg Med.* 2009;10(1):6-10.
14. McGinn MJ, Povlishock JT. Pathophysiology of Traumatic Brain Injury. Neurosurg *Clin N Am.* 2016;27(4):397-407. doi:10.1016/j.nec.2016.06.002
15. McCrory P. Does second impact syndrome exist? *Clin J Sport Med.* 2001;11(3):144-149.
16. Squier W, Mack J, Green A, Aziz T. The pathophysiology of brain swelling associated with subdural hemorrhage: the role of the trigeminovascular system. *Childs Nerv Syst.* 2012;28(12):2005-2015.
17. Ryan LM, Warden DL. Post concussion syndrome. *Int Rev Psychiatry.* 2003;15(4):310-316.
18. Cristofori I, Levin HS. Traumatic brain injury and cognition. *Handb Clin Neurol.* 2015;128:579-611.
19. Anderson-Barnes VC, Weeks SR, Tsao JW. Mild traumatic brain injury update. *Continuum (Minneap Minn).* 2010;16(6 Traumatic Brain Injury):17-26.
20. Dwyer B, Katz DI. Postconcussion syndrome. *Handb Clin Neurol.* 2018;158:163-178.
21. Bramley H, Hong J, Zacko C, Royer C, Silvis M. Mild traumatic brain injury and post-concussion syndrome: treatment and related sequela for persistent symptomatic disease. *Sports Med Arthrosc Rev.* 2016;24(3):123-129.
22. Baandrup L, Jensen R. Chronic post-traumatic headache—a clinical analysis in relation to the International Headache Classification 2nd Edition. *Cephalalgia.* 2005;25(2):132-138.
23. Couch JR, Bearss C. Chronic daily headache in the posttrauma syndrome: relation to extent of head injury. *Headache.* 2001;41(6):559-564.
24. Vargas BB. Posttraumatic headache in combat soldiers and civilians: what factors influence the expression of tension-type versus migraine headache? *Curr Pain Headache Rep.* 2009;13(6):470-473.
25. Sandsmark DK, Elliott JE, Lim MM. Sleep-wake disturbances after traumatic brain injury: synthesis of human and animal studies. *Sleep.* 2017;40(5).
26. Dikmen S, Machamer J, Temkin N. Mild Traumatic brain injury: longitudinal study of cognition, functional status, and post-traumatic symptoms. *J Neurotrauma.* 2017;34(8):1524-1530.
27. Weiss HD, Stern BJ, Goldberg J. Post-traumatic migraine: chronic migraine precipitated by minor head or neck trauma. *Headache.* 1991;31(7):451-456.
28. Matharu MS, Goadsby PJ. Post-traumatic chronic paroxysmal hemicrania (CPH) with aura. *Neurology.* 2001;23;56(2):273-275.
29. Hecht JS. Occipital nerve blocks in postconcussive headaches: a retrospective review and report of ten patients. *J Head Trauma Rehabil.* 2004;19(1):58-71.
30. Zhang L, Plotkin RC, Wang G, Sandel ME, Lee S. Cholinergic augmentation with donepezil enhances recovery in short-term memory and sustained attention after traumatic brain injury. *Arch Phys Med Rehabil.* 2004;85(7):1050-1055.
31. Silver JM. Effort, exaggeration and malingering after concussion. *J Neurol Neurosurg Psychiatry.* 2012;83(8):836-841.

32. Perino C, Rago R, Cicolini A, Torta R, Monaco F. Mood and behavioural disorders following traumatic brain injury: clinical evaluation and pharmacological management. *Brain Inj*. 2001;15(2):139-148.

33. Lucke-Wold BP, Nguyen L, Turner RC, et al. Traumatic brain injury and epilepsy: underlying mechanisms leading to seizure. *Seizure*. 2015;33:13-23.

34. Wei Chen, Ming-De Li, Gui-Fang Wang, Xia-Feng Yang, Liu L, Meng FG. Risk of post-traumatic epilepsy after severe head injury in patients with at least one seizure. *Neuropsychiatr Dis Treat*. 2017;13:2301-2306.

35. Webster KM, Sun M, Crack P, O'Brien TJ, Shultz SR, Semple BD. Inflammation in epileptogenesis after traumatic brain injury. *J Neuroinflammation*. 2017;14(1):1-17.

36. Gupta PK, Sayed N, Ding K, et al. Subtypes of post-traumatic epilepsy: clinical, electrophysiological, and imaging features. *J Neurotrauma*. 2014;31(16):1439-1443.

37. Qian C, Löppönen P, Tetri S, et al. Immediate, early and late seizures after primary intracerebral hemorrhage. *Epilepsy Res*. 2014;108(4):732-739.

38. Ostergard T, Sweet J, Kusyk D, Herring E, Miller J. Animal models of post-traumatic epilepsy. *J Neurosci Methods*. 2016;272:50-55.

39. McKee AC, Alosco ML, Huber BR. Repetitive head impacts and chronic traumatic encephalopathy. *Neurosurg Clin N orth Am*. 2016;27(4):529-535.

40. McKee AC, Robinson ME. Military-related traumatic brain injury and neurodegeneration. *Alzheimers Dement*. 2014;10(suppl 3):S242-S253.

41. Stern RA, Daneshvar DH, Baugh CM, et al. Clinical presentation of chronic traumatic encephalopathy. *Neurology*. 2013;81(13):1122–1129.

Evaluation and Diagnosis

13

Physical Examination, Signs, and Symptoms

BRIAN IM, MD, AND EMMA NALLY, MD

OUTLINE

The goal of the neurological examination for the physiatrist is to confirm the diagnosis and identify deficits that will affect an individual's function. This enables the development of rehabilitation goals and a timeline for the patient to reach those goals. This is important in educating families and caregivers and for providing training to safely care for the patient upon transition either to home or another facility.

Brain injuries can be diffuse or focal, and the deficits are not always consistent with the neurological injury. Phenomena such as diaschisis can also complicate the clinical picture because it can produce deficits in areas distant from the injury. In addition, brain-injured patients often have complicated neurosurgical and medical courses, and their mental status may fluctuate day to day. Cognitive and/or communication deficits also may limit the efficacy of the interview. It is important to perform serial neurological examinations to identify if there is a new focal neurological deficit that warrants acute

intervention, and if the neurological examination is stable, it can be reassuring to the physiatrist and prompt investigation of a non–brain-injury cause for a change in medical stability.

Glasgow Coma Scale

- The Glasgow Coma Scale (GCS) is the primary initial assessment tool in the field or emergency department.[1]
- The score is based on the best visual, verbal, and motor responses (Table 13.1)[1]
- The scores range from 3 to 15, and a score of 3T is given if the patient is intubated (see Table 13.1).
- Used to define severity of injury
  - Mild: 13 to 15
  - Moderate: 8 to 12
  - Severe: 3 to 8

Mental Status Examination

The mental status examination (MSE) describes the mental state and behaviors of the patient and can help discriminate between mood and thought disorders, such as depression and schizophrenia, and cognitive impairment caused by brain injury.[2] This is important because there is a prevalence of psychiatric disorders after traumatic brain injury (TBI).[3] Socioeconomic and cultural factors and language barriers, including aphasia, can affect the MSE and must be taken into account. The physiatric MSE emphasizes the cognitive examination and level of consciousness.

1. Level of consciousness:
   - Consciousness requires an intact pontine reticular activating system.
   - Lethargic: The patient is easy to arouse but with slowing of speech and movement.
   - Obtunded: The patient is difficult to arouse and once aroused is confused.
   - Stuporous: The patient arouses to pain but with minimal response.

TABLE 13.1	Glasgow Coma Scale	
Function		**Rating**
Eye Opening		
Spontaneous		4
To speech		3
To pain		2
No response		1
Best Motor Response		
Obeys commands		6
Localizes to stimuli		5
Withdraws to pain		4
Flexion response		3
Extensor response		2
No response		1
Verbal Response		
Oriented		5
Confused conversation		4
Inappropriate words		3
Incomprehensible sounds		2
No response		1

Adapted from Braddom R. *Physical Medicine and Rehabilitation*. 4th ed. Philadelphia, PA: Elsevier Saunders; 2011:10.

- In acute settings, the GCS can be used to assess consciousness.
2. Orientation: understanding of one's situation in space and time
   - Includes orientation to person, place, time, and situation
   - Orientation to person is usually intact and if impaired may be suspicious for malingering versus a more severe brain injury
3. Attention: ability to focus and direct one's intellect
   - Can test by asking patient to repeat increasing lengths of numbers forward and backward.
   - The average individual should be able to repeat seven numbers forward and five backward.
4. Memory:
   - Testing memory requires first that the patient is able to register the information you are asking them to remember.
   - Registration: the ability to repeat information immediately
   - Short-term memory: recall of three words after 5 minutes
   - Long term memory: recall past details
     - Example: Name past presidents.

5. Speech:
   - Includes assessment of fluency, repetition, comprehension, naming, writing, reading, prosody, and quality of speech
6. Abstract thinking is the understanding of the meaning of words beyond the literal interpretation.
   - Requires a higher intellectual function
   - Example: How are an apple and orange alike?
     - Abstract answer: both fruit
     - Concrete answer: both round
7. Insight:
   - Awareness of impairment and understanding that treatment might be helpful
   - A lack of insight is associated with decreased employability and community integration after brain injury.[4,5]
8. Judgment:
   - Ability to make measured decisions and reach reasonable conclusions
   - Judgment requires insight into one's situation.
9. Mood and affect:
   - Mood: The patient may be able to describe their mood or the evaluator infers from the interview.
   - Anhedonia may also be observed here, which is a decreased ability to feel pleasure or engage in pleasurable activities.
   - Affect is a description of the current emotional state that is observed by the examiner. It includes type, range, reactivity, and appropriateness.
10. Thought process and content:
    - Thought process includes form of thinking and flow of thought and ranges between goal-directed and disconnected thoughts.[2]
      - Common descriptors include logical, tangential, circumstantial, and closely or loosely associated.
    - Thought content is what the patient is thinking about, for example, if they have obsessions, phobias, or delusions.[2]

Communication

1. Left hemisphere communication disorders:
   - Damage to the dominant hemisphere, which is usually the left hemisphere, typically results in aphasia. This is where the language centers are, such as Broca's and Wernicke's area, and damage to these areas or to any of their communications may result in aphasia[1] (Fig. 13.1).
   - Key components of examination include naming, repetition, comprehension, and fluency (Fig. 13.2).
2. Right hemisphere communication disorders:
   - Characterized by cognitive linguistic deficits and are often accompanied by some level of left-sided neglect, which is a phenomenon in which the patient does not recognize the left side of their body or objects in the left field of vision[1]
   - Highlights the effects that attention, memory, problem solving, and interpretive language have on communication

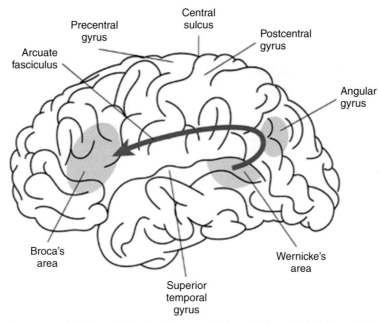

• **Fig. 13.1** Language-related areas in the brain. (From Braddom R. *Physical Medicine and Rehabilitation.* 4th ed. Philadelphia, PA: Elsevier Saunders; 2011:54.)

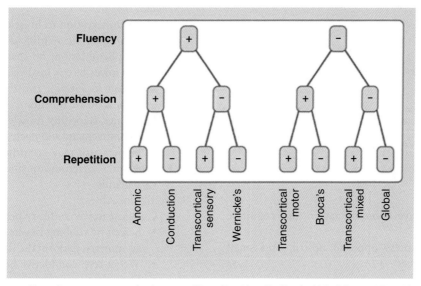

• **Fig. 13.2** Flow chart to assess aphasia types. (From Braddom R. *Physical Medicine and Rehabilitation.* 4th ed. Philadelphia, PA: Elsevier Saunders; 2011:55.)

- The patient may seem socially inappropriate or uninterested in conversation.
- See Table 13.2 for the difference between aphasia (left hemisphere) and right hemisphere communication disorders.
3. Dysarthria:
   - Articulation of speech is impaired with intact content and comprehension.
4. Apraxia of speech:
   - Impairment of oral motor planning in the absence of muscle weakness

- Can be tested by asking the patient to repeat words with increasing number of syllables

Cranial Nerve Examination

1. Olfactory:
   - This is the most commonly injured cranial nerve in mild TBI.[3] It occurs at a higher rate in moderate and severe TBI, but the incidence is difficult to ascertain given the difficulty in examining the nerve in an unresponsive patient and in those who are

<table>
<tr><td colspan="2">TABLE 13.2</td><td>**Comparison Between Aphasia (Left Hemisphere) and Right Hemisphere Communication Deficits**</td></tr>
</table>

Aphasia	Right Hemisphere Disorder
Pure linguistic deficits dominant	Linguistic deficits not dominant
More severe problems in naming, fluency, auditory and comprehension, reading, and writing	Only mild problems
No left-sided neglect	Left-sided neglect
No denial of illness	Denial of illness
Speech generally relevant	Speech often irrelevant, rambling
Generally normal affect	Often lacks affect
Recognizes familiar faces	May not recognize familiar faces
Simplification of drawings	Rotation and left-sided neglect of drawings
No significant prosodic defect	Significant prosodic defect
Appropriate humor	Inappropriate humor
May retell the essence of a story	May retell only nonessential, isolated details
May understand implied meanings	Understands only literal meanings

From Braddom R. *Physical Medicine and Rehabilitation*. 4th ed. Philadelphia, PA: Elsevier Saunders; 2011:58.

conscious but have communication and cognitive impairments.[6]
- Close eyes, compress opposite nostril, and smell common substances
2. Optic:
   - Visual acuity: central vision
   - Ophthalmoscope examination: observe the optic disc, retinal vessels, and fovea.
     - In increased intracranial pressure may see blurring of the optic disc
   - Visual fields: this involves confrontational testing. This can be difficult to do with brain injury patients because cognitive impairments may make it difficult to follow commands for testing.
   - Visual extinction: typically occurs after unilateral brain damage. Patients will be unable to identify two bilateral stimuli presented simultaneously but can identify single stimuli presented in each visual field independently.[7]

3. Oculomotor:
   - The oculomotor nerve innervates all extraocular muscles except superior oblique and lateral rectus.
     - Medial rectus: adducts the eye
     - Superior rectus: elevates the eye
     - Inferior oblique: elevates the eye
     - Inferior rectus: depresses the eye
   - Levator palpebrae: elevates eyelid
   - Pupilloconstrictor muscle: constricts the pupil
   - Ciliary muscle: controls thickness of lens in accommodation
4. Trochlear:
   - Controls the superior oblique muscle: depresses the eye primarily while in adduction
5. Trigeminal:
   - Sensation to face, mucous membranes of nose, mouth, and tongue
     - Consists of three divisions: ophthalmic (V1), maxillary (V2), and mandibular (V3)
     - Test each division with pinprick, light touch, and temperature.
   - Motor muscles of mastication: masseters, pterygoids, and temporalis
6. Abducens:
   - Lateral rectus: abducts the eye
7. Facial:
   - Motor innervation to muscles of facial expression
     - Central lesion: sparing of forehead
     - Peripheral lesion: no sparing of forehead; upper and lower face is involved
   - Sensation to anterior two-thirds of the tongue and external acoustic meatus
   - Innervates stapedius muscle; functions to dampen ossicle movement and decrease volume
     - Hyperacusis may occur in facial nerve palsy
   - Innervates secretomotor fibers to lacrimal and salivary glands
8. Vestibulocochlear:
   - Cochlear nerve: auditory nerve
     - Screen by rubbing fingers near each ear; if there is asymmetry, perform the Rinne and Weber tests.[1,11]
     - Weber test: conductive hearing loss
     - Place the tuning fork on top of the patient's head; it will be louder on the side with conductive hearing loss.
     - Rinne test: air conduction versus bone conduction
     - Place the tuning fork on the mastoid prominence; then place near the ear once the patient can no longer hear it. If the bone conduction is greater than the air conduction, there is a conductive hearing impairment.
     - If there is a sensorineural hearing loss, the vibration is heard substantially longer than usual in the air.
   - Vestibular nerve:
     - Dix-Hallpike maneuver can differentiate between a peripheral or central vestibular dysfunction.

9. Glossopharyngeal:
   - Taste to posterior one-third of tongue; sensation to the pharynx and middle ear[1]
   - Tested together with the vagus nerve by performing the gag reflex
10. Vagus:
    - Innervates the muscles of the larynx and pharynx[1]
      - Damage to this nerve may result in dysphagia.
    - Recurrent laryngeal nerve: Damage can lead to hoarseness.[8]
    - The vagus nerve also supplies parasympathetic fibers.
11. Spinal accessory:
    - Innervates the trapezius and sternocleidomastoid muscles
    - The ipsilateral sternocleidomastoid rotates the head to the contralateral side and brings the ear to ipsilateral shoulder.
12. Hypoglossal:
    - Controls the intrinsic muscles of the tongue
    - Peripheral lesion: Tongue points to side of the lesion.
    - Central lesion: Tongue points away from the lesion.

Cranial Nerve Reflexes

1. Pupillary light reflex[11]:
   - Afferent: optic nerve (cranial nerve [CN] II)
   - Efferent: oculomotor nerve (CN III)
   - Shining light in one eye results in both pupils constricting.
   - Anisocoria up to 1 mm asymmetry is physiological (but it has to be observed in the light and dark).
2. Gag reflex[11]:
   - Afferent: glossopharyngeal nerve (CN IX)
   - Efferent: vagus nerve (CN X)
   - Touching the pharynx with a long Q-tip on both the left and right side should elicit a gag or cough.
3. Corneal reflex[11]:
   - Afferent: trigeminal nerve (V)
   - Efferent: facial nerve (VII)
   - Touching the cornea with a cotton wisp will elicit a blink response in both eyes.

Oculomotor Examination

1. Fixation[12]:
   - Alternately focus on an object 1 m away and then an object 6 m away.
   - Monitor for abnormal eye movements such as nystagmus, which can indicate dysfunction of the vestibular system.
2. Saccadic movements[12]:
   - Voluntary rapid eye movements; patient's gaze fixates alternately on two targets
   - Monitor for saccadic slowing and dysmetria.
   - Saccadic dysmetria occurs with over- or undershooting a target; to a small degree is normal but should decrease with repetitive testing
3. Pursuit movements[12]:
   - Moving an object with the patient's head held still will normally result in smooth movement of the eyes as they track the object.
   - Corrective saccades will be seen if the eyes cannot keep up with the object.
4. Convergence[12]:
   - In the average individual, the location of maximum convergence is approximately 8 to 10 cm.
   - In brain-injured patients, the location of maximum converge is typically longer than this.
5. Opticokinetic nystagmus[12]:
   - This is a normal nystagmus that is elicited by tracking of a movement and is typically performed by observing the patient track a sequence of moving stimuli. A normal response is the eyes tracking the object then rapidly moving in the opposite direction to pick up the next object.
   - When performing this, the examiner should observe regularity, smoothness, and duration of the optokinetic response.
6. Vestibular system[13]:
   - This can be tested by assessing for the vestibulo–ocular reflex. With a normally functioning vestibular system, the patient should have the ability to keep the fovea centered on a target despite movements of the head.

Dysphagia

- Oropharyngeal dysphagia:
  - Commonly a result of weakness or motor apraxia in the muscle of the larynx and pharynx[1]
- Dysphagia can result in aspiration pneumonia, dehydration, and malnutrition.
- Bedside screen for dysphagia:
  - Performed by having the patient drink a small sip of water
  - Observe for any coughing, dyspnea, or change in voice quality.
  - Often misses silent aspiration
- Videofluorographic swallow study (VFSS):
  - The standard of care for assessing dysphagia
  - Observes oral, pharyngeal, and esophageal phases of swallowing and can identify functional or structural abnormalities
- Fiberoptic endoscopic evaluation of swallowing (FEES):
  - Evaluates pharyngeal and laryngeal anatomy and vocal fold function
  - Does not visualize the oral and esophageal phases of swallowing
  - It may be performed if VFSS is contraindicated, if aspiration is still suspected despite normal VFSS, or if vocal cord dysfunction is suspected.

Motor

1. Strength:
   - Manual motor muscle testing[1]:
     - 0: No movement
     - 1: Trace muscle movement is felt when examiner is palpating the muscle
     - 2: Full active range of motion (AROM) with gravity eliminated
     - 3: Full AROM against gravity but not against resistance
     - 4: Full AROM and provides moderate resistance
     - 5: Full AROM and provides maximal resistance
2. Motor apraxia:
   - Impaired motor planning when performing tasks or movements despite understanding of the request or command and without muscular or sensory impairment
3. Involuntary movements
   - This includes tremors, dystonia, myoclonus, choreiform movements, and akathisia.
4. Tone:
   - Spasticity: velocity-dependent involuntary increase in tone; commonly measured using one of two scales:
     A. Modified Ashworth Scale (MAS)[1]
        - See Table 13.3
     B. Modified Tardieu Scale[1]:
        - This is a more objective measurement of spasticity involving measurement of resistance to passive movement at three velocities and at specific positions.
        - Despite being less subjective than the MAS, it is technically more difficult to perform and therefore not routinely performed at the bedside.
        - V1: slowest velocity of the limb
        - V2: speed of the limb falling under gravity
        - V3: speed of the limb moving as fast as possible
        - The degrees of angles at which resistance occurs is measured at each velocity.

TABLE 13.3	The Modified Ashworth Scale
Score	**Description**
0	No increase in muscle tone
1	Slight increase in muscle tone manifested by a catch and release at end range of motion
1+	Slight increase in muscle tone, manifested by a catch followed by minimal resistance throughout the remained of the range of motion
2	More marked increase in tone through most of the range of motion but joint easily moved
3	Considerable increase in muscle tone; passive movement is difficult
4	Affected part is rigid in flexion or extension

From Braddom R. *Physical Medicine and Rehabilitation.* 4th ed. Philadelphia, PA: Elsevier Saunders; 2011:642.

- Rigidity: Tone is constant throughout the entire range of motion regardless of velocity of movement.

Sensation

1. Spinothalamic tract:
   - Rough touch, temperature, and pain sensation
2. Dorsal columns:
   - Fine touch, proprioception, and vibration
3. Dermatomes
   - The spinothalamic tract and dorsal columns should be tested in each dermatome (Fig. 13.3).
4. Extinction:
   - Inability to recognize a stimulus when performed concurrently with a second stimulus[14]
   - Ability to recognize the same stimulus when performed in isolation
5. Graphesthesia:
   - Inability to identify numbers or letters traced on the palm
6. Stereognosis
   - Inability to identify objects placed in the hand[1,11]

Reflexes

1. Superficial:
   - Plantar reflex, abdominal, cremasteric, bulbocavernous, superficial anal reflexes
2. Deep tendon reflexes:
   - Biceps, brachioradialis, triceps, pronator teres, patella, medial hamstrings, Achilles
   - 0 no response, 1+ decreased but present, 2+ usual response, 3+ brisk, 4+ hyperactive
3. Primitive reflexes:
   - Redevelopment of an infantile reflex in an adult
     - Examples: rooting reflex, grasp reflex, palmomental response[1]

Gait

Observe the patient perform these activities:
1. Rise from sitting (timed testing is commonly used)
2. Balance (modified balance error scoring system [mBESS] testing is used in the sports concussion assessment tool [SCAT5])
3. Walking speed (timed testing is commonly used)
4. Stride and step length
5. Tandem gait, heel, and toe walking[1]

Cerebellar Testing

1. Point-to-point movement evaluation:
   - Finger-nose-finger test: over- or underprojecting one's fingers is known as dysmetria
   - Heel-to-shin test: If motor and sensory systems are intact, asymmetry in the heel-to-shin test implies an ipsilateral cerebellar lesion.
2. Rapid alternating movements:
   - Inability to perform rapid alternating movements is known as dysdiadochokinesis.

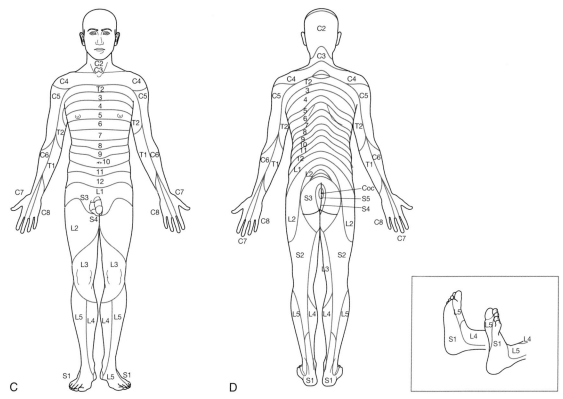

• **Fig. 13.3** A dermatome is supplied by afferent nerve fibers from a single spinal nerve. This figure is a dermatomal map indicating which spinal nerves supply sensation to different areas of the body. Cervical (C2-C8), thoracic (T1-T12), lumbar (L1-L5), and sacral (S1-S5). (From Braddom R. *Physical Medicine and Rehabilitation.* 4th ed. Philadelphia, PA: Elsevier Saunders; 2011:16.)

3. Romberg:
   • This test result is positive if a patient is unable to maintain balance after standing still with their eyes closed but is able to maintain balance with their eyes open.
4. Gait (ataxia) heel, toe, tandem walking:
   • In unilateral cerebellar injury, the patient's gait deviates toward the side of the lesion.
   • Tandem walking detects function of the vermis of the cerebellum.
5. Oculomotor examination:
   • Inability to shift gaze from one target to another with overshooting of the target is ocular dysmetria.[11]

Clinical Signs of Upper Motor Neuron Lesion

• Hypertonia
• Weakness
• Hyperreflexia[1]

Clinical Signs of Lower Motor Neuron Lesion

• Hypotonia
• Weakness
• Hyporeflexia
• Muscle atrophy
• Fasciculations[1]

Examining Patients with Altered Level of Consciousness

The JFK Coma Recovery Scale (CRS) (revised) (Fig. 13.4) can guide assessment:
• The CRS consists of 24 items in six areas addressing auditory, visual, motor, oromotor, communication, and arousal; a higher score indicates improved outcome.
• Identifies minimally conscious patients from those in a vegetative state and monitors emergence from minimally conscious states
• Provides useful prognostication information:
Visual tracking in patients thought to be in a vegetative state correlates with higher rates of recovered consciousness within 12 months of injury than those that do not track.[15]

Agitation

• During recovery from a brain injury, up to 70% of patients exhibit agitation.[16]
• Consistency of reporting is important when assessing agitation and behavioral issues and the efficacy of interventions.
• The agitation behavior scale (ABS) (Fig. 13.5) is an objective assessment of agitation and can be performed serially to assist in determining whether treatments are effective.[17]

JFK COMA RECOVERY SCALE-REVISED
Record Form

Patient:	Date:								
AUDITORY FUNCTION SCALE									
4-Consistent movement to command*									
3-Reproducible movement to command*									
2-Localization to sound									
1-Auditory startle									
0-None									
VISUAL FUNCTION SCALE									
5-Object recognition*									
4-Object localization: Reaching*									
3-Visual pursuit*									
2-Fixation*									
1-Visual startle									
0-None									
MOTOR FUNCTION SCALE									
6-Functional object use†									
5-Automatic motor response*									
4-Object manipulation*									
3-Localization to noxious stimulation*									
2-Flexion withdrawal									
1-Abnormal posturing									
0-None/Flaccid									
OROMOTOR/VERBAL FUNCTION SCALE									
3-Intelligible verbalization*									
2-Vocalization/oral movement									
1-Oral reflexive movement									
0-None									
COMMUNICATION SCALE									
3-Oriented†									
2-Functional: accurate†									
1-Non-functional: Intentional*									
0-None									
AROUSAL SCALE									
3-Attention*									
2-Eye opening w/o stimulation									
1-Eye opening with stimulation									
0-Unarousable									
TOTAL SCORE									

Abbreviation: w/o, without.
*Denotes MCS.
†Denotes emergence from MCS.

• **Fig. 13.4** JFK Coma Recovery Scale revised record form. (From Giacino J, Kalmar K, Whyte J. The JFK Coma Recovery Scale-revised: measurement characteristics and diagnostic utility. *Arch Phys Med Rehabil.* 2004;85[12]:2020-9.)

AGITATED BEHAVIOR SCALE

Patient _____

Observ. environ. _____

Rater/disc. _____

Period of observation:

From: _____ a.m. / p.m. ___/___/___

To: _____ a.m. / p.m. ___/___/___

At the end of the observation period indicate whether the behavior described in each item was present and, if so, to what degree: slight, moderate or extreme. Use the following numerical values and criteria for your ratings.

1 = absent: the behavior is not present.
2 = present to a slight degree: the behavior is present but does not prevent the conduct of other, contextually appropriate behavior. (The individual may redirect spontaneously, or the continuation of the agitated behavior does not disrupt appropriate behavior.)
3 = present to a moderate degree: the individual needs to be redirected from an agitated to an appropriate behavior, but benefits from such cueing.
4 = present to an extreme degree: the individual is not able to engage in appropriate behavior due to the interference of the agitated behavior, even when external cueing or redirection is provided.

DO NOT LEAVE BLANKS.

_____ 1. Short attention span, easy distractibility, inability to concentrate.
_____ 2. Impulsive, impatient, low tolerance for pain or frustration.
_____ 3. Uncooperative, resistant to care, demanding.
_____ 4. Violent and or threatening violence toward people or property.
_____ 5. Explosive and/or unpredictable anger.
_____ 6. Rocking, rubbing, moaning or other self-stimulating behavior.
_____ 7. Pulling at tubes, restraints, etc.
_____ 8. Wandering from treatment areas.
_____ 9. Restlessness, pacing, excessive movement.
_____ 10. Repetitive behaviors, motor and/or verbal.
_____ 11. Rapid, loud or excessive talking.
_____ 12. Sudden changes of mood.
_____ 13. Easily initiated or excessive crying and/or laughter.
_____ 14. Self-abusiveness, physical and/or verbal.

_____ Total Score

• **Fig. 13.5** Agitated Behavior Scale. (From Bogner, J. *The Agitated Behavior Scale.* The Center for Outcome Measurement in Brain Injury; 2000. Available from http://www.tbims.org/combi/abs. Accessed January 19, 2019.)

Review Questions

1. An 87-year-old man sustained a traumatic brain injury 3 weeks ago secondary to a fall that resulted in a right temporal bone fracture and right subdural hematoma. He was treated conservatively and was transferred to your inpatient rehabilitation unit 1 week ago and is now Ranchos Los Amigos Scale V. On morning rounds, you notice he has new right frontalis paralysis and right nasolabial fold flattening. The rest of the physical examination is normal. What is the most likely diagnosis?
a. Acute ischemic stroke
b. Central cranial nerve (CN) VII palsy
c. Lyme disease
d. Peripheralv CN VII palsy

2. You are seeing a patient in your outpatient clinic who was referred for spasticity management. He is 71 years old and had a left ischemic middle cerebral artery infarct 3 months ago, and now he has right spastic hemiplegia. When testing his left forearm extension, you note that there is a slight increase in muscle tone with a catch followed by minimal resistance throughout the remainder of the range of motion. What is his Modified Ashworth Scale score?
a. 1
b. 1+
c. 2
d. 3
e. 4

3. A 76-year-old woman with a right middle cerebral artery infarct is admitted to your inpatient rehabilitation service. On physical examination, you note that she is unable to identify numbers or letters traced into her palm, but she is able to identify objects placed in her hand. She is able to identify sensation correctly when touching both sides of the body at the same time. What is her sensory deficit?
   a. Graphesthesia
   b. Stereognosis
   c. Tactile extinction
   d. Impaired proprioception

Answers on page 388.
Access the full list of questions and answers online. Available on ExpertConsult.com

References

1. Braddom R, ed. *Physical Medicine and Rehabilitation.* 4th ed. Philadelphia, PA: Elsevier Saunders; 2011.
2. Synderman D, Rovner B. Mental status examination in primary care: a review. *Am Fam Physician.* 2009;80(8):809-814.
3. Coello A, Canals AG, Gonzalez JM, Martin JJ. Cranial nerve injury after minor head trauma. *J Neurosurg.* 2010;113(3): 547-555.
4. Sherer M, Bergloff P, Levin E, High WM, Oden KE, Nick TG. Impaired awareness and employment outcome after traumatic brain injury. *J Head Trauma Rehabil.* 1998;13(5):52-61.
5. Ownsworth T, Clare L. The association between awareness deficits and rehabilitation outcome following acquired brain injury. *Clin Psychol Rev.* 2006;26(6):783-795.
6. Zasler N, Katz D, Zafote R. *Brain Injury Medicine.* 2nd ed. New York, NY: Demos Medical Publishing; 2013.
7. Rorden C, Jelson L, Simon-Dack S, Baylis L, Baylis G. Visual extinction: the effect of temporal and spatial bias. *Neuropsychologia.* 2009;47(2):321-329.
8. Garfinkle AM, Danys IR, Nicolle DA, Colohan AR, Brem S. Terson's syndrome: a reversible cause of blindness following subarachnoid hemorrhage. *J Neurosurg.* 1992;76(5):766-771.
9. Amalnath D, Kumar S, Deepanjali S, Dutta TK. Balint syndrome. *Ann Indian Acad Neurol.* 2014;17(1):10-11.
10. Zukic S, Sinanovic O, Zonic L, Hodzic R, Mujagic S, Smajlovic E. Anton's syndrome due to bilateral ischemic occipital lobe strokes. *Case Rep Neurol Med.* 2014;2014:474952.doi:10.1155/2014/474952.
11. Russell S, Triola M. The Precise Neurological Exam. Available at https://informatics.med.nyu.edu/modules/pub/neurosurgery. Accessed January 19, 2019.
12. Walker HK, Hall WD, Hurst JW, eds. Cranial nerves III, IV, and VI: the oculomotor, trochlear, and abducens nerves. In: *Clinical Methods: The History, Physical, and Laboratory Examinations.* 3rd ed. Boston, MA: Butterworths; 1990. Available at https://www.ncbi.nlm.nih.gov/books/NBK406.
13. Kontos A, Deitrick J, Collins M, Mucha A. Review of vestibular and oculomotor screening and concussion rehabilitation. *J Athl Train.* 2017;52(3):256-261.
14. Kluger B, Meador K, Garvan CW, et al. A test of the mechanisms of sensory extinction to simultaneous stimulation. *Neurology.* 2008;70(18):1644-1645.
15. Giacino J, Kalmar K, Whyte J. The JFK Coma Recovery Scale-revised: measurement characteristics and diagnostic utility. *Arch Phys Med Rehabil.* 2004;85(12):2020-2029.
16. Nott MT, Chapparo C, Baguley IJ. Agitation following traumatic brain injury: an Australian sample. *Brain Inj.* 2006;20(11):1175-1182.
17. Bogner J. The agitated behavior scale. The Center for Outcome Measurement in Brain Injury. Available at http://www.tbims.org/combi/abs. Accessed January 19, 2019.

14

Diagnostic Procedures and Electrophysiology

KIRK LERCHER, MD, MBS

OUTLINE

Traumatic brain injury (TBI) is a major cause of morbidity, hospitalization, and disability in the United States. Improvements in high-quality acute care have led to patients surviving longer, even after severe TBI. The emphasis of early intervention includes prevention or mitigation of the effects of secondary injury, mediated by physiological excitotoxicity, inflammation, and neuronal damage that occur after the initial injury. Ongoing efforts to improve our ability to diagnose and classify TBI will give clinicians a tool to prognosticate outcome from a more informed standpoint. Although not standard clinical practice, it is hoped that measures such as cerebrospinal fluid (CSF) analysis, serum biomarkers, functional dynamics such as gait assessment, and electrodiagnostic techniques (quantitative electroencephalography [qEEG] and somatosensory evoked potential [SSEP]) will help provide insight to the etiology of TBI and give the clinician the ability to better understand and predict the trajectory of the patient's overall recovery. The aim of this chapter is to allow the reader to have a better understanding of the current state of research into these diagnostic modalities for TBI and the efforts to improve our understanding of the underlying etiology of TBI and its sequelae.

Diagnostics

Cerebrospinal Fluid Analysis

Secondary injury:
- Follows initial TBI mediated by an inflammatory and excitotoxic cascade leading to further neurological damage and clinical impairments
- Efforts to better understand the mechanism and develop strategies to mitigate its destructive properties are ongoing
- CSF has been used in monitoring inflammatory and cytotoxic mediators

Interleukins (ILs):
- Disruption of the blood-brain barrier after TBI allows infiltration of inflammatory mediators into the brain parenchyma.
- The IL-1 system of proteins have been shown to play an important role in inflammation after a TBI.
  - IL-1B in CSF in patients with severe TBI may have prognostic value and has been shown to be attenuated with hypothermia.[1,2]
  - One study showed IL-1 levels in CSF were elevated in patients with TBI and correlated with worse prognosis.[3]
- IL-8 levels were found to correlate with increased intracranial pressure (ICP) and decreased cerebral perfusion pressure (CPP) in severe TBI and thus is suggested to be predictive of impending secondary injury.[4]

Metabolic:
- Neuronal damage after TBI is mediated by excitatory amino acids such as glutamate.[5]
  - Elevated CSF glutamate levels found in severe TBI, however, are not necessarily correlated with outcome.
- Neuronal recovery after TBI is metabolically demanding.
  - Cerebral damage worsened by an uncoupling of cerebral blood flow with increased energy demand.
  - One study assessed glucose and lactate as a prognostic tool, finding that a low glucose:lactate ratio and high CSF lactate levels may be predictive of poorer outcome.[6]

Neuroproteins

TBI is considered a risk factor for onset of Alzheimer's type dementia with associated abnormal CSF amyloid-B and phosphorylated tau (p-tau).[7]
- Debatable clinical significance of this relationship
- Possible benefit in preventing dementia with targeted immunotherapy
- One study in chronic TBI patients with disorder of consciousness showed differential effect of amyloid-B and p-tau
  - Amyloid-B levels were low, and p-tau levels were normal, suggesting amyloid-B may be a better target of immunotherapy.[7]

CSF neurofilament light (NF-L)chain protein:
- Increased 10-fold at 2 weeks postconcussion and remained elevated at 28 weeks postinjury in a cohort of boxers[8]
  - Subacute axonal injury in absence of overt symptoms, which likely would have cleared the athlete to return to their sport

Serum Analysis

Specific serum biomarkers for TBI with preventative and prognostic value has been of interest given the ease of obtaining a sample, but there has been limited success.
- Few biomarkers have been consistently elevated in the acute phase after TBI.

Glial fibrillary acidic protein (GFAP) and ubiquitin C-terminal hydrolase-L1 (UCH-L1):
- The combination of GFAP, an astroglial biomarker, and UCH-L1, a neuron-specific biomarker, has been found to be elevated early after TBI and helps predict patients who will require neurosurgical intervention.[9]

S100B:
- An astroglial protein sensitive to brain injury but not specific to TBI
- High levels correlated with injury severity and poor outcome[10]
- Normal S100B levels have been correlated with negative intracranial computed tomography findings; helpful in predicting which mild TBI (mTBI) patients may require CT[11]
- Inversely associated with return to work after mTBI[11]

Tau:
- A microtubule-associated protein abundant in neurons and other cells
- Ultrasensitive Quanterix Simoa assay demonstrated acute increase in hockey players after a game than preseason levels[11]
  - Highest levels immediately after a concussion
  - Duration of symptoms correlated with tau levels at 1 hour after concussion
  - Limitations: Assay doesn't distinguish between CNS- and non–CNS-derived tau.

Spectrin N-terminal fragment (SNTF):
- Marker for neurodegeneration prevalent after TBI or cerebral ischemia
- Levels elevated in the serum of patients with severe TBI[11]
  - Elevated levels after mTBI correlate with prolonged cognitive impairments[11]
    - Predicted severity of mTBI and return to play in professional ice hockey players[11]

Gait Analysis

Balance impairments are common after TBI of all severities and are a routine component of the clinical assessment after a concussion.[12]
- Currently, balance assessments are limited to static control of posture.
- Evidence is indicating dynamic balance testing, combining motor tasks with cognitive testing, in a dual task assessment is a better method of detecting more subtle cognitive impairments.

Gait characteristic derangements after a concussion in dual-tasking assessments include[12]:
- Slower walking speed
- Shortened stride length
- Longer period of double-leg stance phase of gait
- Increased medial–lateral displacement of the patient's center of mass (COM)
- Faster velocity of side-to-side movement of the patient's COM

Electrophysiology

Conventional Electroencephalography

Electroencephalography (EEG) was the first clinical diagnostic tool to provide evidence of abnormal brain function after TBI.[11]
- Correlated with functional imaging to provide optimal, noninvasive, monitoring of brain activity
- Portable and inexpensive; appealing diagnostic and prognostic tool
- Common in the acute postinjury critical care setting
- Limitation: need for clinicians skilled in the equipment and software

Nonconvulsive seizures occur in approximately 20% of TBI patients in critical care setting.
- Deleterious impact on neurorecovery and would go undetected without continuous EEG monitoring[11]

Common EEG findings in the early postinjury period after moderate or severe TBI[11]:
- Generalized or focal slowing
- Attenuated posterior alpha
- These findings usually resolve with recovery of consciousness

EEG abnormalities are rare in mTBI and when present are usually associated with loss of consciousness for greater than 2 minutes.[11]
- EEG is not recommended or clinically appropriate for assessment of mTBI.
- EEG-based devices are being marketed as diagnostic tools in the acute setting of mTBI.

- Food and Drug Administration approved only as adjunct tools in the assessment of mTBI.
- EEG abnormalities in mTBI that are noted in the first 24 hours are usually associated with posttraumatic amnesia (PTA) of greater than 30 minutes' duration.
  - Helpful prognostic tool as prolonged and incomplete recovery is more likely in such circumstances[11]
- EEG abnormalities in mTBI are likely to resolve completely within 3 months postinjury.[11]

Factors that can influence the presence and persistence of EEG abnormalities include:
- Early or advanced age
- Comorbid pre- and postinjury conditions:
  - Illicit substance use, anxiety, pain, cooccurring neurological problems, time postinjury, and technical quality[11]

One review showed most studies correlating conventional EEG with TBI were of poor quality and have several methodological limitations, including[13]:
- Inconsistency in clinical case definitions of TBI
- Heterogenous TBI population with various comorbidities
- Inconsistency in time postinjury
- Broad range of recording and data assessment, limiting cross-sectional comparisons
- Confounding effects of psychiatric, neurological, or substance abuse factors

Routine conventional EEG in evaluation of patients with TBI, other than in the neurocritical care setting, is not recommended over a thorough history and physical examination.[11]

Quantitative Electroencephalography

qEEG refers to computer-assisted analysis of EEG data.
- Different methods include comparing frequency and amplitudes of signals to measure differences or changes in connectivity between different areas of the brain that are affected after TBI.[14]

Information can be represented graphically by comparing electrodes in different areas of the scalp, known as *brain electrical activity mapping* (BEAM).

There are typical qEEG findings that are unique to patients with TBI[11]:
- Reduced mean alpha frequency
- Increased theta activity
- Increased theta:alpha ratios

Discriminant functions:
- Refers to statistical functions that were developed by a combination of qEEG findings to probabilistically discriminate individuals with TBI from healthy controls solely with qEEG[11,13]
- Clinical utility is controversial because the discrimination of a patient with TBI from a control is of limited clinical value
- qEEG data rely on information derived from thorough history and physical examination, neuropsychological assessment, and neuroimaging
- May have medico-legal and forensic implications

A qEEG-based TBI severity index was developed to characterize TBI severity retrospectively[14]:
- Overall classification accuracy of 96%
- Retrospectively predicted initial Glasgow Coma Scale score, duration of posttraumatic coma, and post-TBI performance on a broad range of neuropsychological tests
- Further studies to control for confounding variable are needed to validate this measure but is a promising tool with clinical utility

To date available evidence regarding the clinical usefulness of qEEG as a diagnostic tool is low, but it does represent a promising application of electrophysiological techniques to the care and treatment of patients recovering from TBI.

Evoked Potentials

Evoked potentials (EPs) are scalp-recorded responses to external stimuli that reflect automatic preconscious information processing by the nervous system.[11]
- Sensory cortex readings are evident in 1 to 150 ms after stimulus
- Cerebral information processing recordings occur 70 to 500 ms after stimulus

When paired with thorough history, physical, and cognitive evaluation, EPs may help identify neurobiological correlations with sequelae of a TBI and help target treatments.

Short-latency EPs:
- Occur within the first 30 ms of stimulus
- Brainstem auditory, pattern visual, brainstem trigeminal, motor, and somatosensory EPs
- Delayed latency is the most common type of short-latency EP abnormality after mTBI[11]
  - Development of the EP is after stimuli is abnormally delayed
- Somatosensory EPs may be most prognostically useful in severe TBI[11]
  - Assess perseveration of automatic preconscious information processing in patients with disorders of consciousness
  - Controversy regarding utility of their use in clinical decision making

Middle-latency EPs:
- Middle-latency P50 evoked-response abnormalities are associated with impaired auditory processing and correlated with lower hippocampal volumes and may reflect posttraumatic cholinergic deficits.[11]
- Studies have looked at P50 evoked responses to paired auditory stimuli as a means of measuring processing speed among patients with persistent attention and memory impairments after TBI.[11]
- Findings suggest the potential utility of applying EPs to the study of neuropsychiatric symptoms

Long-latency EPs:
- Occur 70 ms or greater after stimulus
- Considered markers of cortically mediated stimulus detection and processing, specifically in cognitive tasks

- Frequently used in the study of cognitive impairments after TBI of all severities[11]
  - Most frequently studied long-latency EPs are auditory mismatch negativity (MMN), auditory N200 (N2), P300 (P300a and P300b), and Contingent Negative Variation, with many used in the study of patients with disorders of consciousness after TBI.[15]
  - Reduced amplitudes or delayed latencies of N2, P300, and CNV have been correlated with reduced processing and attention in mTBI.[16]
  - P300 abnormalities have been used to monitor recovery of function after a TBI because normalization of

these abnormalities correlates with functional recovery after TBI.[11]
- Delayed latency suggests slowed detection of stimuli
- Reduced amplitude suggests inattention
- Exaggerated amplitude suggests distractibility.
  - Possible measure of posttraumatic cholinergic function
  - Reduced amplitude and prolonged latency have been correlated with cholinergic depletion.[11]
  - Abnormalities may normalize with treatment of a cholinesterase inhibitor.[11]

Review Questions

1. Which inflammatory cytokine was found to correlate with increased intracranial pressure (ICP) and decreased cerebral perfusion pressure (CPP) in the acute setting of patients with severe traumatic brain injury (TBI)?
   a. Interleukin (IL)-1
   b. IL-1B
   c. IL-6
   d. IL-8
2. Neurorecovery from TBI is a metabolically demanding process that is believed to be related to a mismatch between cerebral blood flow and metabolic demand. What cerebrospinal fluid (CSF) marker of this metabolic process has been shown to correlate with poorer outcomes after TBI?
   a. High glutamate
   b. Low glucose:lactate ratio

   c. High glucose:lactate ratio
   d. Low lactate
3. Which serum biomarker has been helpful in determining when to obtain a CT after a TBI?
   a. Glial fibrillary acidic protein (GFAP)
   b. S100B
   c. Ubiquitin C-terminal hydrolase-L1 (UCH-L1)
   d. Tau

Answers on page 388.
Access the full list of questions and answers online.
Available on ExpertConsult.com

References

1. Marion DW, Penrod LE, Kelsey SF, et al. Treatment of traumatic brain injury with moderate hypothermia. *N Engl J Med.* 1997;336(8):540-546.
2. Clark RS, Kochanek PM, Chen M, et al. Increases in Bcl-2 and cleavage of caspase-1 and caspase-3 in human brain after head injury. *FASEB J.* 1999;13(8):813-821.
3. Yue Y, Shang C, Dong H, Meng K. Interleukin-1 in cerebrospinal fluid for evaluating the neurological outcome in traumatic brain injury. *Biosci Rep.* 2019;39(4):BSR20181966.
4. Stein DM, Hu PF, Brenner M, et al. Brief episodes of intracranial hypertension and cerebral hypoperfusion are associated with poor functional outcome after severe traumatic brain injury. *J Trauma.* 2011;71(2):364-373.
5. Mazzeo AT, Filippini C, Rosato R, et al. Multivariate projection method to investigate inflammation associated with secondary insults and outcome after human traumatic brain injury: a pilot study. *J Neuroinflammation.* 2016;12(1):157.
6. Lozano A, Franchi F, Seastres RJ, et al. Glucose and lactate concentrations in cerebrospinal fluid after traumatic brain injury. *J Neurosurg Anesthesiol.* 2020;32(2):162-169.
7. Bagnato S, Andriolo M, Boccagni C, Sant'Angelo A, D'Ippolito ME, Galardi G. Dissociation of cerebrospinal fluid amyloid-B and tau levels in patients with prolonged posttraumatic disorders of consciousness. *Brain Inj.* 2018;32(8):1056-1060.
8. Neselius S, Brisby H, Granholm F, Zetterberg H, Blennow K. Monitoring concussion in a knocked-out boxer by CSF biomarker analysis. *Knee Surg Sports Traumatol Arthrosc.* 2015;23(9):2536-2539.
9. Li J, Yu C, Sun Y, Li Y. Serum ubiquitin C-terminal hydrolase L1 as a biomarker for traumatic brain injury: a systematic review and meta-analysis. *Am J Emerg Med.* 2015;33(9):1191-1196.
10. Vos PE, Jacobs B, Andriessen TM, et al. GFAP and S100B are biomarkers of traumatic brain injury: an observational cohort study. *Neurology.* 2010;75(20):1786-1793.
11. Silver JM, McAllister TW, Arciniegas DB. *Textbook of Traumatic Brain Injury.* 3rd ed. Washington, DC: American Psychiatric Association Publishing; 2019.
12. Howell DR, Kirkwood MW, Provance A, Iverson GL, Meehan WP. Using concurrent gait and cognitive assessments to identify impairments after concussion: a narrative review. *Concussion.* 2018;3(1):CNC54.
13. Amyot, F, Aciniegas DB, Brazaitis MP, et al. A review of the effectiveness of neuroimaging modalities in the detection of traumatic brain injury. *J Neurotrauma.* 2015;32(22):1693-1721.
14. Zasler ND, Katz DI, Zafonte RD. *Brain Injury Medicine: Principles and Practice.* 2nd ed. NewYork 2013.
15. Kotchoubey B. Evoked and event-related potentials in disorders of consciousness: a quantitative review. *Conscious Cogn.* 2017;54:155-167.
16. Moore RD, Lepine J, Ellemberg D. The independent influence of concussive and sub-concussive impacts on soccer players' neurophysiological and neuropsychological function. *Int J Psychophysiol.* 2017;112:22-30.

15

Neuroimaging (Structural and Functional)

SAMAN HAZANY, MD, JIMMY C.HUANG, MD, AND ZAID HADDADIN, MD, PhD

Imaging Modalities in Trauma

Radiography

Radiography is not adequately sensitive in the detection of intracranial pathology and doesn't have a role in traumatic brain injury (TBI) (Fig. 15.1).[1,2]

Computed Tomography

Computed tomography (CT) is the imaging modality of choice in acute head trauma for several reasons[1-4]:
- CT is quick and widely available. It can typically be completed in 15 minutes or less.
- CT is highly sensitive for the detection of intra- and extraaxial hemorrhage.
- CT is also superior in the detection of bony details, including fractures of the skull and/or face.[1,3,4]

Magnetic Resonance Imaging

Magnetic resonance imaging (MRI) is inferior to CT in the acute setting for these reasons[1,2]:
- It takes much longer to complete an examination.

- It provides less detailed evaluation of bony structures.
- It's more sensitive to motion artifact.
- It is much more difficult managing sick and potentially crashing patients in an MRI machine compared with a CT scanner.

Primary Effects of Neurotrauma

Extraaxial Hemorrhages

Epidural Hematoma

- On head CT, an epidural hematoma is classically seen as a hyperdense extraaxial collection of blood external to the dura with a biconvex or lentiform shape that does not cross cranial sutures (Fig. 15.2).
- It is typically arterial in origin, and usually the middle meningeal artery is the culprit.[1,2,5]
- It is often associated with skull fracture (90%–95% of the time). When this holds true, the temporal bone is most commonly involved bone (Fig. 15.3).[1,2,5]
- Typically, 30% to 50% have a secondary associated pathology (i.e., mass effect, secondary herniation, contrecoup subdural hematoma, or cerebral contusions).[1]
- Most patients require emergent surgical evacuation. If the size is less than 1 cm with no cerebral edema, some can be managed nonoperatively.[6]

Subdural Hematoma

- Noncontrast CT is the best *initial* study, but MRI is better able to depict extent and age in the nonacute setting.
- On a head CT, a subdural hematoma is seen as an extraaxial collection of blood located between the dura and arachnoid with a crescentic shape that spreads diffusely across cranial convexities, as it can extend across cranial sutures but not dural attachments (Figs. 15.4 and 15.5).
- Findings on brain MRI are variable in appearance secondary to the different appearance of blood on MRI depending on its age (Figs. 15.6 and 15.7).

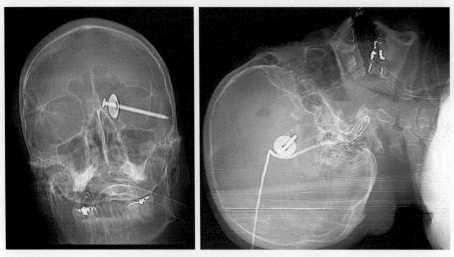

• **Fig. 15.1** Frontal and lateral radiographs of the skull of a 42-year-old male who attempted suicide by shooting a nail gun in his head demonstrate a nail overlying the frontal lobe.

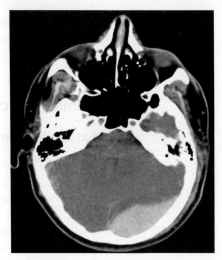

• **Fig. 15.2** Axial noncontrast head computed tomography scan of a 21-year-old man after a motor vehicle accident shows convex hyperintense collection adjacent to the left occipital lobe consistent with an epidural hematoma.

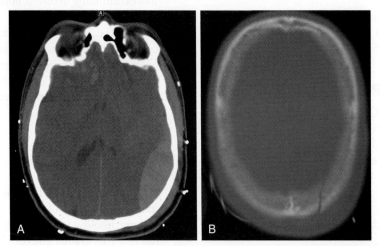

• **Fig. 15.3** **(A)** Axial noncontrast head computed tomography in a 54-year-old man after a high-speed bicycle accident without helmet showing a convex hyperintense collection adjacent to the left occipital lobe consistent with an epidural hematoma. Notice an area of brain parenchymal heterogeneous attenuation with hyperdense and hypodense components within the right orbitofrontal region. This is consistent with contre-coup brain contusion. **(B)** Minimally displaced fracture through the left parietal skull at a more superior cut.

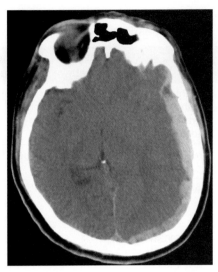

• **Fig. 15.4** Axial noncontrast head computed tomography of a 48-year-old man with headache and no known trauma. The patient was on blood thinners. Concave hyperdense collection along the left cerebral convexity consistent with a subdural hematoma.

Please see Table 15.1 for summary of the appearance of blood products on CT and MRI depending on stage of injury.

• Typically, subdural hemorrhage is secondary to traumatic tearing of bridging cerebral veins. The trauma may be very minor, especially in elderly patients as they are predisposed to tearing secondary to cerebral atrophy.
• Patients with ventricular shunts are at a higher risk because the shunted system does not act as a natural tamponade.[1,7]
• The hematoma can grow slowly with increasing risk for mass effect and herniation if not identified and treated early.[8]

• According to the Brain Trauma Foundation guidelines, patients symptomatic subdural hematomas (SDH) greater than 1 cm in thickness and/or an associated midline shift greater than 5 mm, with decreasing Glasgow Coma Score (GCS) score or showing signs of herniation are treated surgically. Otherwise, patients with av small and/or asymptomatic SDH can be managed nonoperatively.[9]

Subarachnoid Hemorrhage (SAH)

• Trauma is the most common cause. A ruptured aneurysm is the most common nontraumatic cause.[1,2]
• It is thought to be secondary to disruption of small subarachnoid vessels or direct extension into the subarachnoid space.
• Collections of blood can be seen on CT as linear areas within the perisylvian regions, the anteroinferior frontal and temporal sulci, and over the hemispheric convexities.
• Traumatic subarachnoid hemorrhages are commonly seen adjacent to cortical contusions and under acute epidural and subdural hematomas (Fig. 15.8).
• On MRI, the affected cerebrospinal fluid (CSF) spaces with acute subarachnoid hemorrhage will show hyperintense signal on T1 and fluid-attenuated inversion recovery (FLAIR) and hypointense signal on gradient echo (GRE) sequences.
• Clinical presentation of SAH is most often in the form of headache, classically defined as maximal onset and the worst headache of my life. Delayed vasospasm can occur approximately 7 days after onset of SAH and can lead to ischemic symptoms.[1,2,10]
• Supportive therapy is the primary treatment. Oral or intraarterial calcium channel blocker can be given to prevent secondary vasospasm.[1,2,10]

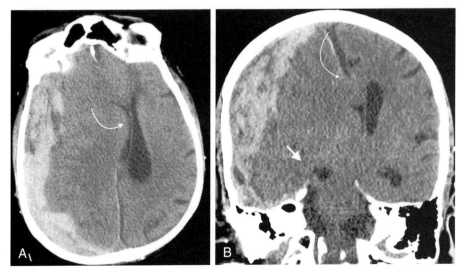

• **Fig. 15.5** Axial **(A)** and coronal **(B)** noncontrast head computed tomography scans of 78-year-old man on Coumadin status post fall with large concave hyperdense collection in the right cerebral convexity with secondary leftward subfalcine herniation *(curved arrow)* and right uncal herniation *(straight arrow)*.

TABLE 15.1	Appearance of stages of hemorrhage on CT and MRI[2]					
Stage	Content	Computed Tomography	T1WI	T2WI	Mass Effect	Time Course
Hyperacute	Oxy-hemoglobin	High density	Mild hyperintensity	High intensity with peripheral low intensity	+++	<6 h
Acute	Deoxy-hemoglobin	High density	Isointense to low intensity	Low intensity	+++	6–72 h
Early Subacute	Intracellular methemoglobin	High density	High intensity	Low intensity	+++/++	<3 days–1 week
Late Subacute	Extracellular methemoglobin	Isodense	High intensity	High intensity with rim of low intensity	±	1–2 weeks to months
Chronic	Hemosiderin	Low density	Low intensity	Low intensity	−	2 weeks–years

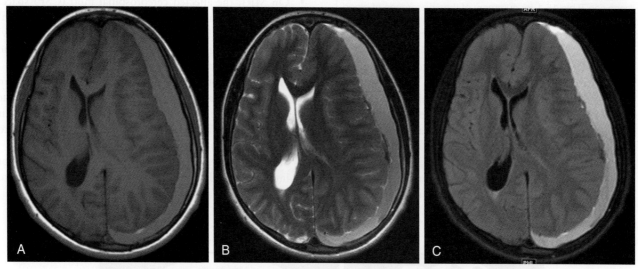

• **Fig. 15.6** **(A)** T1, **(B)** T2, and **(C)** fluid-attenuated inversion recovery (FLAIR) axial noncontrast brain magnetic resonance imaging scans from a 13-year-old male patient who presented with 1-month history of headaches after a fall surfing demonstrate a concave collection along the left cerebral convexity that is hyperintense on T1, T2, and T2-FLAIR weighted images, most consistent with a late subacute subdural hematoma.

Parenchymal Injuries

Cerebral Contusions

- Cerebral contusion is the medical term for a *brain bruise*, which can be hemorrhagic or nonhemorrhagic. It typically involves the gray matter and underlying subcortical white matter.
- The majority of cerebral contusions are secondary to blunt head trauma caused by forceful impact of the cerebrum against the skull surface.[1,11]
- Cerebral contusions are commonly associated with traumatic subarachnoid hemorrhage in the adjacent sulci.

- The most common areas affected are temporal lobes and inferior surfaces of the frontal lobes.[1,2] They are usually multiple, variable in size, and bilateral.
- Contusions 180 degrees opposite the site of a direct impact (coup) are common and called *contrecoup* lesions (Fig. 15.9).
- Petechial hemorrhages with associated surrounding hypodense areas of edema are most common finding on head CT. However, head CT scan of patients with cerebral contusion can commonly appear normal.[1]
- Brain MRI is much more sensitive than CT for detecting cerebral contusions.[1,2]

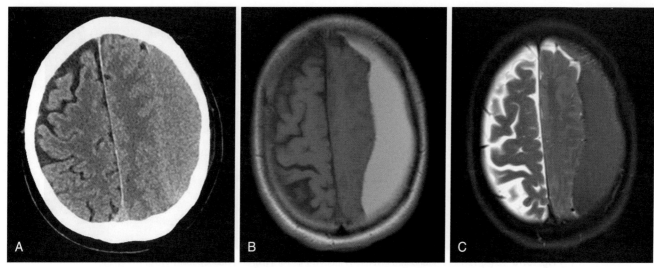

• **Fig. 15.7** Axial noncontrast computed tomography (CT) **(A)**, T1-weighted **(B)**, and T2-weighted **(C)** images of the brain of a 76-year-old man who presented to the emergency department with headache and lower extremity weakness since a fall 2 weeks earlier. Large left cerebral convexity subdural collection is isodense to gray matter on CT, hyperintense (bright) on T1, and hypointense (dark) on T2yw, most compatible with an early subacute subdural hematoma.

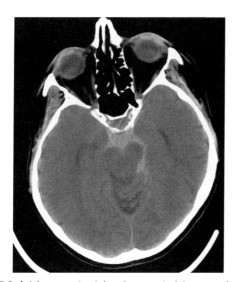

• **Fig. 15.8** Axial noncontrast head computed tomography from a 68-year-old woman after motor vehicle accident with hyperdense attenuation in the interpeduncular and suprasellar cisterns, most consistent with subarachnoid hemorrhage.

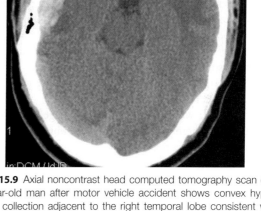

• **Fig. 15.9** Axial noncontrast head computed tomography scan of a 25-year-old man after motor vehicle accident shows convex hyperdense collection adjacent to the right temporal lobe consistent with epidural hematoma (coup injury). Additionally, notice the heterogeneous, predominantly hypodense attenuation within the left temporal lobe compatible with brain contusion and subtle subarachnoid hyperdense blood products (contrecoup injury).

• FLAIR sequence is most sensitive for detecting cortical edema and associated subarachnoid hemorrhage, which appears as hyperintense foci.
• GRE sequence is the most sensitive sequence to detect parenchymal hemorrhages (Fig. 15.10).

Diffuse Axonal Injury

• Diffuse axonal injury (DAI) is caused by axonal shearing secondary to rapid deceleration that exceeds the elastic capacity of the axons.[1,2,12]

• DAI can be subdivided into hemorrhagic and nonhemorrhagic.
• CT is relatively insensitive for detection of DAI and is normal 50% to 80% of the time.[1]
• MRI is much more sensitive for detection of DAI.
    • GRE sequence is most sensitive for hemorrhagic axonal DAI, which shows up as hypointense blooming foci.
    • FLAIR sequence is most sensitive for nonhemorrhagic DAI, which shows up as hyperintense foci.

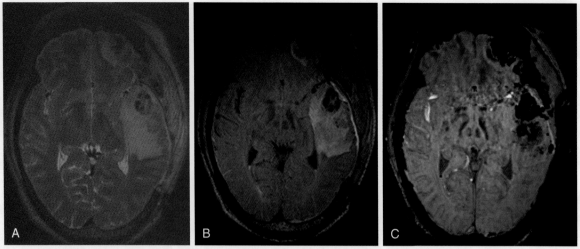

• **Fig. 15.10** T2 **(A)** T2-Fluid Attenuated Inversion Recovery (FLAIR) **(B)**, and Susceptibility Weighted Image (SWI) axial **(C)** noncontrast magnetic resonance imaging scans of the brain from a 56-year-old homeless man who was found down after suspected assault show areas of susceptibility artifact (dark on SWI) and edema (bright on T2 and T2-FLAIR) within the left temporal and frontal lobes and adjacent subarachnoid space compatible with hemorrhagic cerebral contusion and subarachnoid hemorrhage. Also note the postoperative findings of left frontal–parietal–pterional craniectomy and a thin sliver of subdural collection deep to the craniectomy region.

- DAI has historically been classified into grades I to III according to study by Adams et al published in 1989. However, new grading has been published that subdivides the old grade III into stage III and IV depending on if there are lesions in the substantia nigra or mesencephalic tegmentum, as this is a strong predictor of long-term poor outcome.[13]
  - Stage I: axonal damage in white matter of cerebral hemispheres
  - Stage II: white matter axonal damage extending to the corpus callosum
  - Stage III: white matter axonal damage extending to the brainstem but not involving substantia nigra or mesencephalic tegmentum
  - Stage IV: white matter axonal damage extending to the brainstem involving the substantia nigra and/or mesencephalic tegmentum
- It is estimated that 80% of lesions are at the microscopical level and are nonhemorrhagic.[1,12,14]

Diffusion Tensor Imaging

- Diffusion tensor imaging (DTI) is a relatively new MRI technique that takes advantage of the intrinsic property of anisotropic diffusion of water molecules in brain tissues to assess tissue integrity and organization. Because of the highly uniform collinear structure of normal white matter, DTI is uniquely well suited for the assessment of DAI.
- The anatomical orientation of axons, white matter fibers, are color-coded on DTI. Red color signifies transverse orientation, green color signifies anterior–posterior or posterior–anterior orientation, and blue color signifies craniocaudal orientation of fibers.
- Studies in animal models have demonstrated the correlation of DTI findings and TBI pathology. However, these

findings have been harder to demonstrate in human studies.[14-15]
- Recently published review article of the current research on DTI in patients with TBI concluded that DTI is sensitive to a wide range of differences in diffusion metrics but currently lacks the necessary specificity and standardization for meaningful clinical application.[16]
- The utility of DTI in mild TBI remains controversial. DTI findings are more reliable and clinically relevant in setting of moderate to severe TBI, which is often accompanied by abnormalities on structural imaging. In these cases, DTI can demonstrate extent of white matter damage. (Figs. 15.11 and 15.12).

Miscellaneous

Pneumocephalus

- Pneumocephalus is the presence of gas within the intracranial cavity.
- It is most commonly associated with trauma, surgery, and rarely, an infection with a gas-producing organism.[17]
- Although rare, the air can accumulate and cause mass effect on the brain, which is called *tension pneumocephalus*, ultimately leading to rapid neurological deterioration.
- Air can be seen in epidural, subdural, subarachnoid, and intraventricular spaces. The most common location of air is frontal subdural space.[1]
- Air will be extremely hypodense on CT (-1000 HU) and will be seen as a signal void (dark) on MRI (Fig. 15.13).

Penetrating Trauma

- Best imaging modality is a noncontrast head CT preferably accompanied by CT angiogram of the head.[1]

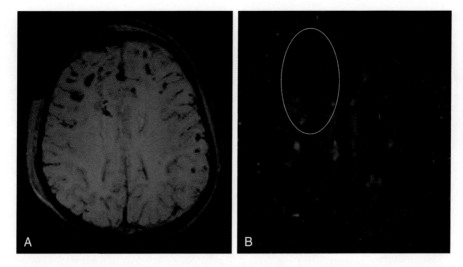

• **Fig. 15.11** Axial SWI **(A)** ND two-dimensional diffusion tractography **(B)** images from a 19-year-old woman after high-speed motor vehicle collision showing multiple bilateral foci of susceptibility artifact (dark/hypointense signal) especially with in the right frontal lobe most compatible with brain parenchymal and subarachnoid blood products and hemorrhagic diffuse axonal injury. Areas of white matter disruption most obvious in the right frontal lobe involving the green fibers (white oval marker) most compatible with posttraumatic axonal injury.

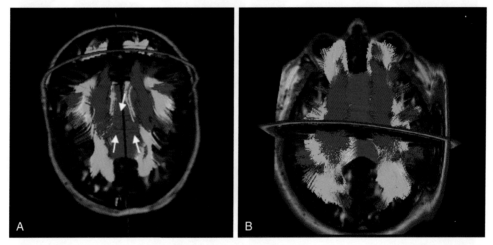

• **Fig. 15.12** **(A)** Three dimensional tractography images in this 54 -year-old status post motor vehicle accident demonstrates subtle apparent transverse bandlike defects in the fibers of the corpus callosum (arrows). Please note that dark anterior-posterior line through the center of corpus callosum represents an overlapping thin sagittal slice that is being views from the superior aspect of the 3 dimensional image. **(B)** three dimensional diffusion tensor images of a normal patient. While these findings can represent white matter injury, they are not specific for traumatic brain injury, especially in absence of structural imaging abnormalities. Other etiologies such as imaging and post-processing technical issues, small vessel ischemic disease, and other potential etiologies of white matter disease have to be considered. (Images courtesy of Dr. Gerald E. York).

- Imaging findings are highly varied and dependent on the mechanism of injury (e.g. size, shape, number, velocity, and course). You will typically see a tract, pneumocephalus, and an entry wound, with or without an exit wound (Figs. 15.14 and 15.15).
- The primary cause of damage is a pressure wave in front of the penetrating object that "crushes" the tissue and creates temporary cavitation.[1]
- The secondary effects of penetrating trauma (e.g., epidural, subdural, and subarachnoid hemorrhage; vascular complications [such as arterial or venous tear, arterial

dissection, occlusion or pseudoaneurysm, and venous thrombosis]; ischemia and infarction; and/or brain herniation) are usually more devastating and often cause severe morbidity and mortality.[1,2]

Abusive Head Trauma

- This is the most common cause of traumatic death in infancy.[1,18]
- The mortality rate is anywhere from 15% to 60%, estimated to be approximately 1200 deaths per year in the United States.[18]

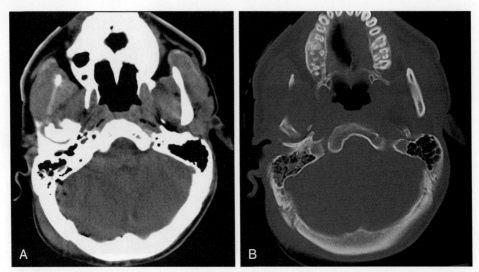

• **Fig. 15.13** Axial noncontrast head computed tomography of a 21-year-old male pedestrian in a pedestrian vs. motor vehicle accident shows **(A)** tiny well-circumscribed hypodense foci of air density within the right occipital convexity most consistent with pneumocephalus. **(B)** Bone window demonstrates minimally displaced fracture through the right occipital skull.

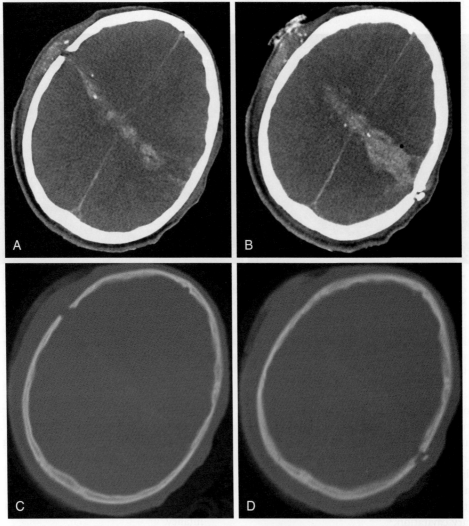

• **Fig. 15.14** Axial noncontrast head computed tomography at sequential levels with brain windows **(A and B)** and bone windows **(C and D)** of a 16-year-old young man after a self-inflicted gunshot wound shows high-velocity penetration injury with site of entrance **(A and C)** and exit **(B and D)**. Brain parenchymal hemorrhage and diffuse cerebral edema are noted. Notice the scattered foci of air consistent with pneumocephalus.

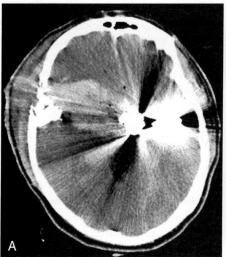
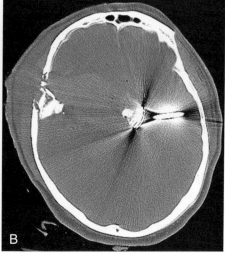

• **Fig. 15.15** Axial brain window **(A)** and bone window **(B)** computed tomography images of the head demonstrate penetrating trauma secondary to a nail gun shot with a nail entering through the right parietal skull and surrounding brain parenchymal, intraventricular, and likely subarachnoid hemorrhage, right to left shift (subfalcine herniation) and diffuse cerebral edema.

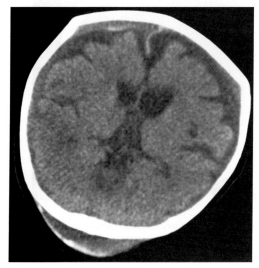

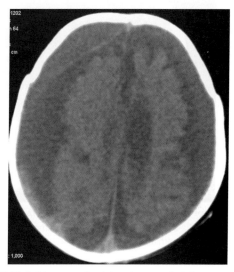

• **Fig. 15.16** Noncontrast head computed tomography scan of an 8-month-old infant who presented with inconsolable crying shows bilateral subacute subdural hematomas, a sliver of more recent/acute blood in the right subdural space (representing blood products of varying ages), and a scalp contusion on the back of the head.

• **Fig. 15.17** Axial noncontrast head computed tomography of a 3-year-old female infant demonstrating chronic bilateral subdural hygromas with layering subacute blood products on the right side.

Secondary Effects of Neurotrauma

Brain Herniation Syndromes

- An important clue that one might be dealing with non-accidental trauma (NAT) is identifying multiple injuries of varying chronicity that are disproportionately severe relative to the given history.
- Subdural hemorrhage is seen in greater than 50% of cases. Subarachnoid hemorrhage is commonly seen but usually is associated with subdural hemorrhage and usually in less than 50% of cases.[1,18]
- Other commonly seen neuroradiological injuries include intraventricular hemorrhage, epidural hemorrhage, shear injuries, cortical contusions, parenchymal brain lacerations, and subdural hygromas (Fig. 15.16 and 15.17).[1,2,18]

- Brain herniation is defined as brain displaced from one compartment into another.
- Trauma is the most common inciting event leading to brain herniation.[1]
- Once the sutures of the skull have fused, there is a very defined volume within the skull for the cerebral blood volume, perfusion, and CSF to coexist. In the case of an intracranial hemorrhage or hematoma, the increase in volume leads to increase in intracranial pressure, which can result in one or more cerebral herniations.

- Many types of herniation are characterized by the area of the brain that is herniating:
  - Subfalcine herniation (Fig. 15.18)
  - Descending transtentorial herniation
  - Second most common cerebral herniation[1,2,19]
    - Can be unilateral or bilateral
  - Unilateral descending transtentorial herniation (also known as *uncal herniation*) occurs when the uncus and hippocampus portions of the temporal lobe are pushed over the edge of the tentorial incisura by an enlarging mass.
    - Bilateral herniation occurs when both temporal lobes are displaced
  - Tonsillar herniation
    - Secondary to enlarging mass in the posterior fossa
    - The cerebellar tonsils are displaced inferiorly into the foramen magnum

- Most common signs/symptoms of brain herniation include focal neurological deficit (e.g., contralateral hemiparesis, ipsilateral pupil cranial nerve III palsy, and ipsilateral hemiplegia) and decreased mental status.[1,2,19,20]
- Treatment includes identifying and treating the primary cause of the elevated intracranial pressure and/or decompressive craniectomy.

Vascular Complications

- They are most commonly seen in penetrating injuries but can be seen in the setting of nonpenetrating injuries and blunt trauma, especially when there is a skull base fracture.
- Complications include arterial tear, dissection, pseudoaneurysm, occlusion, venous tear or thrombosis, and arteriovenous fistula such as carotid-cavernous fistula (Figs. 15.19 and 15.20).

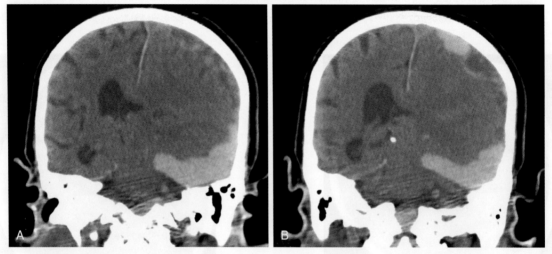

• **Fig. 15.18** Two coronal slices (**A** and **B**) of a noncontrast head computed tomography scans from a 76-year-old man after a fall demonstrating large subdural hematoma with secondary subfalcine and uncal herniation.

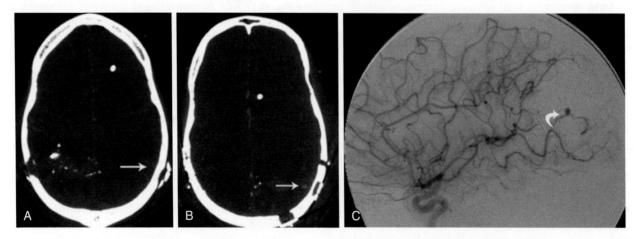

• **Fig. 15.19** Angiographic images in a 28-year-old man after penetrating gunshot injury. (**A**) Normal axial computed tomography angiography (CTA) image with exit wound over the left parietal region *(arrow)*. (**B**) Follow-up CTA image on day 3 demonstrating an interval development of pseudoaneurysm terminal internal carotid artery (TICA) arising from the peripheral branch of the left middle cerebral artery (MCA) at the wound exit site *(arrow)*. (**C**) Sagittal DSA images confirm the CTA findings with TICA *(arrow)*.[21]

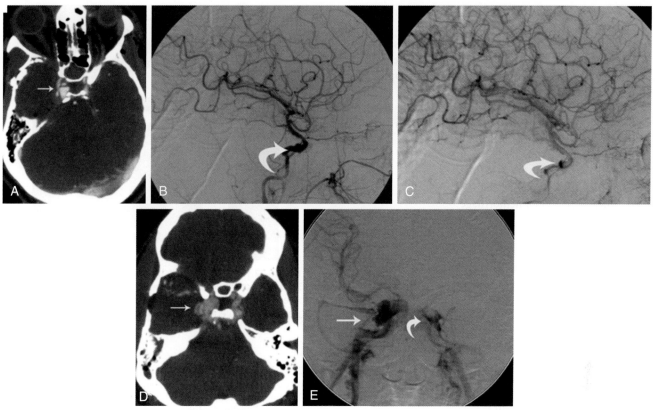

• **Fig. 15.20** Angiographic images in a 36-year-old woman after penetrating gunshot injury. **(A)** Initial axial computed tomography angiography (CTA) image demonstrating a 6-mm terminal internal carotid artery (TICA) pseudoaneurysm arising from the right ICA *(arrow)*. **(B,C)** Sagittal digital subtraction angiography (DSA) images confirming the CTA findings of TICA *(arrow)*. **(D)** Follow-up CTA image on day 10 demonstrating an interval development of carotid–cavernous fistula caused by aneurysmal rupture *(arrow)*. **(E)** Coronal digital subtraction angiography (DSA) image confirming the CTA findings with carotid–cavernous fistula *(straight arrow)* and contrast opacification of the contralateral cavernous sinus *(curved arrow)*.[21]

Review Questions

1. A 78-year-old man with history of multiple prior falls is brought in to the local emergency department (ED) from his care facility because his caretaker noticed his altered mental status. What would be the imaging modality of choice for evaluating this patient's head/brain for underlying pathology?
   a. Skull radiography
   b. Brain magnetic resonance imaging (MRI)
   c. Head computed tomography (CT)
   d. Further imaging is not needed
2. A head CT was obtained for the patient in the previous question. What type of head injury is seen in Fig. 15.21, and what space does this injury involve?
   a. Epidural, extraaxial
   b. Epidural, intraaxial
   c. Subdural, extraaxial
   d. Subdural, intraaxial
   e. Subarachnoid, extraaxial
   f. Subarachnoid, intraaxial

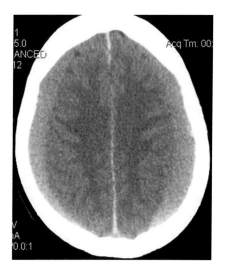

• **Fig. 15.21** Axial noncontrast head computed tomography of a 70-year-old woman with altered mental status demonstrating iso- to hyperdense concave fluid collections bilaterally most consistent with subacute subdural hematomas.

3. A 22-year-old man is brought to the ED after a motor-cycle accident. The patient states he briefly lost consciousness at the time of the accident but was alert and oriented within minutes and able to converse with the emergency medical services (EMS) crew appropriately at the scene. However, en route to the ED, the patient is starting to become more confused and less alert. His head CT is displayed in Fig. 15.22. What is the most likely diagnosis?
   a. Epidural hematoma
   b. Subdural hematoma
   c. Subarachnoid hemorrhage
   d. Intraparenchymal hemorrhage

Answers on page 389.
Access the full list of questions and answers online.
Available on ExpertConsult.com

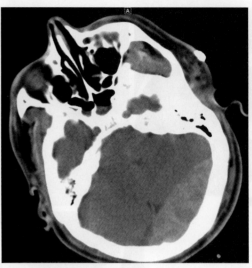

• **Fig. 15.22** Axial noncontrast head computed tomography of an 18-year-old patient after a high-speed skateboarding accident with a convex hyperdense collection in the right posterior convexity most consistent with an epidural hematoma.

References

1. Osborn A, Hedlund G, Salzman K. *Osborn's Brain*. 2nd ed. Philadelphia PA: Elsevier; 2017.
2. Nadgir R, Yousem D. *Neuroradiology*. 4th ed. Philadelphia PA: Elsevier; 2016.
3. Lolli V, Pezzullo M, Delpierre I, Sadeghi N. MDCT imaging of traumatic brain injury. *Br J Radiol*. 2016;89(1061): 20150849.
4. Bodanapally UK, Sours C, Zhuo J, Shanmuganathan K. Imaging of traumatic brain injury. *Radiol Clin North Am*. 2015;53(4): 695-715.
5. Peres C, Caldas J, Puglia P, et al. Endovascular management of acute epidural hematomas: clinical experience with 80 cases. *J Neurosurg*. 2018;128(4):1044-1050.
6. Basamh M, Robert A, Lamoureux J, Saluja RS, Marcoux J. Epidural hematoma treated conservatively: when to expect the worst. *Can J Neurol Sci*. 2015;43(1):74-81.
7. Cepeda S, Gómez PA, Castaño-Leon AM, Martínez-Pérez R, Munarriz PM, Lagares A. Traumatic intracerebral hemorrhage: risk factors associated with progression. *J Neurotrauma*. 2015;32(16):1246-1253.
8. Vega RA, Valadka AB. Natural history of acute subdural hematoma. *Neurosurg Clin North Am*. 2017;28(2):247-255.
9. Bajsarowicz P, Prakash I, Lamoureux J, et al. Nonsurgical acute traumatic subdural hematoma: what is the risk? *J Neurosurg*. 2015;123(5):1176-1183.
10. Harders A, Kakarieka A, Braakman R. Traumatic subarachnoid hemorrhage and its treatment with nimodipine. *J Neurosurg*. 1996;85(1):82-89.
11. Graham D, Adams J, Nicoll J, Maxwell W, Gennarelli T. The nature, distribution and causes of traumatic brain injury. *Brain Pathol*. 1995;5(4):397-406.
12. Davceva N, Sivevski A, Basheska N. Traumatic axonal injury, a clinical-pathological correlation. *J Forensic Leg Med*. 2017;48:35-40.
13. Abu Hamdeh S, Marklund N, Lannsjö M, et al. Extended anatomical grading in diffuse axonal injury using MRI: hemorrhagic lesions in the substantia nigra and mesencephalic tegmentum indicate poor long-term outcome. *J Neurotrauma*. 2017;34(2): 341-352.
14. Zhao W, Ford JC, Flashman LA, McAllister TW, Ji S. White matter injury susceptibility via fiber strain evaluation using whole-brain tractography. *J Neurotrauma*. 2016;33(20):1834-1847.
15. Eierud C, Craddock RC, Fletcher S, et al. Neuroimaging after mild traumatic brain injury: review and meta-analysis. *NeuroImage Clin*. 2014;4:283-294.
16. Asken B, DeKosky S, Clugston J, Jaffee M, Bauer R. Diffusion tensor imaging (DTI) findings in adult civilian, military, and sport-related mild traumatic brain injury (mTBI): a systematic critical review. *Brain Imaging Behav*. 2017;12(2):585-612.
17. Dabdoub C, Salas G, Silveira E, Dabdoub C. Review of the management of pneumocephalus. *Surg Neurol Int*. 2015;6(1):155.
18. Greeley C. Abusive head trauma: a review of the evidence base. *AJR Am J Roentgenol*. 2015;204(5):967-973.
19. Young G. Impaired consciousness and herniation syndromes. *Neurol Clin*. 2011;29(4):765-772.
20. Currie S, Saleem N, Straiton J, Macmullen-Price J, Warren D, Craven I. Imaging assessment of traumatic brain injury. *Postgrad Med J*. 2015;92(1083):41-50.
21. Bodanapally U, Shanmuganathan K, Boscak AR, et al. Vascular complications of penetrating brain injury: comparison of helical CT angiography and conventional angiography. *J Neurosurg*. 2014;121:1275-1283.

16
Functional Evaluation

DANIEL W. KLYCE, PHD, ABPP, RONALD T. SEEL, PHD, AND RICHARD D. KUNZ, MD

Clinical Measurement

Clinical measurement is an important component of treatment during recovery from brain injury. As a means of assessment, clinical measurement may involve the use of various screening tools, rating scales, or standardized tests. The use of these measures among interprofessional rehabilitation providers can facilitate efficient communication, the selection of targets for intervention, and tracking outcomes.

Some measures are better than others, and selecting an appropriate measure for use in practice or research requires familiarity with properties that characterize the utility of a measurement tool. Screening tools used in differential diagnosis may be characterized by their sensitivity to detect a condition and specificity to rule out another condition. The reliability of a rating scale can refer to how well the items work together to measure a construct, the agreement among different providers using the same scale, and the consistency of the scale's performance over time. The validity of a measure describes how well a measure assesses the condition that it purports to measure, how logically the items of a measure relate to its target, and how relatable the measure is to the everyday lives of individuals with brain injury. A brief list of measurement terms and definitions may be found in Table 16.1.

Evaluation of functional status depends on the properties of the measurement tool, appropriate use of the measure, and interpretation of the results. Standardized tests are developed under specific conditions that must be replicated or approximated when administered in clinical practice or research

settings to ensure valid assessment. Normed measures are interpreted after comparing the results of a test to reference groups based on variables such as age, ethnicity, sex, or education level. In general, the results of any test should be interpreted in the context of potentially confounding situational factors such as fatigue, discomfort, emotional state, effects of medication, effort, and sensitivity to evaluation potential.

Domains of Functional Assessment

Global Outcome

Disability Rating Scale

The Disability Rating Scale (DRS)[1] is an eight-item measure that assesses general functional changes through recovery. It

TABLE 16.1	Definition of Measurement Terms
Measurement Term	**Definition**
Diagnostic Likelihood	
Sensitivity	True positive rate
Specificity	True negative rate
Positive predictive value	Probability of diagnosis based on positive screen
Negative predictive value	Probability of no diagnosis based on negative screen
Reliability	
Internal consistency	How well items work together to measure a purported construct
Interrater reliability	Agreement among different raters using the same measure
Test–retest reliability	Stability in measurement using the same test over time
Validity	
Construct validity	How well measure assesses what it purports to measure
Content validity	How logically the items relate to the construct being measured
Ecological validity	How relatable a measure is to everyday life

is commonly used in inpatient rehabilitation settings and can be used to track recovery over time into the community. Admission and discharge DRS scores from inpatient rehabilitation predictive of long-term employment outcomes.

The total scale score may range from 0 to 29, with higher scores indicating greater levels of disability. Item content includes:

- Three items modified from the Glasgow Coma Scale (GCS) (eye opening, communication ability, and motor control)
- Three items measuring cognitive ability relate to feeding, toileting, and grooming
- One global level of functioning item measuring degree of functional independence
- One employability item measuring degree of restrictions on work or school

Glasgow Outcome Scale

The Glasgow Outcome Scale (GOS)[2] is considered the "gold standard" in outcome studies. The GOS categorizes a survivor's function into one of five classifications of function:

- Dead
- Vegetative (unable to interact with the environment)
- Severe disability (able to follow commands but unable to live independently)
- Moderate disability (able to live independently but not return to work or school)
- Good recovery (able to return to work or school)

To allow for additional specificity regarding level of function, an extension of the GOS, the Glasgow Outcome Scale-Extended (GOS-E)[3] split the good recovery, moderate disability, and severe disability categories (e.g., "upper" and "lower" moderate disability) to create a total of eight categories of functioning. The GOS-E is more sensitive to change among individuals with less severe injuries and is administered as a structured interview to increase reliability and consistency.

Adaptive and Daily Living Skills

Functional Independence Measure

The Functional Independence Measure (FIM)[4] is an 18-item instrument assessing level of independent functioning on various physical and cognitive tasks:

- Physical items relate to tasks such as ambulation, toileting, transfers, continence, and grooming.
- Cognitive items relate to problem solving, communication, memory, and social interaction.
- Performance on each item is rated at a level of 7 (complete independence), 6 (modified independence), 5 (supervision), 4 (minimum assistance), 3 (moderate assistance), 2 (maximum assistance), or 1 (total dependence).

The FIM is commonly used in inpatient or subacute rehabilitation centers to assess progress toward functional goals or to communicate to families or other treatment staff the level of care a survivor may require. Accrediting bodies

and third-party payers review FIM scores to determine program effectiveness. Given the FIM's focus on basic activities of daily living (ADLs), its usefulness often diminishes as individuals transition into the community and make further progress in recovery.

Continuity Assessment Record and Evaluation Tool

The Improving Medicare Post-Acute Care Transformation Act of 2014 (IMPACT Act) required that facilities offering rehabilitation services collect and submit standardized data elements to the Centers for Medicare & Medicaid Services (CMS). The rationale for this standardization effort was to improve continuity, outcomes, affordability, and communication among long-term care hospitals (LTCHs), inpatient rehabilitation facilities (IRFs), skilled nursing facilities (SNFs), and home health agencies (HHAs).

- The Continuity Assessment Record and Evaluation (CARE) Tool item set was developed through comparison of its performance to the FIM.
- Items are organized by self-care, functional mobility, and supplemental functional abilities.
- Items are scored as 6 (independent with or without a device), 5 (setup or cleanup with assistance), 4 (supervision or touching assistance), 3 (partial/moderate assistance), 2 (substantial/maximal assistance), and 1 (dependent).

Mayo-Portland Adaptability Inventory–4th Revision

The Mayo-Portland Adaptability Inventory–4th Revision (MPAI-4)[5] is a 35-item instrument that assesses a broad range of brain injury sequelae across three domains of functioning, including an Ability Index, Adjustment Index, and Participation Index.

- Ability Index measures motor functioning, dexterity, speech and communication, sensory issues, and cognitive abilities.
- Adjustment Index measures mood, anxiety, somatic concerns, self-awareness, social cognition, and social functioning.
- Participation Index measures social contacts, leisure and recreational activities, self-care abilities, productivity, and other instrumental ADLs.

The measure may be self-rated or rated by a significant other, a professional provider, or by team consensus. Response options range from 0 (no impairment or normal functioning) to 4 (moderate to severe impairment or interference with normal functioning). The measure may be used with children or adolescents, with the degree of impairment rated based on developmentally normative expectations for an individual's abilities.

Behavioral Functioning

Rancho Level of Cognitive Function Scale

The Rancho Level of Cognitive Function Scale (LCFS)[6] scale is designed to measure cognitive and behavioral function as

individuals with brain injury emerge from coma. An individual's presentation is categorized as:
- Level I: nonresponsive (unresponsive to all stimuli)
- Level II: generalized responses (inconsistent, nonpurposeful responses)
- Level III: localized responses (inconsistent response directly related to stimulus)
- Level IV: confused and agitated
- Level V: confused, inappropriate, and nonagitated
- Level VI: confused, appropriate, with deficits in memory
- Level VII: automatic, appropriate, with deficits in judgment and insight
- Level VIII: purposeful and appropriate, although occasionally requiring supervision
- Level IX: purposeful and appropriate, standby assistance needed upon request
- Level X: purposeful and appropriate with modified independence

The Rancho scale is commonly used in inpatient or subacute rehabilitation centers to guide treatment and behavioral interventions for patients who may be confused, disruptive, or otherwise unable to participate effectively in care. As such, it is effective at communicating a general impression of presentation but may not capture subtle changes over time.

Agitated Behavior Scale

The Agitated Behavior Scale (ABS)[7] is a 14-item measure that assesses behavioral symptoms of agitation after brain injury. Agitation is operationalized as an excess of behavior that occurs during an altered state of consciousness. Response options for each item range from 1 (not present) to 4 (present to an extreme degree). The items of the ABS span three subscales, including (1) disinhibition, (2) aggression, and (3) lability.
- Disinhibition assesses behaviors such as a short attention span, impulsivity, self-stimulation, restlessness, and pulling at tubes or restraints.
- Aggression assesses behaviors such as resistance to care, explosive anger, threatening behaviors, and self-abusiveness.
- Lability assesses behaviors such as excessive talking, sudden changes in mood, and easily initiated crying or laughing.

The ABS is a helpful, objective measure of agitation or behavioral dyscontrol that can be used across the continuum of recovery.

Neuropsychiatric and Psychological Status

Patient Health Questionnaire–9

The Patient Health Questionnaire–9 (PHQ-9)[8] is a nine-item measure that assesses symptoms of depression. Item content is based on the *Diagnostic and Statistical Manual of Mental Disorders* (DSM) criteria for an episode of depressed mood:
- Items related to anhedonia, sadness, guilt, suicidal ideation, sleep, fatigue, appetite, concentration, and psychomotor agitation/retardation

- Respondents rate how much they have been bothered by each symptom over the past 2 weeks
- Response options include 0 (not at all), 1 (several days), 2 (more than half the days), and 3 (nearly every day)
- A total score is derived by summing the responses to each item
- Total scores of 15 or greater indicate treatment for depression is most likely warranted

The PHQ-9 has been validated for use among individuals with brain injury. The recommended criterion for a positive depression screen among individual with TBI is at least five items endorsed at the level of 2 (more than half the days), one of which should be anhedonia or depressed mood item.

Neurobehavioral Symptom Inventory

The Neurobehavioral Symptom Inventory (NSI)[9] is a 22-item measure that assesses postconcussive symptoms.
- Respondents rate how much they have been disturbed by symptoms over the past 2 weeks.
- Response options include 0 (none/rarely present/not a problem), 1 (mild/occasionally present/not disruptive), 2 (moderate/often present/occasionally disruptive), 3 (severe/frequently present/frequently disruptive), and 4 (very severe/almost always present/cannot function without help).

Items content spans four domains, including physical, cognitive, affective, and sensory or vestibular symptoms. Raw scores are calculated for each of the four domains and to create a total score.

Recovery of Consciousness/Memory Recovery

Orientation Log

The Orientation Log (O-Log)[10] is a 10-item measure assessing temporal, spatial, and situation orientation. Responses to orientation prompts are scored based on whether:
- The spontaneous response is correct (3),
- The response is correct after providing a logical cue (2),
- The correct response is identified among three choices (1), or
- No correct/appropriate response is given (0).

A total score is derived by summing the 10 items for a possible range of 0 to 30. Serial administration of the O-Log is used to estimate emergence from posttraumatic amnesia (PTA), and administration is discontinued after obtaining two consecutive scores greater than or equal to 25/30, separated by at least 24 hours but not more than 72 hours. The day of the first score greater than or equal to 25/30 that satisfies the discontinuation criterion is used to denote the date of emergence from PTA. A modified O-Log can be used to assess orientation among individuals with barriers to communication by providing written multiple-choice options for each item. In this paradigm, items are scored dichotomously (correct or not), and a cut-off of 8 of 10 is used to satisfy the discontinuation criterion.

Coma Recovery Scale–Revised

The Coma Recovery Scale–Revised (CRS-R)[11] is a bedside assessment tool for differentiating levels of consciousness.
- Composed of six subscales: auditory, visual, motor, oromotor/verbal, communication, and arousal
- 23 dichotomously scored items
- Items summed to create total score identifying ascending levels of conscious behavior or ability

Combination of items can be used to differentiate vegetative state, minimally conscious state, and emergence from coma based on Multi-Society Task Force and Aspen Workgroup criteria. An American Congress of Rehabilitation Medicine practice parameter recommends use of the CRS-R based on its standardized administration and scoring procedures, item content, and interrater and test–retest reliability.

Social Role Participation and Social Competence

Participation Assessment With Recombined Tools–Objective-17

The Participation Assessment with Recombined Tools–Objective–17 (PART-O-17)[12] is a 17-item measure used to assess social participation. The items assess functioning across three domains, including:
- Productivity (e.g., participation in work, school, or homemaking)
- Social relations (e.g., interactions with friends, family, supportive others, and partners)
- Going out and about (e.g., dining out, shopping, entertainment, religious activities)

Each item is scored on a scale of 0 to 5, with each response option corresponding to time spent engaged in each activity, either based on frequency of occurrence or duration of time throughout the week or month. The items can be combined to create domain scores and total scores (either averaged or balanced). Standard scores are calculated based on reference groups.

Craig Hospital Inventory of Environmental Factors

The Craig Hospital Inventory of Environmental Factors (CHIEF)[13] is a 25-item measure used to assess environmental barriers to social role fulfilment encountered by people with disabilities. The environmental barriers described by the items span five domains, including:
- Policies (e.g., barriers related to government, business, or education/employment policies)
- Physical/structural (e.g., barriers related to the natural or designed environment)
- Work/school (e.g., barriers related to attitudes, help, and support in education or employment settings)
- Attitudes/support (e.g., barriers related to discrimination, community values or beliefs)
- Services/assistance (e.g., access to transportation, medical care, information, community services, or equipment)

For each item, respondents are asked to reflect over the past year and rate how frequently the barrier was encountered and the degree to which each barrier was a problem.
- Frequency is rated on a 0 to 4 scale (0, never; 1, less than monthly; 2, monthly; 3, weekly; and 4, daily)
- Degree of problems is rated from 0 to 2 (0, no problem or never encountered; 1 a little problem, and 2, a big problem)

Neuropsychological Tests

Compared with the screening measures or rating scales described earlier, neuropsychological evaluations represent a more comprehensive assessment of brain-based behavior or performance across domains of cognitive, emotional, and personality functioning. Clinical neuropsychology is a specialty area of professional psychology that focuses on understanding brain-based relationships and the normal and abnormal functioning of the CNS. Clinical neuropsychologists apply principles of assessment and intervention to measure functional abilities and make recommendations to maximize recovery and rehabilitation. "Although neurological diagnoses can validly be established using many other techniques and methods (e.g., computed tomography [CT] and magnetic resonance imaging [MRI]) the *psychological* consequences of cerebral damage are uniquely represented by neuropsychological evaluation[14]."

Neuropsychological evaluations integrate information from a variety of sources, including medical records, clinical interviews, behavioral observations, collateral informants, and the results of neuropsychological tests administered as part of a flexible or fixed battery of assessment tools. Most referral questions for neuropsychological evaluation after brain injury will involve characterizing (1) whether an individual's performance is different from the estimated or known baseline pattern, (2) whether performance is at variance with what would be expected based on known injuries, (3) what an individual's pattern of functioning means for treatment and recovery, (4) the real-word implications of performance for social participation, and (5) what accommodations or interventions would help maximize performance.

Neuropsychological tests are developed through a rigorous process of standardization, and these tests are administered under strictly controlled conditions designed to replicate the protocol for routine administration. The results of neuropsychological tests are interpreted by comparing an individual's performance to that of a normative or reference group. As such, it is important to select a test with adequate normative data, often based on factors such as age, sex, education level, ethnic background, or diagnostic group. Finally, neuropsychological tests are selected based on the quality of their measurement properties (e.g., sensitivity/specificity, reliability, validity, measurement error) and their suitability for measuring the domain of functioning of relevance to the referral question. Tests may assess performance across multiple domains of functioning, including processing speed, attention and concentration, language ability, visuospatial functioning, psychomotor skill, learning and memory, reasoning, and executive functioning. Commonly used neuropsychological tests categorized by domain of functioning are included in Table 16.2.

TABLE 16.2 Common Neuropsychological Tests by Domain of Cognitive Functioning

Academic Abilities

Wechsler Individual Achievement Test–3rd Edition (WIAT-III)
Wide Range Achievement Test–4th Edition (WRAT–4)
Woodcock-Johnson IV Tests of Achievement (WJ-IV-Ach)

Psychomotor Skill

Finger Tapping Test
Grooved Pegboard Test
Luria Motor Test
Tactual Performance Test (TPT)

Attention, Concentration, and Working Memory

Brief Test of Attention
Digit Span (WAIS-IV)
Ruff 2 & 7 Selective Attention Test
Letter Number Sequencing (WAIS-IV)
Arithmetic (WAIS-IV)

Speed of Mental Processing

Trail Making Test–Part A (TMT-A)
Coding (WAIS-IV)
Symbol Search (WAIS-IV)
Digit Symbol Coding (WAIS-IV)
Symbol Digits Modality Test

Language

Boston Naming Test
Boston Diagnostic Aphasia Examination
Controlled Oral Word Association Test (COWA)
Category Fluency Test

Visuospatial Ability and Perceptual Reasoning

Block Design (WAIS-IV)
Visual Puzzles (WAIS-IV)

Learning and Memory (Verbal)

Logical Memory (WMS-IV)
Verbal Paired Associates (WMS-IV)
California Verbal Learning Test – III (CVLT-III)
Rey Auditory Verbal Learning Test (RAVLT)
Buschke Selective Reminding Test (SRT)

Executive Functioning

Trail Making Test–Part B (TMT-B)
Wisconsin Card Sort Test (WCST)
Color Word Interference (DKEFS)
Tower Test (DKEFS)
Design Fluency (DKEFS)

Learning and Memory (Visual)

Visual Memory (WMS-IV)
Visual Reproduction (WMS-IV)
Rey Complex Figure
Brief Visuospatial Memory Test–Revised (BVMT-R)

Personality

Minnesota Multiphasic Personality Inventory–2nd Edition (MMPI–2)
Personality Assessment Inventory
Millon Clinical Multiaxial Inventory–III (MCMI-III)

Effort

Test of Memory Malingering (TOMM)
Word Memory Test (WMT)

DKEFS, Delis Kaplan Executive Function System; *WAIS-IV*, Wechsler Adult Intelligence Scale, 4th ed.; *WMS-IV*, Wechsler Memory Scale, 4th ed.

Review Questions

1. As a physiatrist working with an inpatient rehabilitation team, you are interested in monitoring the effects of an atypical antipsychotic used to manage agitation among patients with traumatic brain injury (TBI). Which of these measures might you consider using to monitor and make modifications to a patient's agitation medication regimen?
   a. Orientation Log (O-Log)
   b. Participation Assessment with Recombined Tools–Objective–17 (PART-O-17)
   c. Craig Hospital Inventory of Environmental Factors (CHIEF)
   d. Agitated Behavior Scale (ABS)

2. John had a severe TBI 2 years ago. He is currently living successfully in a group home environment, which is familiar and in which his day is highly structured. John perform his activities of daily living (ADLs) with minimal assistance. He exhibits decreased insight and can be socially awkward at times. John is unable to participate in gainful employment because of his chronic cognitive impairments. Which of these Rancho Level of Cognitive Function Scale (LCFS) levels best describes John's level of function?
   a. Rancho LCFS III
   b. Rancho LCFS V
   c. Rancho LCFS VII
   d. Rancho LCFS IX

3. A 35-year-old accountant is seen in the outpatient brain injury clinic with cognitive complaints of difficulty concentrating, impaired short-term memory, difficulty multitasking, and low frustration tolerance that have persisted since a moderate TBI approximately 30 months ago. She states that she is concerned about her performance at work, and her supervisor has noted an overall decline in the quality of her work products. The physiatrist performs a complete neurologic examination including the Folstein Mini-Mental Status Exam (MMSE) which she scored 29/30. Neurologic examination is normal. Which of these would be the most appropriate next diagnostic test?
   a. Magnetic resonance imaging (MRI) of the brain with and without contrast
   b. Comprehensive neuropsychological evaluation
   c. Prolonged electroencephalogram (EEG)
   d. Montreal Cognitive Assessment (MoCA)

Answers on page 389.
Access the full list of questions and answers online. Available on ExpertConsult.com

References

1. Rappaport M, Hall KM, Hopkins K, Belleza T, Cope DN. Disability rating scale for severe head trauma: coma to community. *Arch Phys Med Rehabil.* 1982;63(3):118-123.
2. Teasdale GM, Pettigrew LE, Wilson JL, Murray G, Jennett B. Analyzing outcome of treatment of severe head injury: a review and update on advancing the use of the Glasgow Outcome Scale. *J Neurotrauma.* 1998;15(8):587-597.
3. Wilson JL, Pettigrew LE, Teasdale GM. Structured interviews for the Glasgow Outcome Scale and the extended Glasgow Outcome Scale: guidelines for their use. *J Neurotrauma.* 1998;15(8): 573-585.
4. *Guide for the Uniform Data Set for Medical Rehabilitation (including the FIM(TM) instrument), Version 5.1.* Buffalo, NY: State University of New York at Buffalo; 1997.
5. Malec JF. The Mayo-Portland Participation Index: a brief and psychometrically sound measure of brain injury outcome. *Arch Phys Med Rehabil.* 2004;85(12):1989-1996.
6. Gouvier WD, Blanton PD, LaPorte KK, Nepomuceno C. Reliability and validity of the Disability Rating Scale and the Levels of Cognitive Functioning Scale in monitoring recovery from severe head injury. *Arch Phys Med Rehabil.* 1987;68(2):94-97.
7. Corrigan JD. Development of a scale for assessment of agitation following traumatic brain injury. *J Clin Exp Neuropsychol.* 1989;11(2):261-277.
8. Fann JR, Bombardier CH, Dikmen S, et al. Validity of the Patient Health Questionnaire-9 in assessing depression following traumatic brain injury. *J Head Trauma Rehabil.* 2005;20(6):501-511.
9. Cicerone KD, Kalmar K. Persistent postconcussion syndrome: the structure of subjective complaints after mild traumatic brain injury. *J Head Trauma Rehabil.* 1995;10(3):1-17.
10. Jackson WT, Novack TA, Dowler RN. Effective serial measurement of cognitive orientation in rehabilitation: the Orientation Log. *Arch Phys Med Rehabil.* 1998;79(6):718-721.
11. Giacino JT, Kalmar K, Whyte J. The JFK Coma Recovery Scale-Revised: measurement characteristics and diagnostic utility. *Arch Phys Med Rehabil.* 2004;85(12):2020-2029.
12. Whiteneck GG, Dijkers MP, Heinemann AW, et al. Development of the Participation Assessment with Recombined Tools–Objective for use after traumatic brain injury. *Arch Phys Med Rehabil.* 2011;92(4):542-551.
13. Steinfeld EH. Environment as a mediating factor in functional assessment. In: Dittmar S, Gresham G, eds. *Functional Assessment and Outcome Measurement for the Rehab Health Professional.* Gaithersburg, MD: Aspen Publishers; 1997.
14. Reitan RM, Wolfson D. Influence of age and education on neuropsychological test results. *Clin Neuropsychol.* 1995;9(2): 151-158.

17

Intensity of Services, Specialized Rehabilitation Therapies, and Interdisciplinary Team Management

GARY NOEL GALANG, MD AND JUSTIN LOUIS WEPPNER, DO

Intensity of Services

Inpatient Rehabilitation Facility

- Inpatient rehabilitation facilities (IRFs) are hospitals that specialize in intensive rehabilitation.
- IRFs provide the most intensive therapy and the greatest variety of rehabilitation services. These may occur in general rehabilitation units or in dedicated brain injury units that are within acute care facilities or part of freestanding postacute hospitals.
- Medicare has established these following regulatory requirements for IRFs:
1 A rehabilitation physician must review and approve each patient, and the patient must meet these criteria:
  - Require close medical supervision by a rehabilitation physician to manage medical conditions and require

specialized rehabilitative nursing expertise to support participation in an intensive rehabilitation therapy program.
  - Require the active and ongoing therapeutic intervention of multiple therapy disciplines, including physical therapy (PT), occupational therapy (OT), speech language pathology (SLP), or prosthetics and orthotics and at least one therapy discipline must be PT or OT.
  - Require an intensive rehabilitation therapy program uniquely provided in IRFs and must tolerate 3 hours of rehabilitation therapy per day at least 5 days a week or at least 15 hours of intensive rehabilitation therapy within a consecutive 7-day period, beginning with the date of admission.
  - Be sufficiently medically stable to benefit from IRF services.
  - Provided services may result in a measurable and significant improvement in the patient's condition within a reasonable time frame.
2 A postadmission physician evaluation to verify that the patient's preadmission assessment information remains unchanged or documentation of any changes must be completed within 24 hours of admission.
3 Individualized overall plan of care must be completed by the rehabilitation physician within 4 days for each patient, emphasizing the interdisciplinary approach to care provided in IRFs.
4 Interdisciplinary team meetings are required at least once per week throughout the IRF hospitalization.

Long-Term Acute Care Hospital

- Long-term acute care hospitals (LTACHs) take care of medically complex patients who require longer inpatient hospitalizations.
- Although LTACHs provide rehabilitative therapies, their primary focus is on medical and nursing care of complex conditions.

- Medicare mandates the length of stay (LOS) to be greater than 25 days on average, reflecting the expectations of medical complexity.
  - Medical complexity includes the need for respiratory therapy because of ventilator or tracheostomy dependence, prolonged ventilator weaning, intensive respiratory care, parenteral feeding, dialysis, complex wound care, or multiple intravenous medications or transfusions.
- Additionally, a 3-day intensive care unit LOS at the acute care hospital immediately preceding LTACH admission or 96 hours of mechanical ventilation services during the LTACH admission is required by Medicare for admission.
- There is no Medicare requirement for the amount of rehabilitation therapy at LTACHs.

Skilled Nursing Facility

- Skilled nursing facilities (SNFs) provide skilled nursing and rehabilitation care at a less intensive and more variable level than IRFs.
- SNFs provide PT, OT, and SLP therapy and skilled nursing services.
- SNFs must designate a physician to serve as medical director who is responsible for implementation of resident care policies and coordination of medical care in the facility.
- A physician must visit every 30 days for the first 3 months of stay and every 60 days thereafter.
- Medicare patients must have had a 3-day qualifying stay in an acute care hospital within the preceding 30 days and need skilled nursing and/or skilled therapy services.
- There is no requirement for a specific number of hours of therapies per day.
- Medicare covers SNF services on a short-term basis up to 100 days in a benefit period (Table 17.1).
- Patients with a brain injury are usually admitted to this level of care from acute hospital care or after acute inpatient rehabilitation.

Home Health Rehabilitation

- Rehabilitation therapy and nursing services can be provided in a patient's home by a home care agency.
- A doctor sends orders for therapy to the agency, which then visits the patient at home to assess their need for skilled services and provides those services.

TABLE 17.1	Medicare Coverage for Skilled Nursing Facility (SNF) Stays	
SNF Days	Medicare Pays for Covered Services	Patient Responsibility for SNF Services
1–20	Full Cost	Nothing
21–100	All except a daily coinsurance	Up to $176 per day in 2020
>100	Nothing	Full cost

- Home care agencies provide standard PT, OT, SLP, registered nurse (RN), home health aide, medical social services, and necessary medical supplies, excluding durable medical equipment such as wheelchairs.
- The intensity of therapy services is usually one to three times per week for each therapy.
- RN visits may be one to seven times per week for wound care, medication management, bladder catheterization, or other services.
- Home care services are short term. Medicare defines a maximum 60 days for home care services per episode of care. Patients typically receive these services for a few weeks after hospitalization.
- To be covered by Medicare, the patient must be certified as homebound by the referring physician, meaning that the patient must be unable to leave the home, an activity that would require a "considerable and taxing effort."

Outpatient Rehabilitation

- Outpatient therapy services are provided in the outpatient departments of acute care and rehabilitation hospitals, in rehabilitation clinics, and in doctors' offices.
- Besides standard PT, OT, and SLP services, they may offer pool therapy, driving evaluation, orthotic and adaptive technology services, wheelchair clinic, vocational rehabilitation consultation, electrical stimulation, robotic, and virtual reality therapy interventions.
- Therapy frequency is usually one to three times per week.
- In 2018, Congress eliminated the limits on Medicare payments for therapy services in one calendar year.
- For Medicare to pay for services, the law requires the therapist or therapy provider to confirm that therapy services are medically reasonable and necessary when they reach these amounts each calendar year:
  - $2080 for PT and SLP services combined in 2018
  - $2080 for OT services in 2018

Specialized Rehabilitation Therapies

Disorders of Consciousness Program

- Persons with disorders of consciousness (DoC) who are in a coma, vegetative state (VS), or a minimally conscious state (MCS) remain at a high level of medical acuity after intensive care.
- Individuals with DoC recover over a longer period and many regain the ability to function independently. In those who survive severe brain injury, there is a marked variability in long-term medical, cognitive, and physical needs.
- DoC programs determine the patient's level of consciousness and responsiveness, identify barriers preventing effective communication and environmental control, advise on medical stability for continued care, establish prognosis, monitor for recovery, optimize the medication regimen, identify long-term care needs, prevent secondary complications, and ensure proper medical equipment is available.

- Families who are provided comprehensive education and hands-on training with follow-up support are likely willing and able to provide care for medically stable persons with DoC at home.
- Patients may be transitioned to mainstream inpatient rehabilitation programs once they emerge.

Day Program Rehabilitation

- Coordinated form of outpatient rehabilitation may take place in a day program, with PT, OT, and SLP therapies, group treatments and group activities, case management, and team meetings to set goals and review progress.
- The length and intensity of treatment are determined by the patient's needs but are largely constrained by health insurance payer contracts and public funding policies limiting the duration of care and range of covered services.

Supported Living Programs

Slow-to-Recover Program

- The primary goal of this program is supporting patients to prevent complications and avoid physical deterioration such as decubitus ulcers or muscle contractures.
- These typically include pharmacologic and behavioral stimulation interventions designed to increase responsiveness and normal awareness.

Residential Rehabilitation Program

- Group residence programs may provide services at various stages after injury but may be aimed at patients just discharged from acute care hospitalizations, acute inpatient rehabilitation, or for those who require a more structured supervised setting away from their own home setting.
- Residential rehabilitation programs offer individual therapies and group therapies and resources to foster independent living skills.
- The programs usually provide only part-time nursing services with a mix of professional therapists and other professional disciplines.
- Programs may or may not provide physician services.

Long-Term Community Supported Living Program

- A small percentage of individuals with severe and pervasive disabilities after brain injuries are able to live in community-integrated settings, such as family, group homes, or supported apartments but require ongoing supportive services to maintain their maximum level of health, functional ability, and community participation.
- The services provided by community supportive living programs are similar to those provided by residential supportive living programs but are typically not as frequent or intensive.

Interdisciplinary Team Management

Team Models

- Rehabilitation usually denotes that multiple disciplines engage with patients and their families to determine and work toward attainable goals.
- A team comprises different professional disciplines that are needed to provide comprehensive rehabilitation care.
- Almost all rehabilitation programs involve a team of treating providers. However, the team may be configured in different ways, each of which addresses a particular set of treatment goals.
- There are multiple team models:
  - *Multidisciplinary teams* involve multiple professions working in parallel to treat patients who have reasonable awareness of a small set of circumscribed problems. This model is commonly used in the outpatient setting.
  - *Interdisciplinary teams* are a coordinated group of experts from several different fields, working together toward common goals. It is the preferred team delivery system in IRFs, requiring routine communication to achieve these goals.
  - *Transdisciplinary teams* require providers from various disciplines to offer treatment in a coordinated fashion and temporarily adopt each other's roles in treating the patient. Transdisciplinary teams are most common in residential or day treatment programs.

Management Principles

- Team leadership typically is the responsibility of the physiatrist, but there may be shared leadership related to a specific patient issue or program focus.
- It is important to set expectations and know how to delegate.
- Interdisciplinary teams with strong physiatrist leadership and involvement have been associated with high team cohesiveness, showing behaviors that focus on patient services.[1]
- External factors that influence team processes and functions are healthcare facility cultures, hospital-level administration and hierarchy, and supervisory expectations.[1]

Team Interprofessional Relationships

- Five central components of inpatient rehabilitation team functioning are:
1 Physician support
2 Shared leadership
3 Supervisor team support
4 Team cohesiveness
5 Team effectiveness
- A team culture is developed through collaborative leadership, care philosophy, relationships, environmental contexts, and communication.[2]
- Team members often develop alliances within the team, usually among those engaged in the physical

needs of patients or those supporting psychosocial needs.[2]

- Communication within teams is a required interpersonal skill for all team members, especially the team leader.
- Communication is usually complex and often nonlinear, requiring both formal and informal communication among team members.[2]

Development of Therapeutic Alliance

- *Therapeutic alliance* refers to the positive relationship, mutual trust, and shared goals between provider and patient in a treatment program.
- Therapeutic alliance has been identified as a significant variable in enhancing outcomes in posthospital brain injury rehabilitation.[3]
- Rehabilitation programs seek to develop a positive working relationship with their patients with varying degrees of success, with some programs monitoring therapeutic alliance and providing interventions as needed.

The Rehabilitation Team Conference

- The purpose of the IRF interdisciplinary team is to foster frequent, structured, and documented communication among disciplines to establish, prioritize, and achieve treatment goals.
- Team conferences must be held once a week, starting within seven consecutive calendar days that begin on the day of admission.
- Document participation by professionals from these disciplines (who must have current knowledge of the patient as documented in the IRF medical record):
  - A rehabilitation physician with specialized training and experience
  - An RN with specialized training or experience in rehabilitation
  - A social worker or a case manager (or both)
  - A licensed or certified therapist from each discipline involved in treating the patient
- A weekly interdisciplinary team meeting must be led by a rehabilitation physician who is responsible for making the final decisions regarding the patient's treatment in the IRF.

Review Questions

1. A rehabilitation physician must approve each Medicare patient before admission to an inpatient rehabilitation facility (IRF). Which of these criteria would meet the Medicare requirements for inpatient rehabilitation admission?
   a. Require close supervision by a rehabilitation physician.
   b. Require only one therapy discipline.
   c. The patient is able to tolerate 2 hours of therapy 5 days a week.
   d. The patient is able to tolerate 3 hours of therapy 3 days a week.

2. You are consulted for disposition recommendations for a patient with a severe traumatic brain injury (TBI) with high medical complexity. The patient's insurance payer is Medicare. You recommend the patient be transferred to a long-term acute care hospital (LTACH). Which of these is a Medicare requirement for admission to an LTACH?
   a. 2-day intensive care unit length of stay immediately preceding the LTACH admission

   b. 3-day intensive care unit length of stay immediately preceding the LTACH admission
   c. 24 hours of mechanical ventilation services during the LTACH admission
   d. 48 hours of mechanical ventilation services during the LTACH admission

3. What are the Medicare requirements for the amount of rehabilitation therapy services at LTACHs?
   a. 1 hour of therapy 3 days a week
   b. 2 hours of therapy 5 days a week
   c. 3 hours of therapy 5 days a week
   d. There is no Medicare requirement for the amount of rehabilitation therapy at LTACHs.

Answers on page 389.
Access the full list of questions and answers online. Available on ExpertConsult.com

References

1. Smits SJ, Falconer JA, Herrin J, Bowen SE, Strasser DC. Patient-focused rehabilitation team cohesiveness in Veterans Administration hospitals. *Arch Phys Med Rehabil.* 2003;84(9):1332-1338.
2. Sinclair LB, Lingard LA, Mohabeer RN. What's so great about rehabilitation teams? An ethnographic study of interprofessional collaboration in a rehabilitation unit. *Arch Phys Med Rehabil.* 2009;90(7):1196-1201.
3. Evans CC, Sherer M, Nakase-Richardson R, Mani T, Irby JW. Evaluation of an interdisciplinary team intervention to improve therapeutic alliance in post-acute brain injury rehabilitation. *J Head Trauma Rehabil.* 2008;23(5):329-338

Complications and Management

18

Cardiovascular and Pulmonary

JAMES J. BEGLEY, MD, MS AND VICTORIA C. WHITEHAIR, MD

Cardiovascular Complications After Brain Injury

Brain disorders including traumatic brain injury (TBI) have been known to affect the heart directly or indirectly. These conditions may include cardiomyopathy, arrhythmias, or autonomic dysfunction.[1]

Cardiomyopathy

Cardiomyopathies caused by brain injury have been attributed to catecholamine and neuroendocrine excess and as a result of the inflammatory process. There are two described syndromes: Takotsubo cardiomyopathy (TCM) and neurogenic stunned myocardium (NSM). Both share similar mechanisms and have similar clinical manifestations and clinical courses. Some investigators feel that the two syndromes are in fact the same condition.

TCM has also been called *left ventricular apical ballooning syndrome* and *broken heart syndrome*. Its first investigators noted the left ventricle's similar appearance to a Takotsubo or "octopus pot" used by Japan fishermen that has a round bottom and narrow neck. Since its initial identification in 1983, it has been seen worldwide in up to 2% of initially presumed acute coronary syndromes.[2]

The Mayo criteria for TCM include:
- Hypokinesis, akinesis, or dyskinesis of the left ventricular midsegments with or without apical involvement

- Absence of obstructive coronary disease or acutely ruptured plaques
- Presence of new electrocardiogram (ECG) abnormalities (either ST-segment elevation or T-wave inversion)
- Absence of pheochromocytoma or myocarditis[2]

NSM has a very similar presentation to TCM, with the main difference being a global hypokinesis of the left ventricle in NSM rather than the segmental wall dysfunction of TCM.[3] Both TCM and NSM may be difficult to distinguish from acute coronary syndrome (ACS). However, both cardiomyopathy syndromes are notable for wall motions that do not correspond to ischemic ECG changes and troponin levels that are only mildly elevated (<2.8 ng/mL). These findings in patients without known heart disease or in new cardiac dysfunction (ejection fraction <40%) suggests an injury-induced cardiomyopathy over ACS.

Causative mechanisms of TCM and NSM may include transient coronary vasospasm, microvascular dysfunction, or myocyte injury caused by excess of catecholamines. It has been observed in association with several stressful settings, including sudden emotional stress or acute medical illnesses such as asthma. The proposed excess catecholamine mechanism has helped explain the appearance of this syndrome after acute brain syndromes such as stroke, ruptured cerebral aneurysm, seizures, encephalitis, or TBI.

The brain's influence on the heart in this condition stems from damage to the insular cortex and subcortical regions. These areas have central influences on cardiovascular function and the autonomic nervous system. This leads to excess catecholamine release from sympathetic nerve endings in myocardium and autonomic dysfunction and neuroinflammation. The catecholamine release subsequently leads to intracellular calcium elevation and cyclic adenosine monophosphate (cAMP) overload with depletion of adenosine triphosphate (ATP) in the myocyte. The calcium influx also leads to myocardial reperfusion injury. Subsequent mitochondrial dysfunction and cell death ensues. Elevation of circulating catecholamines may last up to 10 days after injury, resulting in a persistent high sympathetic tone.[4]

The patient with TCM typically presents with hypertension from the catecholamine storming followed by hypotension from the vasodilation and cardiac dysfunction. There is

TABLE 18.1	Pharmacologic Classes Implicated in Drug-Induced QT Interval Prolongation	

Pharmacologic Class	Representative Examples
Acetylcholinesterase inhibitors	Donepezil
Analgesics	Methadone
Anesthetics	Propofol, desflurane, isoflurane, sevoflurane
Antibacterials	Azithromycin, clarithromycin, clindamycin, erythromycin, roxithromycin, spiramycin, telithromycin, bedaquiline, ciprofloxacin, gatifloxacin, gemifloxacin, grepafloxacin, levofloxacin, moxifloxacin, ofloxacin, sparfloxacin
Anticholinergic	Tolterodine
Antidepressants	Amitriptyline, nortriptyline, desipramine, citalopram, fluoxetine, venlafaxine, trazodone
Antifungals	Fluconazole, ketoconazole, posaconazole, voriconazole
Antihistamines	Diphenhydramine, hydroxyzine, mizolastine
Antimalarials	Quinidine, quinine, chloroquine, halofantrine, piperaquine
Antineoplastic	Arsenic trioxide, depsipeptide, vorinostat, ivosidenib, lenvatinib, vandetanib
Antivirals	Atazanavir, nelfinavir, saquinavir, efavirenz, foscarnet
Antiarrhythmics	Amiodarone, disopyramide, dofetilide, procainamide, quinidine, sotalol
Neuroleptics	Chlorpromazine, droperidol, haloperidol, pimozide, quetiapine, risperidone, sertindole, thioridazine, ziprasidone, clozapine, olanzapine
Promotility agents and antiemetics	Cisapride, dolasetron, domperidone, ondansetron, metoclopramide
Vasodilators	Cilostazol

no agreed-upon management, and it is guided by the maintenance of normal hemodynamics and cerebral perfusion. Inotropic support with dobutamine will improve cardiac function.[5] Beta blockers in the setting of TBI may be protective, because exposure to this medication class during acute hospitalization has demonstrated better outcomes, including reduced mortality.[6] Generally, the effects of maintaining normal hemodynamics in the early stages will result in excellent cardiac outcomes with return of left ventricle function to normal within several weeks to months.[2]

Arrhythmia

Several arrhythmias have been observed during the first week of brain injury, including sinus tachycardia, atrial fibrillation, premature atrial contractions, premature ventricular contractions, and atrioventricular (AV) dissociation. More severe arrythmias such as ventricular fibrillation are rarer and more commonly seen with cardiac injury. Injury to the insula cortex has been associated with prolongation of the QT interval See Table 18.1. A prolonged QT interval has been associated with the dangerous arrhythmia torsades de pointes, and therefore medications known to prolong the QTc should be avoided in the acute hospital and perhaps into rehabilitation hospitalization.[4] Medications known to prolong QTc include certain antiarrhythmics, antipsychotics, antidepressants and erythromycins.[7,8]

Autonomic Dysfunction

Survivors of TBI have been known to demonstrate alterations in autonomic functions, known as *dysautonomia*, after injury to the autonomic nervous system (ANS). Such injuries upset the normal homeostasis of the sympathetic and parasympathetic divisions of the ANS and lead to abnormalities in cardiac function, blood pressure, heart rate variability, gastrointestinal motility, pupillary contraction, and sphincter control. These alterations have been seen in diffuse axonal injury and with secondary injury from hypoxia and focal injuries to the insula, hypothalamus, and brainstem.[9]

Following acute trauma, there is an increase in sympathetic activity with or without brain injury, but these effects are magnified in many cases of severe TBI. Initial responses include tachycardia, tachypnea, and hypertension, which are seen to some degree in most TBI patients in the intensive care unit (ICU). The release of excess catecholamines after injury appears to be responsible for this activity. In the most severe cases, a state of paroxysmal sympathetic hyperactivity (PSH) will emerge, in which extreme autonomic instability is combined with excess upper motor neuron motor activity, which will be discussed in detail in Chapter 24.

Common cardiopulmonary effects associated with PSH include prolonged hypertension, arrhythmias, and tachypnea. Sympathetic overactivity may be demonstrated by

TABLE 18.2	Modified Berne-Norwood Criteria	
Low Risk	**Moderate Risk**	**High Risk**
No moderate or high-risk criteria for DVT	Small subdural or epidural hematoma	ICP monitor placement
	• Small contusion or intraventricular hemorrhage • Multiple contusions per lobe • Subarachnoid hemorrhage with abnormal CT angiogram • Evidence of progression at 24 h after injury	• Craniotomy • Evidence of progression of hemorrhage on CT head scan at 72 h after injury
Initiate pharmacological prophylaxis if CT is stable at 24 h after injury	Initiate pharmacologic prophylaxis if CT is stable at 72 h after injury	Consider placement of retrievable IVC filter

CT, Computed tomography; DVT, deep venous thrombosis; ICP, intracranial pressure; IVC, inferior vena cava.
In Vendantum A, Gopinath SP, Robertson CS. Acute management of traumatic brain injury. In: Eapen BC, Cifu DX, eds. *Rehabilitation After Traumatic Brain Injury*. Philadelphia, PA: Elsevier, 2018.

heart rate variability in response to noxious stimuli.[1] Persistent hypertension increases the risk of secondary brain injury through cerebral edema or expansion of hemorrhage. Additionally, prolonged hypertension places the patient at risk for cardiac dysfunction and resulting anoxic injury. Common arrhythmias during PSH include supraventricular tachycardia, ectopic beats, and atrial fibrillation.[10]

Dysautonomia may also be seen in the rehabilitation admission or later. Autonomic instability may result in postural orthostatic tachycardia syndrome (POTS), which may be severe enough to cause syncope caused by impairment affecting the baroreflex system. Symptoms include palpitations, dizziness, and fatigue. Sympathetic outflow to afferent input from vagal nerve and carotid bodies is poorly modulated, leading to baroreceptor failure.[9] Treatment includes medications to support blood pressure, which may include fludrocortisone, desmopressin, or midodrine. Selective serotonin reuptake inhibitors (SSRIs) or norepinephrine reuptake inhibitors have also been useful in cardiogenic syncope and may be considered in TBI patients with POTS. Tilt table training in physical therapy should be prescribed.[11] Compression stockings and increased salt intake has also been advised.

Whereas autonomic dysfunction has been mostly associated with severe TBI, there is an increased recognition of abnormalities after concussion or mild TBI. Abnormalities described in this setting include heart rate variability as recorded on a 24-hour Holter monitor, changes in pupillary light reflex, eyeball pressure, and arterial pulse waves. Such symptoms when persistent may require delay in return-to-play protocols in athletes with concussion.[12]

Pulmonary Complications After Brain Injury

Patients with severe TBI may face several pulmonary complications in acute hospital management and extending into rehabilitation: pneumonia, pulmonary embolism, aspiration,

and atelectasis. Many patients will have concomitant chest trauma, placing them at additional risk.[13] Some severely injured patients may obtain tracheostomy tubes to allow for better airway protection, but this will require decisions about management, including decannulation during the rehabilitation phase.[14]

Pneumonia

Pneumonia is a common early complication of severe TBI, with an incidence ranging up to 47%, often related to aspiration at the time of injury or associated with mechanical ventilation.[15-19] Risk factors for an early pneumonia in severe brain injury include nasogastric tube insertion, hemiplegia or hemiparesis, and increased age.[17] Polytrauma, whether caused by additional chest injuries or involvement of other body organs, has been cited as an additional risk factor for ventilator-associated pneumonia (VAP).[16] Early identification of pneumonia is important to prevent secondary brain injury from fever, hypoxemia, or hypercapnia.[17] Furthermore, there is a potential for critically ill patients with pneumonia to develop more severe inflammatory lung conditions including acute lung injury (ALI) or acute respiratory distress syndrome (ARDS).[20] VAP in severe TBI patients has been associated with longer duration of mechanical ventilation, longer ICU length of stay, and higher incidence of tracheostomy placement.[16]

Hospital-acquired pneumonia (HAP) has been cited as an independent predictor of poor global outcome up to 5 years after discharge after a severe TBI according to the TBI Model System outcome data. Lower Glasgow Outcome Scale-Extended (GOS-E) scores were noted in the patients who had acquired HAP (42 patients, mean GOS-E 5) versus those without HAP (99 patients, mean GOS-E 7) at 2 and 5 years postinjury. The cause of the extended effect of pneumonia could not be ascertained in this study because of data limitations, but chronic inflammation and secondary brain injury from hypoxemia were postulated.[21]

Long-term studies have shown that long-term survivors of TBI face a higher risk of aspiration pneumonia and subsequent mortality risk. A large multicenter study revealed that TBI survivors discharged from rehabilitation units were 79 times more likely to die of aspiration pneumonia than the general population. Those with higher risks included persons with more severe disability and those discharged to nursing homes. Additional risk factors were prior aspiration pneumonia, percutaneous endoscopic gastrostomy (PEG) placement during acute or rehabilitation hospital admission, and persistent dysphagia at the time of rehabilitation discharge.[22] A study of TBI mortality of TBI survivors up to 40 years after injury showed that patients were 1.5 times more likely to die of any cause, 4 times more likely to die of pneumonia, and 49 times more likely to die specifically from aspiration pneumonia compared with the general population. Higher mortality was associated with increased age at the time of injury, male sex, lower education level, longer hospital length of stay, and vegetative state.[23]

Tracheostomy Tubes

In severe TBI, endotracheal intubation is often required for airway protection to prevent hypoxia and secondary brain injury. Subsequently tracheostomy tube placement is often performed for patients needing extended ventilator support. In this setting a tracheostomy tube may improve patient comfort and pulmonary hygiene and reduce VAP and the need for sedation. Tracheostomy placement has been associated with improvement in survival rates.[24] Risk factors for obtaining a tracheostomy tube after TBI include failed extubation and multiple operating room (OR) visits.[25] Placement traditionally has been performed after 10 to 14 days after injury, but it has also been advocated earlier. Traditional tracheostomy placement has been associated with longer ICU stays and prolonged mechanical ventilation. However, earlier tracheostomy placement (<10 days) has resulted in reduced duration of mechanical ventilation, reduced incidence of pneumonia, and reduced length of ICU and total hospital days when compared with extended endotracheal intubation.[26,27] Tracheostomy placement is also associated with complications including wound infections, subcutaneous emphysema, esophageal injury, laryngeal nerve injury, and tracheal stenosis. So despite attempts to create protocols for tracheostomy placement, the decision for the procedure ultimately remains with the trauma surgeon.

Following release from the ventilator, decannulation can be considered and when appropriate will facilitate communication and swallowing function. Factors to consider before proceeding with decannulation may include the patient's respirations, tracheal secretions, cough, phonation, and swallowing. Maximal expiratory pressure, spontaneous cough, and cough strength are positive predictors of tracheostomy weaning, whereas excessive secretions and anoxic brain injury have been associated with failures. Glasgow Coma Score (GCS) is not associated with failures, and decannulation can be performed successfully in vegetative patients when a strong cough is present.[28,29]

There are a number of techniques and protocols to progress through the process of decannulation. Typical steps and options during the weaning process include:
- Deflation of the tracheostomy cuff
- Downsizing to a smaller diameter tracheostomy tube
- Replacement with a tube without a cuff when positive pressure respiratory treatments are no longer necessary
- Use of a speaking valve when the cuffed tube is in a deflated position
- Capping a cuffless tracheostomy tube for progressively longer hours of the day while monitoring oxygen saturations and vital signs
- Performing laryngoscopy on patients in whom there is suspicion of subglottic airway stenosis or tracheal granulation[30]
- Tolerance of a closed tracheostomy tube for 72 hours is associated with successful decannulation[29]

Venous Thromboembolic Prophylaxis

Deep venous thrombosis (DVT) and pulmonary embolism (PE) can be seen in up to 20% of patients with severe TBI who do not receive prophylaxis.[31] This high incidence is caused by a combination of immobility, prolonged ventilation, and hypercoagulability. Mechanical and pharmacological interventions have been used to prevent these complications. There is no doubt that pharmacologic chemoprophylaxis reduces the incidence of venous thromboembolic (VTE) complications, but the difficult decision has been the timing of the initiation of medications, which can increase the risk of intracranial bleeding or expand existing hemorrhages. Delayed initiation of chemoprophylaxis beyond 4 days has been associated with a threefold increase in DVT,[32] however, whereas a literature review determined that the rate of DVT climbed from 2.6% if the chemoprophylaxis was started by day 3 postinjury up to 14.1% if it was delayed to day 8.[33]

The use of mechanical prophylaxis is safe for nearly all TBI patients and should be initiated early within 24 hours after TBI or within 24 hours of a craniotomy, but the evidence is considered low quality and is a weak recommendation of the Neurocritical Care Society.[34]

The timing of safe initiation of chemoprophylaxis with either low-molecular-weight heparin (LMWH) or unfractionated heparin (UFH) has been studied in the setting of acute brain injury. Current practice by the American College of Surgeons recommends following the Modified Berne-Norwood Criteria See Table 18.2. In these guidelines, it is safe to initiate chemoprophylaxis if there is a stable head computed tomography (CT) scan at 24 hours without hemorrhage—considered the low-risk group. Moderate-risk patients may have pharmacologic prophylaxis at 72 hours if hemorrhage on earlier CT images is stable. In high-risk patients (those with intracranial pressure [ICP] monitor placement, craniotomy, or with further evidence of hemorrhagic progression on head CT at 72 hours), placement of a retrievable inferior vena cava (IVC) filter should be considered.[35]

Preference of LMWH or UFH remains uncertain. The

American College of Chest Physicians' guidelines suggests LMWH for all trauma patients,[36] but the Neurocritical Care Society, Brain Trauma Foundation, and Eastern Association for the Surgery of Trauma have maintained that studies to date do not demonstrate superiority for either LMWH or UFH in the setting of severe traumatic brain injury.[34-38]

Review Questions

1. The primary distinction between Takotsubo cardiomyopathy (TCM) and neurogenic stunned myocardium (NSM) is
   a. only TCM may demonstrate transient coronary vasospasm.
   b. imaging of NSM reveals global hypokinesis of the left ventricle.
   c. troponin levels are higher in TCM.
   d. elevated sympathetic tone is noted after NSM.

2. A 40-year-old man who sustains a severe traumatic brain injury (TBI) without chest injury or known coronary artery disease is noted on the day after injury to have a troponin I level of 1.1, electrocardiogram (ECG) with nonspecific T-wave inversions, and an echocardiogram revealing dyskinesis of the left ventricle midsegment wall without apical wall involvement. The diagnosis is most consistent with
   a. takotsubo cardiomyopathy.
   b. neurogenic stunned myocardium.

   c. acute coronary syndrome.
   d. restrictive cardiomyopathy.

3. A 41-year-old woman with TBI has an ECG revealing a prolonged QTc interval. One concern for this observation is that the prolonged QTc is associated with
   a. premature atrial contractions.
   b. sinus bradycardia.
   c. sinus tachycardia.
   d. torsades de pointes.

Answers on page 390.
Access the full list of questions and answers online. Available on ExpertConsult.com

References

1. Finsterer J, Wahbi K. CNS-disease affecting the heart: brain-heart disorders. *J Neurol Sci.* 2014;345(1-2):8-14. doi:10.1016/j.jns.2014.07.003.
2. Scantlebury DC, Prasad A. Diagnosis of Takotsubo cardiomyopathy. *Circ J.* 2014;78(9):2129-2139.
3. Biso S, Wongrakpanich S, Agrawal A, Yadlapati S, Kishlyansky M, Figueredo V. A review of neurogenic stunned myocardium. *Cardiovasc Psychiatry Neurol.* 2017;2017:5842182. doi:10.1155/2017/5842182.
4. Gregory T, Smith M. Cardiovascular complications of brain injury. *Contin Educ Anaesth Crit Care Pain.* 2012;12(2):67-71. doi:10.1093/bjaceaccp/mkr058.
5. Cheah CF, Kofler M, Schiefecker AJ, et al. Takotsubo cardiomyopathy in traumatic brain injury. *Neurocrit Care.* 2017;26(2):284-291. doi:10.1007/s12028-016-0334-y.
6. Krishnamoorthy V, Burkhard Mackenson G, Gibbons EF, Vavilala MS. Cardiac dysfunction after neurologic injury: what do we know and where are we going? *Chest.* 2016;149(5):1325-1331. doi:10.1016/j.chest.2015.12.014.
7. Shah RR. Drug-induced QT interval prolongation: does ethnicity of the thorough QT study population matter? *Br J Clin Pharmacol.* 2013;75(2):347-358. doi:10.1111/j.1365-2125.2012.04415.x.
8. Isbister GK, Page CB. Drug induced QT prolongation: the measurement and assessment of the QT interval in clinical practice. *Br J Clin Pharmacol.* 2013;76(1):48-57. doi:10.1111/bcp.12040.
9. Baguley IA, Nott MT. Autonomic dysfunction. In: Zasler ND, Katz DI, Zafonte RD, eds. *Brain Injury Medicine: Principles and Practice.* 2nd ed. New York, NY: Demos Medical; 2013.
10. Lemke DM. Sympathetic storming after severe traumatic brain injury. *Crit Care Nurse.* 2007;27(1):30-37.
11. Kanjwal K, Karabin B, Kanjwal Y, Grubb BP. Autonomic dysfunction presenting as postural tachycardia syndrome following traumatic brain injury. *Cardiol J.* 2010;17(5):482-487.
12. Esterov D, Greenwald BD. Autonomic dysfunction after mild traumatic brain injury. *Brain Sci.* 2017;11:7(8):E100. doi:10.3390/brainsci7080100.
13. Lee K, Rincon F. Pulmonary complications in patients with severe brain injury. *Crit Care Res Pract.* 2012;2012:207247. doi:10.1155/2012/207247.
14. Ivanhoe CB, Durand-Sanchez A, Spier ET. Acute rehabilitation. In: Zasler ND, Katz DI, Zafonte RD, eds. *Brain Injury Medicine: Principles and Practice.* 2nd ed. New York, NY: Demos Medical; 2013.
15. Gaddam SS, Robertson CS. Critical care. In: Zasler ND, Katz DI, Zafonte RD, eds. *Brain Injury Medicine: Principles and Practice.* 2nd ed. New York, NY: Demos Medical; 2013.
16. Zygun DA, Zuege DJ, Boiteau PJ, et al. Ventilator-associated pneumonia in severe traumatic brain injury. *Neurocrit Care.* 2006;5(2):108-114.
17. Wang KW, Chen HJ, Liliang PC, et al. Pneumonia in patients with severe head injury: incidence, risk factors, and outcomes. *J Neurosurg.* 2013;118(2):358-363. doi:10.3171/2012.10.JNS127.
18. Kourbeti IS, Vakis AF, Papadakis JA, et al. Infections in traumatic brain injury patients. *Clin Microbiol Infect.* 2012;18(4):359-364. doi:10.1111/j.1469-0691.2011.03625.x.
19. Bronchard R, Albaladejo P, Brezac G, et al. Early onset pneumonia: risk factors and consequences in head trauma patients. *Anesthesiology.* 2004;100(2):234-239.

20. Raghavendran K, Nemzek J, Napolitano LM, Knight PR. Aspiration-induced lung injury. *Crit Care Med*. 2011;39(4):818-826. doi:10.1097/CCM.0b013e31820a856b.

21. Kesinger MR, Kumar RG, Wagner AK, et al. Hospital-acquired pneumonia is an independent predictor of poor global outcome in severe traumatic brain injury up to 5 years after discharge. *J Trauma Acute Care Surg*. 2015;78(2):396-402. doi:10.1097/TA.0000000000000526.

22. Howle AA, Nott MT, Baguley IJ. Aspiration pneumonia following severe traumatic brain injury: prevalence and risk factors for long-term mortality. *Brain Impair*. 2011;12(3):179-186. doi:10.1375/brim.12.3.179.

23. Harrison-Felix CL, Whiteneck GG, Jha A, DeVivo MJ, Hammond FM, Hart DM. Mortality over four decades after traumatic brain injury rehabilitation: a retrospective cohort study. *Arch Phys Med Rehabil*. 2009;90(9):1506-1513. doi:10.1016/j.apmr.2009.03.015.

24. Humble SS, Wilson LD, McKenna JW, et al. Tracheostomy risk factors and outcomes after severe traumatic brain injury. *Brain Inj*. 2016;30(13-14):1642-1647. doi:10.1080/02699052.2016.1199915.

25. Jenkins R, Morris NA, Haac B, et al. Inpatient complications predict tracheostomy better than admission variables after traumatic brain injury. *Neurocrit Care*. 2019;30(2):387-393. doi:10.1007/s12028-018-0624-7.

26. Alali AS, Scales DC, Fowler RA, et al. Tracheostomy timing in traumatic brain injury: a propensity-matched cohort study. *J Trauma Acute Care Surg*. 2014;76(1):70-76; discussion 76-78. doi:10.1097/TA.0b013e3182a8fd6a.

27. Lu Q, Xie Y, Qi X, Li X, Yang S, Wang Y. Is early tracheostomy better for severe traumatic brain injury? A meta-analysis. *World Neurosurg*. 2018;112:e324-e330. doi:10.1016/j.wneu.2018.01.043.

28. Perin C, Meroni R, Rega V, Braghetto G, Cerri CG. Parameters influencing tracheostomy decannulation in patients undergoing rehabilitation after severe acquired brain injury (sABI). *Int Arch Otorhinolaryngol*. 2017;21(4):382-389. doi:10.1055/s-0037-1598654.

29. Enrichi C, Battel I, Zanetti C, et al. Clinical criteria for tracheostomy decannulation in subjects with acquired brain injury. *Respir Care*. 2017;62(10):1255-1263. doi:10.4187/respcare.05470.

30. Wagner AK, Arenth PM, Kwasnica C, McCullough EH. Traumatic brain injury. In: Cifu DX, ed. *Braddom's Physical Medicine & Rehabilitation*. 5th ed. Philadelphia, PA: Elsevier; 2016.

31. Kaufman HH, Satterwhite T, McConnell BJ, et al. Deep vein thrombosis and pulmonary embolism in head injured patients. *Angiology*. 1983;34(10):627-638. doi:10.1177/000331978303401001.

32. Nathens AB, McMurray MK, Cushieri J, et al. The practice of venous thromboembolism prophylaxis in the major trauma patient. *J Trauma*. 2007;62(3):557-562; discussion 562-563. doi:10.1097/TA.0b013e318031b5f5.

33. Abdel-Aziz H, Dunham CM, Malik RJ, Hileman BM. Timing for deep vein thrombosis chemoprophylaxis in traumatic brain injury: an evidence-based review. *Crit Care*. 2015;19:96. doi:10.1186/s13054-015-0814-z.

34. Nyquist P, Bautista C, Jichici D, et al. Prophylaxis of venous thrombosis in neurocritical care patients: an evidence-based guideline: a statement for healthcare professionals from the neurocritical care society. *Neurocrit Care*. 2016;24(1):47-60. doi:10.1007/s12028-015-0221-y.

35. Vendantum A, Gopinath SP, Robertson CS. Acute management of traumatic brain injury. In: Eapen BC, Cifu DX, eds. *Rehabilitation After Traumatic Brain Injury*. Philadelphia, PA: Elsevier; 2018.

36. Gould MK, Garcia DA, Wren SM, et al. Prevention of VTE in nonorthopedic surgical patients: Antithrombotic Therapy and Prevention of Thrombosis, 9th ed: American College of Chest Physicians Evidence-Based Clinical Practice Guidelines. *Chest*. 2012;141(suppl 2):e227S-e277S. doi:10.1378/chest.11-2297.

37. Rogers FB, Cipolle MD, Velmahos G, Rozycki G, Luchette FA. Practice management guidelines for the prevention of venous thromboembolism in trauma patients: the EAST practice management guidelines work group. *J Trauma*. 2002;53(1):142-164.

38. Brain Trauma Foundation, American Association of Neurological Surgeons, Congress of Neurological Surgeons, et al. Guidelines for the management of severe traumatic brain injury. II. Hyperosmolar therapy. *J Neurotrauma*. 2007;24(suppl 1):S14-S20. doi:10.1089/neu.2007.9994.

19

GI and Nutrition

KELLY M. CRAWFORD, MD

Neurological injury can cause various gastrointestinal GI and nutritional complications. These problems can often affect recovery of patients with traumatic brain injury (TBI). Appropriate recognition and practices regarding treatment and prevention can help minimize the impact of these complications.

Gastrointestinal Complications

Gastrointestinal complications can affect a TBI patient in the acute and chronic phases of injury. These complications often affect the tolerance of feeding and thus the nutritional health of the patient.

Gastritis

Gastritis is the most common GI complication after head injury, with a reported incidence of 74% to 100%.[1,2] Head injury has been shown to be an independent risk factor for gastric stress erosions and is shown to be correlated to severity of injury.[2] Erosive gastritis is the most common lesion and is often found in the first week of injury.[1]

There is an elevated risk of gastric ulceration after TBI secondary to gastric acid hypersecretion caused by elevated serum gastrin levels.[3]

- Cushing's ulcer: gastroduodenal ulcer produced by elevated intracranial pressure (ICP) caused by an intracranial tumor, head injury, or other space-occupying lesion

Prevention

Agents used to control gastric acid hypersecretion:
- Proton pump inhibitors
- Histamine 2 (H2) receptor antagonists
  - Higher incidence of aspiration pneumonia thought to be secondary to bacterial overgrowth[4,5]

Cytoprotectant:
- Sucralfate
  - Protects gastric mucosa
  - Does not alter the gastric pH

Gastrointestinal Dysfunction

Gastrointestinal motility disturbances are very common in patients with TBI. Dysfunction of the different segments of the GI tract, including prolonged transit and decreased peristalsis, will increase the risk of aspiration and often delay the onset of enteral feedings.

Gastroesophageal Reflux

Acute brain injury is associated with low pressure in the lower esophageal sphincter (LES) and reduced LES tone, increasing the rate of regurgitation and aspiration.[6,7] Prolonged stays in bed in the supine position and increased abdominal pressure in patients with severe constipation also increase the risk of gastroesophageal reflux disease (GERD).[8]

Symptoms
- Sharp or burning chest pain in the sternal region
- Tightness in the chest or upper abdomen
- Regurgitation
- Nausea

Management
- Proton pump inhibitors, H2-receptor antagonists, sucralfate
- Esophago-gastroduodenoscopic (EGD) examination may be indicated if further evaluation is needed.

- Jejunostomy may be considered in patients with particularly low LES tone and difficulty with feeding tolerance.

Delayed Gastric Emptying

Traumatic brain injury causes a delayed but significant decrease in intestinal contractile activity leading to delayed transit. A delay in gastric emptying (GE) may be suspected when there is feeding intolerance with high residuals. Feeding intolerance can be manifested by diarrhea, vomiting, abdominal distention, and increased gastric residuals.

Although the exact mechanisms of GI motility disturbances are not fully recognized, several factors have been proposed:

- Suppressed vagal nerve activity caused by elevated ICP inhibits GE.[9]
- Corticotropin-releasing factor (CRF), a hormone involved in response to stress, can significantly inhibit GE and intestinal motility mainly via a CRF2-mediated pathway.[10]
- Changes in the brain-gut peptides such as vasoactive intestinal peptide (VIP) and cholecystokinin (CCK) in both the plasma and small intestine[11]
- Hyperglycemia may alter GE by decreasing vagal efferent activity in the central nervous system (CNS) and releasing nitric oxide from the myenteric plexus.[12]

Management
Prokinetic Agents
- Metoclopramide
  - Limited by its potential for CNS side effects because of its central dopaminergic blocking activity
- Erythromycin
  - Similar to the GI hormone motilin
  - Used effectively as a motility agent
- Combination of erythromycin and metoclopramide therapy exhibited greater benefits—and less tachyphylaxis—than erythromycin or metoclopramide monotherapy.[13,14]

Reduced Gut Absorption

Many severe TBI patients do not tolerate early enteral nutrition because of reduced gut absorptive capacity (GAC). The reasons for reduced GAC are not completely understood but may be related to delayed gastric emptying, intestinal dysmotility, mucosal villous atrophy, or edema and reduced perfusion.[15] Singh et al found that GAC was severely depressed in trauma patients soon after injury but returned to normal 1 to 3 weeks later.[16]

- Rat studies demonstrated that the absorption of proteins, carbohydrates, and lipids significantly decreased within 2 weeks after TBI.[17] Additionally, animal studies found intestinal mucosal epithelium may develop apoptosis at 3 hours after TBI, and at 24 hours postinjury, the villous height and surface area decreased significantly and further declined to the degree of mucosal atrophy within a week after injury.[18]
- Dehydration and overhydration may potentially hamper the absorptive function of the intestinal mucosa because of splanchnic hypoperfusion or edema of the GI tract.[19]

Bowel Complications

Bowel Incontinence

Bowel and bladder incontinence have been observed, especially in lesions involving the frontal lobes. Individuals with TBI have a high incidence of fecal incontinence.[20] Volitional control of bowel function is controlled by the frontal lobes.

Incontinence is most often related to cognitive awareness, with control of bowel movements improving as cognition improves. Reflexes, spinal reflex arc, and sensation are typically intact. Decreased awareness of the need to defecate and decreased control of the external sphincter result in the inability to inhibit defecation.[21]

- In one study, using data from the Traumatic Brain Injury Model Systems National Database, the incidences of fecal incontinence were 68% at admission to an inpatient rehabilitation, 12.4% at the time of discharge from rehabilitation units, and 5.2% at 1-year follow-up[22]

Diarrhea

Diarrhea is not a common finding of the TBI population, although with this population, there are multiple causes that should be considered.

Various Etiologies
- Prolonged hospitalization and/or concurrent use of antibiotics
  - Workup should include stool evaluation, testing for *Clostridium difficile*
- Diarrhea-inducing medications
- Enteral tube feeding
  - Diarrhea is the most common complication of enteral tube feeding
  - Formula composition
  - Rate infusion
  - Enteral formula contamination
- Altered bacterial flora
- Hypoalbuminemia
  - Serum albumin level less than 2.6 g/dL is correlated with diarrhea[23]

Complications
- Electrolyte abnormalities
- Dehydration

Constipation

Constipation often develops in patients who are nonambulatory, who have delayed gastric motility or diabetic autonomic neuropathy, and those who use chronic pain medications such as opioids.[8] It can be a much more serious problem in the TBI and spinal cord injury (SCI) patient population, as it can lead to autonomic dysreflexia, which can be a life-threatening event.

Bowel Regimens/Programs
- High-fiber diet
- Daily stimulant laxative
  - Long-term use of Senna products has been associated with melanosis coli.
- Daily stool softener
- Enema, suppository

Complications
- Poor appetite
- Nausea or vomiting
- Abdominal discomfort
- Bowel obstruction or rupture

Gallbladder Disease

Posttraumatic acute acalculous cholecystitis is a potentially serious complication that may develop among patients hospitalized for trauma. The cause is likely multifactorial, often related to hypotension, sepsis, or biliary stasis with subsequent cystic duct obstruction. Most report symptoms usually begin between 1 week and 1 month after trauma.[24]

Suspicion should be raised if patient exhibits:
- Unexplained fever, vomiting, abdominal distention, ileus, right upper quadrant pain, and/or developing intolerance to oral or tube feedings
- Elevated serum bilirubin, alkaline phosphatase, liver enzymes, and leukocytosis

Best diagnosed with:
- Hydroxy iminodiacetic acid (HIDA) scan
- Ultrasound or abdominal computed tomography (CT) scan

Treatment options:
- Cholecystectomy
- Broad spectrum antibiotics

Pancreatitis

Elevations of serum amylase and lipase have been described in patients with head injury.
- Although no clinical signs or symptoms of pancreatitis may be present, hyperamylasemia has been reported in 19% to 41% of patients with severe head injury and in 45% to 60% of patients with intracranial bleeding.[25,26]
  - Proposed causes have included vagal stimulation, altered modulation of the central control of pancreatic enzyme release, and release of cholecystokinin from the brain.[23,24]

Nutritional Considerations

Metabolic Alterations

Traumatic brain injury can stimulate tremendous changes in metabolism. The degree of this hypermetabolic state is proportional to the severity of injury and motor dysfunction.[27] The result of these alterations is systemic catabolism, which leads to hyperglycemia, protein wasting, and increased energy demand.

The injured brain stimulates the secretion of many hormones that affect metabolic function, including hypothalamic–pituitary axis products such as adrenocorticotrophin releasing hormone (ACTH), growth hormone, prolactin, vasopressin, and cortisol as a natural response to stress. Glucagon and catecholamines are also released in excess.[28]

Additional metabolic demands can be increased by factors such as hyperventilation, increased cardiac output, fever, restlessness, seizures, and infections. Several studies have revealed that patients with head injuries can have an increase of 120% to 200% of resting energy expenditure and twice the normal oxygen consumption.[29]

Hyperglycemia

Catecholamine levels reflect the severity of head injury. Catecholamines help support blood pressure and cardiac output but also increase basal metabolism, oxygen consumption, proteolysis, muscle wasting, glycogenolysis, and hyperglycemia.

Hyperglycemia (>200 mg/dL) is a predictor of poor outcome and is associated with an increased morbidity and mortality in TBI patients.[30] TBI patients, however, have demonstrated some differences in brain glucose metabolism and likely require slightly higher glucose values to ensure appropriate brain metabolism.[31]
- Maintenance of serum glucose values between 80 and 110 mg/dL may result in cerebrospinal fluid (CSF) glucose values below the normal threshold.[32]

The precise goal glucose range is not well defined for TBI patients. In practice, either no guidance at all or excessively aggressive protocols are likely to lead to more hypoglycemia, which may be problematic.
- The American Society for Parenteral and Enteral Nutrition (ASPEN) recommends controlling blood glucose in the range of 100 to 150 mg/dL to improve CSF glucose values and reduce the risk of hypoglycemia.[28,33]

Nutritional Support

Nutrition Assessment

Brain Trauma Foundation guidelines recommend that moderate to severe TBI patients should receive basal caloric replacement at least by the fifth day and at most by the seventh day postinjury to decrease mortality.[34] Prompt assessment of the nutrition requirements is needed to establish goals for optimal calories, protein, and fluids. The hypermetabolic response can be prolonged and is usually correlated with injury severity, thus the measured resting energy expenditure is higher in those patients with more severe brain injury.[35]

Nutritional Assessment: Calories

Accurate assessment of caloric requirements in TBI patients is important in providing adequate nutritional support. Delayed nutritional support may result in negative outcomes such as poor wound healing, malnutrition, impaired organ function, and altered immunological status.[28]

Unfortunately, predicting the nutritional needs of a patient with TBI is not simple. Many of the various equations used to predict energy expenditure are not specific to TBI and have a degree of inaccuracy.[28]

- Indirect calorimetry is the current "gold standard" for determining energy expenditure in TBI patients.[28]

Nutrition status will often fluctuate during recovery and require periodic reassessment of metabolic needs to prevent underfeeding. More calories may also be required if the patient has additional injuries and/or stress, especially long bone fractures or sepsis.

For example:

- Comatose TBI patients have increased resting metabolic expenditure of 120% to 140% because of hypercatabolic response.[31]
- Pharmacologically induced coma patients, however, may have a resting metabolic expenditure as low as 80%.[36]

Close monitoring is also needed to prevent overfeeding. Metabolic needs will often decrease as the patient's medical stability improves. Prolonged or excessive overfeeding can be harmful as well.

Overfeeding can result in metabolic complications such as[28]:

- Hyperglycemia
- Refeeding-like syndrome with electrolyte derangements
- Hepatic steatosis
- Pulmonary compromise with difficulty weaning from the ventilator
- Obesity

Nutritional Assessment: Protein

Inflammatory mediators and catecholamines trigger hypercatabolism in TBI patients, often resulting in protein breakdown. Protein catabolism appears to be related to the severity of injury and appears to peak 8 to 14 days after injury.[37]

- Recommendations suggest protein provision ranging between 1.5 and 2 g/kg per day for acute TBI patients to account for the excess catabolism.[38]

Routine monitoring and adjustment of protein doses should be done during TBI recovery to ensure safety and efficacy.

Nutritional Assessment: Fluids and Electrolytes

Monitoring of blood pressure and volume status is necessary in patients with moderate to severe TBI. TBI patients often require intravenous fluid resuscitation after injury to maintain adequate mean arterial and cerebral perfusion pressures.

Excessive fluid volumes, however, may also be harmful. Excessive fluid resuscitation may decrease cerebral compliance and increase brain edema[39] Large volumes of salt-free water and other hypotonic fluids should be avoided to prevent exacerbation of cerebral edema and hyponatremia[31]

Enteral Versus Parenteral Nutrition Support

Many patients with moderate to severe TBI have feeding intolerance secondary to intubation, dysphagia, or altered mental status and require an alternative means of feeding. Parenteral nutrition (PN) has been associated with increased risk of infection, immunosuppression, hyperglycemia, hepatic steatosis, and diminished gastric mucosa integrity. Enteral nutrition (EN), however, has demonstrated protective effects against infection, a decrease in critical care days, and improved mortality when administered appropriately.[7]

Parenteral nutrition should be considered in those who do not tolerate enteral nutrition or when safe enteral access cannot be achieved.

- Central venous access is required for infusion of the hyperosmolar solutions of parenteral solutions.
- Precaution must be taken to prevent infection and hyperglycemia, particularly in patients receiving PN.

The TBI patient should be reassessed frequently for the ability to swallow and continued need for temporary or longer-term feeding access. The use of a percutaneous endoscopic gastrostomy (PEG) tube is indicated when a patient persists with dysphagia for a prolonged period. TBI patients are likely to tolerate gastric feedings as the acute phase subsides (2–3 weeks).[40] Optimal timing of PEG placement varies pending stabilization of the patient's clinical status, established feeding tolerance, and demonstration of adequate bowel function.

Timing of Nutrition

Early nutritional support is an important goal in treating the TBI patient. The American Society of Parenteral and Enteral Nutrition (ASPEN) and Society of Critical Care Medicine (SCCM) guidelines recommend EN be initiated within 24 to 48 hours for critically ill adults, as long as patients are hemodynamically stable.[33] Early nutritional support can prevent breakdown of protein and fat stores, reduce inflammatory response, decrease infections, and improve neurological outcomes. In addition, early administration of EN promotes gut integrity and motility,[33] whereas a long period of starvation is associated with mucosal atrophy and reduced enzymatic activity.[23]

Feeding to goal within 2 to 3 days has been associated with accelerated neurological recovery and a decreased incidence of death caused by infection.[41] Once feeding access has been established:

- Administer a calorically dense EN product as early as possible.[33]
- Provide at least 18% to 25% of calories as protein to account for protein catabolism.[31]
- Frequently monitor patient tolerance to EN rate and advance as tolerated.
- Reevaluate metabolic needs of the patient throughout recovery.

Nutrient Supplementation

Omega-3

Some animal studies have suggested that docosahexaenoic acid (DHA) and eicosapentaenoic acid (EPA) supplementation may have neuroprotective benefits through inhibition of the central proinflammatory response. However, the role of omega-3 supplementation on the treatment or prevention of the detrimental effects of human neurological injuries is currently undefined.[42]

Zinc

Available clinical data suggest that zinc deficiency should be prevented to enhance the potential for neurological recovery in the acute care setting.[42]
- Moderate to severe TBI
  - Acute increases in urinary zinc excretion and significant decreases in serum zinc levels have been shown to be proportional to the severity of injury.[43]
  - Zinc supplementation has been associated with increased visceral proteins and improvements in Glasgow Coma Scale (GCS) scores 2 weeks after start of treatment.[44]

- Mild TBI
  - There have been no clinical trials to address the efficacy of zinc supplementation in mild TBI.

Vitamin D

Research findings have suggested that vitamin D supplementation may serve as a role in treatment of TBI as a neuroprotective adjuvant with progesterone.
- Severe TBI
  - Treatment with the combination therapy of vitamin D and progesterone demonstrated significantly greater improvements in GCS values and Glasgow Outcome Scale (GOS) values.[45]
- Mild TBI
  - No clinical trials have addressed the efficacy of vitamin D supplementation in mild TBI.

Review Questions

1. A 22-year-old man with traumatic brain injury (TBI) and dysphagia was recently started on bolus tube feedings through his percutaneous endoscopic gastrostomy tube. Following the boluses, he complains of burning pain behind his breastbone and associated nausea. He also has associate coughing after the feeds. What is the most likely etiology of his condition?
   a. Suppressed vagal nerve activity
   b. Reduced lower esophageal sphincter
   c. Reduced gut absorptive capacity
   d. Mucosal villous atrophy

2. A 53-year-old woman with TBI and a history of diabetes mellitus type 2 has been found to have elevated gastric residual volumes, abdominal distention, and nausea. What treatment options have studies shown to be most beneficial in this condition?
   a. Metoclopramide
   b. Erythromycin
   c. Erythromycin and metoclopramide
   d. Cisapride

3. What is the most appropriate approach in attempting to control hyperglycemia during nutritional support for a brain injury patient?
   a. Blood glucose concentrations should be maintained above 200 mg/dL.
   b. Blood glucose concentrations should be maintained at 80 to 100 mg/dL.
   c. Blood glucose concentrations should be maintained at 110 to 180 mg/dL.
   d. During nutritional support, it is not recommended to monitor blood glucose concentrations.

Answers on page 390.
Access the full list of questions and answers online. Available on ExpertConsult.com

References

1. Kamada T, Fusamoto H, Kawano S, Noguchi M, Hiramatsu K. Gastrointestinal bleeding following head injury: a clinical study of 433 cases. *J Trauma.* 1977;17(1):44-47.
2. Brown TH, Davidson PF, Larson GM. Acute gastritis occurring within 24 hours of severe head injury. *Gastrointest Endosc.* 1989;35:37-40.
3. Idjadi F, Robbins R, Stahl WM, Essiet G. Prospective study of gastric secretion in stressed patients with intracranial injury. *J Trauma.* 1971;11(8):681-688.
4. Driks MR, Craven DE, Celli BR, et al. Nosocomial pneumonia in intubated patients given sucralfate as compared with antacids or histamine type 2 blockers. The role of gastric colonization. *N Engl J Med.* 1987;317:1376-1382.
5. Huang J, Cao Y, Lio C, Wu L, Gao F. Effect of histamine-2-receptor antagonists versus sucralfate on stress ulcer prophylaxis among critical care patients: a meta-analysis of 10 randomized controlled trials. *Crit Care.* 2010;14(5):R194.
6. Saxe JM, Ledgerwood AM, Lucas CE, Lucas WF. Lower esophageal sphincter dysfunction precludes safe gastric feeding after head injury. *J Trauma.* 1994;37(4):581-584; discussion 584-586.
7. Kirby DF, Creasey L, Parisian KR. Gastrointestinal and nutritional issues. In: Zasler N, Katz D, Zafont R, eds. *Brain Injury Medicine: Principles and Practice.* New York, NY: Demos Medical Publishing; 2007:283-301.

8. Singal AK, Betesh N, Korsten MA. Gastrointestinal diseases. In: Christian A, ed. *Medical Management of Adults with Neurologic Disabilities*. New York, NY: Demos Medical Publishing; 2009.

9. Norton JA, Ott LG, McLain C, et al. Intolerance to enteral feeding in the brain-injured patient. *J Neurosurg*. 1988;68(1):62-66.

10. Stengel A, Tache Y. Neuroendocrine control of the gut during stress: corticotropin-releasing factor signaling pathways in the spotlight. *Annu Rev Physiol*. 2009;71:219-239.

11. Hang CH, Shi JX, Li JS, Wu W, Li WQ, Yin HX. Levels of vasoactive intestinal peptide, cholecystokinin and calcitonin gene-related peptide in plasma and jejunum of rats following traumatic brain injury and underlying significance in gastrointestinal dysfunction. *World J Gastroenterol*. 2004;10 (6):875-880.

12. Horowitz M, Jones KL, Wishart JM, Maddox AF, Harding PE, Chatterton BE. Relationships between gastric emptying, intragastric meal distribution and blood glucose concentrations in diabetes mellitus. *J Nucl Med*. 1995;36(12):2220-2228.

13. Dickerson RN, Mitchell JN, Morgan LM, et al. Disparate response to metoclopramide therapy for gastric feeding intolerance in trauma patients with and without traumatic brain injury. *JPEN J Parenter Enteral Nutr*. 2009;33(6):646-655.

14. Nguyen NQ, Chapman M, Fraser RJ, Bryant LK, Burgstad C, Holloway RH. Prokinetic therapy for feed intolerance in critical illness: one drug or two? *Crit Care Med*. 2007;35(11): 2561-2567.

15. Chapman MJ, Fraser RJL, Matthews G, et al. Glucose absorption and gastric emptying in critical illness. *Crit Care*. 2009;13(4):R140.

16. Singh G, Harkema JM, Mayberry AJ, Chaudry IH. Severe depression of gut absorptive capacity in patients following trauma or sepsis. *J Trauma*. 1994;36(6):803-809.

17. Yu XY, Yin HH, Zhu JC. Increased gut absorptive capacity in rats with severe head injury after feeding with probiotics. *Nutrition*. 2011;27(1):100-107.

18. Hang CH, Shi JX, Sun BW, Li JS. Apoptosis and functional changes of dipeptide transporter (pepT1) in the rate small intestine after traumatic brain injury. *J Surg Res*. 2007;137(1):53-60.

19. Btaiche IF, Chan LN, Pleva M, Kraft MD. Critical illness, gastrointestinal complications, and medications therapy during enteral feeding in critically ill adult patients. *Nutr Clin Pract*. 2010;25(1):32-49.

20. Nakayama H, Jorgensen HS, Pedersen PM, Raaschou HO, Olsen TS. Prevalence and risk factors of incontinence after stroke. The Copenhagen Stroke Study. Stroke 1997;28(1): 58–62.

21. Cifu DX, Caruso D. Chapter 26, Bladder Issues In: Buschbacher RM, ed. Rehabilitation Medicine Quick Reference: *Traumatic Brain Injury*. New York, NY: Demos Medical Publishing; 2010.

22. Foxx-Orenstein A, Kolakowsky-Hayner S, Marwitz JH, et al. Incidence, risk factors, and outcomes of fecal incontinence after acute brain injury: findings from the Traumatic Brain Injury Model Systems national database. *Arch Phys Med Rehabil*. 2003;84(2):231-237.

23. Tan M, Zhu JC, Yin HH. Enteral nutrition in patients with severe traumatic brain injury: reasons for intolerance and medical management. *Br J Neurosurg*. 2011;25(1):2-8.

24. Branch Jr CL, Albertson DA, Kelly DL. Post-traumatic acalculous cholecystitis on a neurosurgical service. *Neurosurgery*. 1983; 12(1):98-101.

25. Bouwman DL, Altshuler J, Weaver DW. Hyperamylasemia: a result of intracranial bleeding. *Surgery*. 1983;94(2):318-323.

26. Liu KJ, Atten MJ, Lichtor T, et al. Serum amylase and lipase elevation is associated with intracranial events. *Am Surg*. 2001;67(3):215-220.

27. Fruin AH, Taylor C, Pettis MS. Caloric requirements in patients with severe head injuries. *Surg Neurol*. 1986;25:25-28.

28. Cook AM, Peppard A, Magnuson B. Nutrition considerations in traumatic brain injury. *Nutr Clin Pract*. 2008;23:608-620.

29. Kaufman HH, Timberlake G, Voelker J. Medical complications of head injury. *Med Clin North Am*. 1993;77(1):43-60.

30. Young B, Ott L, Dempsey R, Haack D, Tibbs P. Relationship between admission hyperglycemia and neurologic outcome of severely brain-injured patients. *Ann Surg*. 1989;210(4):466-472.

31. Cook AM, Magnuson BW. Nutritional considerations. In: Zollman F, ed. *Manual of Traumatic Brain Injury Assessment and Management*. 2nd ed. New York, NY: Demos Medical Publishing; 2016:202-213.

32. Vespa P, Boonyaputthikul R, McArthur DL, et al. Intensive insulin therapy reduces microdialysis glucose values without altering glucose utilization or improving the lactate/pyruvate ratio after traumatic brain injury. *Crit Care Med*. 2006;34:850-856.

33. McClave SA, Martindale RG, Vanek VW, et al. Guidelines for the provision and assessment of nutrition support therapy in the adult critically ill trauma patient: Society of Critical Care Medicine (SCCM) and American Society for Parenteral and Enteral Nutrition (ASPEN). *JPEN J Parenter Enteral Nutr*. 2009;33(3):277-316.

34. Brain Trauma Foundation. Guidelines form the management of severe traumatic brain injury. *Neurosurgery*. 2017;80(1):6-15.

35. Clifton GL, Robertson CS, Grossman RG, Hodge S. Foltz R, Garza C. The metabolic response to severe head injury. *J Neurosurg*. 1984;60(4):687-696.

36. McCall M, Jeejeebhoy K, Pencharz P, Moulton R. Effect of neuromuscular blockade on energy expenditure in patients with severe head injury. *J Parenter Enteral Nutr*. 2003;27(1):27-35.

37. Young B, Ott L, Yingling B, McClain C. Nutrition and brain injury. *J Neurotrauma*. 1992;9(suppl 1):S375-S383.

38. Hatton J, Ziegler TR. Nutritional support of the neurosurgical patient. In: Tindall G, Cooper PR, Barrow DL, eds. *The Practice of Neurosurgery*. Baltimore, MD: Williams & Wilkins; 1998:381-396.

39. Hariri RJ, Firlick AD, Shepard SR, et al. Traumatic brain injury, hemorrhagic shock, and fluid resuscitation: effects on intracranial pressure and brain compliance. *J Neurosurg*. 1993;79:421-427.

40. Ward EC, Green K, Morton AL. Patterns and predictors of swallowing resolution following adult traumatic brain injury. *J Head Trauma Rehabil*. 2007;22:184-191.

41. Borzotta AP, Pennings J, Papsadero B, et al. Enteral versus parenteral nutrition after severe closed head injury. *J Trauma*. 1994;37:459-468.

42. Scrimgeour AG, Condlin ML. Nutritional treatment for traumatic brain injury. *J Neurotrauma*. 2014;31:989-999.

43. McClain CJ, Twyman DL, Ott LG, et al. Serum and urine zinc response in head-injured patients. *J Neurosurg*. 1986;64:224-230.

44. Young B, Ott L, Kasarskis E, et al. Zinc supplementation is associated with improved neurologic recovery rate and visceral protein levels of patients with severe closed head injury. *J Neurotrauma*. 1996;13:25-34.

45. Aminmansour B, Nikbakht H, Ghorbani A, et al. Comparison of the administration of progesterone versus progesterone and vitamin D in improvement of outcomes in patients with traumatic brain injury: a randomized clinical trial with placebo group. *Adv Biomed Res*. 2012;1:58.

20
Genitourinary

KELLY M. CRAWFORD, MD

Voiding disorders are common among patients with traumatic brain injury (TBI). Such voiding disorders are referred to as *neurogenic bladder dysfunction*. Urological disorders in TBI can range from 32% to 70% depending on the location of the injury within the brain.[1]

Neuroanatomy

The neuroanatomy of normal voiding can be divided into the central and peripheral nervous systems. The relevant central nervous system structures include:

- Frontal lobe of the brain
- Pontine micturition center (PMC)
- Spinal cord

The frontal lobe maintains bladder continence by preventing bladder contraction. This is accomplished by inhibitory signals sent from the frontal lobe to the detrusor muscle, preventing bladder contraction and deactivating signals to the PMC, which diminishes the urge to urinate. The PMC is a major relay center between the brain and the bladder. PMC stimulation is an excitatory response that results in efficient voiding by coordinating simultaneous bladder contraction and sphincter relaxation. Involuntary voiding is suppressed by a cascade of inhibitory signaling initiated by the brain.[2]

Neurogenic Bladder

The most common bladder abnormality after brain injury is incontinence.[3] The incidence of urinary incontinence is 62%,[4] and that of urinary retention is 8% to 9%.[4,5] Urinary incontinence is associated with poorer admission and discharge functional status and longer rehabilitation length of stay.[4]

Urinary dysfunction in TBI patients varies based on the area of brain or brainstem involved. Initial voiding dysfunction may be caused by a cerebral shock with an initial period of detrusor areflexia. With lesions above the PMC, the most common chronic urinary dysfunction is involuntary bladder contractions (detrusor hyperactivity). Patients will have detrusor hyperreflexia (spastic bladder) because of an uninhibited and intact reflex pathway. Voiding is characterized by urgency with or without incontinence because of the loss of cortical tonic inhibition to the bladder. In patients with more isolated brainstem injuries involving areas at or below the PMC, detrusor sphincter dyssynergia (DSD) may also occur. DSD is characterized by intermittent or sustained failure of relaxation of the urinary sphincter during a bladder contraction.[2] Patients with lesions in only the basal ganglia or thalamus have normal sphincter function and may gain urinary control.[2] True urgency incontinence with reduced bladder sensation is associated with global underperfusion of the cerebral cortex, especially the right frontal areas.[6]

Clinical Features

- When caused by unawareness with poor volitional control, there will most commonly be bladder accidents when the bladder is filled (approximately 250 cc).

- Increased control of urinary continence is typically seen as cognition, communication, and behavior improve.
- A spastic bladder will often result in significant urinary retention caused by a spastic external sphincter. Without intervention, the bladder will only empty at large volumes (>500 cc) related to overflow incontinence, and there will be an elevated risk of hydronephrosis.[3]

Assessment

Postvoid residual (PVR) measurements
- PVR urine can be determined by catheterization or by using a bedside ultrasound machine.

Anorectal examination:
- Should include an assessment of trauma, perirectal sensation, and the presence or absence of volitional rectal sphincter contraction, as well as an evaluation of sacral reflexes (anal wink and bulbocavernosus reflex)
- Is useful in predicting the potential for regaining bladder control and classifying upper or lower motor neuron patterns[2,3]

Medication review:
- Retention can often be related to medications

Blood urea nitrogen and serum creatinine:
- Measure kidney function

Diagnostic testing:
- Urinalysis with culture and sensitivity
- Renal and bladder sonography to evaluate for the presence of vesicoureteral reflux or stones.
- Urodynamic testing measures pressure within the bladder during both storage and voiding[2]

Management of Neurogenic Bladder

Bladder Management

Clean Intermittent Catheterization

- Clean intermittent catheterization (CIC) is generally accepted as the best and safest long-term bladder management method short of controlled urination.[7]
- CIC is typically performed four to six times daily with a goal to obtain 500 cc or less per catheterization by adjusting the frequency.
- Patients with adequate cognition and hand function should be educated on how to perform self-CIC. Others may need to rely on the assistance of caregivers.
- The patient should be monitored for return of voiding.
- If spontaneous voiding does return, PVRs should be measured to verify adequate bladder emptying. PVR volumes should be less than 100 cc.[2]
- The most common problems associated with CIC are urinary tract infection (UTI), urethral trauma, and incontinence between catheterizations, but studies have shown no significant increase in urinary complications when proper cleaning techniques are practiced.[8]

Timed Voiding

- Schedule for regular bladder emptying, typically every 3 to 4 hours.
- Timed voiding may assist with behavioral training in cognitively impaired patients.

Reflex Voiding

- Reflex voiding requires intact sacral reflexes, and voiding occurs at inappropriately low bladder volumes and may occur without voluntary control.
- In persons with lesions above the PMC, coordinated relaxation of the sphincter mechanism is present and voiding is generally efficient, even if uncontrolled.
- A condom catheter may be indicated for male patients who are incontinent between scheduled voids but must be monitored closely for penile skin breakdown.

Indwelling Catheters

- There is a limited role for indwelling Foley catheterization in the TBI population.
- Indwelling catheters may be indicated for acute management or short-term management of urinary retention or if fluid output must be closely monitored.
- Complications from Foley catheters have been well documented, including UTI, epididymitis and prostatitis, urethral strictures, traumatic hypospadias, urethral incompetence in women, urethritis, bladder calculi, and development of a small, poorly compliant bladder.[9]

Medications to Manage Neurogenic Bladder

Pharmacotherapy is rarely indicated for voiding dysfunction in TBI. Medications, however, have been used occasionally to treat the effects of neurogenic bladder in the TBI population. These include anticholinergic agents, alpha blockers, antispasmodics, tricyclic antidepressants, and rarely cholinergic agents.

Anticholinergic Agents

- Hyoscyamine, oxybutynin, tolterodine, darifenacin, solifenacin, trospium
- Used in the treatment of hyperreflexic bladder or urge incontinence by inhibiting involuntary bladder contractions
- Muscarinic cholinergic receptor antagonists that prevent uninhibited bladder contractions
- Potential adverse effects:
  - Dry mouth
  - Blurred vision
  - Palpitations
  - Drowsiness
  - Constipation
  - Dry Eyes
  - Dizziness
  - Cognitive Changes (confusion)
  - Urinary retention

- Caution in TBI patients given potential negative effect on cognition

Alpha-1 Blockers

- Tamsulosin, terazosin, doxazosin, prazosin
- Used for smooth muscle inhibition at the bladder neck and in the prostate
- Help open the bladder neck, especially with the reflex voiding management method
- Potential adverse effects:
  - Orthostatic hypotension
  - Dizziness, rhinitis
  - Retrograde ejaculation

Tricyclic Antidepressants

- Amitriptyline, imipramine
- Inhibit reuptake of norepinephrine and serotonin at presynaptic neurons; have both peripheral alpha-adrenergic and central anticholinergic properties, enabling urine storage by reducing bladder contractility and increasing outlet resistance
- In some cases have been used in the treatment of hyperreflexic bladder with incontinence and may have multiple benefits when used in patients with depression or chronic neuropathic pain[2]
- Potential adverse effects:
  - Dry mouth
  - Excessive drowsiness
  - Constipation
  - Blurred vision
  - Tachycardia
  - Urinary retention

Antispasmodic Agents

- Baclofen, diazepam, botulinum toxin
- Used for bladder spasticity with DSD
- Potentially relax both the urinary bladder, by exerting a direct spasmolytic action on the smooth muscle of the bladder, and the striated external sphincter
- Reported to increase bladder capacity and decrease urge incontinence
- Potential adverse effects:
  - Sedation
  - Muscle weakness
  - Confusion
- Caution in TBI patients given sedation and potential negative effect on cognition

Cholinergic Agents

- Bethanechol
- Used in the treatment of areflexic or underactive bladder
- Typically, limited role in TBI patient given that the most common voiding dysfunction in this population is bladder hyperactivity
- Muscarinic cholinergic receptor agonists that stimulate the bladder to empty

- Potential adverse effects:
  - Dizziness/lightheadedness
  - Diarrhea
  - Bradycardia
  - Increased salivation
  - Sweating
  - Watery eyes
- They should not be used in patients with bladder outlet obstruction, including enlarged prostate or DSD, as it may lead to elevated intravesical pressure.

Medical Complications of Neurogenic Bladder

The treatment and prevention of medical complications are essential in the management of neurogenic bladder. Urological complications include skin irritation and breakdown, UTI, urinary stone disease, vesicoureteral reflux, renal failure, bladder cancer, and urethral strictures and trauma.

Skin Irritation and Breakdown

There is an elevated risk with incontinence and/or with use of condom catheter:
- Must monitor skin integrity closely and frequently
- Meticulous perineal care
- Protective skin agents and interventions should be used.

Urinary Tract Infections

A neurogenic bladder with incomplete bladder emptying can lead to increased frequency of UTIs and hydronephrosis.
- A UTI can lead to confusion, agitation, and increased neurological symptoms.

Symptoms

- Urinary retention
- Urinary incontinence
- Urinary frequency/urgency
- Burning with urination
- Suprapubic tenderness
- Cloudy or foul-smelling urine

Testing

- Urinalysis with culture and sensitivities
- Complete blood count, basic metabolic panel, hepatic profile

Treatment

- Antibiotics (intravenous or oral)
- Supportive measures
  - Hydration
  - Analgesia for pain (phenazopyridine)
  - Measure postvoid residuals to ensure adequate emptying
  - Catheterization for urinary retention

Vesicoureteral Reflux and Renal Failure

Vesicoureteral reflux may result from high detrusor pressures, which are typically related to severe DSD.[7]

- Vesicoureteral reflux can lead to pyelonephritis and renal failure, particularly in the presence of recurrent infections.[10]
- The occurrence of renal failure in patients with neurogenic bladder has substantially decreased because of improvements in bladder management.[2]

Urinary Stone Disease

Patients with longstanding neurogenic bladder are predisposed to the development of urinary stone disease, especially in the presence of vesicoureteral reflux and recurrent infections.[11]

- Additional risk factors:
  - Hypercalcemia
  - Associated complete spinal injury
  - History of prior stones
  - Sepsis
  - Advanced age
  - Use of indwelling catheter(s)

- Struvite stones and calcium oxalate stones account for 90% of calculi in patients with neurogenic bladder.[12]
- The incidence of kidney stone formation is highest in patients with indwelling catheters.[2]
- Bladder stones are significantly associated with indwelling catheters: 2.3% of intermittent catheter users had bladder stones in the first month, whereas 8.8% of indwelling catheter users developed bladder stones in their first month.[8]

Cancer

Bladder cancer is associated with chronic indwelling catheters.[13] The risk of bladder cancer has been related to the duration of chronic indwelling catheter use and attributed to chronic irritation of the bladder wall and infection of the bladder leading to dysplastic change and squamous metaplasia.[13,14]

- Squamous cell carcinoma is the most common type of bladder cancer seen in this population. It is aggressive and is often metastatic at diagnosis with an associated poor prognosis.[13]
- Screening
  - Cystoscopy is recommended after 5 to 10 years of indwelling catheter use, then every other year.[2]

Review Questions

1. Which of these statements is true regarding neurogenic bladder in a patient with traumatic brain injury (TBI)?
   a. It most commonly presents as urinary retention in the brain-injured patient.
   b. It will often involve detrusor hyporeflexia because of an uninhibited and intact reflex pathway.
   c. Voiding dysfunction is characterized by varying degrees of urge incontinence.
   d. It is often best treated with an indwelling Foley catheter.

2. A 46-year-old man with TBI recently had his Foley catheter removed before transferring to the inpatient rehabilitation unit. He has started to void spontaneously but also has intermittent episodes of recorded urinary incontinence throughout the day. What is the most appropriate initial assessment of his urinary incontinence?
   a. Perform urodynamic testing to assess bladder pressures.
   b. Order blood urea nitrogen and serum creatinine to assess kidney function.

   c. Order urinalysis and urine culture to assess for infection.
   d. Measure postvoid residuals to verify adequate bladder emptying.

3. A 25-year-old woman with severe TBI has been having frequent episodes of urinary incontinence throughout the day. Her recorded postvoid residuals have been less than 100 cc. These episodes, however, have caused disruptions in her inpatient rehabilitation therapy sessions. What is the best initial bladder management program for this patient?
   a. Start a clean intermittent catharization program every 6 hours.
   b. Start a timed voiding schedule with nursing every 3 to 4 hours.
   c. Place an indwelling Foley catheter.
   d. Start patient on an antispasmodic medication

Answers on page 391.
Access the full list of questions and answers online.
Available on ExpertConsult.com

References

1. Wein AJ, Kavoussi LR, Novick AC, Partin AW, Peters CA. *Campbell–Walsh Urology.* 9th ed. Philadelphia, PA: Saunders; 2007.
2. Schneider H, Stein A. Genitourinary system. In: Christian A, ed. *Medical Management of Adults with Neurologic Disabilities.* New York, NY: Demos Medical Publishing; 2009.
3. Cifu DX, Caruso D. Chapter 26, Bladder Issues In: Buschbacher RM, ed. Rehabilitation Medicine Quick Reference: Traumatic Brain Injury. New York, NY: Demos Medical Publishing; 2010.
4. Chua K, Chuo A, Kong KH. Urinary incontinence after traumatic brain injury: incidence, outcomes and correlates. *Brain Inj.* 2003;17(6):469-478.

5. Mysiw WJ, Fugate LP, Clinchot DM. Assessment, early rehabilitation intervention, and tertiary prevention. In: Zasler N, Katz D, Zafont R, eds. *Brain Injury Medicine: Principles and Practice.* New York, NY: Demos Medical Publishing; 2007:283-301.

6. Griffiths D. Clinical studies of cerebral and urinary tract function in elderly people with urinary incontinence. *Behav Brain Res.* 1998;92(2):151-155.

7. Weld KJ, Graney MJ, Dmochowski RR. Differences in bladder compliance with time and association of bladder management with compliance in spinal cord injured patients. *J Urol.* 2000;163:1228-1233.

8. Braddom RL. *Physical Medicine and Rehabilitation.* 3rd ed. Philadelphia, PA: Saunders; 2007.

9. Weld KJ, Wall BM, Mangold TA, et al. Influences on renal function in chronic spinal cord injured patients. *J Urol.* 2000;164(5):1490-1493.

10. Hackler RH, Katz PG. Management of common problems in spinal cord injured patients. *Am Urol Assoc Update Ser.* 1991;10(6):42-47.

11. Hall MK, Hackler RH, Zampieri TA, et al. Renal calculi in spinal cord-injured patients: association with reflux, bladder stones, and Foley catheter drainage. *Urology.* 1989;34:126-128.

12. Griffith DP, Khonsari F, Skurnick JH, et al. A randomized trial of acetohydroxamic acid for the treatment and prevention of infection-induced urinary stones in spinal cord injury patients. *J Urol.* 1988;140(2):318-324.

13. Kaufmann JM, Fam B, Jacobs SC, et al. Bladder cancer and squamous metaplasia in spinal cord injury patients. *J Urol.* 1977;118:967-971.

14. Goble NM, Clarke TJ, Hammonds JC. Histological changes in the urinary bladder secondary to urethral catheterization. *Br J Urol.* 1989;63:354-357.

Soft Tissue and Orthopedic Conditions

G. Sunny Sharma, MD, AND Sanjog Pangarkar, MD

This chapter identifies common soft tissue and musculoskeletal conditions that may be encountered in the treatment of patients with traumatic brain injury (TBI). An overview is provided on these topics:
- Background, diagnosis, and treatment strategies for heterotopic ossification
- Fracture implications and healing
- Musculoskeletal injuries of the shoulder and low back
- Use of musculoskeletal imaging

Heterotopic Ossification

The formation of mature lamellar bone in ectopic extraskeletal regions is termed *heterotopic ossification* (HO). This condition can occur in periarticular and soft tissue areas and be further divided into traumatic HO and neurogenic HO (NHO).
- Etiologies of traumatic HO include fracture, joint replacement, and soft tissue injury.
- Etiologies of NHO may include TBI and spinal cord injury (SCI).
- The incidence of HO after TBI is estimated at 4% to 28% [1-3] and can occur in more than one location, especially in patients with long bone fractures. [2,3]

Pathophysiology and Risk Factors

The pathophysiology of HO is not well understood and is believed to be the result of a complex interplay between neurohumoral factors that produce differentiation of pluripotent mesenchymal stem cells into osteoblasts. [1,4] Patients with severe TBI have demonstrated elevated serum osteogenic factors and neuropeptides that create an optimal environment for bone formation and mineralization. [2,4-6] Bone morphogenetic protein (BMP) and transforming growth factor β1 (TGF-β1) are also implicated in allowing abnormal bone formation. Other factors such as substance P, leptin, platelet-derived growth factor, interleukin-1, and interleukin-6 are felt to be potential mediators in experimental models. [4]

Risk factors for the development of HO include:
- Higher severity TBI, immobility, limb spasticity, and associated fractures [1]
- Military personnel involved in blast-related injuries have an incidence as high as 60% to 64%. [7]
- Coma duration, use of mechanical ventilation, and clinical signs of autonomic dysregulation are also associated with the development of HO in TBI. [8]

Clinical Presentation and Diagnosis

Heterotopic ossification typically progresses through three stages of development, starting with immature bone matrix formation. This is followed by an intermediate stage of inflammation and progressive calcification that ends with the final stage of maturation. Symptoms of HO are variable throughout these stages and are further outlined in Table 21.1. HO commonly develops within the first few months of injury but can be difficult to recognize as symptoms appear similar to deep venous thrombosis, septic joint, hematoma, cellulitis, and pressure injury.
- HO may affect upper and lower extremities but most commonly involves the hip and thigh, which can occur in two-thirds of cases. [4,9]
- In these patients, HO can develop inferomedial to the hip and be associated with adductor spasticity.

TABLE 21.1 Common Presenting Symptoms of Heterotopic Ossification
- Decreased range of motion and pain
- Local swelling and warmth adjacent to the involved joint
- Generalized edema and guarding of the involved limb
- Low-grade fevers and decreased joint mobility

- Scherbal et al. demonstrated upregulation of BMP in muscle specimens around the hip in rat models exposed to TBI and tibia fracture compared with tibia fracture alone.[10] This may lend support to why HO develops around the hip.
- The elbow is the second most common location for HO in TBI,[4] with the shoulder and knee affected to a lesser extent.[3,4]

Diagnostic Tests
- In the initial stage, HO is primarily a clinical diagnosis.
- Elevated serum alkaline phosphatase may be the earliest laboratory indication but is nonspecific and may be present in other conditions, including fractures and liver dysfunction.
- Serum levels usually increase over the first 6 to 12 weeks after injury and may be helpful in patients unable to provide clinical history or participate in physical examination.[9]
- Alkaline phosphatase levels do not correlate with maturation of HO.

Imaging Modalities
- Imaging modalities such as x-rays may not identify HO in the early stages because of a lack of calcium deposition.
- Bone scan may be the most sensitive test for early detection and can identify HO as early as 2 weeks after symptom onset.[4]
- Magnetic resonance imaging (MRI) and ultrasound have also been used for early detection.
- Argyropoulou et al. demonstrated MRI recognized knee HO almost simultaneously with clinical symptom onset.[11]
- Rosteius et al. used ultrasound for screening HO in SCI patients and showed a sensitivity of 88%.[12]
- In comparison, plain x-rays may not recognize HO for 3 to 6 weeks after symptom onset but can be useful in confirming maturity of HO.

Treatment Modalities
Prevention
Methods believed to slow progression of HO include range of motion exercises, medications, and radiation therapy.
- Physical therapy can help preserve joint range of motion and mobility.
- Nonsteroidal antiinflammatory drugs (NSAIDs) such as indomethacin significantly reduce development of HO in SCI patients.[4] Comparable results have been seen in patients undergoing total joint replacement.[1]
- Although NSAIDs are believed to decrease HO in TBI patients, their specific effects are not well described in the literature, and some studies have only evaluated them in combination with other treatments.[1,13]

- NSAIDs also may have adverse effects on the gastrointestinal system and potentially inhibit bone healing after fracture.
- Radiation therapy is thought to prevent differentiation of mesenchymal stem cells into osteoblasts and has demonstrated less HO formation in patients undergoing surgery around the hip. Still, radiation is not commonly used because dosing guidelines aren't standardized, and the long-term effects are largely unknown.[4]

Medications
- Patients who develop HO typically begin treatment with NSAIDs, which interfere with bone formation.
- Bisphosphonates have also been shown to reduce HO in early and late stages of maturation,[4] with etidronate believed to reduce HO by inhibiting mineralization of organic osteoid.
- Better results are expected if bisphosphonates are started before HO detection on plain film[4] and continued for 6 months.

Surgical Treatment
- Surgical resection of HO may be considered if joint mobilization is severely restricted or if functional tasks and self-care are inhibited.[14]
- Excision is traditionally delayed until maturation of the disease, up to 1.5 years after TBI.[4]
- Recent evidence suggests resection of immature HO may not increase the rate of recurrence.[3,4] As such, surgery can be an effective treatment to improve range of motion, prevent ankylosis, reduce pain, and prevent impingement of neurovascular structures.

Future Considerations
Future research may identify therapeutic targets that aid in the diagnosis and treatment of HO, including neuropeptides and signaling pathways such as substance P, macrophages, BMP, and retinoic acid receptor agonists.[6,7]

Fractures

Traumatic brain injury may be accompanied by skeletal trauma that results in long bone fractures. These fractures may go undetected in the acute setting in brain injury patients who have cognitive impairments, speech dysfunction, absent sensation, or are unable to participate in physical examination. In a prospective study by Sobus et al., bone scans completed before inpatient rehabilitation revealed 25 undetected fractures in 60 children with TBI.[15]

Normal fracture healing is completed through a series of continuous steps including inflammation, repair, and remodeling.[16]
- The inflammatory phase is generally the shortest stage of healing and allows for migration of chemical mediators to the injury site to create an optimal environment.
- During the reparative process, damaged bone is resorbed, and fibroblasts begin to build a new osteoid matrix. This resorption allows for the detection of fracture lines on plain films. A soft callus then begins to form to bridge the

fracture gap. Chondrocytes and osteoblasts then begin to mineralize the fracture callus to assist with union.

- The final stage of remodeling can take months and reshapes immature bone to provide strength and stability to the fracture site.

Patients who have sustained TBI often show an alteration in normal fracture healing. This can include enhanced osteogenesis, resulting in increased callus volume, accelerated callus formation, and higher mineral density.[2,17,18] One study found the time for bone union decreased by almost half in patients with TBI compared with fracture alone.[2] Although not confirmed, this is believed to be related to multiple signaling cascades that allow release of osteogenic factors.

Although there may be enhanced fracture healing and bone formation in the acute stages after TBI, these same pathways may contribute to long-term impairment in bone metabolism. Patients with TBI have been shown to have decreased bone mineral density, resulting in increased risk of osteopenia and osteoporosis, which can increase fracture risk over time.[17] This is thought to be influenced by variations in parathyroid hormone after TBI, which can result in decreased vitamin D levels. Additionally, systemic inflammation in the chronic stages of TBI may promote osteoclastic activity.

Soft Tissue and Nerve Injuries

Musculoskeletal injuries are common in patients with TBI. They may result from the injury itself or develop over time because of overuse. Like fractures, these soft tissue injuries may go undetected after acute TBI, as Sobus et al. noted 24 areas of soft tissue trauma in 60 children with TBI.[15] Over the long term, TBI patients often report musculoskeletal pain causing limited function and quality of life. A study by Brown et al. contacted patients for follow-up approximately 26 years after their initial injury and found 79% reported some type of musculoskeletal complaint.[19]

Falsetti et al. evaluated 163 patients with acquired brain injury and signs or symptoms of musculoskeletal pathology with ultrasound.[20] Patients included had diagnoses of stroke and severe brain injury, which included TBI. Musculoskeletal complications were seen in approximately half of these patients, with shoulder pain found in more than 25%. Diagnoses included shoulder subluxation, rotator cuff pathology, and frozen shoulder. Contractures and spasticity were noted in 18% of the patients.

Musculoskeletal Problems of the Shoulder

Musculoskeletal injuries to the shoulder commonly include impingement syndrome, rotator cuff injury, adhesive capsulitis, and glenohumeral instability.

- Impingement syndrome is a frequent cause of shoulder pain, with the supraspinatus tendon most commonly involved.

- Poor blood supply in a hypovascular zone along the articular surface of the tendon may be responsible for this phenomenon.[1]
- Anatomical changes such as a hooked acromion, weak scapular stabilizers, or glenohumeral joint capsule tightness also may contribute.
- Patients typically report pain along the anterior and lateral shoulder that is worsened with overhead activity. Examination of the shoulder with maneuvers compressing the region between the acromion and humeral head can reproduce symptoms.
- Cervical spine pathology may also refer pain to the shoulder and is often included in workup of shoulder pain.
- Nonoperative treatment of this condition focuses on rehabilitation therapies that emphasize scapular stabilization exercises,[1] including strengthening agonists and stretching antagonistic muscles.

General principles of rehabilitation after injury follow three broad stages that include acute, recovery, and functional phases.

- During the acute phase, emphasis is placed on reducing symptoms, core strengthening, and maintenance of aerobic conditioning. When the patient has pain-free range of motion and can participate in strengthening exercises, they may advance to the recovery phase.
- The recovery phase involves restoration of flexibility, strength, and proprioception of the injured limb.[1] Once full strength is regained, the patient can then progress to the functional phase.
- The functional phase works on task-specific activities and emphasizes return to normal activity.

Radiculopathies

Radiculopathy is caused by mechanical compression of a nerve root that results in a variety of symptoms, including pain, paresthesia, numbness, tingling, or weakness.[21] Mechanical compression is commonly caused by disk herniation but may also result from spinal stenosis, facet joint arthropathy, synovial cyst, or neoplasm.

- In the lumbar region, the most common disk herniations are at L4–L5 and L5–S1, with the L5 and S1 nerve roots most commonly involved.[1]
- In the cervical region, the C7 and C6 nerve roots are most commonly implicated.
- Radiculitis can occur in the absence of mechanical compression and is felt to be a result of chemically induced inflammation of the nerve.

Clinically, patients may report symptoms within a dermatomal distribution. Weakness or atrophy may also be present in a given myotome.

- For example, an L4–L5 disk herniation causing mechanical compression of the L5 nerve root may produce radiating pain along the posterolateral thigh and anterolateral leg. Numbness in the lateral leg and first web space may be appreciated in classic presentations.

- Diminished reflexes may also be found, such as a depressed patellar reflex in patients with L4 nerve root compression.
- Red flag symptoms may alert clinicians to conditions that require further diagnostic workup and may include the presence of constitutional symptoms, systemic illness, gait disturbance, and bowel or bladder dysfunction.
- Clinicians should also be aware of signs and symptoms of myelopathy, such as the presence of upper motor neuron signs, which may warrant urgent evaluation and possible intervention.

The natural history of radiculopathy tends to favor resolution of symptoms over time.[1] If symptoms are causing functional impairments and limiting quality of life, then conservative treatments may include NSAIDs, therapy, and epidural steroid injections.

Musculoskeletal Imaging

Imaging modalities are commonly used to assist in the diagnosis of various musculoskeletal injuries. Advancements in these technologies have allowed for improved anatomical visualization and in some instances dynamic and functional evaluation.

- Traditional plain radiography allows for evaluation of bony anatomy, which can assist in diagnosing fractures, bony deformities, ossification, and arthritic changes.
- Computed tomography (CT) generates overlapping contiguous images of the scanned area and offers better visualization of fractures and organs.[21]
- MRI doesn't use radiation but instead uses a magnetic field to create images that are a few body layers thick at a time. This allows for improved visualization of soft tissue structures and organs.

- Many consider MRI the gold standard in spinal imaging and for soft tissue pathology.

The use of ultrasound has also increased because of advances in technology that have improved image resolution, accessibility, and portability. Musculoskeletal ultrasound has assisted in the diagnosis of soft tissue and nerve injuries and is commonly used for needle guidance in procedures. Musculoskeletal ultrasound has many advantages compared with other imaging modalities.

- For example, it does not use radiation and provides improved patient comfort.
- It also allows for dynamic evaluation of ligaments and tendons during examination.
- Warden et al. found ultrasound to have a higher sensitivity and equivalent specificity to MRI in confirming clinically diagnosed patellar tendinopathy.[22]
- During ultrasound-guided procedures, real-time visualization of vascular structures and nerves also allows for improved safety.

Musculoskeletal structures have characteristic features when visualized with ultrasound[23]:

- Normal tendons have a hyperechoic appearance with a fibrillar echotexture and organized linear strands.
- Muscle and cartilage both appear hypoechoic, and cartilage may appear anechoic at times.
- Ligaments have a hyperechoic and striated appearance that is usually more compact compared with tendons.[23]
- Nerves have a fascicular appearance with a hyperechoic rim that is described as a honeycomb pattern.

Abnormal features visualized with ultrasound may include tendons with hypoechoic areas and a loss of the normal fibrillar echotexture.[24] Neovascularity may also be seen within injured tendons and can be assessed with color Doppler. Nerve compression syndromes may cause nerve swelling with increased circumference appreciated on ultrasound.

Review Questions

1. You are consulted to evaluate a 25-year-old male patient with a history of seizure disorder who was involved in a motor vehicle accident resulting in a severe traumatic brain injury (TBI) and facial fracture. The patient is currently in a coma and receiving total parenteral nutrition. Which of these patient characteristics is a risk factor for the development of heterotopic ossification (HO)?
   a. History of seizure disorder
   b. Prolonged coma duration
   c. Male gender
   d. Presence of facial fracture

2. Which of these is the most common location for the development of HO in patients with TBI?
   a. Knee
   b. Wrist
   c. Hip
   d. Shoulder

3. A 50-year-old woman with a recent history of TBI is currently admitted in the acute rehabilitation unit. She has developed HO of the left hip with severely restricted range of motion that is limiting her self-care and functional tasks. The patient is being considered for surgical excision of the HO. Which of these is the best tool to evaluate for maturity of the HO?
   a. Bone scan
   b. Plain x-ray
   c. Dual-energy x-ray absorptiometry (DEXA)
   d. Alkaline phosphatase level

Answers on page 391.
Access the full list of questions and answers online.
Available on ExpertConsult.com

References

1. Braddom R, Cifu D. *Braddom's Physical Medicine and Rehabilitation.* 5th ed. Philadelphia, PA: Elsevier; 2016.
2. Fuller D, Mani U, Keenan M. Heterotopic ossification of the shoulder in patients with traumatic brain injury. *J Shoulder Elbow Surg.* 2013;22(1):52-56.
3. Almangour W, Schnitzler A, Salga M, Debaud C, Denormandie P, Genêt F. Recurrence of heterotopic ossification after removal in patients with traumatic brain injury: a systematic review. *Ann Phys Rehabil Med.* 2016;59(4):263-269.
4. Sullivan M, Torres S, Mehta S, Ahn J. Heterotopic ossification after central nervous system trauma. *Bone Joint Res.* 2013;2(3):51-57.
5. Davis E, Davis A, Gugala Z, Olmsted-Davis E. Is heterotopic ossification getting nervous? The role of the peripheral nervous system in heterotopic ossification. *Bone.* 2018;109:22-27.
6. Brady R, Shultz S, McDonald S, O'Brien T. Neurological heterotopic ossification: current understanding and future directions. *Bone.* 2018;109:35-42.
7. Edwards D, Kuhn K, Potter B, Forsberg J. Heterotopic ossification: a review of current understanding, treatment, and future. *J Orthop Trauma.* 2016;30:S27-S30.
8. van Kampen P, Martina J, Vos P, Hoedemaekers C, Hendricks H. Potential risk factors for developing heterotopic ossification in patients with severe traumatic brain injury. *J Head Trauma Rehabil.* 2011;26(5):384-391.
9. Roberts P. Heterotopic ossification complicating paralysis of intracranial origin. *J Bone Joint Surg Br.* 1968;50-B(1):70-77.
10. Scherbel U, Riess P, Khurana J, Born C, De Long W. Expression of bone morphogenic proteins in rats with and without brain injury and a tibia fracture. *Orthop J (Univ PA).* 2001;14:85-89.
11. Argyropoulou M, Kostandi E, Kosta P, et al. Heterotopic ossification of the knee joint in intensive care unit patients: early diagnosis with magnetic resonance imaging. *Crit Care.* 2006;10(5):R152.
12. Rosteius T, Suero E, Grasmücke D, et al. The sensitivity of ultrasound screening examination in detecting heterotopic ossification following spinal cord injury. *Spinal Cord.* 2016;55(1):71-73.
13. Aubut JA, Mehta S, Cullen N, Teasell RW, ERABI Group, SCIRE Research Team. A comparison of heterotopic ossification treatment within the traumatic brain and spinal cord injured population: an evidence based systematic review. *NeuroRehabilitation.* 2011;28(2):151-160.
14. Huang H, Cheng W, Hu Y, Chen J, Zheng Z, Zhang P. Relationship between heterotopic ossification and traumatic brain injury. *J Orthop Translat.* 2018;12:16-25.
15. Sobus KM, Alexander MA, Harcke HT. Undetected musculoskeletal trauma in children with traumatic brain injury or spinal cord injury. *Arch Phys Med Rehabil.* 1993;74:902-904.
16. Eiff M. *Fracture Management for Primary Care.* 3rd ed. Philadelphia, PA: Elsevier; 2018.
17. Bajwa N, Kesavan C, Mohan S. Long-term consequences of traumatic brain injury in bone metabolism. *Front Neurol.* 2018;9:115.
18. Locher RJ, Lünnemann T, Garbe A, et al. Traumatic brain injury and bone healing: radiographic and biomechanical analyses of bone formation and stability in a combined murine trauma model. *J Musculoskelet Neuronal Interact.* 2015;15(4):309-315.
19. Brown S, Hawker G, Beaton D, Colantonio A. Long-term musculoskeletal complaints after traumatic brain injury. *Brain Inj.* 2011;25(5):453-461.
20. Falsetti P, Acciai C, Carpinteri F, Palilla R, Lenzi L. Bedside ultrasonography of musculoskeletal complications in brain injured patients. *J Ultrasound.* 2010;13(3):134-141.
21. Benzon H, Raja S, Fishman S, Liu S, Cohen S, Hurley R. *Essentials of Pain Medicine E-Book.* 4th ed. Philadelphia, PA: Elsevier Health Sciences; 2017.
22. Warden S, Kiss Z, Malara F, Ooi A, Cook J, Crossley K. Comparative accuracy of magnetic resonance imaging and ultrasonography in confirming clinically diagnosed patellar tendinopathy. *Am J Sports Med.* 2007;35(3):427-436.
23. Jacobson J. *Fundamentals of Musculoskeletal Ultrasound.* 2nd ed. Philadelphia, PA: Elsevier/Saunders; 2013.
24. James S, Ali K, Pocock C, et al. Ultrasound guided dry needling and autologous blood injection for patellar tendinosis. *Br J Sports Med.* 2007;41(8):518-521.

22

Pain

MORGAN O'CONNOR, MD, AND SANJOG PANGARKAR, MD

OUTLINE

This chapter discusses some of the common causes of pain that occur after a traumatic brain injury (TBI) and includes the topics of posttraumatic headache, complex regional pain syndrome (CRPS), and myofascial pain.

Posttraumatic Headache

Background and Epidemiology

- Headache is the most common physical symptom of TBI.
- The prevalence of headache after TBI is approximately 58% to as high as 90%.[1]
- The International Headache Society (IHS) defines post-traumatic headache (PTH) as:
  - "When a new headache occurs for the first time in close temporal relation to trauma or injury to the head and/or neck, it is coded as a secondary headache attributed to the trauma or injury. This remains true when the new headache has the characteristics of any of the primary headache disorders classified in Part One of ICHD-3."[2]
  - "When a preexisting headache with the characteristics of a primary headache disorder becomes chronic or is made significantly worse (usually meaning a two-fold or greater increase in frequency and/or severity) in close temporal relation to such trauma or injury, both the initial headache diagnosis and a diagnosis of [PTH]. Headache attributed to trauma or injury to the head and/or neck (or one of its types or subtypes) should be given, provided that there is good evidence that the disorder can cause headache."[2]
- This new headache or exacerbation of preexisting headache occurs within 7 days of trauma to the head.
- If headache symptoms persist for less than 3 months, it is termed *acute*. If symptoms persist for greater than 3 months, the headache is termed *persistent*.[2]
- The IHS uses a 7-day window for diagnosis of posttraumatic headache, but PTH may develop beyond this window[3]—commonly referred to as *delayed onset*.
- PTH, although common in isolation, evaluation should be considered for other symptoms of postconcussive syndrome symptoms:
  - Fatigue, memory deficits, dizziness, insomnia, impaired concentration, irritability, blurred vision, anxiety, light, and sound sensitivity[4]
- Patients with preexisting headache and female gender are more likely to report PTH.
- Severity of TBI is not felt to be related to the incidence of posttraumatic headache.[5]
- Posttraumatic seizures and intracranial hemorrhage do, however, correlate with increased severity of headaches reported at 36 months.[6]
- Migraine-type headache is the most common category of posttraumatic headache and accounts for approximately 35% of posttraumatic headache types.
- Probable migraine type headaches account for approximately 25% of PTH.
- Tension-type headaches account for approximately 20% and cervicogenic headache approximately 10%.[7]
- Often more than one headache type is identified.

Mechanism

- The mechanisms of PTH are not fully understood but are hypothesized to occur through central and peripheral factors.
- Proposed peripheral mechanisms include damage to cranial tissues such as arteries, dura mater, bone, muscle, cranial nerves, skin, and fascia, which creates an inflammatory state vis-a-vis release of cytokines and chemokines.
  - Activation of this cascade results in local monocyte and glial cell activation along with release of nociceptive neuropeptides resulting in spontaneous pain, hyperalgesia, and allodynia.
- Proposed central mechanisms include damage to spinothalamic and thalamocortical pathways resulting in hyperexcitability of central neurons and a possible decrease in descending inhibitory pain control.[8]
- Psychological factors such as posttraumatic stress disorder, anxiety, and depression may also be associated with PTH.[9,10]

Treatment

- At this time, there are no US Food and Drug Administration–labeled medications approved for management of posttraumatic headache.[11]
- Some practitioners have successfully used treatment strategies focused on the primary headache.
  - This includes abortive and preventive migraine medications used off label.
- Care should be taken when using these pharmacologic treatment strategies to avoid precipitating rebound or medication overuse headaches.
- Understanding the initial mechanism of injury may be beneficial in decision making because the presence of occipital neuralgia, cervicogenic headache, or oculomotor or vestibular dysfunction may allow another treatment strategy.

Posttraumatic Headache Summary Points

- Most common physical symptom after TBI
- Either a new headache or exacerbation of existing headaches after trauma
- May be part of a postconcussive syndrome; consider evaluation for other symptoms
- Mechanisms not well understood; likely involves both central and peripheral mechanisms
- Migraine-type headaches most common
- Consider tailoring treatment strategies based on primary headache type

Complex Regional Pain Syndrome

Background and Epidemiology

- CRPS is a clinical syndrome that often occurs after trauma.
- The hallmark of this disorder is pain and typically includes sensory, autonomic, motor, and trophic changes.

- Gellman et al found that patients with severe TBI had a 12% incidence of CRPS (primarily in limbs with spasticity).
  - Among these patients, 75% had an injury to the affected limb.[12]
- CRPS has a peak incidence between 37 and 50 years of age.
- CRPS affects women more commonly than men, at a ratio of 2:1 to 4:1
- CRPS affects the upper extremities more commonly than lower extremities.[13]

Diagnosis

- CRPS is a clinical diagnosis relying on a thorough clinical history and examination.
- The International Association for the Study of Pain has adopted the Budapest Criteria for diagnosis of CRPS, in which there is a sensitivity of 0.99 and specificity of 0.68.[14]
- The diagnostic criteria are as follows:
  - "Continuing pain which is disproportionate to any inciting event.
  - At least one symptom in three of four of the following categories:
    1. Sensory: Reports of hyperalgesia and/or allodynia.
    2. Vasomotor: Reports of temperature asymmetry and/or skin color changes and/or skin color asymmetry.
    3. Sudomotor/Edema: Reports of edema and/or sweating changes and/or sweating asymmetry.
    4. Motor/Trophic: Reports of decreased range of motion and/or motor dysfunction (weakness, tremor, dystonia) and/or trophic changes (hair, nails, skin).
  - Must display at least one sign at time of evaluation in two or more of the following categories:
    1. Sensory: Evidence of hyperalgesia (to pinprick) and/or allodynia (to light touch and/or deep somatic pressure and/or joint movement).
    2. Vasomotor: Evidence of temperature asymmetry ($>1°C$) and/or skin color changes and/or asymmetry
    3. Sudomotor/Edema: evidence of edema and/or sweating changes and/or sweating asymmetry
    4. Motor/Trophic: Evidence of decreased range of motion and/or motor dysfunction (weakness, tremor, dystonia) and/or trophic changes (hair, nails, skin).
  - There is no other diagnosis that better explains the signs and symptoms."[15]
- Pain associated with CRPS is often described as burning, continuous, and exacerbated by movement, stress, or pressure.
- Temperature changes and swelling may be seen in the affected limb.

- The pain may not follow a specific dermatome or peripheral nerve distribution and often has more distal than proximal involvement.
- If the symptoms develop after an injury not identifiable as trauma to a specific nerve, it is classified as CRPS type I (previously known as *reflex sympathetic dystrophy*).
- If symptoms develop after damage to a peripheral nerve, it is classified as CRPS type II (previously known as *causalgia*).
  - CRPS type II symptoms may initially be confined to a specific peripheral nerve distribution but can become more diffuse over time.[15]
- Additional diagnostic testing may be performed but is not required for making the diagnosis and should be directed at excluding other possible diagnoses.
- These studies have been used in the past to support a diagnosis of CRPS:
  - Triple phase bone scan: The uptake phase may demonstrate a characteristic pattern of subcutaneous blood pool changes.[16]
  - Radiography may demonstrate patchy bone demineralization.
  - Sudomotor testing, which is not commonly available, may reveal side-to-side asymmetry.

Pathophysiology and Treatment

- The pathophysiology of CRPS is not well understood but is believed to stem from peripheral and central sensitization mechanisms and abnormal coupling of peripheral nociceptive afferents and sympathetic efferent neurons.
- The treatment of CRPS in patients with TBI is similar to that of non–brain-injured individuals.
- The mainstay of treatment of CRPS is a gradual and progressive rehabilitation program that uses pharmacology, physical therapy, and pain interventions, if necessary.
- Initial therapy should be focused on reactivation of the affected extremity, contrast baths, desensitization/contrast textures, mirror-box therapy, and graded motor imagery.
- As the patient's symptoms improve, careful progression from low-intensity stimuli, such as isometric strengthening, to more intense stimuli, such as aerobic conditioning and movement therapies, is recommended.[17]

Pharmacological Treatment

- Evidence-based pharmacologic management of CRPS is limited because of an incomplete understanding of the underlying pathophysiology.
- Ideally, monotherapy reduces risk of adverse drug effects, drug interactions, and improves compliance, but is rarely effective clinically.
- Oral steroids have been shown to be of benefit early in the course of CRPS (<6 months), but benefit diminishes afterward.[18]

- Gabapentinoids, defined as alpha (2)-delta subunit voltage gated calcium channel antagonists such as gabapentin or pregabalin, have been used successfully to treat neuropathic pain conditions such as painful diabetic neuropathy and have shown a small benefit in CRPS.[19]
- Tricyclic antidepressants and serotonin norepinephrine reuptake inhibitors (SNRI) have been used with some benefit in other neuropathic pain conditions, and their use has been extended to CRPS.
  - Despite the frequency of use, there is a paucity of data on the benefits of these medications in CRPS.[20]
- Calcium regulating medications, including bisphosphonates and calcitonin, may provide benefit in CRPS cases refractory to other treatment modalities.[21,22]
- Trial of analgesics may include nonsteroidal antiinflammatory medications (NSAIDs) and, if necessary, opioid-based medications at the lowest effective dose.
- Ketamine infusions have been used for cases of CRPS refractory to conventional treatment.
  - Ketamine is an N-methyl-D-aspartate (NMDA) receptor antagonist most commonly used as an anesthetic and may be beneficial in chronic pain states, including CRPS.
  - Some studies demonstrate ketamine may provide short-term benefit (<3 months), but long-term efficacy has not been established.[23]

Procedural Interventions

- Sympathetic plexus blocks have been shown to be beneficial for short-term pain relief and may help by interrupting sympathetic coupling/outflow that likely occurs in CRPS.[24,25]
  - Although these blocks may provide short-term benefit, they are unlikely to completely manage symptoms of CRPS in isolation.
  - The combination of physical and/or occupational therapy with multimodal care may improve outcomes.
- There are relatively few randomized controlled trials designed to evaluate the efficacy of spinal cord stimulation in CRPS, but spinal cord stimulation and dorsal root ganglion stimulation[26] have been used as a treatment option for refractory CRPS.
  - Symptom improvement in CRPS with spinal cord stimulation tends to be greatest in the first year, with subsequent reduction in pain relief by year five.[27,28]

Complex Regional Pain Syndrome Summary Points

- Clinical diagnosis by Budapest Criteria; additional diagnostic testing is not required
- Pathophysiology not well understood; involves central and peripheral mechanisms and may involve abnormal coupling of peripheral nociceptive afferents and sympathetic efferent neurons
- Treatment should include therapy disciplines with inclusion of sensitization exercises.

- Evidence for various pharmacologic and interventional treatment strategies in CRPS is limited, and clinical practice is often based on extrapolation of data from other neuropathic pain conditions.

Myofascial Pain

Background and Epidemiology

- Myofascial pain arises from the muscles and/or fascia and can be associated with taut bands of skeletal muscle called *trigger points*.
- There are no accepted diagnostic criteria for this disorder, and a broad differential should be considered before making the diagnosis.
- After headache, the neck, shoulders, back, and limb are the most frequent sites of pain in brain injury, which in part may be myofascial in nature.[29]

Pathophysiology

- Causes of myofascial pain may be varied and should be fully evaluated.
- In the acute setting of TBI, consider the mechanisms involved and potential for unrecognized bony, ligamentous, or tendinous injury.
- Chronically consider:
  - Deconditioning related to prolonged hospitalization and recovery may alter patient mobility and contribute to pain.
  - Alterations in biomechanics, postural changes, and heterotopic ossification may contribute to patient discomfort over time.
  - In the setting of TBI, spasticity may be an additional contributor to patient discomfort.

Treatment

- Treatment for myofascial pain may include physical therapy for stretching, posture training, massage, myofascial release, and modalities such as heat, ultrasound, and transcutaneous electrical nerve stimulation.
- Medication options: Begin with over-the-counter NSAIDs and/or acetaminophen.
- If symptoms are refractory to these treatments, consideration may be given to SNRIs, such as duloxetine.
- If clinical examination suggests spasticity, then medications such as baclofen and tizanidine should be considered.
  - Diazepam may serve a role in the treatment of spasticity, but risks and benefits should be considered carefully in light of risks of sedation and dependence.
- If trigger points are found on exam (taut bands of muscle that produce a characteristic radiating pain when palpated), consideration may be given for trigger point injection or dry needling.
  - This injection involves identifying the trigger point and inserting a needle into the area of pain, often resulting in a muscle twitch or spasm, which may reduce pain for a period.[30]

Myofascial Pain Summary Points

- Pain arising from muscles/fascia; may be associated with trigger points
- No diagnostic criteria; consider a broad differential prior to making this diagnosis
  - In the acute setting, consider bone, ligament, or tendon injury.
  - Chronically, consider effects of deconditioning, biomechanical changes, spasticity, and heterotopic ossification.
- Treatment should include physical therapy and therapeutic modalities.
- Medication, if necessary, should primarily be with NSAIDs and/or acetaminophen.
- Trigger points, if present, may be amenable to treatment with trigger point injections.

Review Questions

1. What is the most common physical symptom experienced after a traumatic brain injury (TBI)?
   a. Trigger points
   b. Muscle spasms
   c. Weakness
   d. Headache
   e. Cognitive deficits
2. Which group is more likely to experience posttraumatic headache?
   a. Individuals without preexisting headache
   b. Women
   c. Individuals who suffered a severe traumatic brain injury
   d. Men

3. The most common headache type associated with posttraumatic headache is:
   a. Migraine
   b. Cervicogenic
   c. Tension
   d. Cluster
   e. Trigeminal neuralgia

Answers on page 391.
**Access the full list of questions and answers online.
Available on ExpertConsult.com**

References

1. Nampiaparampil DE. Prevalence of chronic pain after traumatic brain injury: a systematic review. *JAMA*. 2008;300(6):711-719. doi:10.1001/jama.300.6.711.

2. International Headache Society. Headache attributed to trauma or injury to the head and/or neck. In: *ICHD-3 The International Classification of Headache Disorders*. 3rd ed. Available at: https://www.ichd-3.org/5-headache-attributed-to-trauma-or-injury-to-the-head-andor-neck/. Accessed November 26, 2018.

3. Theeler BJ, Erickson JC. Mild head trauma and chronic headaches in returning us soldiers. *Headache*. 2009;49:529-534. doi:10.1111/j.1526-4610.2009.01345.x.

4. Kobeissy FH, Lucas S. Characterization and *Management of Headache after Mild Traumatic Brain Injury. Brain Neurotrauma*: Molecular, Neuropsychological, and Rehabilitation Aspects. Hoboken, NJ: Taylor & Francis; 2015.

5. Hoffman JM, Lucas S, Dikmen S, et al. Natural history of headache after traumatic brain injury. *J Neurotrauma*. 2011;28:1719-1725. doi:10.1089/neu.2011.1914.

6. Hong CK, Joo JY, Shim YS, et al. The course of headache in patients with moderate-to-severe headache due to mild traumatic brain injury: a retrospective cross-sectional study. *J Headache Pain*. 2017;18(1):48. doi:10.1186/s10194-017-0755-9.

7. Lucas S, Hoffman JM, Bell KR, Walker W, Dikmen S. Characterization of headache after traumatic brain injury. *Cephalalgia*. 2012;32:600-606. doi:10.1177/0333102412445224.

8. Defrin R. Chronic post-traumatic headache: clinical findings and possible mechanisms. *J Man Manip Ther*. 2013;22:36-43. doi:10.1179/2042618613y.0000000053.

9. Bryant RA, Marosszeky JE, Crooks J, Baguley IJ, Gurka JA. Interaction of posttraumatic stress disorder and chronic pain following traumatic brain injury. *J Head Trauma Rehabil*. 1999;14:588-594. doi:10.1097/00001199-199912000-00007.

10. Defrin R, Ginzburg K, Solomon Z, et al. Quantitative testing of pain perception in subjects with PTSD–implications for the mechanism of the coexistence between PTSD and chronic pain. *Pain*. 2008;138:450-459. doi:10.1016/j.pain.2008.05.006.

11. Watanabe TK, Bell KR, Walker WC, Schomer K. Systematic review of interventions for post-traumatic headache. *PM R*. 2012;4:129-140. doi:10.1016/j.pmrj.2011.06.003.

12. Gellman H, Keenan MAE, Stone L, Hardy SE, Waters RL, Stewart C. Reflex sympathetic dystrophy in brain-injured patients. *Pain*. 1992;51:307-311. doi:10.1016/0304-3959(92)90214-v.

13. Sandroni P, Benrud-Larson LM, McClelland RL, Low PA. Complex regional pain syndrome type I: incidence and prevalence in Olmsted county, a population-based study. *Pain*. 2003;103:199-207. doi:10.1016/s0304-3959(03)00065-4.

14. Harden NR, Bruehl S, Perez RS, et al. Validation of proposed diagnostic criteria (the "Budapest Criteria") for Complex Regional Pain Syndrome. *Pain*. 2010;150:268-274. doi:10.1016/j.pain.2010.04.030.

15. IASP Terminology Working Group. *Classification of Chronic Pain*. 2nd ed. (Revised). IASP Terminology–IASP. Available at: http://www.iasp-pain.org/PublicationsNews/Content.aspx?ItemNumber=1673. Accessed November 15, 2018

16. Kreitler S. *The Handbook of Chronic Pain*. New York, NY: Nova Biomedical Books; 2007.

17. Harden RN, Oaklander AL, Burton AW, et al. Complex regional pain syndrome: practical diagnostic and treatment guidelines, 4th edition. *Pain Med*. 2013;14:180-229. doi:10.1111/pme.12033.

18. Braus DF, Krauss JK, Strobel J. The shoulder-hand syndrome after stroke: a prospective clinical trial. *Ann Neurol*. 1994;36:728-733. doi:10.1002/ana.410360507.

19. van de Vusse AC, Stomp-van den Berg SG, Kessels AH, Weber WE. Randomised controlled trial of gabapentin in complex regional pain syndrome type 1. *BMC Neurol*. 2004;4:13. doi:10.1186/1471-2377-4-13.

20. Resmini G, Ratti C, Canton G, Murena L, Moretti A, Iolascon G. Treatment of complex regional pain syndrome. *Clin Cases Miner Bone Metab*. 2016;12(suppl 1):26-30.

21. Gobelet C, Waldburger M, Meier JL. The effect of adding calcitonin to physical treatment on reflex sympathetic dystrophy. *Pain*. 1992;48:171-175. doi:10.1016/0304-3959(92)90055-g.

22. Manicourt DH, Brasseur JP, Boutsen Y, Depreseux GV, Devogelaer JP. Role of alendronate in therapy for posttraumatic complex regional pain syndrome type I of the lower extremity. *Arthritis Rheum*. 2004;50:3690-3697. doi:10.1002/art.20591.

23. Zhao J, Wang Y, Wang D. The effect of ketamine infusion in the treatment of complex regional pain syndrome: a systemic review and meta-analysis. *Curr Pain Headache Rep*. 2018;22(2):12. doi:10.1007/s11916-018-0664-x.

24. Gungor S, Aiyer R, Baykoca B. Sympathetic blocks for the treatment of complex regional pain syndrome: a case series. *Medicine (Baltimore)*. 2018;97(19):e0705.

25. Yucel I, Demiraran Y, Ozturan K, Degirmenci E. Complex regional pain syndrome type I: efficacy of stellate ganglion blockade. *J Orthop Traumatol*. 2009;10:179-183. doi:10.1007/s10195-009-0071-5.

26. Deer TR, Levy RM, Kramer J, et al. Dorsal root ganglion stimulation yielded higher treatment success rate for complex regional pain syndrome and causalgia at 3 and 12 months: a randomized comparative trial. *Pain*. 2016;158(4):669-681.

27. Kemler MA, De Vet HC, Barendse GA. Effect of spinal cord stimulation for chronic complex regional pain syndrome Type I: a five–year final follow-up of patients in a randomized controlled trial. *J Neurosurg*. 2008;108:292-298.

28. Picarelli H, Neto HS, Oliveira MLD, Teixeira MJ. Neuromodulation in treating complex regional pain syndrome: a critical review of the evidence. *J Neurol Neurosci*. 2017;8:1. doi:10.21767/2171-6625.1000173.

29. Irvine KA, Clark JD. Chronic pain after traumatic brain injury: pathophysiology and pain mechanisms. *Pain Med*. 2017;19:1315-1333. doi:10.1093/pm/pnx153.

30. Desai MJ, Saini V, Saini S. Myofascial pain syndrome: a treatment review. *Pain Ther*. 2013;2(1):21-36.

23

Neuroendocrine, Metabolic and Hormonal Conditions

ONDREA MCKAY, MD, AND NEIL JASEY, MD

Incidence and Prevalence

- Pituitary damage because of brain trauma was first recognized in 1918 and was initially thought to be relatively rare. It has only been with increased awareness that it has been found to be more prevalent. Schneider et al reported that it occurred in approximately 27% of patients who were screened with chronic traumatic brain injury (TBI) and subarachnoid hemorrhage (SAH) and that it had an impact on functional recovery and morbidity.[1]
- Approximately two-thirds of patients who have died from severe head injuries have been found to have structural abnormalities in the pituitary stalk, pituitary, or hypothalamus.[2]
- In 2000, Benvenga and colleagues published a large review of posttraumatic hypopituitarism (PTH) that helped to further classify the relationship between TBI and PTH. They were able to identify hundreds of cases described in the literature and add new cases of patients identified by the authors that further recognized the presence of PTH in mild injuries and found that multiple hormonal abnormalities can occur at once.[3]
- Although multiple hormonal abnormalities can exist simultaneously, growth hormone deficiency appears to be the most prevalent hormone deficiency in those screened 6 months or more postevent.[4,5]

Anatomy Review

The pituitary gland is a small pea-sized structure located in the base of the brain in the middle cranial fossa. It is composed of two lobes (anterior and posterior) that are connected to the hypothalamus by the infundibulum. The anterior lobe produces and secretes hormones, whereas the posterior lobe only secretes them. The posterior lobe hormones (antidiuretic hormone, oxytocin) are produced by nerve cells in the hypothalamus and then stored and secreted by the posterior pituitary. Pituitary anatomy and the essential role the hypothalamus plays in regulating pituitary function is illustrated in Figure 23.1.

There are many theories regarding the pathophysiology behind PTH. Generally, it is believed that the unique structure of the pituitary, its anatomical location within the sella turcica, and the complex it forms with the hypothalamus through the infundibulum place it at risk for a variety of injuries. Subsequently, the pituitary is susceptible to direct injury, edema, and ischemic insult. Ischemia is felt to be a result of direct injury to the tenuous hypophyseal portal veins that supply blood to the gland and secondary effects of injury such as hypoxia and hypotension. The connection to the hypothalamus by the infundibulum makes these structures prone to shearing forces or transection in the setting of TBI. Additionally, the bony encasement of the sella turcica does not accommodate for edema that can occur postinjury, further compromising the gland.[6]

Pituitary Hormones

Anterior Pituitary

- **Thyroid-stimulating hormone (TSH):** Thyroid function is strongly regulated by the hypothalamic–pituitary–thyroid complex. Thyrotropin-releasing hormone (TRH) is released from the hypothalamus and causes the release of TSH subunits. Mature TSH is released from the pituitary

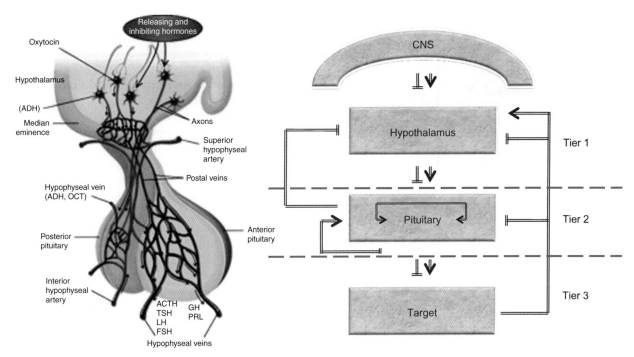

• **Fig. 23.1** Hypothalamic–pituitary anatomy and intricate feedback mechanisms that regulate hormonal levels. (Reprinted from: Melmed S. *The Pituitary*. 4th ed. London, UK: Elsevier/Academic Press; 2017:23-45).

and then reaches the thyroid gland, where it stimulates thyroid hormone production and release. Figure 23.2 illustrates how thyroid hormones eventually reach the hypothalamus and pituitary, where they inhibit the production and secretion of TRH and TSH, contributing to the axis. Due to the potential confounding effects of nonthyroidal illness (sick euthyroid syndrome) and the long half-life of thyroxine, it has been suggested that screening for thyroid dysfunction can reasonably be deferred for several (>4–6) weeks after TBI—assuming there is no suspicion of prior thyroid dysfunction—and then treated if necessary.[6]

• **Adrenocorticotropic hormone (ACTH):** In response to ACTH stimulation, the adrenal cortex produces three major classes of steroids: mineralocorticoids, glucocorticoids, and adrenal androgens. The adrenal androgens are responsible for secondary sexual characteristics in females. The glucocorticoids modulate metabolism and the immune responses. The mineralocorticoids are responsible for the modulation of blood pressure, vascular volume, and electrolytes and are also critical in the stress response.[2] Acute ACTH deficiency can be life threatening and should be treated. Otherwise dynamic screening for deficiency should only be done if suspected.[7]

• **Follicle-stimulating hormone/luteinizing hormone (FSH/LH):** The gonadotrophins make up approximately 10% of what? function? volume? of the anterior pituitary. In the acute phase, it has been found there is a transient suppression of gonadotropin release that typically recovers to normal levels; therefore, treatment should be considered only in the chronic phase. Decreased levels are associated with fatigue, fertility issues, and decreased bone mineral density.[8] There may also be a link with testosterone levels and rehabilitation outcomes. Young et al, in a small retrospective study, found that low rehab admission testosterone levels correlated with longer lengths of stay and decreased Functional Independence Measure efficiency, although these findings were not significant. Although testosterone replacement can be relatively easy to treat, any suspicion of prolonged gonadotropin deficiency should be worked up in conjunction with an endocrinologist. No large studies have examined the effects of female sex hormone replacement in TBI.[9]

• **Growth hormone (GH):** Long-term GH deficiency (GHD) is associated with decreased quality of life, impaired cognition, decreased lean body mass, reduced bone mineral density, and impaired cardiac function. A serum/plasma IGF-I level below the reference range for age and gender is suggestive of GHD, although it is not diagnostic. Low levels require referral to an endocrinologist for dynamic testing to investigate for GHD and coincident ACTH/cortisol deficiency. However, referral for dynamic testing of GHD in a subject with an IGF-I level in the normal range in most instances can be deferred to greater than 12 months after TBI. GH replacement would generally not be considered until this time point because spontaneous recovery may occur in some subjects.

• **Prolactin (PRL):** PRL induces and maintains lactation, suppresses sexual drive, and decreases reproductive function. It can be elevated because of many disease states, including TBI, and its elevation is considered a nonspecific finding. No relation has been made to prolactin levels and outcomes post TBI.

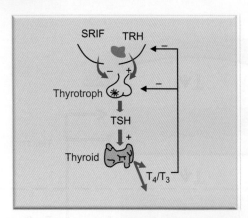

• **Fig. 23.2** Thyroid hormone regulation. (Reprinted from Melmed S. *The Pituitary.* 4th ed. London, UK: Elsevier/Academic Press; 2017:23-45.)

Posterior Pituitary

• **Oxytocin:** Oxytocin stimulates milk production and is not of clinical relevance in TBI management at this time, therefore it has not been studied.
• **Antidiuretic hormone (ADH):** ADH is synthesized in the paraventricular and supraoptic nuclei of the hypothalamus and stored in the secretory granules of the posterior pituitary. In response to the body's feedback mechanism, it is then released into the bloodstream to maintain circulating blood volume and serum osmolality. It does this by promoting water reabsorption in the distal collecting tubules and collecting ducts of the kidney. Secretion of ADH is controlled by two principal negative-feedback mechanisms: osmoregulation and baroregulation. Osmoregulation is the mechanism used by the body to maintain water balance. Normal serum osmolality is 280 to 295 mOsm/kg. Even slight changes in serum osmolality can markedly affect ADH release. In general, ADH is mostly secreted based on concentration of body fluids, but in cases of severe volume depletion such as hypotension or blood loss, which can occur with TBI, baroregulation takes precedence and can cause excessive stimulation of ADH.
• **Diabetes insipidus (DI):** Studies have shown that when diagnosed by using the water deprivation test, the prevalence of DI is as high as 26% in the acute phase and 6.9% among long-term survivors.[10] DI is characterized by an abnormal increase in urine output, an increase in fluid intake and thirst caused by decreased secretion of ADH, resulting in elimination of extracellular fluid. In trauma patients, DI is typically caused by damage to the posterior part of the pituitary gland where ADH is stored and secreted. It has been consistently linked to more severe injuries, cerebral edema, lower Glasgow Coma Scale (GCS) scores, and higher mortality rates. The occurrence of DI has also been associated with brain death as it is present in 80% of brain-dead patients. The

overall mortality ate of TBI patients with PTDI ranges between 57% to 69% and increases to 86% to 90% in those with early onset of diabetes insipidus in the first 3 days from injury.[11]
• **Syndrome of inappropriate antidiuretic hormone (SIADH):** Hyponatremia is the most common electrolyte abnormality in patients with neurologic problems and is particularly common after TBI; up to 33% of patients with TBI have hyponatremia at some point in their recovery. SIADH is characterized by abnormally high levels or continuous secretion of ADH, causing renal reabsorption and retention of water. Water is continually being reabsorbed by the kidneys, leading to concentrated urine, fluid retention, and hyponatremia. The treatment of SIADH is focused on fluid restriction and slow, careful replacement of sodium with an intravenous hypertonic solution of sodium chloride and/or diuretics. Medications to suppress ADH activity (demeclocycline hydrochloride) or inhibit renal response to ADH (lithium carbonate) are also options.[12]
• **Cerebral salt wasting (CSW):** Unlike SIADH, CSW is characterized by a true hyponatremia, specifically hyponatremia that results from a loss of both sodium and extracellular fluid. Even though ADH levels are elevated in patients with CSW, the body loses extracellular fluid and plasma volume decreases, resulting in decreased body weight (volume-contracted state). The pathophysiology of CSW syndrome is unclear but is thought to be caused by multiple mechanisms that affect sodium and water balance. It can be difficult to distinguish from SIADH, so extracellular fluid status is important to better differentiate between these two causes of hyponatremia. CSW usually requires replacement of fluid volume with physiological saline but can also be treated with hypertonic saline when more rapid correction is needed. As in treatment of SIADH, hypertonic solutions must be administered slowly to avoid rapid correction, which can result in central pontine myelinolysis. In patients who tolerate oral intake, fluid can be replaced orally, often with salt tablet supplements. Restriction of fluids is contraindicated in patients with CSW. If fluids are restricted, patients will be at risk for cerebral vasospasm, cerebral ischemia, and/or infarction.

Screening Recommendations

• Screening for neuroendocrine dysfunction in mild TBI (mTBI) remains controversial because the exact prevalence is unknown. Screening should be considered for more complicated cases.
• Posttraumatic hypopituitarism happens frequently in the moderate to severe TBI population. Therefore, it's suggested that all patients with moderate to severe TBI should have a hormonal assessment screening in the postacute phase, usually at 3 to 6 months post TBI or by 12 months

at the latest.[13] Logistically, this may be challenging, and often clinicians defer to a more pragmatic approach of screening those with clinical symptomatology of hypopituitarism.

- Early acute care screening for pituitary dysfunction is not recommended for the purpose of detecting post-TBI hypopituitarism. There is also no evidence that replacement of pituitary hormones in the acute phase is beneficial, and therefore it is not recommended except in rare cases.[6]
- Consensus guidelines suggest that for individuals in a permanent vegetative state or at an extremely low level of functioning, the evaluation and treatment should be limited to hypoadrenalism, DI, SIADH, and thyroid dysfunction.[2]
- Prospective studies examining pituitary dysfunction after TBI have demonstrated that hormonal dysfunction is often transient and usually recovers within 3 to 12 months of injury.[6]

Treatment

- Many studies have shown that some neuroendocrine deficits may be transient and that there is no reliable way to predict the future of hormonal integrity after injury. However, PTH is felt to be permanent at 12 months.
- All patients 6 to 12 months postinjury should undergo immediate replacement of all pituitary deficiencies except for GH deficiency. GH deficiency may occur only in response to other hormonal deficiencies, so other hormonal replacements should be done before treating GH deficiency to avoid unnecessary expense.

- Gonadotrophin deficiencies may occur as a result of stress-induced impairment; because it is not a clinical emergency, the recommendation is to retest before initiation of hormonal replacement.[2]
- If significant hormonal abnormalities are suspected, referral to endocrinology is indicated for dynamic testing and treatment.[6]

Summary

- Growth hormone is the most common hormonal deficiency post TBI.
- Hormonal abnormalities in the acute setting are often transient;; therefore, screening should occur in the post-acute setting unless clinically indicated.
- Hyponatremia is the most common electrolyte abnormality after neurologic injuries and is very common after TBI.
- The presence of diabetes insipidus early in the acute care stay is associated with increased mortality.
- PTH can occur in mTBI, but currently there are no guidelines or recommendations regarding screening in the mild TBI population, and it should only be done if the patient is symptomatic.[7]
- There remains some controversy about the appropriate time for screening for PTH and treatment, but if any clinical suspicion exists, the patient should be screened and treated. The appropriate timing for screening and treatment for PTH remains controversial, but should take place if there is clinical suspicion of dysfunction.

Review Questions

1. A 59-year-old woman was admitted to your inpatient service, and you have noticed that on the second day of admission, she is lethargic and confused on morning rounds. Initial laboratory studies from admission have returned and show serum sodium of 124 mEq/L, serum osmolality of 230 mOsm/kg, and urine osmolality of 285 mOsm/kg. Nurses report low urine output but are unsure of how much she drank overnight. What is the most likely diagnosis?
   a. Syndrome of inappropriate antidiuretic hormone (SIADH)
   b. Diabetes insipidus
   c. Cerebral salt wasting (CSW) syndrome
   d. Psychogenic polydipsia

2. You are seeing a patient who sustained a moderate traumatic brain injury (TBI) in a motor vehicle crash 6 months ago for a follow-up visit in your outpatient office to review laboratory studies. At the last appointment, your patient reported fatigue, hair loss, and weight gain. You obtained laboratory studies including thyroid function tests. What laboratory studies would support your hypothesis of hypothyroidism?
   a. High thyroid-stimulating hormone (TSH) and high free T4
   b. Low TSH and high free T4
   c. High TSH and low free T4
   d. Low TSH and high free T3

3. You are giving a lecture on pituitary dysfunction after TBI to physical medicine and rehabilitation residents, and one of them asks what's the most common hormonal abnormality after traumatic brain injury. You reply
   a. thyroid hormone deficiency.
   b. gonadotropin deficiency.
   c. hyponatremia.
   d. growth hormone deficiency.

Answers on page 392.
Access the full list of questions and answers online.
Available on ExpertConsult.com

References

1. Schneider HJ, Kreitschmann-Andermahr I, Ghigo E, Stalla GK, Agha A. Hypothalamopituitary dysfunction following traumatic brain injury and aneurysmal subarachnoid hemorrhage: a systematic review. *JAMA*. 2007;298(12):1429-1438.

2. Zasler ND, Katz DI, Zafonte RD. *Brain Injury Medicine: Principles and Practice*. 2nd ed. New York, NY: Demos Medical Pub.; 2013.

3. Benvenga S, Campenní A, Ruggeri RM, Trimarchi F. Clinical review 113: hypopituitarism secondary to head trauma. *J Clin Endocrinol Metab*. 2000;85(4):1353-1361.

4. Kozlowski Moreau O, Yollin E, Merlen E, Daveluy W, Rousseaux M. Lasting pituitary hormone deficiency after traumatic brain injury. *J Neurotrauma*. 2012;29(1):81-89.

5. Tanriverdi F, Senyurek H, Unluhizarci K, Selcuklu A, Casanueva FF, Kelestimur F. High risk of hypopituitarism after traumatic brain injury: a prospective investigation of anterior pituitary function in the acute phase and 12 months after trauma. *J Clin Endocrinol Metab*. 2006;91(6):2105-2111.

6. Tan CL, Alavi SA, Baldeweg SE, et al. The screening and management of pituitary dysfunction following traumatic brain injury in adults: British Neurotrauma Group guidance. *J Neurol Neurosurg Psychiatry*. 2017;88(11):971-981.

7. Quinn M, Agha A. Post-traumatic hypopituitarism-who should be screened, when, and how? *Front Endocrinol (Lausanne)*. 2018;9:8.

8. Agha A, Rogers B, Mylotte D, et al. Neuroendocrine dysfunction in the acute phase of traumatic brain injury. *Clin Endocrinol (Oxf)*. 2004;60(5):584-591.

9. Rosario ER, Aqeel R, Brown MA, Sanchez G, Moore C, Patterson D. Hypothalamic-pituitary dysfunction following traumatic brain injury affects functional improvement during acute inpatient rehabilitation. *J Head Trauma Rehabil*. 2013;28(5):390-396.

10. Agha A, Thornton E, O'Kelly P, Tormey W, Phillips J, Thompson CJ. Posterior pituitary dysfunction after traumatic brain injury. *J Clin Endocrinol Metab*. 2004;89(12):5987-5992.

11. Capatina C, Paluzzi A, Mitchell R, Karavitaki N. Diabetes insipidus after traumatic brain injury. *J Clin Med*. 2015;4(7): 1448-1462.

12. Kirkman MA, Albert AF, Ibrahim A, Doberenz D. Hyponatremia and brain injury: historical and contemporary perspectives. *Neurocrit Care*. 2013;18(3):406-416.

13. Ghigo E, Masel B, Aimaretti G, et al. Consensus guidelines on screening for hypopituitarism following traumatic brain injury. *Brain Inj*. 2005;19(9):711-724.

24

Paroxysmal Sympathetic Hyperactivity

VICTORIA C. WHITEHAIR, MD, AND JAMES J. BEGLEY, MD, MS

Autonomic Pathophysiology

The autonomic nervous system (ANS) unconsciously controls critical body functions and coordinates our responses to stimuli. The two main branches of the ANS are the sympathetic system, which drives the "fight or flight" response, and the parasympathetic system, which produces the "rest and digest" response. These branches are integrated with the Central Nervous System (CNS) through the central autonomic network (CAN), an internal regulation system consisting of subcortical and cortical structures that coordinates the various responses.[1] The pathophysiology behind autonomic disorders after acquired brain injury remains unknown, but the most frequently cited theories suggest disconnection within the CAN and include the excitatory:inhibitory ratio model, which proposes that injury at the brainstem or above leads to reduced higher-level inhibitory input and results in overamplification of even mild afferent input and the development of allodynic hypersensitivity.[2-4] It is important to note that although radiographic evidence often shows brainstem damage or diffuse axonal injury in patients with severe forms of autonomic dysfunction, no single lesion location has been identified as the cause of the dysfunction, and syndromes can been seen after both focal and diffuse injury.[5]

A Spectrum of Autonomic Dysfunction Syndromes

Although the autonomic dysfunction at the most severe end of the range is the most widely recognized of the post-brain injury autonomic disorders, a spectrum of autonomic disorders ranging in severity and symptoms has been noted corresponding with the variation in brain injury severities and patterns. A number of case reports and case series have showed that a subset of patients develop autonomic dysfunction after even mild traumatic brain injury (mTBI). The most frequently cited abnormalities include heart rate variability, abnormal tilt testing, baroreflex dysfunction, and syncope.[6] Development of postural orthostatic tachycardia syndrome (POTS) has also been reported after TBI.[7] Some post-TBI symptoms, such as temperature dysregulation and excessive or gustatory sweating, are also seen in non-TBI autonomic disorders and may be a result of mild autonomic dysfunction. More exploration of the mild range of autonomic dysfunction after acquired brain injury is needed to better understand the prevalence and impact of these disorders.

Paroxysmal Sympathetic Hyperactivity

The most widely recognized and most severe type of autonomic dysfunction after traumatic brain injury is paroxysmal sympathetic hyperactivity (PSH). PSH is a syndrome of paroxysmal, transient increases in sympathetic activity that can occur after severe brain injury.[8] It is characterized by episodes of catecholamine elevation, severe hemodynamic alterations, and motor overactivity in response to even minor stimulation.[9] This syndrome has been previously known by several other names, including *sympathetic storming*, *autonomic dysfunction syndrome*, and *paroxysmal autonomic instability with dystonia*, but increasingly preference has been given to the term *PSH* because of its specificity and more accurate portrayal of the clinical syndrome.[4,8,10]

Epidemiology

A review of published cases of PSH by Perkes et al. showed that most occurred after TBI (79.4%) followed by hypoxic brain injury (9.7%) and then stroke (5.4%).[11] Hemorrhagic stroke was associated with four times as many cases of PSH as ischemic stroke.[11] The incidence of PSH after severe TBI is variable, with reports of 8% to 33%.[10,12-16] This variability in incidence is likely a result of differences in diagnostic criteria and time since injury. As an example, one study showed 92% of patients had some degree of sympathetic hyperactivity within the first week after injury, but only 24% of patients met criteria for PSH at day 7 postinjury, and only 8% continued to meet criteria for PSH at day 14.[12] Time to PSH onset varies, but emergence of signs and symptoms is often noted after sedation withdrawal.[5] Although the majority of patients show reduction in sympathetic hyperactivity within the first few weeks after injury, studies have shown that a subset of patients develops a chronic form of PSH in which a degree of sympathetic hyperactivity can last as long as 2.5 to 6 months.[5]

Diagnosis and Clinical Features

Despite development of diagnostic assessment tools and a consensus statement, diagnosis of PSH remains one of exclusion. The signs and symptoms of PSH overlap with those of seizures, sepsis, neuroleptic malignant syndrome, serotonin syndrome, malignant hyperthermia, untreated pain, and alcohol or sedative withdrawal, and these potential diagnoses must be considered before attributing all symptoms to PSH.[2,4,8] Although there is no single standard set of criteria used consistently to diagnosis PSH, there is a key group of features that are common among assessment measures.[4,5,8,10,17] These common clinical features are episodic tachycardia, tachypnea, hypertension, hyperthermia, diaphoresis, and posturing. Common ranges for these parameters are noted in Table 24.1.

Additional factors that increase the diagnostic likelihood of PSH include[8,17]:
- Episodes begin after brain injury
- Symptoms occur simultaneously
- Symptoms are paroxysmal
- Symptoms are triggered by even benign or mildly nociceptive stimuli
- Symptoms are severe
- Duration of syndrome 3 or more consecutive days
- Duration of syndrome 2 or more weeks after brain injury
- Two or more episodes daily
- Syndrome persists after treatment of other potential diagnoses
- No other presumed etiology
- No parasympathetic features during episodes

Motor overactivity commonly fluctuates with paroxysms, may be asymmetrical, and includes varying patterns, such as decorticate and/or decerebrate posturing, spasticity, rigidity, and dystonia.

Additional features that may be seen in PSH include:
- Poor gastrointestinal tract absorption
- Elevated white blood cell count without infection
- Elevated catecholamine levels
- Asymptomatic arrhythmias
- Neurogenic lung disease
- Pupillary dilatation
- Excessive salivation
- Crying
- Hiccups
- Yawning
- Sighing

Complications

There are both individual and population-level implications caused by PSH. Compared with symptoms seen in other severe TBI patients, PSH is associated with longer comas, lower Functional Independence Measure scores at

TABLE 24.1 **Signs and Symptoms of Paroxysmal Sympathetic Hyperactivity With Graded Severity**

Symptom	Normal	Mild	Moderate	Severe
Heart rate	<100	100–119	120–139	≥140
Respiratory rate	<18	18–23	24–29	≥30
Systolic blood pressure	<140	140–159	160–179	≥180
Temperature	<37.0	37.0–37.9	38.0–38.9	≥39.0
Sweating	None	Mild	Moderate	Severe
Posturing	None	Mild	Moderate	Severe

Adapted from Rehabilitation After Traumatic Brain Injury by Eapen and Cifu[32] (Original adaptation from Baguley IJ, Perkes IE, Fernandez-Ortega JF, et al. Paroxysmal sympathetic hyperactivity after acquired brain injury: consensus on conceptual definition, nomenclature, and diagnostic criteria. *J Neurotrauma.* 2014;31[17]:1515-1520.[8])

discharge, longer hospital stays, greater healthcare costs, and increased morbidity and mortality rates.[5,8,10,15,18]

Factors such as arrhythmia, tachypnea, hyperglycemia, hyperthermia, and hypernatremia increase the risk for impaired cerebral tissue oxygenation and secondary brain injury.[19] Persistent hypertension increases the risk of secondary brain injury through cerebral edema, expansion of hemorrhage, or anoxic injury from cardiac dysfunction. Cardiopulmonary disorders after TBI are discussed in depth in Chapter 18.

Many additional complications after severe TBI arise because of the sympathetic overactivity of PSH. Fluid loss from diaphoresis can cause hypernatremia, renal insufficiency, and thickened pulmonary secretions. If appropriate dietary supplementation is not maintained, the elevated metabolic state can cause weight loss, malnutrition, muscle atrophy, renal failure, and pressure injuries.[19] Untreated motor overactivity can cause permanent contractures. The relative risk of developing symptomatic heterotopic ossification is 59 times higher in TBI patients with PSH compared with those without.[20]

Management

The primary goal of PSH management is to reduce secondary morbidity and mortality after TBI. As part of that goal, an important first step in management of PSH is to establish the appropriate diagnosis. Other potential diagnoses such as seizures, sepsis, substance withdrawal, and overlap syndromes must be considered, treated, and excluded in tandem with treatment for presumed PSH.

Guidance for PSH management is currently limited by incomplete understanding of the underlying pathophysiology and the lack of large prospective studies on the subject. Management of PSH remains focused on symptom treatment and often includes both pharmacologic and nonpharmacologic interventions.[21]

Nonpharmacologic Management

Nonpharmacologic treatment to prevent secondary complications includes physical and occupational therapy and dietary consultation. Environmental modifications can be used to prevent common triggers of episodes, including touching, repositioning, passive movement, endotracheal tube suctioning, constipation, urinary retention, catheter manipulation, and pressure injuries.[22]

Environmental modifications to prevention and treat triggers include:
- Appropriate positioning
- Preventing and treating constipation and urinary retention
- Managing and preventing pain
- Preventing pressure injury
- Limiting unnecessary environmental stimuli
- Cooling blankets

Pharmacologic Management

Pharmacologic management is often categorized into abortive and preventive treatments. A comparison of pharmacological treatment options is shown in Table 24.2.

Abortive medications are typically used early in the course, have a rapid onset of action, and have a short half-life.[21] The choice in medication depends on the symptom to be treated, but common treatments and indications include:
- Antipyretics for hyperthermia
- Short-acting benzodiazepines or atypical antipsychotics for agitation
- Morphine for pain
- Antihypertensive agents for hypertension

Symptom prevention can be achieved with the use of targeted scheduled medications such as nonselective beta blockers, alpha-2 agonists, long-acting benzodiazepines, baclofen, bromocriptine, gabapentin, and dantrolene.[21]

Opioid receptor agonists are used primarily to suppress allodynic responses.[23] Morphine, a potent μ-opioid receptor agonist, is the most widely used and most efficacious in this class. Morphine is believed to modulate central pathways involved in sympathetic paroxysms in addition to its analgesic properties.[21,24] It is often used as an abortive agent for breakthrough episodes because of its rapid onset and short half-life.

Nonselective beta blockers have been shown to reduce the frequency and severity of PSH episodes.[22] Propranolol, which has good blood-brain penetration because of its lipophilic nature, is the most commonly used within the class and has shown the most efficacy in treatment. Propranolol reduces catecholamine levels, hemodynamic parameters such as heart rate, blood pressure, respiratory rate and temperature, cardiac work load, and metabolic rate and improves Glasgow Coma Scale (GCS), diaphoresis, and posturing.[21,22,25] Propranolol is associated with a lower mortality rate after PSH compared with other beta blockers.[26] Selective beta-1 blockers like metoprolol do not appear to have the same effect as nonselective agents. Labetalol, a beta 1, beta-2, and alpha-2 blocker, has also shown improvement of PSH in case reports but has not been as widely studied as propranolol.[27]

Clonidine is an alpha-2 receptor agonist that acts through both central and peripheral pathways to suppress adrenergic outflow.[22] It reduces blood pressure, heart rate, and circulating levels of catecholamines in PSH.[28] Clonidine does not exhibit much effect on hyperthermia, often requires high doses to achieve improvement, and may cause hypotension and bradycardia between paroxysms.[22]

Benzodiazepines are gamma-aminobutyric acid (GABA_A) receptor agonists and have shown mixed outcomes in the treatment of PSH. Midazolam, lorazepam, and diazepam are the most frequently used, but longer-acting medications such as clonazepam have also been used.[22,23] They can be beneficial in the treatment of motor overactivity, and there is some evidence that they may reduce tachycardia and hypertension.[22,23] However, their negative side effect profile and risk of withdrawal limit their use.[21]

TABLE 24.2	**Medications for the Treatment of Paroxysmal Sympathetic Hyperactivity**					

Medication	Mechanism of Action	Dosing	Symptoms Treated	Contraindications	Adverse Effects
Opioid					
Morphine	μ-Opioid receptor agonist	1–10 mg IV	Hypertension Tachycardia Pain/allodynia	Morphine allergy	Respiratory depression, sedation, hypotension, ileus, risk for withdrawal
Beta Blockers					
Propranolol	Nonselective beta-1 and beta-2 adrenergic blocker	20–60 mg every 4–6 h PO	Hypertension Tachycardia Hyperthermia Diaphoresis	COPD, atrioventricular block, heart failure, severe bradycardia	Bradycardia, bronchospasm, hypotension, sleep disturbances
Labetalol	Beta-1, beta-2, alpha-2 adrenergic blocker	100–200 mg every 12 h PO	Hypertension Tachycardia		
alpha-2 agonist					
Clonidine	Alpha-2 adrenergic agonist	0.1–0.3 mg every 8 h PO	Hypertension Tachycardia	Severe bradycardia	Hypotension, bradycardia, sedation, rebound hypertension, constipation, depression
Benzodiazepines					
Midazolam	GABA$_A$ agonist	1–2 mg bolus IV	Hypertension Tachycardia Agitation Posturing Spasticity	Acute narrow-angle glaucoma, caution with concomitant use of opioids	Sedation, hypotension, respiratory depression, paradoxical reaction
Lorazepam	GABA$_A$ agonist	2–4 mg bolus IV			
Diazepam	GABA$_A$ agonist	5–10 mg IV, PO			
Clonazepam	GABA$_A$ agonist	0.5–5 mg PO every 8–12 h			
Neuromodulators					
Baclofen	GABA$_B$ agonist	5 mg every 8 h PO (max. dose 80 mg/day) Intrathecal: test dose then titrate	Pain Clonus Rigidity Spasticity Posturing	Baclofen hypersensitivity	Elevated hepatic function tests, muscle weakness, sedation, withdrawal syndrome
Bromocriptine	Dopamine agonist	1.25 mg every 12 h PO (max. 40 mg/day)	Dystonia Posturing Hyperthermia Diaphoresis	Hypersensitivity to ergot alkaloids	Confusion, agitation, dyskinesias, nausea, hypotension, may lower seizure threshold
Gabapentin	Inhibition at dorsal horn of spinal cord	300 mg – 900 mg every 8 h PO (max. 3600 mg/day)	Allodynia Spasticity	Hypersensitivity to gabapentin	Mild sedation, edema
Other					
Dantrolene	Interferes with calcium release from sarcoplasmic reticulum	0.25–2 mg/kg every 6–12 h IV (max. 10 mg/kg/day)	Posturing Rigidity Spasticity	Active hepatic disease (hepatitis, cirrhosis)	Hepatotoxicity, weakness

COPD, Chronic obstructive pulmonary disease; *GABA,* gamma aminobutyric acid; *IV,* intravenously; max., maximum; *PO,* enteral.

Baclofen is a GABA$_B$ receptor agonist that provides inhibitory input at spinal cord interneurons and is especially useful for motor overactivity treatment. Although more invasive than the enteral route, intrathecal baclofen appears to be more effective in treating PSH paroxysms and motor symptoms.[29] Abrupt discontinuation must be avoided, as the withdrawal syndrome can be severe.

Bromocriptine is a dopamine D2 agonist whose use is based on similarities between PSH and neuroleptic malignant syndrome, for which bromocriptine is the agent of choice. Case reports have shown blood pressure reduction, but its primary use remains for reduction in motor overactivity.[30]

Gabapentin modulates reactivity of neurologic circuits in the spinal cord through action at presynaptic voltage-gated calcium channels. A case series reported reduction in the frequency and severity of paroxysms in six patients with PSH.[31]

Dantrolene is a ryanodine receptor antagonist that reduces dystonia, spasticity, rigidity, and posturing through interference with calcium release from the sarcoplasmic reticulum. Although it is commonly used for treatment of spasticity evidence is lacking regarding improvement in other aspects of PSH. It is contraindicated in active hepatic disease, and hepatic function must be monitored during treatment.

Review Questions

1. Paroxysmal sympathetic hyperactivity (PSH) has been shown to be associated with
   a. shorter length of hospital stay.
   b. higher morbidity and mortality rates.
   c. absence of functional improvement in rehabilitation.
   d. lower healthcare costs.
2. Common clinical features of PSH episodes include all of these except
   a. hypertension.
   b. tachypnea.
   c. bradycardia.
   d. hyperthermia.

3. Which of these injury types can result in autonomic dysfunction?
   a. Mild TBI
   b. Severe TBI
   c. Hypoxic brain injury
   d. All of the above

Answers on page 392.
Access the full list of questions and answers online.
Available on ExpertConsult.com

References

1. Benarroch EE. The central autonomic network: functional organization, dysfunction, and perspective. *Mayo Clin Proc.* 1993; 68(10):988-1001.
2. Baguley IJ, Heriseanu RE, Cameron ID, Nott MT, Slewa-Younan S. A critical review of the pathophysiology of dysautonomia following traumatic brain injury. *Neurocrit Care.* 2008;8(2): 293-300.
3. Baguley IJ, Nott MT, Slewa-Younan S, Heriseanu RE, Perkes IE. Diagnosing dysautonomia after acute traumatic brain injury: evidence for overresponsiveness to afferent stimuli. *Arch Phys Med Rehabil.* 2009;90(4):580-586.
4. Lump D, Moyer M. Paroxysmal sympathetic hyperactivity after severe brain injury. *Curr Neurol Neurosci Rep.* 2014;14(11):494.
5. Baguley IJ, Nicholls JL, Felmingham KL, Crooks J, Gurka JA, Wade LD. Dysautonomia after traumatic brain injury: a forgotten syndrome? *J Neurol Neurosurg Psychiatry.* 1999;67(1):39-43.
6. Pertab JL, Merkley TL, Cramond AJ, Cramond K, Paxton H, Wu T. Concussion and the autonomic nervous system: an introduction to the field and the results of a systematic review. *NeuroRehabilitation.* 2018;42(4):397-427.
7. Kanjwal K, Karabin B, Kanjwal Y, Grubb BP. Autonomic dysfunction presenting as postural tachycardia syndrome following traumatic brain injury. *Cardiol J.* 2010;17(5):482-487.
8. Baguley IJ, Perkes IE, Fernandez-Ortega JF, Rabinstein AA, Dolce G, Hendricks HT. Paroxysmal sympathetic hyperactivity after acquired brain injury: consensus on conceptual definition, nomenclature, and diagnostic criteria. *J Neurotrauma.* 2014;31(17):1515-1520.
9. Fernandez-Ortega JF, Baguley IJ, Gates TA, Garcia-Caballero M, Quesada-Garcia JG, Prieto-Palomino MA. Catecholamines and paroxysmal sympathetic hyperactivity after traumatic brain injury. *J Neurotrauma.* 2017;34(1):109-114.
10. Fernandez-Ortega JF, Prieto-Palomino MA, Garcia-Caballero M, Galeas-Lopez JL, Quesada-Garcia G, Baguley IJ. Paroxysmal sympathetic hyperactivity after traumatic brain injury: clinical and prognostic implications. *J Neurotrauma.* 2012;29(7):1364-1370.
11. Perkes I, Baguley IJ, Nott MT, Menon DK. A review of paroxysmal sympathetic hyperactivity after acquired brain injury. *Ann Neurol.* 2010;68(2):126-135.
12. Baguley IJ, Slewa-Younan S, Heriseanu RE, Nott MT, Mudaliar Y, Nayyar V. The incidence of dysautonomia and its relationship with autonomic arousal following traumatic brain injury. *Brain Inj.* 2007;21(11):1175-1181.
13. Hendricks HT, Heeren AH, Vos PE. Dysautonomia after severe traumatic brain injury. *Eur J Neurol.* 2010;17(9):1172-1177.
14. Lv LQ, Hou LJ, Yu MK, et al. Prognostic influence and magnetic resonance imaging findings in paroxysmal sympathetic hyperactivity after severe traumatic brain injury. *J Neurotrauma.* 2010;27(11):1945-1950.
15. Fernandez-Ortega JF, Prieto-Palomino MA, Munoz-Lopez A, Lebron-Gallardo M, Cabrera-Ortiz H, Quesada-Garcia G. Prognostic influence and computed tomography findings in dysautonomic crises after traumatic brain injury. *J Trauma.* 2006;61(5):1129-1133.
16. Rabinstein AA. Paroxysmal sympathetic hyperactivity in the neurological intensive care unit. *Neurol Res.* 2007;29(7):680-682.
17. Perkes IE, Menon DK, Nott MT, Baguley IJ. Paroxysmal sympathetic hyperactivity after acquired brain injury: a review of diagnostic criteria. *Brain Inj.* 2011;25(10):925-932.
18. Mathew MJ, Deepika A, Shukla D, Devi BI, Ramesh VJ. Paroxysmal sympathetic hyperactivity in severe traumatic brain injury. *Acta Neurochir (Wien).* 2016;158(11):2047-2052.
19. Lemke DM. Sympathetic storming after severe traumatic brain injury. *Crit Care Nurse.* 2007;27(1):30-37; quiz 8.
20. Hendricks HT, Geurts AC, van Ginneken BC, Heeren AJ, Vos PE. Brain injury severity and autonomic dysregulation accurately predict heterotopic ossification in patients with traumatic brain injury. *Clin Rehabil.* 2007;21(6):545-553.
21. Samuel S, Allison TA, Lee K, Choi HA. Pharmacologic management of paroxysmal sympathetic hyperactivity after brain injury. *J Neurosci Nurs.* 2016;48(2):82-89.
22. Rabinstein AA, Benarroch EE. Treatment of paroxysmal sympathetic hyperactivity. *Curr Treat Options Neurol.* 2008;10(2):151-157.
23. Baguley IJ, Cameron ID, Green AM, Slewa-Younan S, Marosszeky JE, Gurka JA. Pharmacological management of Dysautonomia following traumatic brain injury. *Brain Inj.* 2004; 18(5):409-417.
24. Meyfroidt G, Baguley IJ, Menon DK. Paroxysmal sympathetic hyperactivity: the storm after acute brain injury. *Lancet Neurol.* 2017;16(9):721-729.
25. Ammar MA, Hussein NS. Using propranolol in traumatic brain injury to reduce sympathetic storm phenomenon: a prospective randomized clinical trial. *Saudi J Anaesth.* 2018;12(4):514-520.
26. Schroeppel TJ, Sharpe JP, Magnotti LJ, et al. Traumatic brain injury and beta-blockers: not all drugs are created equal. *J Trauma Acute Care Surg.* 2014;76(2):504-509; discussion 509.
27. Do D, Sheen VL, Bromfield E. Treatment of paroxysmal sympathetic storm with labetalol. *J Neurol Neurosurg Psychiatry.* 2000;69(6):832-833.
28. Payen D, Quintin L, Plaisance P, Chiron B, Lhoste F. Head injury: clonidine decreases plasma catecholamines. *Crit Care Med.* 1990;18(4):392-395.
29. Cuny E, Richer E, Castel JP. Dysautonomia syndrome in the acute recovery phase after traumatic brain injury: relief with intrathecal Baclofen therapy. *Brain Inj.* 2001;15(10):917-925.
30. Russo RN, O'Flaherty S. Bromocriptine for the management of autonomic dysfunction after severe traumatic brain injury. *J Paediatr Child Health.* 2000;36(3):283-285.
31. Baguley IJ, Heriseanu RE, Gurka JA, Nordenbo A, Cameron ID. Gabapentin in the management of dysautonomia following severe traumatic brain injury: a case series. *J Neurol Neurosurg Psychiatry.* 2007;78(5):539-541.
32. Eapen BC, Hong S, Subbarao B, Jaramillo CA. Chapter 3 - Medical Complications After Moderate to Severe Traumatic Brain Injury. Ed: Eapen BC, Cifu CX. In Rehabilitation After Traumatic Brain Injury, Elsevier, 2019; 23-36, ISBN 9780323544566.

25

Spasticity and Contractures

KATHERINE LIN, MD, SAURABHA BHATNAGAR, MD, FAAPMR, AND
BLESSEN C. EAPEN, MD

Benefits of Spasticity

- Helps maintain muscle bulk
- Facilitates ambulation, standing, and transfers
- Helps promote venous return and decreases edema
- Helps prevent deep venous thrombosis (DVT)
- Helps prevent osteoporosis
- Decreases the risk of orthostatic hypotension
- Helps awareness of potentially noxious stimuli

Disadvantages of Spasticity

- Pain
- Risk of contractures
- Risk of heterotopic ossification
- Risk of joint subluxation and dislocation
- Interference in activities of daily living (ADLs) and nursing care
- Skin breakdown
- Masks volitional movement
- Negatively affects ambulation, bed positioning, sitting, standing, and transfers
- Bowel/bladder dysfunction
- Sleep disturbances

Clinical Presentation

Tables 25.1 and 25.2 include the most common upper and lower extremity presentations after traumatic brain injury (TBI).[2]

Physical Examination

Inspection

- Resting body position and use of orthotics
- Muscle spasms associated with movement
- Gait assessment
- Skin integrity

Overview

Definition

Spasticity is a motor disorder characterized by a velocity-dependent increase in tonic stretch reflex (muscle tone) to passive muscle stretch.

Pathophysiology

- Motor dysfunction secondary to lesions proximal to the alpha motor neuron
- Loss of descending inhibitory influences on the 1A interneuron[1]

TABLE 25.1   Common Upper Extremity Patterns

Upper Extremity Pattern	Involved Muscles
Shoulder adduction and internal rotation	Latissimus dorsi, teres major, pectoralis major, subscapularis.
Elbow flexion	Brachioradialis, biceps brachii, brachialis.
Wrist flexion	Flexor carpi radialis, flexor carpi ulnaris, FDS, FDP
Forearm pronation	Pronator teres, pronator quadratus
Clenched fist	FDP, FDS
Thumb in palm deformity	Adductor pollicis, FPL, FPB

FDP, Flexor digitorum profundus—results in flexion at the distal interphalangeal joint (DIP); *FDS,* flexor digitorum superficialis—results in flexion at the proximal interphalangeal joint (PIP); *FPB,* flexor pollicis brevis; *FPL,* flexor pollicis longus.

TABLE 25.2   Common Lower Extremity Patterns

Lower Extremity Pattern	Involved Muscles
Hip flexion and adduction	Iliopsoas, rectus femoris, adductors
Knee flexion	Biceps femoris, semitendinous, semimembranous
Equinovarus	Gastroc-soleus complex, tibialis anterior/posterior
Toe curling	FDL, FDP, FHL, FHB

FDL, Flexor digitorum longus; *FDP,* flexor digitorum profundus; *FHB,* flexor hallucis brevis; *FHL,* flexor hallucis longus.

Physical Maneuvers

- Perform a passive motion maneuver across the joint of the affected limb to elicit an involuntary velocity-dependent tonic stretch reflex.
- Exaggerated phasic stretch reflexes—tendon jerks and clonus—can also often be elicited because of hyperexcitability of the stretch reflex.
- Depending on the degree of spasticity, the muscles will exhibit varying degrees of resistance.

Grading Scales

- Help qualify the spasticity and aid in determining response to treatment[1]

TABLE 25.3   Modified Ashworth Scale

0	No increase in muscle tone with ROM
1	Slight increase in tone with a catch and release at end ROM
1+	Slight increase in tone followed by catch and slight resistance throughout remainder of ROM
2	More marked increase in muscle tone through most of ROM, but affected part easily moved
3	Considerable increase in tone, passive movement is difficult
4	Affected part held in rigid flexion or extension

ROM, Range of motion.

- Two main grading scales qualify the degree of spasticity: Modified Ashworth Scale (MAS) and Tardieu Scale (Table 25.3)

Workup

Increases in spasticity should prompt further evaluation:
- Initial workup should begin with a thorough history and physical examination to assess for exacerbating factors along with basic laboratory studies to rule out underlying infection.
- Common precipitants are urinary tract infections, kidney stones, bladder distension, stool impaction, wounds, DVT, pain, restrictive clothing, psychological or emotional stressors, and changes in temperature.[1]

Treatment

Treatment Goals

- Balance out the benefits and disadvantages of spasticity
- Increase patient comfort
- Facilitate caretaker management
- Optimize function

Prevention of Spasticity

- Avoid noxious stimuli
- Maintain proper positioning
- Maintain a daily stretching and range of motion program

Nonpharmacological Management: Physiotherapy and Modalities*

- Physiotherapy: stretching, splinting, serial casting[4]
- Cryotherapy

*Use of modalities in TBI patients should be performed with caution, because they may be insensate or present with impaired communication, limiting their ability to convey adverse effects of treatment.

TABLE 25.4   Oral Medications for Spasticity

Medication	Dosing	Mechanism of Action	Common Side Effects	Cautions
Diazepam	Starting dose, 2 mg TID Max. 60 mg/day	Modulates postsynaptic effects of gamma aminobutyric acid (GABA) A transmission	Somnolence, muscle weakness, cognitive impairment	May worsen cognition in TBI, respiratory, or CNS depression
Baclofen	Starting dose, 5 mg TID Max. 80 mg/day	GABA B receptor agonist	Somnolence, lowered seizure threshold, confusion	Sudden withdrawal can cause seizures, hallucinations, fever
Tizanidine	Starting dose, 2 mg TID Max. 36 mg/day	Alpha-2 adrenergic receptor agonist	Hypotension, somnolence, xerostomia, asthenia, hepatotoxicity	LFT monitoring (on initiation and at 1, 3, and 6 months); contraindicated in concurrent use with IV ciprofloxacin because of inhibition of CYP1A2
Clonidine	Starting dose, 0.1 mg BID	Alpha-2 adrenergic receptor agonist	Hypotension, xerostomia, headache, somnolence	Withdrawal may result in hypertensive crisis
Dantrolene	Starting dose, 25 mg daily Max. 400 mg/day	Inhibits Ca2+ from the sarcoplasmic reticulum	Flushing, diarrhea, hepatotoxicity	Hepatotoxic: Monitor LFTs weekly in first month and every other month in first year

BID, twice a day; *IV*, intravenous; *LFT*, liver function test; *Max.*, maximum; *TBI*, traumatic brain injury; *TID*, three times a day.

- Local heat
- Ultrasound
- Transcutaneous electrical nerve stimulation[4]
- Electromyographic biofeedback
- Vibration[4]

Pharmacological Management

Oral Route of Administration

See Table 25.4 includes information on commonly used oral medications for spasticity.[1,3]

Local Interventions: Nerve Blocks, Chemical Neurolysis, and Chemodenervation

Nerve Blocks and Chemical Neurolysis

- The agent is injected directly next to a nerve or at the motor point, identified through use of a variable-intensity stimulator for localization, to induce neurolysis.[5]
- Local anesthetics bupivacaine and lidocaine can be used to disrupt the nerve signal for short-term evaluation and diagnostic purposes.
- Neurolytic agents phenol and ethanol are used to achieve more permanent effects and can last from months to years.
- Phenol nerve block of the tibial nerve has shown efficacy in reducing ankle plantarflexion inversion spasticity for up to 6 months[5] (Table 25.5).

Chemodenervation

- Clostridium botulinum is a gram-positive anaerobic bacterium that produces a family of neurotoxins with seven serotypes (A–G).[6]
- In the United States, three type A toxins are currently approved for clinical use in spasticity.
- Botulinum toxin is injected directly into the muscle belly as close to the motor end plate as possible.
- Time of onset is 24 to 72 hours, peak effect at 4 to 6 weeks, and duration of effect is 2 to 6 months.
- Injections should be spread out by a minimum of 3-month intervals to prevent antibody formation, which can lead to secondary nonresponse to treatment[3,6] (Table 25.6).

Intrathecal Baclofen Treatments

- Allows direct delivery of high concentrations of baclofen directly into the intrathecal space without the unwanted CNS effects (lethargy, confusion) of oral baclofen
- Indicated in patients with widespread spasticity that is unresponsive to conservative treatments or who are unable to tolerate medication side effects at their therapeutic dosage[7]

Complications

- Pump hardware malfunction

TABLE 25.5 Neurolytic Agents

Medication	Dosage	Mechanism of Action	Complications	Cautions
Phenol	Common concentration: 2%–7% >5% results in chemodenervation	Induces axonal destruction via nonselective protein denaturation at concentrations >3%–5%	Dysesthesia, muscle weakness, muscle pain/tenderness, skin sloughs	Intravascular injection can lead to convulsions, CNS depression, cardiovascular collapse
Ethyl alcohol	Concentration of 45%–100% required to achieve neurolytic effects	See above	See above	Intravascular injection has little to no systemic side effects

CNS, Central nervous system.

TABLE 25.6 Chemodenervation

Medication	Dosage	Mechanism of Action	Contraindications	Cautions
Botulinum toxin	Dosing varies based on targeted muscles, clinician experience, and serotype used	Prevents the presynaptic release of ACH at the NMJ by cleaving the SNAP-25 protein within the nerve terminal Prevents exocytosis of ACH-containing vesicles leading to chemical denervation	Infection at planned site of injection Known sensitivity to botulinum toxin	Caution use in neuromuscular diseases as may increase risk for dysphagia and respiratory depression Effects may spread beyond the targeted muscles

ACH, Acetylcholine; *NMJ*, neuromuscular junction.

- Programming error
- Medication overdose or withdrawal

Baclofen Withdrawal Signs[1,3,7]
- Fever
- Altered mental status
- Seizures
- Hallucinations
- Pruritus
- Tachycardia
- Exaggerated rebound spasticity

Surgical Management

Permanent surgical interventions are generally reserved in cases of refractory spasticity and contracture formation.

Orthopedic Interventions

- Tendon lengthening and tendon transfer procedures
- Split anterior tibial tendon transfer (SPLATT)
- Achilles lengthening procedure

Neurosurgical Interventions

- Surgical sectioning at the level of peripheral nerves and nerve rootlets
- Central electrical stimulators
- Neuroablative procedures
- Selective dorsal root rhizotomy[8]

Review Questions

1. Compared with botulinum toxin, the use of phenol for spasticity management is NOT associated with
   a. an increased risk of dysesthesia.
   b. lower cost.
   c. need for frequent administration.
   d. greater technical difficulty in administration.

2. On passive motion maneuver across the elbow joint, you note these findings: slight increase in tone followed by catch and slight resistance throughout remainder of range of motion (ROM). What Modified Ashworth Score (MAS) does this represent?
   a. 1
   b. 1+
   c. 2
   d. 3

3. On passive motion maneuver across the elbow joint, you note these findings: marked increase in muscle tone throughout ROM, but the joint is easily moved. What MAS does this represent?
   a. 1
   b. 1+
   c. 2
   d. 3

Answers on page 392.

Access the full list of questions and answers online. Available on ExpertConsult.com

References

1. Elovic E, Baerga E, Escaldi SV, et al. Associated topics in physical medicine and rehabilitation: spasticity. In: Cuccurullo SJ, ed. *Physical Medicine and Rehabilitation Board Review.* New York, NY: Demos Publishing; 2015:861-874.
2. Thibaut A, Chatelle C, Ziegler E, et al. Spasticity after stroke: physiology, assessment, and treatment. *Brain Inj.* 2013;27:1093-115.
3. Ripley D, Driver S, Stork R, et al. Pharmacologic management of the patient with traumatic brain injury. In: Eapen B, Cifu D, eds. *Rehabilitation After Traumatic Brain Injury.* St. Louis, MO: Elsevier; 2018:133-156.
4. Nair KP, Marsden J. The management of spasticity in adults. *BMJ.* 2014;349:g4737.
5. Anwar F, Mee H, Ramanathan S. Phenol nerve blocks for ankle plantar flexor and invertor spasticity in upper motor neuron lesions. A case series. *J Int Soc Phys Rehabil Med.* 2018:1:55-60.
6. Intiso D. Therapeutic use of botulinum toxin in neurorehabilitation. *J Toxicol.* 2011;2012:802893.
7. Francisco GE, Yablon SA, Schiess MC, Wiggs L, Cavalier S, Grissom S. Consensus panel guidelines for the use of intrathecal baclofen therapy in poststroke spastic hypertonia. *Top Stroke Rehabil.* 2006;13(4):74-85.
8. Aquilina K, Graham D, Wimalasundera N. Selective dorsal rhizotomy: an old treatment re-emerging. *Arch Dis Child.* 2015;100:798.
9. Coffey RJ, Edgar TS, Francisco GE. Abrupt withdrawal from intrathecal baclofen: recognition and management of a potentially life-threatening syndrome. *Arch Phys Med Rehabil.* 2002;83: 735-741.

26

Post-Traumatic Hydrocephalus

NEIL JASEY, MD, AND LAURIE DABAGHIAN, MD

Hydrocephalus is "an active distention of the ventricular system of the brain related to inadequate passage of cerebrospinal fluid (CSF) from its point of production within the ventricular system to its point of absorption into the systemic circulation."[1] It is broadly categorized as communicating or non-communicating. It is caused by:

- Excess CSF production
- Obstruction of CSF flow in the ventricles or subarachnoid space
- Decrease in absorption via the arachnoid granulations

Hydrocephalus ex vacuo is a compensatory enlargement of CSF space including cerebral ventricles and subarachnoid spaces in response to brain parenchyma loss.[2]

Pathophysiology

The choroid plexus produces 80% of CSF, and 20% is produced by the transependymal flow of fluid to the ventricles from parenchyma.[3]

CSF circulates from the lateral ventricles foramina of Monro, third ventricle aqueduct of Sylvius fourth ventricle foramina of Luschka and Magendie subarachnoid space (Fig. 26.1).

It is reabsorbed by arachnoid granulations in the dural venous sinuses.[4]

The underlying pathophysiology of posttraumatic hydrocephalus is primarily caused by a disruption of CSF flow.

Communicating or nonobstructive hydrocephalus is caused by impaired reabsorption of CSF at the arachnoid granulations after infection, inflammation, or hemorrhage. These processes cause scarring and fibrosis of the subarachnoid space, impairing re-absorption leading to enlargement of the ventricles.[4]

The dysfunction of the arachnoid villa is thought to be caused by subarachnoid blood; its metabolic products including hemoglobin, iron, and transforming growth factor-ß1 (TGF-β1) released from platelets. TGF-β1 and thrombin cause mechanical blockage and fibrosis of the arachnoid granulations, preventing CSF absorption and outward CSF flow from the subarachnoid space to the venous circulation.[3,5] Additionally, iron and thrombin cause ciliary dysfunction and destruction and ependymal cell damage in the ventricles impairing CSF circulation and causing hydrocephalus.[3,6]

Noncommunicating or obstructive hydrocephalus is caused by a blockage preventing the flow of CSF to the subarachnoid space. The obstruction can happen anywhere along the pathway of CSF flow, including the foramen of Monro, aqueduct of Sylvius, fourth ventricle, or the foramen of Luschka or Magendie. This causes accumulation of CSF proximal to the blockage, leading to increased ventricle size and increased CSF pressure.[4]

There are emerging hydrodynamic models looking at the role of pulsatile pressure and flow of CSF in the pathophysiology of hydrocephalus. These concepts are challenging the current theories of hydrocephalus.[7]

Incidence

Within 2 months after moderate to severe traumatic brain injury (TBI), 70% of patients develop ventriculomegaly caused by any etiology.[8] Studies excluding other causes of hydrocephalus, such as atrophy, have shown an incidence of posttraumatic hydrocephalus (PTH) ranging from 3.7% to 45%.[9-12] Variation may be caused by underdiagnosis and differences in diagnosing criteria.[13] In patients with decompressive craniectomy, a metaanalysis of retrospective studies determined that the rate of PTH is 6.3% to 54%,[14] similar to that reported by De Bonis et al. (0.7%–51.4%).[15]

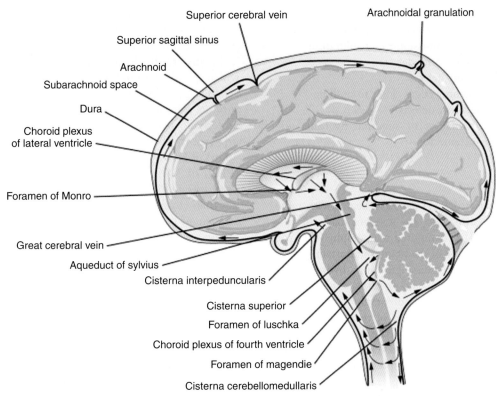

Superior cerebral vein

Superior sagittal sinus

Arachnoid

Subarachnoid space

Dura

Choroid plexus
of lateral ventricle

Foramen of Monro

Great cerebral vein

Aqueduct of sylvius

Cisterna interpeduncularis

Cisterna superior

Foramen of luschka

Choroid plexus of fourth ventricle

Foramen of magendie

Cisterna cerebellomedullaris

Arachnoidal granulation

• **Fig. 26.1** Anatomy of the ventricular system with cerebrospinal fluid flow. (From Abou-Hamden A, Drake J. Hydrocephalus and arachnoid cysts. In: Swaiman K, Ashwal S, Ferriero D, et al., eds. *Swaiman's Pediatric Neurology.* Philadelphia, PA: Elsevier; 2017:e561-e576.)

In the postacute period, patients may be diagnosed with hydrocephalus up to 8 weeks into their rehabilitation stay, with most diagnosed earlier. In some cases, patients may be diagnosed even a year after their injury.[11]

Presentation

The classic triad of symptoms present in a patient with hydrocephalus include incontinence, ataxia, and confusion—also known as *wet, wild, and wobbly.* The gait abnormality can be described as *magnetic* and resembles the type of ambulation noted in those with frontal lobe[16] or subcortical injury.[17] The cognitive deficits may manifest as impaired memory and confusion.[13]

In PTH, the presentation is often subtler. As described by Ivanhoe, "patients may present with abulia, emotional lability, perseveration, mutism, apraxia, or change in bladder or bowel function not related to infection[18]." The citation for this quote is the same as that following- It is Clinicians must be wary of a decline in function, plateau in improvement, or less improvement than expected as potential signs of PTH.[18] Additional symptoms include headache, nausea, increased spasticity, epileptic seizures, aggressiveness and parkinsonian features such as bradykinesia, rigidity, and postural instability.[9,16,19,20]

The most telling findings on physical examination are the characteristic gait of hydrocephalus (wide based, unsteady, small steps),[21] papilledema, focal neurological findings,[13]

and an abducens nerve palsy presenting as a mild decrease in lateral horizontal eye movement.[16] The lateral rectus palsy has been described as a component of Parinaud's syndrome, in which dilation of the third ventricle causes a downward compression on the collicular plate of the midbrain.[16]

In patients with severe TBI, diagnosis of PTH may be more difficult. A combination of radiographic imaging, CSF dynamics, and clinical deterioration during rehabilitation are used to assist the diagnosis of PTH.[11]

PTH has been shown to prevent and delay recovery after TBI and impair outcomes.[9] With CSF diversion, significant clinical improvement has been reported both acutely and long term, with positive impact seen in the Glasgow Outcome Scale, Functional Independence Measure (FIM), Disability Rating Scale (DRS), and Neurobehavioral Rating Scale at follow-up.[9,10]

Risk Factors

Risk factors for subsequent development of PTH include[9,11,15,22-24]:
- Older age
- Traumatic subarachnoid hemorrhage and intraventricular hemorrhage (Fisher grades III or IV)
- Posterior circulation bleeds
- More severe injury
  - Longer posttraumatic amnesia
  - Lower GCS scores

- Vegetative state
- Length of coma greater than or equal to 1 week
- Lower FIM scores on admission to rehabilitation
- Decompressive craniectomy defects
  - Larger craniectomy defects
  - Superior craniectomy edges closer to midline
  - Bilateral craniectomy defects
  - Extracranial herniation or subdural hygroma after decompressive craniectomy

Evaluation

Evaluation of suspected PTH typically begins with radiographic evaluation consisting of a standard magnetic resonance imaging (MRI) or computed tomography (CT) scan of the brain. Visualization of the brain is important in identifying ventriculomegaly, distinguishing hydrocephalus from hydrocephalus ex vacuo, and assessing shunt function. Multiple methods exist to standardize evaluation, including the Evans index, which is a marker of ventricular enlargement, or the enlargement of the anterior horns of the lateral ventricles, temporal horns, and third ventricle, and periventricular interstitial edema in the presence of normal or absent sulci[22] (Fig. 26.2).

Ventriculomegaly alone is not a reliable predictor of positive response to shunt placement.[17] More specialized radiographic techniques and invasive testing have been explored to aid in diagnosis and predict response to intervention. Examples include T2-weighted and proton density MRI scans that show a fast fluid flow in the cerebral aqueduct in association with increased ventricular size.[20] Additionally, Mazzini et al. demonstrated that single-photon emission computerized tomography (SPECT) scan had a higher sensitivity than MRI and CT in showing signs of hypoperfusion in the temporal lobes, distinguishing between PTH and ventricular enlargement caused by cortical atrophy.[10] Although used in the past, there is insufficient evidence supporting the use of radioisotope cisternography.[25]

Invasive testing is useful in determining which patients will respond to shunt insertion. These include different versions of CSF removal via lumbar puncture (LP) in varying volumes to transiently relieve the effects of the underlying hydrocephalus and evaluate for clinical improvement. These tests include tap tests—in which 30 to 50 mL is removed or prolonged external lumbar drainage (ELD) of 300 mL or repeated LPs are done. These tests demonstrate higher sensitivity and positive predictive values than clinical examination alone. The posttap clinical assessment is often subjective, with the most reliable predictor of clinical improvement being gait analysis.[18] Within gait, the most sensitive aspects are walking speed, steps needed for turning, and tendency toward falling.[21] Overall, positive responses to ELD and tap tests are the most well supported predictors of clinical improvement after shunt implantation.[25]

Treatment

The decision to treat PTH is typically subjective, based on clinical evaluations and dependent on the relationship with the neurosurgeon. Definitive treatment involves CSF diversion before the point of obstruction or impaired absorption via endoscopic third ventriculostomy (ETV) or a shunt connecting the ventricular system to a low-pressure cavity.[9] The most common shunts are ventriculoperitoneal shunt (VPS) (Fig. 26.3) followed by ventriculoatrial shunts with lumbar and pleural shunts reserved for unusual circumstances.[26] ETV has seen a rise in popularity as a treatment option given the rates of shunt failure and complications. The ventriculostomy is placed between the

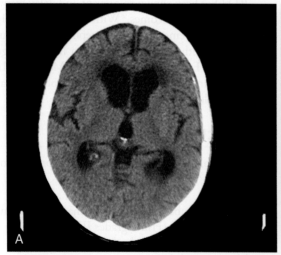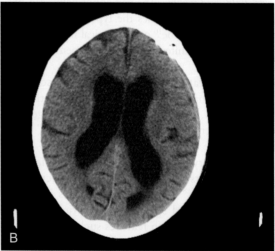

• **Fig. 26.2 (A and B)** Computed tomography (CT) scan of a 74-year-old woman with a history of traumatic brain injury and left subdural hemorrhage secondary to a fall with "moderate ventriculomegaly out of proportion to sulcal prominence suggestive of communicating hydrocephalus." This is an original photo.

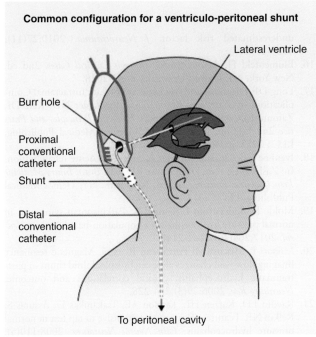

Common configuration for a ventriculo-peritoneal shunt

Lateral ventricle

Burr hole

Proximal
conventional
catheter

Shunt

Distal
conventional
catheter

To peritoneal cavity

• **Fig. 26.3** Ventriculoperitoneal shunt. (From Corns R, Martin A. Hydrocephalus. *Surgery*. 2012; 30[3]:142-148.)

floor of the third ventricle and the prepontine cistern midway between the mammillary bodies and the infundibular recess.[27] In 2015 Grand et al. reported in a retrospective review that ETV had been used successfully to treat hydrocephalus of varying etiologies, including aqueduct

stenosis, intraventricular hemorrhage, normal-pressure hydrocephalus, communicating hydrocephalus, remote head trauma, obstruction from tumor or cyst, and VPS obstruction.[27]

Types of Shunts

A full review of the different types of available shunts is beyond the scope of this chapter. Since the unidirectional valve was developed to prevent backflow of blood and clogging, subsequent generations of valves have been designed to limit overshunting. Newer valves are typically adjustable or use an antisiphon or gravitational design so that too much fluid is not removed in the vertical position.[26] Programmable shunts allow adjustment for different opening pressures without reoperation and are typically controlled by a magnet.[17]

Complications After Shunt Placement

Complication rates after shunt insertion for PTH are typically reported to be between 6% to 12%[9,25] and 11% for idiopathic hydrocephalus.

The most commonly encountered issues include:
• Postplacement seizures (12%)
• Shunt malfunction (12%)
• Shunt infection (6%)[9]

Other complications are a result of hydraulic mismanagement caused by overshunting, including positional headaches, subdural and hygroma formation, symptomatic slit ventricle, or skull deformations.[26]

Review Questions

1. You are taking care of a patient who sustained a traumatic brain injury (TBI). She is no longer making gains in therapy and is now regressing and requiring more assistance with transfers. Additionally, she is not tolerating her feeds and has been having increased episodes of emesis. You have also noticed increased spasticity in her limbs. Laboratory work and clinical picture otherwise have been stable. What would be your next step in management of this patient?
   a. Repeat labs and send urine-.
   b. Order a video electroencephalogram (EEG).
   c. Repeat head computed tomography (CT) or magnetic resonance imaging (MRI).
   d. Start a neurostimulant.
2. A patient developed hydrocephalus while in your care and underwent ventriculoperitoneal shunt (VPS) placement. Postprocedure, the patient showed improvement in his gait and mental status but since yesterday has started to become increasingly confused and is complaining of a headache that is not relieved with change

in position. What is the most common cause of his symptoms?
   a. Disconnection of the shunt components
   b. Distal shunt obstruction
   c. Proximal ventricular catheter occlusion
   d. Postsurgical headache
3. You admit a 28-year-old patient who sustained a TBI to your acute inpatient rehabilitation unit. In the emergency department, he had a Glasgow Coma Scale (GCS) score of 11, and head CT showed large right frontal subarachnoid hemorrhage and intraventricular hemorrhage. No neurosurgical intervention was performed. What puts him at highest risk for developing posttraumatic hydrocephalus?
   a. Age
   b. GCS score
   c. CT head findings
   d. No neurosurgical intervention

Answers on page 392.
Access the full list of questions and answers online.
Available on ExpertConsult.com

References

1. Rekate HL. A contemporary definition and classification of hydrocephalus. *Semin Pediatr Neurol.* 2009;16(1):9-15.

2. Denes Z, Barsi P, Szel I, Boros E, Fazekas G. Complication during postacute rehabilitation: patients with posttraumatic hydrocephalus. *Int J Rehabil Res.* 2011;34(3):222-226.

3. Chen Q, Feng Z, Tan Q, et al. Post-hemorrhagic hydrocephalus: Recent advances and new therapeutic insights. *J Neurol Sci.* 2017;375:220-230.

4. Oreskovic D, Klarica M. Development of hydrocephalus and classical hypothesis of cerebrospinal fluid hydrodynamics: facts and illusions. *Prog Neurobiol.* 2011;94(3):238-258.

5. Chen S, Luo J, Reis C, Manaenko A, Zhang J. Hydrocephalus after subarachnoid hemorrhage: pathophysiology, diagnosis, and treatment. *Biomed Res Int.* 2017;2017:8584753.

6. Gao F, Liu F, Chen Z, Hua Y, Keep RF, Xi G. Hydrocephalus after intraventricular hemorrhage: the role of thrombin. *J Cereb Blood Flow Metab.* 2014;34(3):489-494.

7. Tomycz LD, Hale AT, George TM. Emerging insights and new perspectives on the nature of hydrocephalus. *Pediatr Neurosurg.* 2017;52(6):361-368.

8. Poca MA, Sahuquillo J, Mataro M, Benejam B, Arikan F, Baguena M. Ventricular enlargement after moderate or severe head injury: a frequent and neglected problem. *J Neurotrauma.* 2005;22(11):1303-1310.

9. Weintraub AH, Gerber DJ, Kowalski RG. Posttraumatic hydrocephalus as a confounding influence on brain injury rehabilitation: incidence, clinical characteristics, and outcomes. *Arch Phys Med Rehabil.* 2017;98(2):312-319.

10. Mazzini L, Campini R, Angelino E, Rognone F, Pastore I, Oliveri G. Posttraumatic hydrocephalus: a clinical, neuroradiologic, and neuropsychologic assessment of long-term outcome. *Arch Phys Med Rehabil.* 2003;84(11):1637-1641.

11. Kammersgaard LP, Linnemann M, Tibaek M. Hydrocephalus following severe traumatic brain injury in adults. Incidence, timing, and clinical predictors during rehabilitation. *NeuroRehabilitation.* 2013;33(3):473-480.

12. Guyot LL, Michael DB. Post-traumatic hydrocephalus. *Neurol Res.* 2000;22(1):25-28.

13. Schultz BA, Bellamkonda E. Management of medical complications during the rehabilitation of moderate-severe traumatic brain injury. *Phys Med Rehabil Clin N orth Am.* 2017;28(2):259-270.

14. Fattahian R, Bagheri SR, Sadeghi M. Development of posttraumatic hydrocephalus requiring ventriculoperitoneal shunt after decompressive craniectomy for traumatic brain injury: a systematic review and meta-analysis of retrospective studies. *Med Arch.* 2018;72(3):214-219.

15. De Bonis P, Pompucci A, Mangiola A, Rigante L, Anile C. Posttraumatic hydrocephalus after decompressive craniectomy: an

16. underestimated risk factor. *J Neurotrauma.* 2010;27(11):1965-1970.

16. Blumenfeld H. *Neuroanatomy Through Clinical Cases.* 2nd ed. New York, NY: Oxford University Press; 2018.

17. Long DF. Diagnosis and Management of Late Intracranial Complications of Traumatic Brain Injury. In: Zasler ND, Katz DI, Zafonte RD, editors. *Brain Injury Medicine Principles and Practice* 2nd Edition. New York, NY: Demos Medical Publishing, LLC.; 2013. p. 726-47.

18. Ivanhoe CB, Durand-Sanchez A, Spier ET. Acute rehabilitation. In: Zasler ND, Katz DI, Zafonte RD, eds. *Brain Injury Medicine Principles and Practice.* 2nd ed. New York, NY: Demos Medical Publishing, LLC.; 2013.

19. Molde K, Soderstrom L, Laurell K. Parkinsonian symptoms in normal pressure hydrocephalus: a population-based study. *J Neurol.* 2017;264(10):2141-2148.

20. Missori P, Miscusi M, Formisano R, et al. Magnetic resonance imaging flow void changes after cerebrospinal fluid shunt in posttraumatic hydrocephalus: clinical correlations and outcome. *Neurosurg Rev.* 2006;29(3):224-228.

21. Ravdin LD, Katzen HL, Jackson AE, Tsakanikas D, Assuras S, Relkin NR. Features of gait most responsive to tap test in normal pressure hydrocephalus. *Clin Neurol Neurosurg.* 2008;110(5):455-461.

22. Chen H, Yuan F, Chen SW, et al. Predicting posttraumatic hydrocephalus: derivation and validation of a risk scoring system based on clinical characteristics. *Metab Brain Dis.* 2017;32(5):1427-1435.

23. Di G, Hu Q, Liu D, Jiang X, Chen J, Liu H. Risk factors predicting posttraumatic hydrocephalus after decompressive craniectomy in traumatic brain injury. *World Neurosurg.* 2018;116:e406-e413.

24. Xie Z, Hu X, Zan X, Lin S, Li H, You C. Predictors of shunt-dependent hydrocephalus after aneurysmal subarachnoid hemorrhage? A systematic review and meta-analysis. *World Neurosurg.* 2017;106:844-60.e6.

25. Halperin JJ, Kurlan R, Schwalb JM, Cusimano MD, Gronseth G, Gloss D. Practice guideline: Idiopathic normal pressure hydrocephalus: Response to shunting and predictors of response: Report of the Guideline Development, Dissemination, and Implementation Subcommittee of the American Academy of Neurology. *Neurology.* 2015;85(23):2063-2071.

26. Aschoff A, Kremer P, Hashemi B, Kunze S. The scientific history of hydrocephalus and its treatment. *Neurosurg Rev.* 1999;22(2-3):67-93; discussion 94-95.

27. Grand W, Leonardo J, Chamczuk AJ, Korus AJ. Endoscopic third ventriculostomy in 250 adults with hydrocephalus: patient selection, outcomes, and complications. *Neurosurgery.* 2016;78(1):109-119.

27
Cranial Nerve Disorders

GARY NOEL GALANG, MD, AND JUSTIN LOUIS WEPPNER, DO

OUTLINE

Twelve pairs of cranial nerves (CNs) emerge from the brain and radiate from its surface. CN injuries occur before, during, or after passing through the skull from compression secondary to increased intracranial pressure, traction, transection, ischemic event, acceleration–deceleration injury, shearing, skull fracture, intracranial hemorrhage, vascular occlusion, or brainstem herniation (Table 27.1). CN injuries are a relatively common complication of traumatic brain injury (TBI), but their incidence is difficult to estimate, and they have been shown to occur in mild to severe TBI. CN injury diagnosis is often based on physical examination, which may initially be complicated by the patient's mental status. A complete CN examination is necessary to assess for CN injury during recovery from TBI. The CNs most susceptible to injury in TBI are CN I followed by CN VII and CN VIII. Trigeminal (CN V) and lower CN (CN IX–XII) injuries are rare.

Olfactory (CN I)

- Olfactory stimuli are detected by specialized chemoreceptors on bipolar primary sensory neurons of the olfactory nerve.

- Axons of these bipolar neurons travel via short olfactory nerves that traverse the cribriform plate of the ethmoid bone to synapse in the olfactory bulbs.
- From the olfactory bulbs, sensory information travels via olfactory tracts that communicate with the brain through the olfactory processing areas.
- Injury occurs from direct bony disruption, from olfactory bulb compression, or from a rapid shift in the position of the brain relative to the skull base, shearing the fixed olfactory receptor axons from the mobile olfactory bulb.
- Higher incidences of olfactory injury are associated with increased TBI severity, with anosmia in 25% to 30%, 15% to 19%, and 0% to 16% of patients with severe, moderate, and mild head injuries, respectively.[1]
- Injury to the olfactory nerve is the only CN injury commonly associated with mild TBI.
- No treatments are available for CN I injury, and reversible confounding diagnoses—including nasal obstruction, polyps, injury to the nasal passages, rhinitis, sinusitis, medications, and seizures—should be identified and managed.
- Alterations in the sense of smell may also alter the sense of taste, which can result in anorexia.
- Inability to detect spoiled food and gas leakage are the two predominant adverse effects involving personal safety.
- Approximately one-third of patients may experience some degree of spontaneous recovery, which usually occurs within 6 to 12 months after injury.[2]

Optic (CN II)

- The optic nerve provides the special sense of sight.
- It transmits visual information from the retina to the thalamus and then to the extrageniculate pathways.
- The reported incidence of optic nerve injury is 0.7% to 2.5%.[3-5]
- Sphenoid bone fracture or optic nerve compression can result in unilateral blindness. Optic chiasm insults can lead to bitemporal hemianopsia.
- Treatment options include (1) systemic steroids, (2) surgical decompression of the optic canal, (3) combination of steroids and surgery, and (4) observation alone.

TABLE 27.1	Cranial Nerve (CN) Examination and Diagnostic Evaluation	
CN	**Examination**	**Diagnostic Evaluation**
I	Test ability to identify familiar odors, one naris at a time with eyes closed	CT of the paranasal sinuses MRI may be used especially if intracranial pathology is suspected in the olfactory bulbs or tracts
II	Test visual acuity, test visual fields, and perform ophthalmoscopic examination	Electroretinography and visual evoked potentials EEG may be used to assess for occipital seizures
III	Inspect eyelids for drooping Inspect pupils for equality and their direct and consensual response to light and accommodation Test extraocular eye movements in the six cardinal positions with convergence on near targets, pursuit movements, and saccades Doll's eye maneuver may be used for unconscious patients	CT is ideal for ruling out bony lesions such as fractures and evaluating for herniation in acute trauma
IV	Assess adduction in conjunction with downward gaze of the involved eye	CT or MRI may localize an inciting lesion
V	Inspect face for muscle atrophy and tremors Palpate jaw muscles for tone and strength as the patient clenches teeth Test superficial pain and sensation in each of the three branches Assess corneal reflex	EMG and NCS may provide diagnostic information
VI	Assess for deficiency in lateral gaze when testing eye movement through full horizontal gaze	CT or MRI may localize an inciting lesion
VII	Inspect symmetry of facial features with various facial expressions (e.g., smile, frown, wrinkle forehead, puff cheeks, close eyes tightly) Test ability to identify sweet and salty tastes on each side of the tongue	CT is useful for assessing bony structures EMG and NCS offer insights into prognosis and therapeutic options
VIII	Test sense of hearing with whisper screening test Compare bone and air conduction of sound via Rinne and Weber tests Examine tympanic membrane for perforation Test eye movements for nystagmus	Audiogram Auditory brainstem response has value for assessing brainstem and CN integrity in patients unable to participate in an audiogram
IX	Test gag reflex and swallowing ability Test ability to identify sour and bitter tastes	MRI is the standard imaging modality for CN IX, X, and XI nerve injuries For CN XI injuries, EMG/NCS may aid diagnosis and provide prognostic information
X	Inspect palate and uvula for symmetry with speech sounds and gag reflex Assess for dysphagia	
XI	Test trapezius muscle strength by shrugging shoulders against resistance Test sternocleidomastoid muscle strength by turning head to each side against resistance	
XII	• Inspect tongue in mouth and while protruding for symmetry, tremors, and atrophy	• MRI is ideal for assessing lesions near the medulla • Moving distally, CT assesses for bony lesions

CT, computed tomography; *EEG,* electroencephalography; *EMG,* electromyography; *MRI,* magnetic resonance imaging; *NCS,* nerve conduction study.

- A visual recovery rate of 40% to 60% has been reported, with baseline visual acuity being an important predictor of final outcome. Negative predictors of vision recovery include presence of blood in the posterior ethmoidal cells, age above 40 years, loss of consciousness, and absence of recovery after 48 hours of steroid treatment.[6,7]

Oculomotor (CN III)

- The oculomotor nerve supplies somatic motor innervation to the levator palpebrae superior; superior, medial, and inferior rectus; and inferior oblique.
- CN III provides parasympathetic nerve fibers that innervate the sphincter muscle of the iris and the ciliary

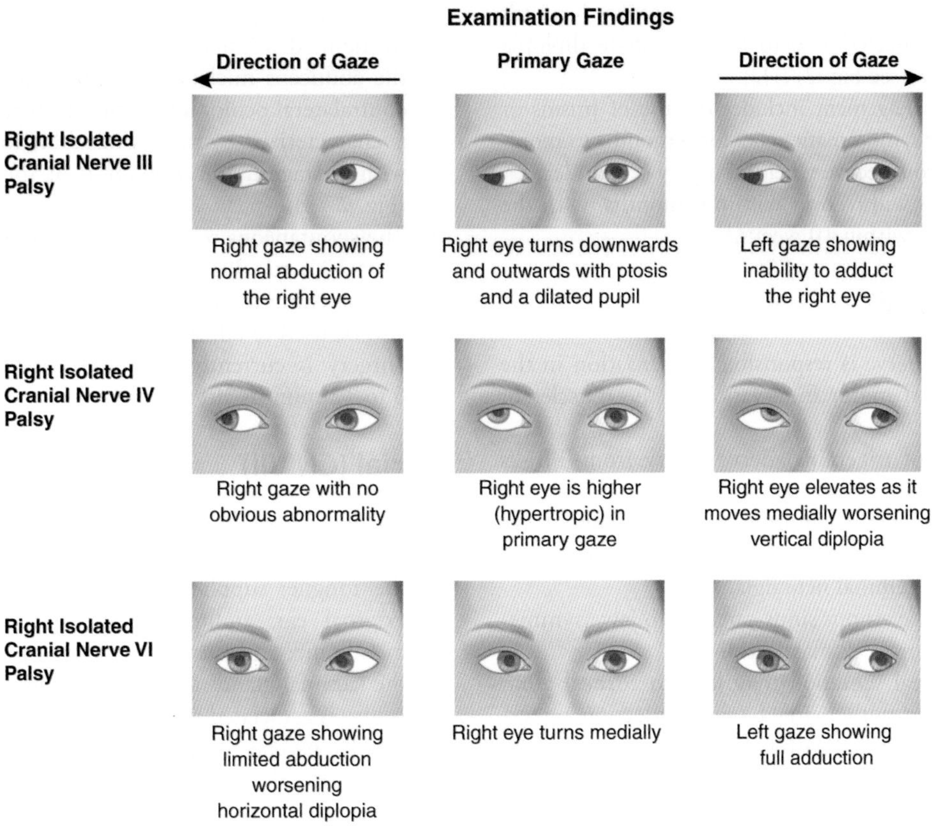

Examination Findings

	← Direction of Gaze	Primary Gaze	Direction of Gaze →
Right Isolated Cranial Nerve III Palsy	Right gaze showing normal abduction of the right eye	Right eye turns downwards and outwards with ptosis and a dilated pupil	Left gaze showing inability to adduct the right eye
Right Isolated Cranial Nerve IV Palsy	Right gaze with no obvious abnormality	Right eye is higher (hypertropic) in primary gaze	Right eye elevates as it moves medially worsening vertical diplopia
Right Isolated Cranial Nerve VI Palsy	Right gaze showing limited abduction worsening horizontal diplopia	Right eye turns medially	Left gaze showing full adduction

• **Fig. 27.1** Examination findings for isolated cranial nerve III, IV, and VI palsies.

muscle, which controls the shape of the lens during accommodation.

- A complete oculomotor nerve palsy will result in exotropia with a characteristic down-and-out position in the affected eye, ptosis, and mydriasis (Fig. 27.1).
- This nerve is often injured at the point of exit through the dura or from compression caused by uncal herniation related to increased intracranial pressure (Fig. 27.2).

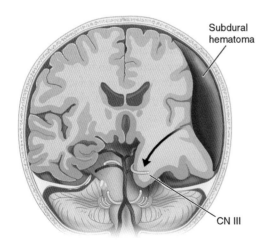

• **Fig. 27.2** The first structure to herniate is usually the uncus on the medial temporal lobe. As the uncus herniates, it compresses the midbrain, resulting in ipsilateral third nerve palsy. The parasympathetic fibers are on the outside of cranial nerve (CN) III, and the first sign of uncal herniation is usually pupillary dilatation followed by paralysis of the extraocular muscles.

- Direct oculomotor nerve injury occurs in 1.1% of TBI cases.[8]
- Occlusion therapy provides symptomatic relief of diplopia while the patch is on but does not provide long-term therapeutic benefit.
- Strabismus surgery is delayed 6 to 9 months to allow spontaneous recovery, which may correct the cosmetic deformity without improving the underlying cause.
- Most patients will experience functional recovery within 6 to 12 months of injury, with a 40% chance of complete recovery.[9]
- Aberrant reinnervation may occur in patients recovering from CN III palsy:
  - Eyelid-gaze dyskinesis: elevation of the involved eyelid on downgaze
  - Pupil-gaze dyskinesis: pupil constriction on downgaze or adduction

Trochlear (CN IV)

- The trochlear nerve provides somatic motor innervation to the superior oblique muscle, which provides eye intorsion, depression, and abduction.
- Unilateral traumatic lesion of the trochlear nerve has a reported incidence of 0.23% to 3.20%.[10,11]
- The primary complaint is diplopia, which is often vertical and worse with reading or walking down the stairs.
- There is deficient inferior movement of the affected eye when attempting to look down and inward. The involved

eye is superior in primary gaze. Compensatory head tilt away from the affected side to help eliminate diplopia may be observed (see Fig. 27.1).

- Symptomatic management includes the use of prisms or eye patching for symptomatic relief for 6 months to monitor for spontaneous recovery before surgery is considered.
- 50% of patients will recover within 6 months, with the average recovery within 10 weeks.[12]

Trigeminal (CN V)

- The trigeminal nerve is responsible for sensation in the face, cornea, and motor innervation of the muscles of mastication.
- The incidence of trigeminal nerve injury from TBI is 1.4% to 2.0%.[13]
- Patients with trigeminal injuries may complain of eye pain, decreased facial sensation, or facial dysesthesias and symptoms of trigeminal neuralgia.
- A lesion in the cavernous sinus can lead to jaw asymmetry on opening or weak mastication.
- Decreased corneal sensation may lead to corneal abrasions and drying with marked scleral injection on examination and is treated with frequent eye irrigation and lubricating gel.
- Patients with facial dysesthesias may respond to anticonvulsant medications such as carbamazepine, which may be combined with nerve blocks.
- If conservative measures fail, neurectomy and decompressive surgery may be considered.

Abducens (CN VI)

- The abducens is a somatic motor nerve that provides innervation to the lateral rectus muscle.
- Injury is reported to occur in 1.0% to 2.7% of all head traumas.[14,15]
- It is vulnerable to increased intracranial pressure and may serve as an early indicator of increased intracranial pressure.
- Injury caused to the cavernous sinus or skull base fractures can result in abducens palsy, resulting in medial deviation of the ipsilateral eye and diplopia that improves when the contralateral eye is abducted (see Fig. 27.1).

- Internuclear ophthalmoplegia (INO) arises from a lesion to the medial longitudinal fasciculus, which arises from the abducens nucleus in the pons and traverses to the contralateral oculomotor nucleus in the midbrain. INO is characterized by paresis of adduction on lateral gaze, with nystagmus on abduction of the contralateral eye (Fig. 27.3).
- The spontaneous recovery rate for CN VI injury ranges from 12% to 73% at 6 months.[16,17]
- Eye patching for symptomatic cases or prism lenses can also be used to alleviate diplopia.
- Surgery is currently indicated for nonrecovery within 6 to 12 months after injury.

Facial (CN VII)

- The facial nerve controls the muscles of facial expression; provides taste sensation from the anterior two-thirds of the tongue; supplies tactile sensation to parts of the external ear, auditory canal, and external tympanic membrane; and furnishes visceral motor innervation to the lacrimal glands and salivary glands.
- Injury is associated with a transverse temporal bone fracture (transverse to the long axis of the petrous pyramid), with CN VII injuries occurring in half of patients with a transverse fracture.
- Of all temporal bone fractures, 80% to 90% are longitudinal, and 10% to 20% are transverse.
- Upper motor neuron (UMN) lesions above the motor nucleus of CN VII cause contralateral paralysis of the face below the eyes.
- Lower motor neuron (LMN) lesions damaging the facial nucleus or its axons along its course after leaving the nucleus cause ipsilateral paralysis of the entire face on one side, with flattening of the forehead and inability to close the eye.
- Temporal bone fractures are associated with LMN injury.
- Injury to the facial nerve is the second most common CN injury, with a 5% incidence.[18]
- When the onset of nerve palsy is delayed, the nerve is frequently structurally intact and recovers within 8 weeks.[19]
- Spontaneous recovery occurs in up to 30% of cases.[18]
- The primary ocular complication of facial palsy is corneal exposure caused by decreased ability to close the

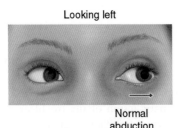
Looking left

Normal abduction

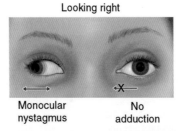
Looking right

Monocular nystagmus

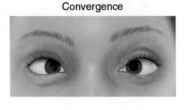
Convergence

No adduction

• **Fig. 27.3** Internuclear ophthalmoplegia is caused by a lesion of the medial longitudinal fasciculus and is clinically characterized by total or partial failure to adduct one eye in lateral gaze and a monocular nystagmus of the abducting eye. Convergence is usually preserved.

eye, which may be treated with artificial tears, lubricating ointments, temporary or permanent tarsorrhaphy, or an eyelid gold weight to facilitate eyelid closure.

- Synkinesis is aberrant CN VII reinnervation during nerve regeneration causing crocodile tears in which tears replace salivation during eating.

Vestibulocochlear (CN VIII)

- This sensory nerve is made up of a vestibular division that transmits information regarding head positioning and rotation and a cochlear division, which receives auditory stimuli.
- In cochlear nerve injuries, patients complain of hearing loss and high-frequency tinnitus, whereas injuries to the vestibular division result in complaints of vertigo.
- Sensorineural hearing loss is the most common form in TBI and is caused by disruption of the transmission of auditory pathway impulses, whereas conductive hearing loss results from disruption of sound transmission from damage to the tympanic membrane, ossicles, or cochlea.
- CN VIII injury is common in temporal bone fractures.
- Transverse temporal bone fractures have been reported to result in a high incidence of sensorineural hearing loss, with this injury unamenable to surgical repair.
- Longitudinal fractures (parallel to the long axis of the petrous pyramid) result in conductive hearing loss or mixed conductive and sensorineural hearing loss.
- Conductive deafness usually shows useful recovery and is amenable to surgical intervention.
- Vestibular dysfunction may manifest clinically with vertigo, nystagmus, or ataxia.
- Distinguishing peripheral from central vestibular lesions may be challenging. Peripheral lesions may be accompanied by ipsilateral hearing loss and tinnitus, whereas central lesions may be associated with motor and sensory disturbances of the limbs, dysarthria, dysphagia, or diplopia.

Glossopharyngeal (CN IX)

- The glossopharyngeal nerve controls movement of the pharynx during speech and swallowing, gustatory sensation from the posterior one-third of the tongue, and detection of blood pressure and arterial oxygen.
- The incidence of glossopharyngeal dysfunction after trauma is 0.5% to 1.6%.[13]

- Symptoms include loss of taste over the posterior one-third of the tongue, deviation of the uvula toward the contralateral side, decreased salivation, and mild dysphagia.
- Glossopharyngeal nerve injury symptoms are usually mild and generally require no treatment or symptomatic treatment alone.
- CN IX, X, and XI traverse the jugular foramen together. *Jugular foramen syndrome* (Vernet syndrome) refers to injury of CN IX, X, and XI, usually secondary to a skull base fracture, and may result in significant dysphagia secondary to CN X injury.

Vagus (CN X)

- CN X provides motor innervation to the pharynx and soft palate and parasympathetic innervation to the heart, lungs, and digestive tract.
- The incidence of CN X involvement in TBI is 0.05% to 0.16%.[13]
- Vagus nerve injury may be associated with hoarse voice, absent gag reflex, dysphagia, and hypophonia or aphonia secondary to ipsilateral vocal fold paralysis.

Spinal Accessory (CN XI)

- CN XI provides somatic motor innervation to the sternocleidomastoid muscle and upper half of the trapezius.
- In the setting of TBI, CN XI injury is the often secondary to trauma to the lateral neck.
- Symptoms include inability to turn the head to the opposite side and ipsilateral shoulder depression, resulting in shoulder dysfunction.
- Once CN XI injury is identified, physical therapy should be initiated promptly to strengthen the neck and shoulder muscles.

Hypoglossal (CN XII)

- The hypoglossal nerve provides somatic motor function, innervating the ipsilateral intrinsic tongue musculature.
- Tongue protrusion deviation toward the lesion indicates LMN injury and tongue deviation away from the lesion indicates UMN injury.
- Injury to CN XII is commonly associated with penetrating wounds to the neck.
- Dysarthria and dysphagia may result, necessitating swallowing precautions and oral motor exercises.
- Most unilateral lesions resolve by 6 months, and LMN injuries have a better prognosis.

Review Questions

1. A 27-year-old male patient with a history of recent mild traumatic brain injury (TBI) presents for evaluation with a complaint that all foods taste bland, weight loss, and anorexia. What is the most likely cranial nerve (CN) injury that should be considered in the differential diagnosis for the patient?
   a. CN I (olfactory nerve)
   b. CN XII (hypoglossal nerve)
   c. CN IX (glossopharyngeal nerve)
   d. CN X (vagus nerve)
2. Which CN is the most susceptible to injury in the setting of TBI?
   a. CN V (trigeminal nerve)
   b. CN XII (hypoglossal nerve)
   c. CN VIII (vestibulocochlear nerve)
   d. CN I (olfactory nerve)
3. A 35-year-old female patient presents after a motor vehicle collision in which she was a restrained passenger.

She experiences a brief loss of consciousness with retrograde amnesia and continues to have headaches, horizontal diplopia, and dizziness. Ophthalmologic examination revealed normal visual acuity, and ophthalmoscopy also revealed normal findings. However, on rightward gaze, her left eye does not adduct past the midline, and horizontal nystagmus is noted in the right eye. Upward and downward gaze are normal. What is the diagnosis?
   a. CN III (oculomotor nerve) injury
   b. Horner syndrome
   c. Internuclear ophthalmoplegia (INO)
   d. CN VI (abducens nerve) injury

Answers on page 393.
Access the full list of questions and answers online.
Available on ExpertConsult.com

References

1. Costanzo R, Zasler N. Epidemiology and pathophysiology of olfactory and gustatory dysfunction in head trauma. *J Head Trauma Rehabil.* 1992;7(1):15-24.
2. Welge-Lüssen A, Hilgenfeld A, Meusel T, Hummel T. Long-term follow-up of posttraumatic olfactory disorders. *Rhinology.* 2012;50(1):67-72.
3. Cockerham GC, Goodrich GL, Weichel ED, et al. Eye and visual function in traumatic brain injury. *J Rehabil Res Dev.* 2009; 46(6):811-818.
4. Nau HE, Gerhard L, Foerster M, Nahser HC, Reinhardt V, Joka T. Optic nerve trauma: clinical, electrophysiological and histological remarks. *Acta Neurochir (Wien).* 1987;89(1-2):16-27.
5. Pirouzmand F. Epidemiological trends of traumatic optic nerve injuries in the largest Canadian adult trauma center. *J Craniofac Surg.* 2012;23(2):516-520.
6. Levin LA, Beck RW, Joseph MP, Seiff S, Kraker R. The treatment of traumatic optic neuropathy: the International Optic Nerve Trauma Study. *Ophthalmology.* 1999;106(7):1268-1277.
7. Carta A, Ferrigno L, Salvo M, Bianchi-Marzoli S, Boschi A, Carta F. Visual prognosis after indirect traumatic optic neuropathy. *J Neurol Neurosurg Psychiatry.* 2003;74(2):246-248.
8. Memon MY, Paine KW. Direct injury of the oculomotor nerve in craniocerebral trauma. *J Neurosurg.* 1971;35(4):461-464.
9. Tokuno T, Nakazawa K, Yoshida S, et al. Primary oculomotor nerve palsy due to head injury: analysis of 10 cases. *No Shinkei Geka.* 1995;23(6):497-501.
10. Jin H, Wang S, Hou L, et al. Clinical treatment of traumatic brain injury complicated by cranial nerve injury. *Injury.* 2010;41(9):918-923.
11. Li G, Zhu X, Gu X, et al. Ocular movement nerve palsy after mild head trauma. *World Neurosurg.* 2016;94:296-302.
12. Mansour AM, Reinecke RD. Central trochlear palsy. *Surv Ophthalmol.* 1986;30(5):279-297.
13. Keane JR, Baloh RW. Posttraumatic cranial neuropathies. *Neurol Clin.* 1992;10(4):849-867.
14. Arias MJ. Bilateral traumatic abducens nerve palsy without skull fracture and with cervical spine fracture: case report and review of the literature. *Neurosurgery.* 1985;16(2):232-234.
15. Marconi F, Parenti G, Dobran M. Bilateral traumatic abducens nerve palsy. Case report. *J Neurosurg Sci.* 1994;38(3):177-180.
16. Mutyala S, Holmes JM, Hodge DO, Younge BR. Spontaneous recovery rate in traumatic sixth-nerve palsy. *Am J Ophthalmol.* 1996;122(6):898-899.
17. Holmes JM, Droste PJ, Beck RW. The natural history of acute traumatic sixth nerve palsy or paresis. *J AAPOS.* 1998;2(5):265-268.
18. Odebode TO, Ologe FE. Facial nerve palsy after head injury: case incidence, causes, clinical profile and outcome. *J Trauma.* 2006;61(2):388-391.
19. Berrol S. *Cranial Nerve Dysfunction.* Philadelphia, PA: Hanley & Belfus; 1989.

28

Posttraumatic Seizure and Epilepsy

JUSTIN SUP HONG, MD

Posttraumatic seizure (PTS) and posttraumatic epilepsy (PTE) are potential complications of traumatic brain injury (TBI). PTS is defined as a single seizure resulting from head trauma in exclusion of other causes.[1] PTE is defined as a posttraumatic recurrent seizure disorder with each event being separated by more than 24 hours.[2] For clarification purposes, when referring to *TBI* in this chapter, the author is not including concussion.

Classification

PTS types include[3]:
- Generalized seizures (other terms include *grand mal* or *tonic–clonic seizures* when there is motor involvement or *absence seizures* when there is not)
- Focal seizures without or with alteration of consciousness and awareness (other terms are *simple partial* and *complex partial seizures*, respectively)
  - Focal seizures can progress to generalized seizures (secondary generalization).
  - Most PTS are the focal seizure type (partial)[1,2,4]
- PTS is classified temporally as[1,2,4]:
  - Immediate (occurring within 24 hours posttrauma)
  - Early (between 24 hours and 1 week posttrauma)
  - Late (after 1 week posttrauma)

Epidemiology

Incidence rates of immediate, early, and late PTS are 1% to 4%, 4% to 25%, and 9% to 42%, respectively.[1] Depending on TBI severity, 2% to 50% of patients may develop PTE.[5] In the general population, for 10% to 20% of patients with symptomatic epilepsy, it is attributed to PTE.[1,2,5] Eighty-percent of patients with PTE have their first seizure within 1 year postinjury, 90% within 2 years postinjury.[1] Patients with moderate or severe TBI are at increased risk for seizures for 10 to 20+ years postinjury.[1,6]

Risk Factors for Late-onset Posttraumatic Epilepsy

PTE probability within 5 years postinjury depends on TBI severity: mild TBI (0.7%), moderate TBI (1.2%), severe TBI (10%).[2] Late-onset PTE risk factors include[1,2,5-8]:
- Injury type/location: Biparietal contusions (66%), dural penetration with fragments (62.5%), multiple intracranial operations (36.5%), subcortical contusions (33.4%), evacuated subdural hematoma (27.8%), greater than 5 mm midline shift (25.8%), multiple or bilateral cortical contusions (25%)[7]
- Depressed skull fracture
- Loss of consciousness longer than 30 minutes
- Posttraumatic amnesia longer than 24 hours
- Early PTS
- Alcohol
- Increasing age: Adolescents and adults at higher risk than children.
- Genetics

Pathophysiology

The pathophysiology of PTS and PTE is an area of ongoing research.[1,2,5] Multiple mechanisms have been proposed for PTS. Immediate or early PTS is thought to result from TBI primary injury and late PTS from secondary injury. Seizures result in increased intracranial pressure and neurometabolic demand and can lead to further neurologic injury.[9]

Diagnosis

Making the diagnosis of PTE can be challenging. Depending on the type and location of seizures, the presentation of patients with PTE can range from diffuse tonic–clonic movements to subtle, repetitive alterations in sensation, cognition, and behavior (i.e., partial seizures). Patient signs and symptoms may overlap with other diagnoses, so it is important to approach workup carefully. Although there are diagnostic testing options, the diagnosis of PTE is ultimately made on a clinical basis.

Diagnostic Tests

Consider workup of other medical issues (e.g., acute intracranial process, electrolyte abnormality, infection).[1]

- Electroencephalogram (EEG): Types include standard, sleep, sleep-deprived, ambulatory, or video-monitored. Of the different testing options, video-EEG monitoring is the gold standard. There are limitations to EEG testing. It has limited sensitivity to rule out seizures. It can result in normal findings. Additionally, depending on their neurobehavioral status, patients may not be able to cooperate with the procedure.[10-11]
- Serum prolactin: Can be elevated after a seizure. This laboratory test could be used as an adjunct test to help differentiate between an epileptic and nonepileptic event, but a normal serum prolactin value does not rule out seizure.[12]
- Consider neurology consult.

Treatment Options

- Medication: Current guidelines are to treat TBI patients with 7 days of antiepileptic drug (AED) for seizure prophylaxis. Long-term AED treatment is not recommended for patients with immediate PTS. Studies have not demonstrated efficacy in reduction of late-onset seizures or mortality with long-term AED treatment in the absence of early or late PTS. Patients who have early or late PTS are to be treated with AED long term. *If stable from a seizure standpoint for at least 2 years, taper of AED could be considered.* Superiority of individual AED agents in PTE has not been supported in studies. *All AEDs, especially older agents such as phenytoin and phenobarbital, have potential for cognitive and motor side effects.* In patients with neurocognitive issues, AED adverse effect should be considered in the differential diagnosis. Medication choice should be based on factors including side effect profile, potential drug-drug interactions, patient tolerability, dosing schedule, need for monitoring, and expected patient medication compliance. Female TBI patients with potential for pregnancy should be counseled on potential teratogenic effects of AEDs. Additionally, consider the potential therapeutic effects of individual AEDs (e.g., mood stabilization and migraine prophylactic effects of valproic acid).[1,4,13-14]
- Surgical: Consider neurosurgical consult. Although less extensively studied in the diagnosis of PTE, there are surgical options for patients with intractable epilepsy: Resection can be considered if a seizure focus or area can be localized. In cases in which the seizure foci cannot be localized, vagal nerve stimulator placement is another option, but this intervention is expected, at best, to decrease seizure frequency.[15-16]

Driving and Work

There is variation from state to state in how driving is managed in regards to epilepsy.[17] Patients will need to be stable from a seizure standpoint for a period of time (typically ranging from 3–12 months) and have forms completed by their healthcare provider to request reinstatement of driving privileges by the state board. Restoration of a commercial driver's license may be challenging because of restrictions on medications with potential psychotropic effects.

In regards to work, it is recommended that the employer obtain a comprehensive job description, along with potential for schedule or work accommodations, to maximize safety in returning to work.

Review Questions

1. A late posttraumatic seizure (PTS) occurs during which time frame?
   a. Within 24 hours
   b. Between 1 and 7 days
   c. After 1 week
   d. After 1 month
2. A patient is admitted to the hospital after witnessed fall off a ladder onto his head with loss of consciousness and generalized tonic–clonic movements that resolved after a couple minutes. Head computed tomography (CT) reveals intraparenchymal hematoma without significant mass effect. How long should he be treated with an antiepileptic drug (AED)?
   a. No AED treatment is indicated
   b. 1 week
   c. 3 months
   d. 1 year

3. You are managing a patient in the acute rehabilitation TBI unit. She is presenting with intermittent periods of confusion and irritability manifested as shouting, pulling at lines, and aggression toward staff. This is interfering with her therapy program participation. Recent imaging and laboratory workup have ruled out acute intracranial process, electrolyte abnormality, and ongoing infection. Intermittent seizures are suspected. What is the next reasonable step in care?
   a. Clinically observe
   b. Order standard electroencephalogram (EEG)
   c. Order serum prolactin level
   d. Treat empirically with AED and monitor patient response

Answers on page 394.
Access the full list of questions and answers online. Available on ExpertConsult.com

References

1. Agrawal A, Timothy J, Pandit L, Manju M. Post-traumatic epilepsy: an overview. *Clin Neurol Neurosurg*. 2006;108(5):433-439. doi:10.1016/j.clineuro.2005.09.001.

2. Lucke-Wold BP, Nguyen L, Turner RC, et al. Traumatic brain injury and epilepsy: underlying mechanisms leading to seizure. *Seizure*. 2015;33:13-23. doi:10.1016/j.seizure.2015.10.002.

3. Fisher RS, Cross JH, French JA, et al. Operational classification of seizure types by the International League Against Epilepsy: Position Paper of the ILAE Commission for Classification and Terminology. *Epilepsia*. 2017;58(4):522-530. doi:10.1046/j.1528-1157.2001.35100.x.

4. Zimmermann L, Martin RM, Girgis F. Treatment options for posttraumatic epilepsy. *Curr Opin Neurol*. 2017;30(6):580-586. doi:10.1097/WCO.0000000000000505.

5. Saletti PG, Ali I, Casillas-Espinosa PM, et al. In search of antiepileptogenic treatments for post-traumatic epilepsy. *Neurobiol Dis*. 2019;123:86-99. doi:10.1016/j.nbd.2018.06.017.

6. Temkin NR. Risk factors for posttraumatic seizures in adults. *Epilepsia*. 2003;44(suppl 10):18-20. doi:10.1046/j.1528-1157.44.s10.6.x.

7. Englander J, Bushnik T, Duong TT, et al. Analyzing risk factors for late posttraumatic seizures: a prospective, multicenter investigation. *Arch Phys Med Rehabil*. 2003;84:365-373. doi:10.1053/apmr.2003.50022.

8. Kumar RG, Breslin KB, Ritter AC, Conley YP, Wagner AK. Variability with astroglial glutamate transport genetics is associated with increased risk for post-traumatic seizures. *J Neurotrauma*. 2019;36:230-238. doi:10.1089/neu.2018.5632.

9. Vespa PM, Miller C, McArthur D, et al. Nonconvulsive electrographic seizures after traumatic brain injury result in a delayed, prolonged increase in intracranial pressure and metabolic crisis. *Crit Care Med*. 2007;35(12):2830-2836. doi:10.1097/01.CCM.0000295667.66853.BC.

10. Desai B, Whitman S, Bouffard DA. The role of the EEG in epilepsy of long duration. *Epilepsia*. 1988;29(5):601-606. doi:10.1111/j.1528-1157.1988.tb03768.x.

11. Cuthill FM, Espie CA. Sensitivity and specificity of procedures for the differential diagnosis of epileptic and non-epileptic seizures: a systematic review. *Seizure*. 2005;14:293-303. doi:10.1016/j.seizure.2005.04.006.

12. Chen DK, So YT, Fisher RS. Use of serum prolactin in diagnosing epileptic seizures: Report of the Therapeutics and Technology Assessment Subcommittee of the American Academy of Neurology. *Neurology*. 2005;65:668-675. doi:10.1212/01.wnl.0000178391.96957.d0

13. Wilson CD, Burks JD, Rodgers RB, Evans RM, Bakare AA, Safavi-Abbasi SS. Early and late posttraumatic epilepsy in the setting of traumatic brain injury: a meta-analysis and review of antiepileptic management. *World Neurosurg*. 2018;110:E901-E906. doi:10.1016/j.wneu.2017.11.116.

14. Thompson K, Pohlmann-Eden B, Campbell LA, Abel H. Pharmacological treatments for preventing epilepsy following traumatic head injury. *Cochrane Database Syst Rev*. 2015;8:CD009900. doi:10.1002/14651858.CD009900.pub2.

15. Spencer S, Huh L. Outcomes of epilepsy surgery in adults and children. *Lancet Neurol*. 2008;7:525-537. doi:10.1016/S1474-4422(08)70109-1.

16. Panebianco M, Rigby A, Weston J, Marson AG. Vagus nerve stimulation for partial seizures. *Cochrane Database Syst Rev*. 2015;3(4):CD002896. doi:10.1002/14651858.CD002896.pub2.

17. Krumholz A, Hopp JL, Sanchez AM. Counseling epilepsy patients on driving and employment. *Neurol Clin*. 2016;34(2):427-442. doi:10.1016/j.ncl.2015.11.005.

29
Motor Control

MIRIAM SEGAL, MD

Motor Control

Motor control—the process by which the central nervous system produces purposeful, coordinated movements of the body—can be disrupted in a variety of ways by acquired brain injury:

- This can be described partially as upper motor neuron (UMN) syndrome, which is a collection of features resulting from injury to the corticospinal tracts, otherwise known as the *pyramidal tracts*.[1]
- In terms of coordination, motor control is affected when damage is inflicted on the basal ganglia, cerebellum, and associated tracts—the so-called *extrapyramidal system*.[2]
- Functional movement is hampered by injury to the vestibular system or the visual system.

Motor Learning

The current neurorehabilitation of movement is increasingly imbued with the science of motor skill acquisition or motor learning.[3]

- Motor learning is a complex cognitive process that involves the interaction between cortical and subcortical structures to acquire, retain, and retrieve motor plans to execute actions with speed, accuracy, coordination, and consistency to achieve task goals.[4]
- Several pharmacologic agents are under investigation to enhance motor recovery.

- Both serotonergic and dopaminergic drugs have been suggested to possibly enhance motor outcomes particularly after stroke.[5]
- In 2011 the results of the FLuoxetine for motor recovery After acute ischaeMic stroke (FLAME) trial suggested that fluoxetine enhanced motor recovery after stroke.[6]
- More recently, the Fluoxetine or Control Under Supervision (FOCUS) trial demonstrated no such effect of fluoxetine on motor recovery.[7]

Upper Motor Neuron Syndrome

The upper motor neuron syndrome has been described in terms of both positive signs, negative signs, and rheologic changes—referring to changes involving the physical properties of muscle and soft tissue[1] (Table 29.1).

- Although the negative features of the UMN syndrome are associated with more disability than positive features, they are also less treatable.[8]
- The positive signs of UMN syndrome are unified by the fact that they all involve involuntary muscle overactivity.
- Spasticity, which was defined by Lance in 1980 as "velocity dependent increase in the tonic stretch reflex,"[9] is often used in reference to all positive signs collectively, although this is not semantically correct. These various phenomena each have differing pathophysiology, different functional consequences, and different treatments.

Movement Disorders

Just as the *motor* disorders, which occur with pyramidal tract injury, can be described in terms of positive and negative signs, *movement* disorders can be discussed in terms of the duality of hypokinesia and hyperkinesia.

- The term *dyskinesia* also refers to abnormal involuntary movements.
- The label of *extrapyramidal* has begun to fall out of favor because the corticospinal pathways (i.e., pyramidal tracts) and basal ganglia pathways have turned out to be somewhat entangled, and disorders of movement do exist that are not associated with basal ganglia pathology.

TABLE 29.1	Characteristics of Upper Motor Neuron Syndrome[a]	
Negative	**Positive**	
Weakness/impaired force production	Hyperreflexia and reflex irradiation	
Loss of dexterity	Clonus	
Loss of selective movement control	Spasticity	
Fatigue	Positive Babinski and other primitive reflexes	
Impaired motor planning	Extensor spasms	
Impaired motor control	Flexor spasms	
	Positive support reaction	
	Spastic cocontraction	
	Associated reactions (synkinesis)	
	Spastic dystonia	
Rheologic		
Fixed decrease in muscle length		
Shortening of soft tissue other than muscle		
Increased muscle stiffness		

[a]Characteristics of the upper motor neuron syndrome are divided into negative, positive, and rheologic.

- The classification systems of movement disorders, both as a group of disorders and as individual conditions, are now based on phenomenology as opposed to anatomical localization.[10]
  - **Tremor** is defined as an involuntary, rhythmic, oscillatory movement of a body part.[11] Tremors are classified on two main axes: axis I, clinical features, and axis II, etiology[11] (Table 29.2).

- **Dystonia**, which is characterized by sustained or intermittent muscle contractions causing abnormal, often repetitive movements, postures, or both, is also classified on two such axes[12] (Table 29.3).
- **Parkinsonism** is characterized by bradykinesia, rigidity, resting tremor, and postural instability.[10]
- **Chorea**, **athetosis**, and **ballism** represent a spectrum of disorders that overlap in phenomenology, pathophysiology, and etiology.[13]
  - Athetosis consists of slow, nonrhythmic, writhing movements, predominating in the distal limbs with alternating postures of the proximal limbs.
  - Patients with chorea demonstrate nonrhythmic, jerky nonsuppressible movements of the distal limbs and face.
  - Hemiballismus is a unilateral, rapid, nonrhythmic, nonsuppressible movement observed in the proximal limb.[13] Because it involves the proximal limb, it can resemble wild, flinging, high-amplitude movements.

In posttraumatic movement disorders after severe traumatic brain injury (TBI), the reported incidence has been rather variable, quite possibly because of the fact that they are often delayed in their appearance.[14]

- Krauss et al. studied 398 patients admitted with severe TBI and found that among survivors who were followed up:
  - 50 (22.6%) developed movement disorders.
  - These movement disorders were transient in 23 patients (10.4%).
  - They were persistent in 27 patients (12.2%).
  - Only 12 patients (5.4%) experienced disability as a result.[15]
- Tremor was the most common movement disorder reported, followed by dystonia.[15]

TABLE 29.2	Classification of Tremor[a]		
Axis I: Clinical Features			
Historical features	**Tremor Characteristics**	**Associated Signs**	**Laboratory Tests**
Age at onset	Body distribution	Systemic signs	Electrophysiological tests
Temporal evolution	• Focal, segmental, hemi, generalized	Neurological signs	Structural neuroimaging
Medical history	Activation conditions	• Isolated tremor: no other abnormal signs	Receptor imaging
Family history	• Rest versus action	• Combined tremor: other signs present	Biomarkers
Alcohol/drug sensitivity	• Action tremors: postural versus kinetic		
	• Postural: position dependent versus independent		
	• Kinetic: simple, intention, task specific		
	Tremor frequency		
	• 4 Hz, 4–8 Hz, 8–12 Hz, or >12 Hz		
Axis II: Etiology			
Acquired	Genetically defined	Idiopathic	
		• Familial	
		• Sporadic	

[a]The axis I classification of tremor is based in clinical features of the patient's history and physical examination and possibly additional tests. Axis II classification is based on etiology. A syndrome in axis I may have more than one etiology, and one etiology may result in several syndrome.

TABLE 29.3	**Classification of Dystonia**[a]

Axis I: Clinical Features

Age at Onset	Body Distribution	Temporal Pattern	Associated Features
Infancy: birth–2 years Childhood: 3–12 years Adolescence: 13–20 years Early adulthood: 21–40 years Late adulthood: >40 years	Focal Segmental Multifocal Generalized Hemidystonia	Disease course • Static • Progressive Variability • Persistent • Action specific • Diurnal • Paroxysmal	Isolated versus combined with another movement disorder Presence of any cooccurring neurological or systemic manifestations

Axis II: Etiology

Nervous system pathology	Inherited	Idiopathic
• Evidence of degeneration • Evidence of structural lesions • No structural lesion or degeneration	• Autosomal dominant • Autosomal recessive • X-linked recessive • Mitochondrial Acquired • Perinatal brain injury • Infection • Drug/toxin induced • Vascular • Neoplastic • Brain injury • Psychogenic	• Familial • Sporadic

[a]The Axis I classification of dystonia is based in clinical features of the patient's history and physical examination. Axis II classification is based on etiology.

- The disabling posttraumatic tremors tended to be high-amplitude postural and kinetic tremors of the upper extremity.[15]
  A word on injury mechanism:
- Posttraumatic tremors are usually seen in *severe* closed head injury, most commonly motor vehicle accidents with deceleration injury or in pedestrians who were struck by vehicles and suffered severe closed head injury.[2]
- The association with deceleration trauma suggests that diffuse axonal injury plays a role in posttraumatic tremor, and this has been supported by imaging data.[2]
  In terms of mild to moderate TBI, Krauss's group also conducted a similar study looking at 158 patients, finding that:
- 16 patients (10.1%) had developed movement disorders at approximately 5 years follow-up.
- But only four patients (2.6%) experienced persistent movement disorders.
- None of the movement disorders were disabling or required treatment.[16]
- The most common finding in this group was a postural or intention tremor similar to essential tremor.[16]

Posttraumatic Dystonia

- Hemidystonia is the most common presentation of posttraumatic dystonia.
- It is usually associated with ipsilateral hemiparesis.

- Hemidystonia can be acquired by way of stroke, trauma, or perinatal injury, most commonly caused by a lesion of the contralateral basal ganglia or thalamus.[17]
- Acquired hemidystonia is more likely in patients younger than 25 years of age, and there is often a delay in its appearance from the time of injury, which can be up 40 years.[17]

Treatments for Posttraumatic Tremor and Dystonia

- For both posttraumatic tremor and posttraumatic dystonia, medical treatments are often ineffective.[2]
- Focal chemodenervation procedures can be useful, particularly for dystonia.[4]
- In patients with disabling posttraumatic movement disorders, neurosurgical treatment with deep brain stimulation can be effective and has shown improved tolerance compared with radiofrequency lesioning.[2]
- Evidence also supports the use of intrathecal baclofen for the treatment of generalized dystonia.[18]

Parkinsonism

- Parkinsonism can occur after repeated subclinical head trauma in professional sports, most commonly boxing. This is also referred to as *pugilistic parkinsonism*.[4]

- The severity of this correlates with the length of boxing career and number of bouts.[4] Aside from pugilistic parkinsonism, the epidemiological relationship between parkinsonism and TBI has been difficult to elucidate as far as its role as a risk factor versus a manifestation.[4]

Myoclonus

- *Myoclonus* is defined as sudden involuntary movements caused by muscle contractions or muscle tone lapses, also termed *positive* and *negative myoclonus*.[19]
- The major categories of myoclonus are physiological, essential, epileptic, and symptomatic (secondary).[20]
- One type of symptomatic myoclonus was described by Lance and Adams in 1963 as "myoclonus in patients after severe hypoxic episodes."[21]
  - Since then, many cases of Lance-Adams syndrome have been described, and it is characterized by multifocal action myoclonus that appears after resolution of coma.[22]
- This is also referred to as *chronic posthypoxic myoclonus* and is significantly disabling.[22]
- It is important that this be distinguished from the epileptic myoclonus that can occur almost immediately after cardiac arrest/resuscitation ,which is termed *acute posthypoxic myoclonus* or *myoclonic status epilepticus* and is considered strongly indicative of poor prognosis, particularly in the first 24 hours.[23]

In conclusion, brain injury can affect motor control in a variety of ways. Motor disorders, movement disorders, and visual and vestibular deficits can often coexist and can coexist with cognitive deficits that interfere with motor learning. Clearly characterizing these various phenomena provides an important framework for evaluation and treatment of the functional deficits that result from them.

Review Questions

1. Which of these factors most influence motor learning?
   a. Pyramidal tract integrity
   b. Hyperkinetic movement disorders
   c. Serotonergic and dopaminergic medications
   d. Cognitive capacity
2. Regarding medications to enhance motor recovery after stroke, which of these statements is correct?
   a. The FLAME trial showed that fluoxetine did enhance motor recovery in stroke patients, but the treatment group had an increased rate of fractures.
   b. The FOCUS trial, a small retrospective study of ischemic stroke patients on fluoxetine, suggested a benefit of fluoxetine on motor recovery, but FLAME, a larger randomized controlled trial that was published more recently, refuted that finding.
   c. The FLAME trial suggested that treatment with fluoxetine improved motor recovery but FOCUS, which was published more recently and was much larger, did not show any benefit of fluoxetine versus placebo.
   d. Both FLAME and FOCUS trials suggested that fluoxetine may play a role in promoting motor recovery after ischemic stroke.
3. Which is the most common movement disorder seen in severe traumatic brain injury (TBI)?
   a. Severe generalized spasticity
   b. Hemidystonia
   c. Tremor
   d. Parkinsonism

Answers on page 394.
Access the full list of questions and answers online. Available on ExpertConsult.com

References

1. Segal M. Muscle overactivity in the upper motor neuron syndrome. *Phys Med Rehabil Clin North Am.* 2018;29(3):427-436.
2. Krauss JK. Movement disorders secondary to craniocerebral trauma. *Handb Clin Neurol.* 2015;128:475-496.
3. Winstein C, Lewthwaite R, Blanton SR, Wolf LB, Wishart L. Infusing motor learning research into neurorehabilitation practice: a historical perspective with case exemplar from the accelerated skill acquisition program. *J Neurol Phys Ther.* 2014;38(3):190-200.
4. Zasler ND, Katz DI, Zafonte RD. *Brain Injury Medicine: Principles and Practice.* Demos Medical; 2013:1480.
5. Cramer SC. Drugs to enhance motor recovery after stroke. *Stroke.* 2015;46(10):2998-3005.
6. Chollet F, Tardy J, Albucher JF, et al. Fluoxetine for motor recovery after acute ischaemic stroke (FLAME): a randomised placebo-controlled trial. *Lancet Neurol.* 2011;10(2):123-130.
7. Dennis M, Mead G, Forbes J, et al. Effects of fluoxetine on functional outcomes after acute stroke (FOCUS): a pragmatic, double-blind, randomised, controlled trial. *Lancet.* 2019;393(10168):265-274.
8. Brashear A, Elovic E. *Spasticity: Diagnosis and Management.* Demos Medical Pub; 2016:495.
9. Lance JW. The control of muscle tone, reflexes, and movement: Robert Wartenberg Lecture. *Neurology.* 1980;30(12):1303-1313.
10. Fahn S. Classification of movement disorders. *Mov Disord.* 2011;26:947-957. Available from: http://doi.wiley.com/10.1002/mds.23759.
11. Bhatia KP, Bain P, Bajaj N, et al. Consensus Statement on the classification of tremors. from the task force on tremor of the International Parkinson and Movement Disorder Society. *Mov Disord.* 2018;33(1):75-87.
12. Albanese A, Bhatia K, Bressman SB, et al. Phenomenology and classification of dystonia: A consensus update. *Mov Disord.* 2013;28:863-873. Available at: https://www.movementdisorders.org/MDS-Files1/PDFs/Task-Force-Papers/mdsDystoniaPaper2014.pdf. Accessed April 7, 2019.

13. Biglan KM. Chorea, athetosis, and ballism. In: Kurlan R, Greene P, Biglan K, eds. *Hyperkinetic Movement Disorders*. Oxford University Press; 2015:63-85. Available at: http://oxfordmedicine.com/view/10.1093/med/9780199925643.001.0001/med-9780199925643-chapter-5. Accessed April 7, 2019.

14. Krauss JK, Jankovic J. Head injury and posttraumatic movement disorders. *Neurosurgery*. 2002;50(5):927-939; discussion 939-940.

15. Krauss JK, Tränkle R, Kopp KH. Post-traumatic movement disorders in survivors of severe head injury. *Neurology*. 1996;47(6):1488-1492.

16. Krauss JK, Tränkle R, Kopp KH. Posttraumatic movement disorders after moderate or mild head injury. *Mov Disord*. 1997;12(3):428-431.

17. Chuang C, Fahn S, Frucht SJ. The natural history and treatment of acquired hemidystonia: report of 33 cases and review of the literature. *J Neurol Neurosurg Psychiatry*. 2002;72(1):59-67.

18. Shah H. Intrathecal baclofen infusion for the treatment of movement disorders. *Neurosurg Clin North Am*. 2019;30(2):203-209.

19. Caviness JN, Brown P. Myoclonus: current concepts and recent advances. *Lancet Neurol*. 2004;3(10):598-607.

20. Fahn S, Marsden CD, Van Woert MH. Definition and classification of myoclonus. *Adv Neurol*. 1986;43:1-5.

21. Lance JW, Adams RD. The syndrome of intention or action myoclonus as a sequel to hypoxic encephalopathy. *Brain*. 1963;86:111-136.

22. Gupta HV, Caviness JN. Post-hypoxic myoclonus: current concepts, neurophysiology, and treatment. *Tremor Other Hyperkinet Mov (N Y)*. 2016;6:409. Available at: http://www.ncbi.nlm.nih.gov/pubmed/27708982. Accessed April 7, 2019.

23. American Academy of Neurology. *Prediction of Outcome in Comatose Survivors After Cardiopulmonary Resuscitation AAN Summary of Evidence-based Guideline for Clinicians Recommendations for the Prognostic Value of the Clinical Examination*. Available at: www.aan.com. Accessed April 7, 2019.

30

Pressure Injuries, Bed Rest, and Deconditioning

FABIENNE SAINT-PREUX, MD, EMMA NALLY, MD, AND HEIDI FUSCO, MD

Pressure injuries (PIs) and deconditioning are complications of bed rest, which can occur after brain injury. These complications increase morbidity and mortality and have a negative impact on functional outcome after illness or injury. PIs and deconditioning create a burden for caregivers and longer length of stays, and they increase healthcare costs. Patients with brain injury are at greater risk Keywords: pressure injuries, wound care, therapy modalities, aging from the complications of bed rest, PIs, and deconditioning. It is important to identify risks of these complications and be aware of prevention and treatment measures.

Pressure Injuries

Formerly called *pressure ulcers*, PIs are defined by the National Pressure Ulcer Advisory Panel (NPUAP) as: "localized injury to the skin and/or underlying soft tissue over a bony prominence or related to a medical or other device. The injury occurs as a result of intense and/or prolonged pressure or pressure in combination with shear".[7]

Incidence and Prevalence

In the United States, prevalence ranges between 3% and 69%[1] with an incidence of 23.5% in acute healthcare settings and slightly higher numbers in nursing homes.[2]

Physiology and Stages of Healing

- Anatomy of normal skin:
  - Epidermis
  - Dermis
  - Subcutaneous tissue
- Function of normal skin:
  - Protect from trauma, dehydration, microorganisms
  - Excretion of waste (perspiration)
  - Sensory perception
  - Vitamin D production
  - Thermoregulation (vasoconstriction and dilation of blood vessels in dermis)
- Four phases of wound healing[3] (Fig. 30.1):
  - Phase 1: Hemostasis: prevent further blood loss
    - Immediate
    - Activation of coagulation cascade and creation of blood clot
  - Phase 2: Inflammation: contain injurious process
    - Early
    - Late
  - Phase 3: Proliferation
    - Granulation, angiogenesis, and reepithelialization
    - Extracellular matrix remodeling
    - Collagen deposition: reaches maximum 21 days after the wound is created
  - Phase 4: Tissue remodeling

Sites

PIs are more common at bony prominences and sites of pressure or shear.
- Most frequently injured sites
  - Ischium (28%)
  - Sacrum (17%–27%)

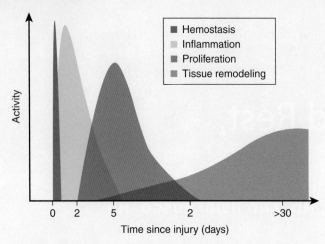

• **Fig. 30.1** Phases of normal wound healing. (From Ho CH, Bogie, K. In Frontera W, DeLisa J, eds. *Physical Medicine and Rehabilitation: Principles and Practice.* 5th ed. Philadelphia, PA: Wolters Kluwer/ Lippincott Williams; Wilkins Health, 2013:1394.)

• Trochanter (12%%–19%)
• Heel (9%%–18%)
• Higher risk associated with different positions (Fig. 30.2)
  • Supine: occiput, scapula, sacrum, ischium
  • Side lying: lateral malleolus, trochanter, elbow, temporal head
  • Wheelchair sitting: scapula, sacrum, ischium, heel
  • Prone: forehead, elbow, knee, toes

Risk Factors

• Extrinsic: external to the patient's body (Table 30.1)
• Intrinsic: within the patient's body
• Populations with:
  • Increased age

• Reduced mobility
• Complex medical conditions
• Cognitive impairments
• Motor and sensory impairment (e.g., spinal cord and brain injury)

Assessment

• PI risk assessment scales
  • Braden scale: most widely used and validated (Fig. 30.3)[5]
  • Has six subscales that quantify sensation, skin moisture, activity, mobility, shear force, and nutritional status
  • A score of 12 and under indicates high risk for PI
  • Norton Scale Fig. 30.4.[6]
    • Five subscales quantify physical and mental condition, activity, mobility, incontinence
    • Total score from 5 to 20; lower score indicates higher risk; score of 14 or less indicates at risk status
    • Greater than 18: low risk
    • Between 18 and 14: medium risk
    • Between 14 and 10: high risk
    • Less than 10: very high risk
  • Waterlow Scale (Fig. 30.5)[13]
    • 10 risk categories for assessment: build (body mass index [BMI]), continence, skin type, mobility, sex, age, appetite and special risks of malnutrition, neurological deficit, major surgery/trauma, medication
    • Scores:
    • 10–14: at risk
    • 15–10: high risk
    • 20+: very high risk
• Staging of PIs
  • Six-stage system proposed by NPUAP (Table 30.2)
  • Note: Stages do not reverse (e.g., a stage IV PI does not become a stage II but rather a healing stage IV).

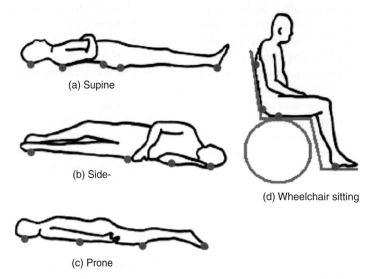

• **Fig. 30.2** Pressure injury sites based on position. (From Ho CH, Bogie, K. In Frontera W, DeLisa J, eds. *Physical Medicine and Rehabilitation: Principles and Practice.* 5th ed. Philadelphia, PA: Wolters Kluwer/Lippincott Williams; Wilkins Health, 2013:1395.)

TABLE 30.1	Extrinsic and Intrinsic Risk Factors of Pressure Injuries
Intrinsic Risk Factors	**Extrinsic Risk Factors**
Muscle atrophy	Applied pressure
Impaired nutritional status	Surface shear
Anemia	Friction
Impaired vascular status	Local microenvironment
Impaired mobility	Psychosocial/lifestyle
Impaired sensation	
Incontinence	

Adapted from Ho CH, Bogie, K. In Frontera W, DeLisa J, eds. *Physical Medicine and Rehabilitation: Principles and Practice.* 5th ed. Philadelphia, PA: Wolters Kluwer/Lippincott Williams; Wilkins Health, 2013:1395.

Treatment

NPUAP Guidelines

- Step 1: Correct risk factors
  - Replace nutritional deficits, especially protein and micronutrient intake.
  - Compensate for impaired mobility.
    - Close monitoring of specific pressure-bearing areas
    - Position change every 2 hours and orthosis or pillows to relieve pressure from heels
    - Pressure reliefs every 15 minutes when sitting
- Step 2: Wound care (Fig. 30.6)
  - Correct moisture balance
    - Excessively moist wounds—cause maceration
    - Excessively dry wounds—prevent granulation and reepithelization
  - Debride necrotic tissue (slough and eschar) with sharps, wet-to-dry, and chemical dressings.
  - Cleanse wound to facilitate removal of necrotic material, exudates, and metabolic wastes.
  - Protect wound from further exposure and trauma with dressings

Adjuvant Therapeutic Modalities (Table 30.3)

- Hydrotherapy: whirlpool, pulsatile lavage
  - Uses: Cleansing and debridement of stage III and IV
  - Risks: Contamination of other wounds/patients
- Electrical stimulation
  - Uses: Grade III and IV
  - Risks: No standardized regimens
- Negative pressure wound therapy
  - Uses: Decrease bacterial load increases circulation, increases granulation
  - Risks: Lack of clinical guidelines

- Therapeutic ultrasound
  - Uses: Deep heating though to improve vascularity
  - Risks: No guidelines
- Electromagnetic therapy
  - Uses: Thought to increase proliferation phase
  - Risks: No guidelines

External Factors: Seating Systems and Pressure Relief Mattresses

- Seating
  - Focuses on cushion material (foam viscoelastic foam, gel, and flotation)
  - Directed by a specialized clinic
- Pressure relief mattresses: static and dynamic
  - Static: same materials as cushion
  - Dynamic: low air loss mattresses

Surgical Management

- Considered in setting of nonhealing stage III and IV despite optimal care or if osteomyelitis is present

Bed Rest and Deconditioning

Bed rest and immobilization were previously theorized to be beneficial treatments and management after trauma and illness. However, studies have demonstrated the benefits of early mobilization and enegative effects of immobilization.[8] The negative effects associated with bed rest and immobilization are catastrophic in patients with neurologic impairments, because they may have paresis and medical complications from the comorbid brain injury.[9] Bed rest has global effects on body systems, causing weakness atrophy, decreased endurance, reduced oxygen utilization, orthostasis osteoporosis, and deconditioning defined as the reduced functional capacity of total body systems.

Effects of Immobility

Disuse Atrophy

- By day 10 of bed rest, there is a 50% decrease of muscle weight.[10]
- By day 14 of bed rest, muscle protein synthesis is reduced by 50%.
- Type I and IIa muscle fibers atrophy more quickly than type IIb fibers.[11]
- Decline in collagen and muscle synthesis.[12]

Loss of Strength and Endurance

- 10% to 15% loss of strength over the first week of bed rest
- 35% to 50% loss of strength over 4 weeks
- Loss of adenosine triphosphate (ATP) and glycogen storage sites and decline in mitochondria density
- Decline in VO_2 max, or maximal oxygen uptake and utilization during exercise.

Functional Impairments

- Decreased mobility and activities of daily living (ADLs)

Patient's Name_____ Evaluator's Name_____ Date of Assessment

SENSORY PERCEPTION ability to respond meaning-fully to pressure-related discomfort	1. Completely Limited Unresponsive (does not moan, flinch, or grasp) to painful stimuli, due to diminished level of consciousness or sedation OR limited ability to feel pain over most of body.	2. Very Limited Responds only to painful stimuli. Cannot communicate discomfort except by moaning or restlessness OR has a sensory impairment which limits the ability to feel pain or discomfort over ½ of body.	3. Slightly Limited Responds to verbal commands, but cannot always communicate discomfort or the need to be turned OR has some sensory impairment which limits ability to feel pain or discomfort in 1 or 2 extremities.	4. No Impairment Responds to verbal commands. Has no sensory deficit which would limit ability to feel or voice pain or discomfort				
MOISTURE degree to which skin is exposed to moisture	1. Constantly Moist Skin is kept moist almost constantly by perspiration, urine, etc. Dampness is detected every time patient is moved or turned.	2. Very Moist Skin is often, but not always moist. Linen must be changed at least once a shift.	3. Occasionally Moist: Skin is occasionally moist, requiring an extra linen change approximately once a day.	4. Rarely Moist Skin is usually dry, linen only requires changing at routine intervals.				
ACTIVITY degree of physical activity	1. Bedfast Confined to bed.	2. Chairfast Ability to walk severely limited or non-existent. Cannot bear own weight and/or must be assisted into chair or wheelchair.	3. Walks Occasionally Walks occasionally during day, but for very short distances, with or without assistance. Spends majority of each shift in bed or chair.	4. Walks Frequently Walks outside room at least twice a day and inside room at least once every two hours during waking hours.				
MOBILITY ability to change and control body position	1. Completely Immobile Does not make even slight changes in body or extremity position without assistance.	2. Very Limited Makes occasional slight changes in body or extremity position but unable to make frequent or significant changes independently.	3. Slightly Limited Makes frequent though slight changes in body or extremity position independently.	4. No Limitation Makes major and frequent changes in position without assistance.				
NUTRITION usual food intake pattern	1. Very Poor Never eats a complete meal. Rarely eats more than ⅓ of any food offered. Eats 2 servings or less of protein (meat or dairy products) per day. Takes fluids poorly. Does not take a liquid dietary supplement OR is NPO and/or maintained on clear liquids or IV's for more than 5 days	2. Probably Inadequate Rarely eats a complete meal and generally eats only about ½ of any food offered. Protein intake incudes only 3 servings of meat or dairy products per day. Occasionally will take a dietary supplement OR receives less than optimum amount of liquid diet or tube feeding.	3. Adequate Eats over half of most meals. Eats a total of 4 servings of protein (meat, dairy products) per day. Occasionally will refuse a meal, but will usually take a supplement when offered OR is on a tube feeding or TPN regimen which probably meets most of nutritional needs.	4. Excellent Eats most of every meal. Never refuses a meal. Usually eats a total of 4 or more servings of meat and dairy products. Occasionally eats between meals. Does not require supplementation.				
FRICTION & SHEAR	1. Problem Requires moderate to maximum assistance in moving. Complete lifting without sliding against sheets is impossible. Frequently slides down in bed or chair, requiring frequent repositioning with maximum assistance. Spasticity, contractures or agitation leads to almost constant friction.	2. Potential Problem Moves feebly or requires minimum assistance. During a move skin probably slides to some extent against sheets, chair, restraints or other devices. Maintains relatively good position in chair or bed most of the time but occasionally slides down.	3. No Apparent Problem Moves in bed and in chair independently and has sufficient muscle strength to lift up completely during move. Maintains good position in bed or chair.					

Total Score

• **Fig. 30.3** Braden Scale. (From Bergstrom N, Braden J, Laguzza A, et al. The Braden Scale for predicting pressure sore risk. *Decubitus.* 1988:1[2];18-19.)

- Pain and stiffness
- Cardiovascular disease caused by inactivity, increasing coronary artery disease, and metabolic syndrome

Contracture
- Lack of joint mobilization throughout full range of motion (ROM)

- Three contributors: myogenic, arthrogenic, and soft tissue contractures
- Negatively affects
  - Mobility: gait pattern, transfers, wheelchair use
  - ADLs and nursing care: bed positioning, perineal hygiene, and skin care; accentuates areas of increased pressure/PIs

		Physical Condition	Mental Condition	Activity	Mobility	Incontinent	TOTAL SCORE
		Good 4	Alert 4	Ambulant 1	Full 4	Not 4	
		Fair 3	Apathetic 3	Walk/help 3	Slightly Impaired limited 3	Occasional 3	
		Poor 2	Confused 2	Chair bound 2	V limited 2	Usually/urine 2	
		V Bad 1	Stupor 1	Bed 1	Immobile 1	Doubly 1	
Name	Date						

• **Fig. 30.4** Norton Risk Assessment Scale. [Adapted from Norton D, McLaren R, Exton-Smith AN. *An Investigation of Geriatric Nursing Problems in Hospital.* Edinburgh, Scotland: Churchill Livingstone; 1962 (reissue 1975)]

Weight/size relationship:
0. Standard
1. Above standards
2. Obese

3. Below standards

Skin type and visual aspect of risk areas:
0. Healthy
1. Frail
1. Dry
2. Edematous
1. Cold and humid
2. Alterations in color
3. Wounded

Sex/Age:
1. Male
2. female
1. 14–49 years
2. 50–64 years
3. 65–74 years
4. 75–80 years
5. Over 81 years

Special risks:

Tissue malnutrition:
8. Terminal/cachexia
5. Cardiac insufficiency
6. Peripheral vascular insufficiency
2. Anemia
1. Smoker

Continence:
0. Complete, urine catheter
1. Occasional incontinence
2. Urine catheter/fecal incontinence
3. Double incontinence

Mobility:
0. Complete
1. Restless
2. Apathy
3. Restricted
4. Inert
5. On chair

Appetite:
0. Normal
1. Scarce/feeding tube
2. Liquid intravenous
3. Anorexia/Absolute diet

Neurological deficit:
5. Diabetes, paraplegic, ACV

Surgery:
5. Orthopedic surgery below waist
5. Over 2 hours in surgery

Medication:
4. Steroids, cytotoxics, anti-inflammatory drugs in elevated dosage

Scoring: Over 10 points: at risk. Over 16 points: high risk. Over 20 points: very high risk.

• **Fig. 30.5** Waterlow Scale. (From Waterlow J. Pressure sores: a risk assessment card. *Nursing Times.* 81[48]:1985;49-55.)

TABLE 30.2	Staging Skin Injuries
Stage 1	Nonblanchable erythema of intact skin
Stage 2	Partial-thickness skin loss with exposed dermis
Stage 3	Pressure injury: full-thickness skin loss
Stage 4	Full-thickness skin and tissue loss
Unstageable	Obscured (e.g., slough, eschar) full-thickness skin and tissue loss; depth unknown
Suspected deep tissue injury	Nonblanchable discoloration, depth unknown

Adapted from National Pressure Ulcer Advisory Panel, European Pressure Ulcer Advisory Panel and Pan Pacific Pressure Injury Alliance. Emily Haesler, ed. *Prevention and Treatment of Pressure Ulcers: Clinical Practice Guideline.* Osborne Park, Western Australia: Cambridge Media; 2014:44-45.

Cardiovascular Dysfunction

- Increased inflammation and atherosclerosis
- Resting heart rate increases by 1 beat/min every 2 days
- Orthostasis
- Decreased VO_2 max
- Decreased blood volume
- Increased blood viscosity
- Deep vein thrombosis and pulmonary embolus
  - Virchow's triad: hypercoagulability, hemodynamic changes (stasis, turbulence), endothelial injury/dysfunction

Pulmonary Dysfunction

- Decrease in vital capacity and functional residual capacity
- Impaired clearance of secretions
- Loss of strength and endurance of intercostal and axillary respiratory muscles

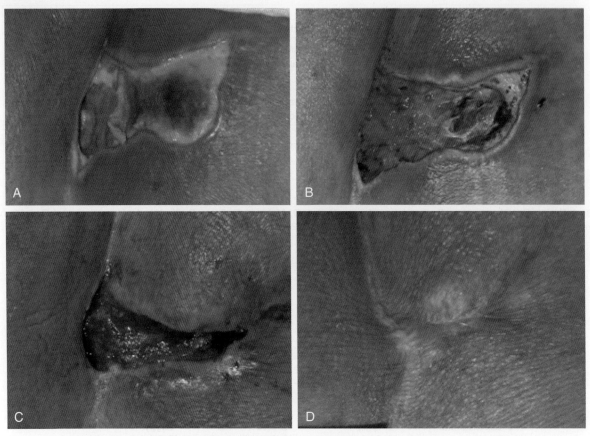

• **Fig. 30.6** Healing pressure injury. Initially an unstageable pressure injury until slough and eschar removed (A). Wound debrided, was a 4×8 cm and 2.5 cm deep, stage IV, full-thickness tissue injury. Treated with pressure-relieving surface, nutritional interventions, sharp debridement, wet to dry dressings. (B) At 3 weeks. (C) At 9 weeks. (D) Closure at 28 weeks. (From Braddom R. *Physical Medicine and Rehabilitation.* 4th ed. Philadelphia, PA: Elsevier Saunders; 2011:697.)

Metabolism and Endocrine System Alterations

- Decreased lean body mass
- Gain in body fat
- Hypercalcemia and hypercalciuria
- Glucose intolerance
- Parathyroid hormone response to hypercalcemia
- Thyroid-stimulating hormone and adrenocorticotrophin releasing hormone alterations
- Catecholamine secretion

Disuse Osteoporosis

- Risk factors
  - Prolonged bed rest
  - Immobility and prolonged nonweight-bearing status
  - Disuse osteopenia
  - Estrogen and calcium deficiency
  - Greatest risk in elderly and spinal cord injury/paraplegic/hemiplegic/quadriplegic population

Genitourinary and Gastrointestinal Side Effects

- Bladder or renal stones
- Urinary tract infection
- Incomplete voiding

- Loss of appetite, slower rate of absorption
- Reduced peristalsis and constipation

Immune System Alteration

- Chronic physical and psychological stresses
  - Reduce tumor rejection
  - Increases tumor growth factors
  - Worsen autoimmune conditions

The Nervous System Mood and Immobility

- Sensory deprivation results in social isolation and psychiatric/behavioral consequences

Prevention and Treatment of Effects From Deconditioning and Bed Rest

- Progressive resistive exercise, stretching, and aerobic exercise
- Flexibility exercises to maintain full ROM
- Strengthening (resistance) exercises
  - Once a day muscle contraction at 30% to 50% of max strength for 3 to 5 minutes three times a week
  - Concentric, isometric, isotonic exercise

<table>
<tr><td colspan="5">**TABLE 30.3 Adjuvant Therapeutic Modalities**</td></tr>
<tr><td>**Modality**</td><td>**What**</td><td>**Advantages**</td><td>**Disadvantages**</td></tr>
<tr>
<td>Hydrotherapy: whirlpool</td>
<td>Extremity is submersed in water at 92°–96°F for 10–20 minutes with or without agitation and antimicrobial agents</td>
<td>Cleansing and mechanical debridement of stage III and IV wounds</td>
<td>
• Cross contamination between patients
• *Pseudomonas* infections
• Potential skin infections for caregivers in contact with contaminated water
</td>
</tr>
<tr>
<td>Hydrotherapy: pulsatile lavage</td>
<td>Portable device delivers pulsed jet streams of water at a known, preset pressure</td>
<td>
• Cleansing and mechanical debridement of stage III and IV wounds
• Less labor intensive
• Single patient use only
</td>
<td>Clinical efficacy under investigation</td>
</tr>
<tr>
<td>Electrical stimulation</td>
<td>Electric stimulation is delivered using surface electrodes placed on or near the wound using frequency of 10–100 Hz</td>
<td>Treatment of severe grade III or IV pressure ulcers</td>
<td>
• Mechanisms of wound healing not fully understood
• Stimulation and treatment paradigms highly variable
</td>
</tr>
<tr>
<td>Negative-pressure wound therapy</td>
<td>Suction pump with foam and occlusive dressing creates negative pressure on wound</td>
<td>
• Decreases bacterial load
• Decreases edema
• Promotes improved local circulation
• Increases granulation
</td>
<td>
• Lack of official guidelines
• Contraindicated when wounds are dry, patient has uncontrolled pain, untreated infection, malnutrition, or poor hemostasis
</td>
</tr>
<tr>
<td>Therapeutic ultrasound</td>
<td>Deep heating administered via ultrasound</td>
<td>Improves vascularity of wound tissue</td>
<td>Limited evidence from clinical trials</td>
</tr>
<tr>
<td>Electromagnetic therapy</td>
<td></td>
<td>Increased blood flow, collagen formation, granulocyte infiltration</td>
<td>Limited evidence from clinical trials</td>
</tr>
</table>

From Ho CH, Bogie, K. In Frontera W, DeLisa J, eds. *Physical Medicine and Rehabilitation: Principles and Practice.* 5th ed. Philadelphia, PA: Wolters Kluwer/Lippincott Williams; Wilkins Health, 2013:1402-1404.

• Eccentric exercise but use caution because it may produce muscle damage in untrained individuals
• Electrical stimulation
• Endurance and fitness exercises
  • Requires daily exercise at target heart rate of 60% to 80% of VO_2 max for 8 weeks to restore/improve endurance
• Prevention and treatment of contractures
  • Proper bed and wheelchair positioning
  • Proper mattress
  • Early mobilization
  • Bed mobility training, active ROM, passive ROM with terminal stretch
  • Continuous passive motion (CPM) machines
  • Strengthening exercise for opposing muscle groups
  • Modalities with heat, progressive splinting (dynamic, casting with or without alcohol, or botulinum injections)
  • Surgery: Tendon lengthening with or without muscle transfer procedures
• Vitamin D and calcium supplementation

Summary

Patients with brain injuries are more likely to be at risk for complications of bed rest, deconditioning, and PI. Close attention to prevention and treatment is warranted.

• Prolonged bed rest and immobility can lead to physical deconditioning, development of contractures, multisystem complications, and development of PIs.
• The most common sites of pressure ulcers are the occiput, sacrum, ischia, trochanter, and heel.
• Assessment of risk for PI is determined using the Braden Scale. NPUAP is used to grade PIs that have already developed.
• Management of PIs include assessment and correction of risk factors, wound care, adjuvant therapeutic modalities, and surgical management.
• Immobility results in physiological impairment, including disuse atrophy, loss of strength and endurance, and functional impairments, including decreased mobility and ADLs, muscle pain/stiffness, and cardiovascular disease.
• Progressive resistance exercise, stretching, aerobic exercise, flexibility, strengthening, endurance, and fitness

exercise can prevent and treat muscle weakness secondary to immobility.
- There are three types of contractures: myogenic, arthrogenic, and soft tissue. These can lead to functional limitations in mobility and ADLs and the development of PIs.

- Management of contracture includes prevention and treatment with passive ROM, heat therapy, progressive splinting, and surgery.
- Immobility and inactivity result in adverse multisystem involvement of the musculoskeletal, cardiopulmonary, genitourinary, gastrointestinal, endocrine/metabolic, immune, and nervous systems.

Review Questions

1. Which patient is at risk of developing a pressure injury?
   a. A young patient with a traumatic shoulder fracture
   b. A hospitalized individual with complex medical condition, cognitive impairment, and motor/sensory impairment
   c. A patient who suffers from eczema
   d. A patient with vitamin D deficiency
2. Which of these is *not* a risk factor for poor wound healing?
   a. Incontinence
   b. Muscle atrophy
   c. Complete spinal cord Injury
   d. Race
   e. Poor nutrition

3. Which of these areas is not a common location for pressure injury?
   a. Ischial tuberosity
   b. Sacrum
   c. Iliac crest
   d. Trochanter
   e. Heels

Answers on page 394.
Access the full list of questions and answers online.
Available on ExpertConsult.com

References

1. Gerson LW. The incidence of pressure sores in active treatment hospitals. *Int J Nurs Stud*. 1975;12(4):201-204.
2. Bergstrom N, Braden B, Kemp M, Champagne M, Ruby E. Multi-site study of incidence of pressure ulcers and the relationship between risk level, demographic characteristics, diagnoses, and the prescription of preventive interventions. *J Am Geriatr Soc*. 1996;44(1):22-30.
3. Eming SA, Brachvogel B, Odorisio T, et al. Regulation of angiogenesis: wound healing as a model. *Prog Histochem Cytochem*. 2007;42:115-170.
4. Ho CH, Bogie, K. Pressure ulcers. In: Frontera WR, DeLisa JA, eds. *Physical Medicine and Rehabilitation: Principles and Practice*. 5th ed., Vol I. Philadelphia, PA: Wolters Kluwer/Lippincott Williams; Wilkins Health, 2013;1393-1409.
5. Bergstrom N, Braden J, Laguzza A, Holman V. The braden scale for predicting pressure sore risk. *Decubitus*. 1988;1(2):18-19.
6. Norton D, McLaren R, Exton-Smith AN. *An Investigation of Geriatric Nursing Problems in Hospitals*. London: National Corporation for the Care of Old People; 1962.
7. National Pressure Ulcer Advisory Panel, European Pressure Ulcer Advisory Panel and Pan Pacific Pressure Injury Alliance. *Prevention and Treatment of Pressure Ulcers: Clinical Practice Guideline*. Emily Haesler (Ed.). Osborne Park, Western Australia: Cambridge Media; 2014.
8. Hashem MD, Parker AM, Needham DM. Early mobilization and rehabilitation of patients who are critically ill. *Chest*. 2016;150(3):722-731. doi:10.1016/j.chest.2016.03.003.
9. Langhorne P, Wu O, Rodgers H, Ashburn A, Bernhardt J. A Very Early Rehabilitation Trial after stroke (AVERT): a Phase III, multicentre, randomised controlled ºtrial. *Health Technol Assess*. 2017;21(54):1-120. doi:10.3310/hta21540.
10. Ferrando A, Lane H, Stuart C, Davis-Street J, Wolfe R. Prolonged bed rest decreases skeletal muscle and whole body protein synthesis. *Am J Physiol*. 1996;270(4 Pt 1):E627-E633.
11. Nonaka I, Miyazawa M, Sukegawa T, Yonemoto K, Kato T. Muscle fiber atrophy and degeneration induced by experimental immobility and hindlimb suspension. *Int J Sports Med*. 1997;18(suppl 4):S292-S294.
12. Clarke M, Bamman M, Feeback D. Bed rest decreases mechanically induced myofiber wounding and consequent wound-mediated FGF release. *J Appl Physiol (1985)*. 1998;85(2):593-600.
13. Waterlow J. Pressure sores: a risk assessment card. *Nurs Times*. 1985;81(48):49-55.
14. Braddom R. *Physical Medicine and Rehabilitation*. 4th ed. Philadelphia, PA: Elsevier Saunders; 2011.
15. Kruger EA, Pires M, Ngann Y, Sterling M, Rubayi S. Comprehensive management of pressure ulcers in spinal cord injury: current concepts and future trends. *J Spinal Cord Med*. 2013:36(6):572-585. doi:10.1179/2045772313Y.0000000093.

31
Dysphagia and Aspiration

LAUREN E. FULKS, MD, AND BENJAMIN N. NGUYEN, MD

OUTLINE

A traumatic brain injury (TBI) can lead to problems with cognition, behavior, and physical functions, with each domain playing a crucial role in swallowing. Normal control of swallowing requires appropriate integration of the brainstem, basal ganglia, thalamus, limbic system, cerebellum, and the motor and sensory nerves (Fig. 31.1).[1] These systems work together to control afferent/efferent, anticipatory/preparatory, and voluntary/automatic processes in the more than 30 muscles involved in swallowing cortices (Fig. 31.2).[1,2] One of the most common challenges faced by clinicians in TBI patients is dysphagia.[3]

Dysphagia

Dysphagia is difficulty in swallowing because of congenital or structural abnormalities or impairment in neuromuscular control. Dysphagia caused by neurologic dysfunction (such as after TBI) may result from abnormalities in any of the four phases of swallowing: oral preparatory phase, oral phase, pharyngeal phase, or esophageal phase.

Risk Factors That Put Patients at Highest Risk of Aspiration Pneumonia

- Glasgow Coma Scale (GCS) score of less than 9
- Rancho Los Amigos Scale (RLAS) score less than 3
- No oral intake on admission
- Intubation
- Tracheostomy
- Oropharyngeal spasticity
- Myoclonus

As such, careful evaluation for dysphagia needs to be a key component of acute rehabilitation for patients after a neurological dysfunction, because impaired swallowing may result in aspiration, decreased epiglottis movement, or impaired laryngeal elevation.[4] Swallowing characteristics of patients with dysphagia after TBI were comparable to patients with dysphagia after stroke in videofluoroscopic swallowing study (VFSS), with findings of aspiration or penetration, decreased laryngeal elevation, and reduced epiglottis inversion.[4]

Without proper attention and intervention, patients are at risk for dehydration, malnutrition, weight loss, aspiration, and pneumonia.[4] These consequences can lead to prolonged hospitalization and worsened functional status limiting improvement in the acute period after injury. There remains limited research and development of dysphagia treatment protocols, leading to a high level of variability based on provider preference and background.

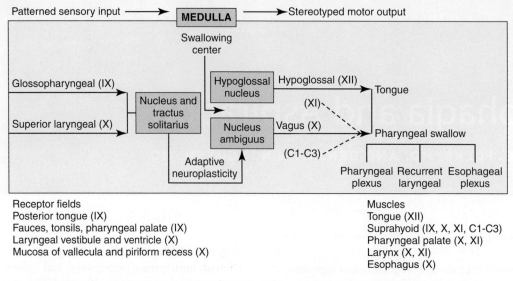

Patterned sensory input ──────→ **MEDULLA** ──────→ Stereotyped motor output

Swallowing center

Glossopharyngeal (IX)

Superior laryngeal (X)

Nucleus and tractus solitarius

Hypoglossal nucleus → Hypoglossal (XII) → Tongue

Nucleus ambiguus → Vagus (X)

(XI) ─ ─ ─

(C1-C3) ─ ─ ─ → Pharyngeal swallow

Adaptive neuroplasticity

Pharyngeal plexus   Recurrent laryngeal   Esophageal plexus

Receptor fields
Posterior tongue (IX)
Fauces, tonsils, pharyngeal palate (IX)
Laryngeal vestibule and ventricle (X)
Mucosa of vallecula and piriform recess (X)

Muscles
Tongue (XII)
Suprahyoid (IX, X, XI, C1-C3)
Pharyngeal palate (X, XI)
Larynx (X, XI)
Esophagus (X)

• **Fig. 31.1** Components of pharyngeal swallow as sensory cued, stereotyped behaviors. (From Groher ME, Crary MA. *Dysphagia Clinical Management in Adults and Children.* St. Louis, MO: Elsevier; 2016.)

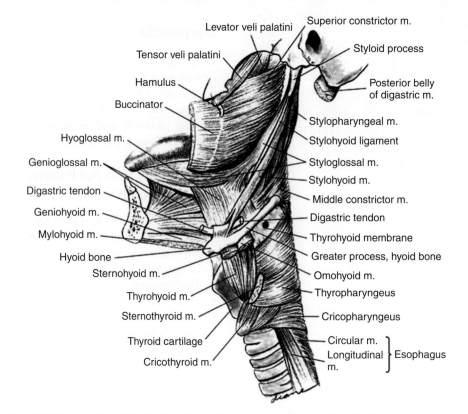

• **Fig. 31.2** Key muscles of the head and neck in swallowing. (From Groher ME, Crary MA. *Dysphagia Clinical Management in Adults and Children.* St. Louis, MO: Elsevier; 2016.)

Summary

- A TBI will lead to problems with cognition, behavior, and physical functions, which all play a crucial role in swallowing.
- Three factors putting patients at highest risk of aspiration pneumonia: GCS score of less than 9, RLAS score less than 3, and no oral intake on admission.[3]
- Other risk factors for dysphagia after TBI include intubation, tracheostomy, oropharyngeal spasticity, or myoclonus.
- Consequences of undiagnosed dysphagia include dehydration, malnutrition, weight loss, aspiration, and pneumonia, which can lead to worsened functional status and prolonged hospitalizations.[4]

Four Phases of Swallowing

Normal swallowing in humans was first described with a three-stage sequential model that depended on the position of the bolus: the oral, pharyngeal, and esophageal stages. Known as the *Process Model*, it describes the mechanism of eating and swallowing solid food.[5,6] Because this model does not describe the mechanism of swallowing liquid food, a four-phase model was developed to describe the biomechanics and bolus movement during command swallows of liquids.[7] In the four-phase model, the oral stage was subdivided into the oral preparatory stage and the oral propulsive stage, whereas the pharyngeal stage and the esophageal stage remain the same. During swallowing, the bolus of food or liquid is manipulated by muscles and reflexes involving the nasopharynx, oropharynx, and hypopharynx.

Oral Preparatory Stage

- This stage starts when liquid bolus is in the anterior part of mouth floor or on the tongue surface enclosed by the hard palate and upper dental arch.
- The oral cavity is sealed posteriorly by the soft palate and tongue to prevent the liquid bolus from leaking into the oropharynx before the swallow.
- An imperfect seal may allow leakage of liquid into the pharynx, which becomes more common with aging.

Oral Propulsive Stage

- This stage helps to prepare the bolus; it includes mastication of the bolus and the use of tongue movements to help with positioning.
- The soft palate moves forward to close the oral cavity.
- The tongue closes the anterior portion of the oral cavity and moves the bolus toward the oropharynx.
- Velopharyngeal closure is needed to protect the bolus from entering the nasopharynx.
- Problems with this phase result in drooling, pocketing, and possibly a compensatory head tilt.[8]

Pharyngeal Stage

- This is a reflexive coordination of events that result in the bolus being moved from the mouth to the esophagus.
- The risk of aspiration is greatest in this phase despite a coordinated inhibition of breathing to prevent aspiration.[8]
- During this phase, the soft palate propels the bolus toward the esophagus, accompanied by elevation of the larynx with anterior hyoid bone movement to help with epiglottis placement over the entry of the airway.
- The true and false vocal cords are adducted to provide additional airway protection.
- A coordinated constriction of the pharynx and relaxation of the cricopharynx or upper esophageal sphincter help the bolus to enter the esophagus smoothly.
- Problems with this phase can result in coughing, choking, a sensation that food is stuck, or aspiration.
- A systemic review of physiological factors related to aspiration in oropharyngeal dysphagia found measurement of tongue strength, hyoid movement, bolus time in the pharynx while the larynx stays open, respiratory rate,

and respiratory swallow phasing help determine aspiration risks.[9]

Esophageal Stage

- Also reflexive in nature, this is the longest phase of swallowing.[8]
- The bolus passes from the pharynx to the esophagus and eventually arrives in the stomach.
- Relaxation of the gastroesophageal sphincter is required even if the patient is in a seated or upright position.
- Problems with this phase can lead to acid reflux symptoms such as frequent burping, throat irritation, or the sensation that food is sticking.

Summary

- Four stages of swallowing: Oral preparatory, oral propulsive, pharyngeal, and esophageal[7]
- Oral preparatory stage: Bolus is in anterior portion of mouth. An imperfect seal will lead to leakage into pharynx, which is more common in aging.
- Oral propulsive: Bolus is positioned and moved toward oropharynx. Problems can result in drooling, pocketing, and head tilt.
- Pharyngeal phase: Greatest risk of aspiration is in this phase and requires a coordinated inhibition of breathing to prevent aspiration. Problems in this phase result in coughing, choking, aspiration, or sensation that food is stuck.
- Esophageal phase: Longest phase of swallowing. Problems can lead to acid reflux symptoms such as frequent burping, throat irritation, or sensation that food is sticking.

Evaluation

Many bedside and instrumental tools have been developed for the diagnosis and treatment of dysphagia with varying degrees of sensitivity and specificity. Testing ranges from dysphagia screening to diagnostic evaluation of dysphagia using bedside and instrumental assessment. Screening is used to assess the possibility of aspiration (overt or silent) and risk for complications.

Screening Tools[2]

- Burke Dysphagia Screening Test
- Standardized Swallowing Assessment
- Timed tests of Hinds and Wiles
- Bedside Swallow Assessment
- Toronto Bedside Swallowing Screening Test (TOS-BSST)
- Clinical Examination
- Modified Mann Assessment of Swallowing Ability
  Screening tests are considered positive if any of the following are present:
- Dysphonia
- Dysarthria
- Abnormal gag
- Abnormal volitional cough

- Cough after swallowing
- Voice change after swallow

Although bedside screening protocols are commonly used, a systemic review of seven databases including Medline, Embase, and Scopus concluded that no bedside screening protocol provides adequate predictive value for the presence of aspiration.[10]

Other Swallowing Evaluations

Videofluorographic Swallowing Study

- This is also known as the *Modified Barium Swallow* (MBS) and is the "gold standard" for evaluation and treatment of oropharyngeal dysphagia.[11,12]
- It involves providing a patient with a variety of consistencies and textures of liquid and foods mixed with barium.
- As the patient eats or drinks these substances, the provider can observe the anatomy and physiology of the patient's swallow in real time.
- It can help diagnose an anatomical abnormality (Zenker's diverticulum, cricopharyngeal bar, stricture, achalasia) that may contribute to the patient's dysphagia.
- MBS is both diagnostic and therapeutic and allows the provider to have the patient preform compensatory strategies or altered consistencies to see if it helps improve the patient's swallow.
- Aspiration can be seen easily on the MBS as demonstrated by penetration of contrast material below the true vocal cords (Fig. 31.3).[13]

Fiber Optic Endoscopic Evaluation

- This is used to evaluate the pharyngeal phase of swallowing.
- A fiber optic camera is passed through the nasal passage to the oropharynx for direct visualization.
- This allows for a direct examination of the patient's anatomy that could be inhibiting the passage of the bolus.

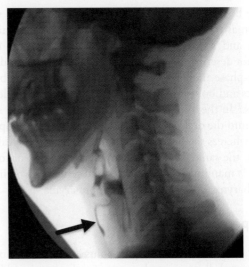

• **Fig. 31.3** Aspiration seen on Modified Barium Swallow (MBS). Thin layer of barium (*arrow*) on the anterior wall of the trachea. (From Chhetri DK, Dewan K. *Dysphagia Evaluation and Management in Otolaryngology.* St. Louis, MO: Elsevier; 2019.)

- There is a limitation: no visualization of aspiration because the camera is only viewing passage of the bolus from the oropharynx to the pharynx.
- It can detect secretions in the oropharynx suggestive swallowing dysfunction (Fig. 31.4).[13]

Manometry

Manometry measures the pressure in the pharynx and esophagus during swallowing to evaluate a patient's esophageal motility and identify potential issue with peristalsis.

Summary

- Bedside evaluation and screening tools often require instrumental assessment as confirmation since silent aspiration can be missed on bedside exam.

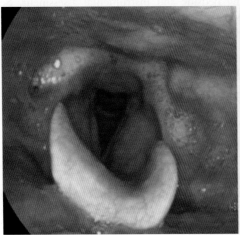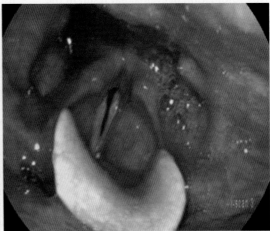

• **Fig. 31.4** Piriform sinus residue. Secretions in the oropharynx are highly suggestive of swallowing dysfunction. Pooling of saliva seen before feeding *(left panel)*. Piriform sinus residue collects during flexible endoscopic evaluation of swallowing. (From Chhetri DK, Dewan K. *Dysphagia Evaluation and Management in Otolaryngology.* St. Louis, MO: Elsevier; 2019.)

- Videofluorographic swallowing study (MBS) is the gold standard for evaluation and treatment.
- MBS is therapeutic as provider can have patient use compensatory strategies or altered consistencies to see if patient's swallow improves.
- Fiberoptic endoscopic evaluation evaluates pharyngeal phase of swallowing only.
- Manometry evaluates a patient's esophageal motility and identifies issues with peristalsis.

Treatment

Treatment for dysphagia includes both compensatory and rehabilitative approaches.[14]

Compensatory Strategies

These reduce symptoms of dysphagia without altering the physiology.

Rehabilitative Strategies

- These improve the swallowing physiology and swallowing safety of the least restrictive diet.[15]
- Exercises include working on lip and tongue strength and movement, range of motion, and voice production.

Compensatory Strategies[16]

- Supraglottic swallow
- Superglottic swallow
- Head Position changes
- Best observed under videofluorographic evaluation to assess/prevent aspiration

Rehabilitative Strategies

- Tongue-strengthening exercises
- Mendelsohn maneuver
- Shaker exercise
- Modified liquid consistency and food texture
  - Best practice: identify a safe way for the patient to eat.
  - Altering the consistency of liquids (honey and nectar thick) and/or change a patient's diet texture (mechanical soft or purée).
  - Increasing the thickness of liquids can decrease the rate of aspiration and penetration, but it leads to larger volume of residual, which poses an increased risk of secondary aspiration in patients.[17]

A systematic review recommends against routine use of modified liquid consistencies but supports the use of modified food consistency, whereby the use of modified food textures helps transition a patient from enteral feeding to oral nutrition. Because the benefit of using a variation of liquid consistencies is unreproducible and has a poor risk/benefit comparison, it is suggested that "in the acute phase, individual counseling with follow up and adjustment of the consistency of texture modified food and thickened liquid should be given."[18]

Neuromuscular Electrical Stimulation

- Neuromuscular electrical stimulation (NMES) has been used to retrain pharyngeal musculature and improve swallow function by promoting reorganization of the motor cortex.[19]
- Electrical stimulation of oral and pharyngeal muscles is used to help reinitiate proper timing of muscle contractions to improve swallowing.

A small pilot study that used an electrical stimulation protocol to help with dysphonia after stroke and TBI described significant improvement in the pharyngeal phase of swallowing and attributed it to improvement in laryngeal elevation from suprahyoid. Because of small sample size and mixed tolerance of electrical stimulation, it concluded that "further research [is] required to discover protocol for treatment and to evaluate effectiveness in other phases of swallowing."[20]

Biofeedback methods such as surface electromyography (sEMG) are used in conjunction with traditional therapy to "increase awareness of swallowing patterns and to help the patient modify, monitor, and challenge performance while executing swallowing maneuvers."[21]

- Surface EMG increases the rate of progress when combined with traditional dysphagia therapy for a group of 45 patients with chronic swallowing problems.[22]
- NMES was found to have a positive impact on swallow function, with NMES having slightly better outcomes[23] or a better outcome that did not reach statistical significance.[19]
- In some studies, NMES was found to have negatively affected laryngeal elevation, resulting in increased risk of aspiration.[24]
- Given the inconsistencies of effectiveness, it is unclear if NMES is effective for the treatment of dysphagia.

Nonoral

If patients are not able to safely pass any bolus besides their own secretions, then they should be taught to use oral or vocal exercises to help begin the recovery process.

These patients will require a secondary mean of nutrition (percutaneous endoscopic gastrostomy [PEG] tube, nasogastric [NG] tube, gastrostomy-jejunostomy tube, or Dobhoff tube), although placement of a feeding tube may not remove all of the risk of aspiration.[25,26]

The risk of developing pneumonia after TBI complicated by dysphagia is high. One study documented that up to 81% of the patients with TBI complicated by dysphagia who developed pneumonia were fed by only a feeding tube, with the risk for aspiration coming from their own secretions or the regurgitated contents of the stomach.[3]

This suggests that with the use of feeding tubes, there still need to be strict precautions to prevent aspiration in this highly susceptible patient group.

Summary

- Dysphagia treatment should include compensatory and rehabilitative strategies.[27]
- Modified liquid consistency and food texture can help promote patient's continuing to practice swallow, but research is controversial about efficacy and risk of secondary aspiration.
- NMES helps retrain pharyngeal musculature and improve swallow function by reorganizing the motor cortex.
- With severe dysphagia, patients may require a secondary mean of nutrition (PEG, NG tube, or Dobhoff tube) although this doesn't eliminate the risk of aspiration.
- A patient can use physical maneuvers to help prevent dysphagia.

Complications

Aspiration

- Aspiration occurs when part of the bolus enters the airway below the true vocal cords into the trachea.
- It can produce symptoms but is commonly asymptomatic and referred to as *silent*.
- Aspiration can be missed easily on bedside examinations and often requires more in-depth evaluation.
- Aspiration puts the patient at risk for developing pneumonia, which occurs in about one-third of stroke patients.[28]
- Patients with an altered level of consciousness, tracheostomy patients, and patients with persistent emesis and reflux symptoms are at a higher risk of developing aspiration pneumonia.
- TBI patients are at higher risk because of the presence of cognitive and sensorimotor impairments.

Dehydration and Malnutrition

- Patients who have trouble with oral intake are at high risk for dehydration and malnutrition.
- The slow recovery of dysphagia results in patients at risk for not meeting their nutritional needs, which leads to decreased overall functional recovery.
- Those who require the usage of thickening agents may not be getting the same free water and hydrating effect from an equivalent amount of unthickened liquid.
- Thickening agent may have an unintended side effects that contribute to dehydration and potential subtherapeutic medication levels.[29]
- Use of thickeners is not without harm, because thickeners may increase amounts of oral and/or pharyngeal residues and may lead to postswallow airway invasion, reduce palatability of thickened liquids, and contribute to noncompliance.[17]
- Patients with dysphagia usually require an extended amount of time to safely consume their meal because of safe swallowing techniques.
- It is important to have a dietitian evaluate every patient with dysphagia and develop an individualized plan to help meet their nutritional requirements through supplements and diet modifications.

Summary

- Complications from dysphagia include aspiration and dehydration and malnutrition.
- TBI patients are at higher risk for aspiration pneumonia due to presence of cognitive and sensorimotor impairments.
- The slow recovery of dysphagia can lead to patients not meeting their nutritional needs for a prolonged period.
- It is important to discuss with a dietician about caloric needs to ensure adequate intake and nutrition to promote overall patient recovery and healing.

Recovery

- Dysphagia treatment must be continued after acute hospitalization and rehabilitation.
- There is varying data in literature about recovery of swallow function after TBI, with some predictive factors that can help guide providers about severity and possibility of recovery and return to regular diet.
- Patients who have a severe injury (low initial GCS score, large amount of neurologic involvement), impaired tongue movement/function, absent oropharyngeal reflex, or increased pharyngeal delay time observed on videofluoroscopic study have all been associated with slower recovery of their dysphagia.[30]
- Another study found that swallowing characteristics of patients with dysphagia after TBI were comparable to those of patients with dysphagia after stroke, with common MBS findings of aspiration or penetration, decreased laryngeal elevation, and reduced epiglottis inversion.[4]
- Patients who underwent surgical intervention after TBI were more likely to be fed nonorally, suggesting a more careful and long-term VFSS may be warranted.[4]
- Patients receiving appropriate and optimal speech therapy treatment should continue to progress and advance toward oral feeding without increased risk of respiratory complication.[30]
- Most patients with dysphagia after TBI will recover swallowing abilities over the first 3 to 5 months after their injury,[3] although some will require a much longer period for their swallow function to return.[31]
- The chance of returning to an unrestricted diet depends on the severity of the brain injury as assessed by GCS, RLAS, the Functional Independent Measure (FIM) score, and functional oral intake on admission.[32]

Summary

- Recovery of dysphagia requires continued therapy and treatment after acute hospitalization and rehabilitation.
- Patients with severe TBI (low initial GCS score, large amount of neurologic involvement), impaired tongue movement/function, absent oropharyngeal reflex, or

increased pharyngeal delay time are associated with slower recovery.

- Most patients with dysphagia following TBI will recover swallowing abilities over the first 3 to five months following their injury, although some will require a much longer period of time for their swallow function to returns.
- A chance of returning to an unrestricted diet depends on the severity of the brain injury with greater likelihood of success correlates with lesser severity of their brain injury as measured by commonly used scales to assess brain injury (GCS score, RLAS score, FIM score, and functional oral intake on admission).

Summary

Swallowing requires a highly coordinated and controlled sequence of events that requires protection of the airway during the bolus transit to the stomach. In a patient with TBI, the anatomical and physiological swallowing mechanisms may be impaired. Cognitive and behavioral impairments among patients with TBI make rehabilitation of dysphagia more challenging.

Most patients with brain injury recover safe and efficient swallowing with therapy during the first 5 months after their injury, although some will need maintenance therapy or nonoral feeding. Unfortunately, clinical trials for specific strategies for patients after TBI are lacking because of a wide variety and high variability between patients in this population. Common variables among studies assessing dysphagia among TBI patient stress the importance of an interdisciplinary approach in which all team members are consistent in their methods for the patient and engage the family to learn and use compensatory strategies.

Review Questions

1. For patients with traumatic brain injury (TBI), the factors that put the patient at greatest risk of aspiration pneumonia are
   a. intubation, tracheostomy, and oropharyngeal spasticity.
   b. Glasgow Coma Scale (GCS) score <9, Rancho Los Amigos Scale (RLAS) <3, nothing by mouth (NPO) status.
   c. Diffuse axonal injury (DAI), facial fracture, and laryngeal swelling.
   d. midbrain injury, depth of coma, and jaw fracture.
2. Common findings on Modified Barium Swallow (MBS) studies between patients with TBI and stroke at risk for dysphagia are
   a. Impaired level of consciousness, presence of tracheostomy, and laryngeal swelling.
   b. Spastic laryngeal muscles, laryngeal swelling, and copious secretions.
   c. Aspiration/penetration, decreased laryngeal elevation, and reduced epiglottis inversion.
   d. Laryngeal depression, piriform sinus residue, and copious secretions in the oropharynx.

3. The differences between the process model and the four phases of swallowing model are
   a. aspiration is more commonly seen in the Four Phases of Swallowing Model.
   b. the Four Phases of Swallowing Model includes the esophageal propulsive phase to describe food transit from the esophagus into the stomach.
   c. the Process Model describes the mechanism of eating and swallowing solid food.
   d. the Process Model includes the oral preparatory stage, the oral propulsive stage, the pharyngeal stage, and the esophageal stage.

Answers on page 395.
Access the full list of questions and answers online. Available on ExpertConsult.com

References

1. Groher ME, Crary MA. *Dysphagia Clinical Management in Adults and Children.* St. Louis, MO: Elsevier; 2016.
2. González-Fernández M, Ottenstein L, Atanelov L, Christian AB. Dysphagia after stroke: an overview. *Curr Phys Med Rehabil Rep.* 2013;1(3):187-196.
3. Hansen TS, Larsen K, Enberg AW. The association of functional oral intake and pneumonia in patients with severe traumatic brain injury. *Arch Phys Med Rehabil.* 2008;89(11):2114-2120.
4. Lee WK, Yeom J, Lee WH, Seo HG, Oh BM, Han TR. Characteristics of dysphagia in severe traumatic brain injury patients: a comparison with stroke patients. *Ann Rehabil Med.* 2016;40(3):432-439.
5. Palmer JB, Rudin NJ, Lara G, Crompton AW. Coordination of mastication and swallowing. *Dysphagia.* 1992;7(4):187-200.
6. Dodds WJ, Stewart ET, Logemann JA. Physiology and radiology of the normal oral and pharyngeal phases of swallowing [see comment]. *AJR Am J Roentgenol.* 1990;154(5):953-963.
7. Matsuo K, Palmer JB. Anatomy and physiology of feeding and swallowing: normal and abnormal. *Phys Med Rehabil Clin N orth Am.* 2008;19(4):691-707.
8. Goyal R, Mashimo H. Physiology of oral, pharyngeal, and esophageal motility. *GI Motility.* 2006.
9. Steele CM, Cichero JA. Physiological factors related to aspiration risk: a systematic review. *Dysphagia.* 2014;29(3):295-304.

10. O'Horo JC, Rogus-Pulia N, Garcia-Arguello L, Robbins J, Safdar N. Bedside diagnosis of dysphagia: a systematic review. *J Hosp Med.* 2015;10(4):256-265.

11. Palmer JB, Tanaka E, Ensrud E. Motions of the posterior pharyngeal wall in human swallowing: a quantitative videofluorographic study. *Arch Phys Med Rehabil.* 2000;81(11):1520-1526.

12. Martin-Harris B, Brodsky MB, Michel Y, et al, MBS measurement tool for swallow impairment-MBSImp: establishing a standard. *Dysphagia.* 2008;23(4):392-405.

13. Chhetri DK, Dewan K. *Dysphagia Evaluation and Management in Otolaryngology.* St. Louis, MO: Elsevier; 2019.

14. Huckabee M, Pelletier C. *Management of Adult Neurologic Dysphagia. 1.* San Diego: Singular Publishing Group; 1999.

15. Carnaby-Mann G, Lenius K, Crary M. Update on assessment and management of dysphagia post stroke. *Northeast Fla Med.* 2007;58(2).

16. van der Kruis JG, Baijens LW, Speyer R, Zwijnenberg I. Biomechanical analysis of hyoid bone displacement in videofluoroscopy: a systematic review of intervention effects. *Dysphagia.* 2011;26(2):171-182.

17. Newman R, Vilardell N, Clave P, et al, Effect of bolus viscosity on the safety and efficacy of swallowing and the kinematics of the swallow response in patients with oropharyngeal dysphagia: White Paper by the European Society for Swallowing Disorders (ESSD). *Dysphagia.* 2016;31(2):232-249.

18. Beck AM, Kjaersgaard A, Hansen T, Poulsen I. Systematic review and evidence based recommendations on texture modified foods and thickened liquids for adults (above 17 years) with oropharyngeal dysphagia - An updated clinical guideline. *Clin Nutr.* 2018;37(6)1980-1991.

19. Bülow M, Speyer R, Baijens L, et al, Neuromuscular electrical stimulation (NMES) in stroke patients with oral and pharyngeal dysfunction. *Dysphagia.* 2008;23(3):302-309.

20. Ko KR, Park HJ, Hyun JK, et al, Effect of laryngopharyngeal neuromuscular electrical stimulation on dysphonia accompanied by dysphagia in post-stroke and traumatic brain injury patients: a pilot study. *Ann Rehabil Med.* 2016;40(4):600-610.

21. Burkhead LM, Sapienza CM, Rosenbek JC. Strength-training exercise in dysphagia rehabilitation: principles, procedures,

22. Crary MA, Carnaby Mann GD, Groher ME, et al. Functional benefits of dysphagia therapy using adjunctive sEMG biofeedback. *Dysphagia.* 2004;19(3):160-164.

23. Permsirivanich W, Tipchatyotin S, Wongchai M, et al. Comparing the effects of rehabilitation swallowing therapy vs. neuromuscular electrical stimulation therapy among stroke patients with persistent pharyngeal dysphagia: a randomized controlled study. *J Med Assoc Thai.* 2009;92(2):259-265.

24. Ludlow CL, Humbert I, Saxon K, et al, Effects of surface electrical stimulation both at rest and during swallowing in chronic pharyngeal Dysphagia. *Dysphagia.* 2007;22(1):1-10.

25. Mizock BA. Risk of aspiration in patients on enteral nutrition: frequency, relevance, relation to pneumonia, risk factors, and strategies for risk reduction. *Curr Gastroenterol Rep.* 2007;9(4):338-344.

26. Gomes GF, Pisani JC, Macedo ED, et al, The nasogastric feeding tube as a risk factor for aspiration and aspiration pneumonia. *Curr Opin Clin Nutr Metab Care.* 2003;6(3):327-333.

27. Cabib C, Ortega O, Kumru H, et al. Neurorehabilitation strategies for poststroke oropharyngeal dysphagia: from compensation to the recovery of swallowing function. *Ann N Y Acad Sci.* 2016;1380(1):121-138.

28. Sellars C, Bowie L, Bagg J, et al. Risk factors for chest infection in acute stroke: a prospective cohort study. *Stroke.* 2007;38(8):2284-2291.

29. Cichero JA. Thickening agents used for dysphagia management: effect on bioavailability of water, medication and feelings of satiety. *Nutr J.* 2013;12:54.

30. Terré R, Mearin F. Evolution of tracheal aspiration in severe traumatic brain injury-related oropharyngeal dysphagia: 1-year longitudinal follow-up study. *Neurogastroenterol Motil.* 2009;21(4):361-369.

31. Burke D, Alexander K, Baxter M, et al, Rehabilitation of a person with severe traumatic brain injury. *Brain Inj.* 2000;14(5):463-471.

32. Hansen TS, Engberg AW, Larsen K. Functional oral intake and time to reach unrestricted dieting for patients with traumatic brain injury. *Arch Phys Med Rehabil.* 2008;89(8):1556-1562.

and directions for future research. *Dysphagia.* 2007;22(3):251-265.

32

Speech and Language

DAVID L ENG, MD, AND BENJAMIN N NGUYEN, MD

This chapter focuses on the impairments to speech and language that occur after brain injury. These impairments can be grouped into four main categories:
- Aphasia
- Dysarthria
- Apraxia of speech
- Cognitive communication disorders.

It is common for these language impairments to occur together, but they can occur separately as well.

Aphasia

Aphasia is the impairment in the ability to produce and/or comprehend spoken or written language caused by damage affecting one or more areas of the brain responsible for language.[1] Aphasia can develop suddenly after a stroke or head injury or slowly secondary to a brain tumor or a progressive neurologic disease such as Alzheimer's disease. It may include impairments in auditory comprehension, verbal expression, reading comprehension, and/or written expression and may cooccur with other speech disorders, such as dysarthria or apraxia of speech.
- Types of aphasia can be categorized based on three main aspects of communication (Table 32.1, Fig. 32.1):

Epidemiology

- Stroke is the most common cause of aphasia, affecting up to 40% to 60% of stroke patients.[2]
- About 1 million people in the United States currently live with aphasia, with 180,000 Americans developing aphasia annually.[1]
- Poststroke aphasia can significantly affect a person's quality of life and has been shown to have a greater negative effect than common conditions such as cancer and Alzheimer's and Parkinson's diseases.[3]

Functional Neuroanatomy

- The language center of the brain is located in the dominant hemisphere—the left hemisphere in the vast majority of individuals. Even in left-handed individuals, approximately 70% have left hemispheric dominance.[4]
- Broca's aphasia is named after the French scientist Paul Broca who first related deficits associated with this type of aphasia to localized brain damage in 1861.[5] Individuals have difficulty accurately forming the words they want to say. Although they may understand speech and know what they want to say, they frequently speak in short phrases with halting, effortful speech, with imprecise articulation and paraphasia. The lesion is localized to the lateral frontal/suprasylvian area of the frontal lobe, commonly known as *Broca's area* (Fig. 32.2). Those with Broca's aphasia often have right-sided weakness or paralysis because the frontal lobe also plays a role in motor control.
- In Wernicke's—or fluent—aphasia, individuals often speak in long, complete phrases that have no meaning. They have a fluent jargon speech with normal prosody, poor auditory comprehension and repetition, and difficulty understanding speech. The lesion localizes to damage to the posterior third of the superior gyrus in the temporal lobe (see Fig. 32.2).
- The arcuate fasciculus—a bundle of axons that connects Wernicke's area to the motor and premotor cortex

TABLE 32.1	**Types of Aphasia**			
Type of Aphasia	Fluency	Comprehension	Repetition	Area of Injury
Global	−	−	−	Left middle cerebral artery stroke
Mixed transcortical	−	−	+	Border zones between parietal, temporal, and frontal lobes
Broca's	−	+	−	Left posterior inferior frontal lobe
Transcortical motor	−	+	+	Frontal lobe, anterior or superior to Broca's area
Wernicke's	+	−	−	Left superior temporal gyrus
Transcortical sensory	+	−	+	Posterior temporal lobe
Conduction	+	+	−	Arcuate fasciculus
Anomia	+	+	+	Angular gyrus
Crossed	+/−	+/−	+/−	Rare occurrence when lesion in the right hemisphere mirrors those seen in the left hemisphere

Adapted from *Braddom's Physical Medicine and Rehabilitation*[46] and *Principles of Rehabilitation Medicine.*[47]

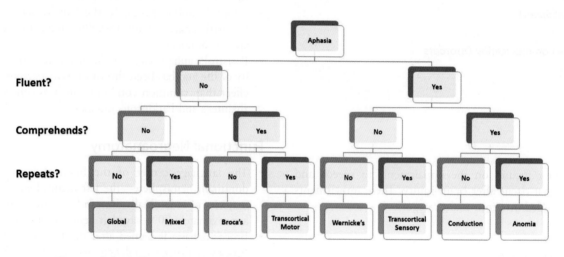

• **Fig. 32.1** Aphasia Tree Diagram (Adapted with permission from the National Aphasia Association.[49])

(including Broca's area)—allows for speech repetition. Damage to this group of neurons results in a conduction aphasia, where speech is fluent (although there may be word-finding pauses) and repetition is impaired. Damage to Broca's area, Wernicke's area, or arcuate fasciculus will result in impaired repetition because the connection between the areas has been affected.

• Lesions affecting the anterior frontal paramedian area anterosuperior to Broca's area will result in impaired initiation of verbal output in a condition known as *transcortical motor aphasia*.

• Lesions located in the posterior parietotemporal area sparing Wernicke's area will lead to anomia with poor auditory comprehension, with intact repetition resulting in a condition called *transcortical sensory aphasia*.

• Damage to both the motor and comprehension centers of the brain, such as after a large left middle cerebral artery stroke, will result in a global deficit in language. Patients will have profound anomia with very poor auditory comprehension with stereotypic utterances.

• Damage to the right hemisphere may lead to cognitive communication disorders such as neglect, affecting reading and writing ability, impairments in memory, attention, perception, and learning.[6]

Treatment

Speech pathologists are experts at assessing and treating the areas and severity of language deficit, including auditory comprehension, fluency, reading, and writing.

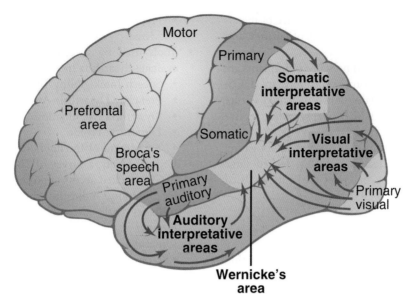

• **Fig. 32.2** Basic neuroanatomy of the language centers of the brain. (Reprinted with permission from Hall J. *Guyton and Hall Textbook of Medical Physiology.* 12th ed. Philadelphia, PA: Saunders Elsevier; 2011.)

• Diagnostic evaluation tools: Western Aphasia Battery[7] and Boston Diagnostic Evaluation of Aphasia[8]
• Studies have shown that intense speech therapy leads to better improvement than intermittent or less structured therapy[9] and that early intense therapy may promote cortical reorganization leading to persistent improvements in language.[10]
• Constraint-induced aphasia therapy (CIAT) focuses on overcoming learned nonuse of language deficits and has been shown to improve aphasia when used in intensive therapy.[11] This form of therapy prohibits the patient from communicating nonverbally to encourage the use of verbal communication.
• Melodic intonation therapy also has been shown to have some benefit in patients with Broca's aphasia in the acute setting after stroke.[12]
• Another strategy to improve communication is augmentative and alternative communication (AAC). These focus on restorative and compensatory strategies, which range in complexity from the use of basic pictures and word boards to computerized communication devices.[13]

Pharmacologic Treatment

Brain injury, whether from trauma or stroke, causes disruptions in the noradrenergic, cholinergic, serotonergic, and dopaminergic pathways from the brainstem to the language cortex.[14] Pharmacologic treatment of aphasia has been studied, but the quality of these studies varies, the patient populations are small, and the results have been inconclusive.[14]

• Catecholaminergic drugs such as bromocriptine, levodopa, dextroamphetamine, and amantadine have been studied but have not shown clear and lasting benefits in improving aphasia.[14]

• Cholinergic drugs such as ameridin, donepezil, bifemelane, aniracetam, galantamine, and physostigmine have also been studied, with donepezil showing some short-term benefit in treating chronic poststroke aphasia.[14]
• Memantine, an NMDA receptor antagonist, may have some lasting benefit when combined with CIAT.[15]
• Piracetam, a nutritional supplement derived from gamma-aminobutyric acid (GABA), may have some short-term benefit in the acute phase when combined with speech therapy.[14]

Noninvasive Brain Stimulation

A range of nonpharmacologic treatments for aphasia exists as an adjunct to speech therapy. These include the use of use of electrical current to modify brain activity, a phenomenon first mentioned more than 200 years ago.[16,17]

Two such methods include:
• Transcranial direct current stimulation (tDCS)
• Transcranial magnetic stimulation (TMS)
  • tDCS: electrodes are placed on the scalp to produce a static electrical field in the underlying brain structures. This has been shown to produce prolonged and sustainable shifts in cortical excitability and functioning when studied in conjunction with functional magnetic resonance imaging (fMRI), positron emission tomography (PET), and electroencephalogram (EEG).[18,19]
  • TMS: an electrical coil is placed over the patient's scalp to induce a fluctuating magnetic wave that creates a dynamic electrical field in the underlying brain.[20]
• Both methods have shown promising results in treating chronic aphasia and are safe procedures with very few side effects.

- Contraindications to TMS are the presence of metallic or cochlear implants, increased risk of seizures, and unstable medical conditions.[21]
- Increased risk of seizures and presence of implants are also considered relative contraindications in tDCS, but studies have not actually shown increased seizure frequency in patients with epilepsy who receive tDCS.[22]
- Despite promising results, the studies investigating the efficacy of these techniques have lacked large sample sizes, and these practices are still not used widely.[14,23,24]

Recovery

Those with aphasia will have the greatest recovery within the first 3 months poststroke. If the symptoms of aphasia last longer than 2 or 3 months after a stroke, a complete recovery is unlikely, although some continue to improve over years or even decades.[1,25]

Dysarthria

Dysarthria is an acquired motor speech disorder after a neurologic injury leading to muscle weakness or incoordination, resulting in impaired phonation, articulation, respiration, and resonance. Dysarthria can be caused by both upper and motor neuron injuries, which include stroke, traumatic brain injury (TBI), amyotrophic lateral sclerosis, Parkinson's disease, and multiple sclerosis.
- Dysarthria can be categorized into types according to the area of deficit[26] (Table 32.2):
  - Flaccid
  - Spastic
  - Ataxic
  - Hypokinetic
  - Hyperkinetic
  - Mixed
- Tools used by speech-language pathologists (SLP) to evaluate dysarthria include[27]:
  - Speech Intelligibility Test
  - Frenchay Dysarthria Assessment
  - Dysarthria Examination Battery
  - Dysarthria Profile
  - Assessment of Intelligibility of Dysarthric Speech
- Unfortunately, a survey of 269 SLPs showed that 35% of SLPs lacked access to any standardized assessment of intelligibility, indicating the need to increase SLP familiarity with currently available standardized assessments.[27]
- Other diagnostic tools include[28]:
  - Computerized aerodynamic assessment to measure the intraoral pressure, nasal airflow, and soft palate closure
  - Endoscopy to observe velopharyngeal function
  - Computerized voice analysis programs to identify and quantify vocal aspects that are impaired
- The impact of dysarthria goes beyond the ability to communicate and often affects psychosocial functioning.

Treatment

Treatment of dysarthria depends on the underlying cause but focuses mainly on improving coordination and muscle control.
- Poor respiratory support can be treated with abdominal binders, biofeedback, and breathing exercises.[29]
- Velopharyngeal dysfunction can be treated with palatal lifts and prostheses.[30]
- Parkinson's patients with hypokinetic dysarthria respond well to the Lee Silverman Voice Treatment Program (also known as *LOUD*).[31]

TABLE 32.2 Classifications of Dysarthria

Type	Site of the Lesion	Symptoms	Speech Characteristics
Spastic	Pyramidal and extrapyramidal	Increased muscle tone, decreased range of motion	Strain-strangled voice quality, hypernasality
Flaccid	Lower motor neuron	Weakness, decreased tone	Slurred speech, breathiness, hypernasality
Hyperkinetic	Basal ganglia, subcortical structures	Quick unsustained involuntary movements	Altered rhythm and rate caused by involuntary speech movements
Hypokinetic	Basal ganglia, subcortical structures	Slow movements	Low volume, reduced movements, festinating speech
Ataxic	Cerebellum	Slow and inaccurate	Slow rate, imprecise articulation, irregular articulatory breakdowns
Mixed	Upper and lower motor neuron	Varies	Variable combination of the above

Adapted from *Braddom's Physical Medicine and Rehabilitation*.[48]

- Dysarthric patients may also benefit from treatment with the SpeechVive device, allowing even those with significant cognitive impairments to speak louder and clearer.[32]
- Constraint-induced therapy, commonly used for motor recovery and aphasia after stroke, has been described as helping recovery for dysarthria after stroke.[33]
- For moderate to severe dysarthria, the use of augmentative and alternative means of communication is indicated.

Despite numerous interventions and clinical trials with attempts to improve dysarthria, two Cochrane review studies found there is no evidence to support or refute the effectiveness of speech and language therapy interventions for dysarthria after nonprogressive brain damage.[34,35]

Apraxia of Speech

Apraxia of speech (AOS) is a motor speech disorder in coordinating and executing the movements necessary in speech production despite normal muscle function and tone. It coexists in patients with aphasia or dysarthria but can occur on its own.
- Location of lesion: left hemisphere, particularly in the region of the left posterior inferior frontal gyrus.[36]
- Characteristics include slow speaking rate, lengthened sounds, lengthened pause between sounds, articulatory groping, difficulty initiating speech, and a preference for automatic phrases, with articulatory distortion errors such as sound substitution and addition[37]
- Diagnostic tool: Apraxia Battery for Adults[37]

Treatment

Treatment focuses on intense and repetitive behavioral therapy. Articulatory–kinematic therapy has shown to be beneficial in these patients and involves following steps repeatedly to produce accurate speech.[38] These patients also benefit from auditory and visual feedback, and the use of tablet and smartphone applications has been shown to improve repetition and naming in patients with AOS.[37] As with all other communication disorders, AAC is indicated in patients with moderate to severe AOS.

Cognitive Communication Disorders

TBI can cause cognitive and social communication impairments that are separate from the previously discussed language impairments.
- Impairments: concentration, attention, naming, processing speed, memory, difficulty with narration, maintaining conversations, and other higher-level forms of complex communication[39]
- Cognitive communication disorders commonly can be misdiagnosed as aphasia
- Areas of the brain usually affected: the nondominant hemisphere and the prefrontal cortex and temporoparietal junction[40]

The degree of cognitive communication impairment is often described in conjunction with the Rancho Los Amigos Levels of Cognitive Functioning[41]:
- Posttraumatic amnesia (PTA) and lower Rancho levels: Assessment of language impairment can be difficult because patients are confused and disoriented and may have a decreased level of consciousness.
  - Intervention with speech therapy typically occurs after the patient has emerged from PTA.[42] Early intervention at these stages usually focuses on the ability to follow simple commands.
- Rancho levels IV to V: Patients are more cognitively aware. Many patients will become verbal communicators, but those who do not may require the use of AAC for short- or long-term use.[43] Therapy at this stage focuses on reorienting the patient and improving memory and learning.
- Rancho levels VI to VIII: Patients may be capable of abstract thought and can progress to more complex and higher-level communication.[42]
- During late recovery and with mild TBI, patients can continue to have cognitive and social communication disorders that can last for years and if left untreated can lead to significant psychosocial impairment and difficulties returning to work or maintaining relationships.[44]

A comprehensive review of cognitive rehab will be discussed elsewhere, but briefly, therapy targeted toward social communication usually follows two approaches: impairment-specific versus context-sensitive or holistic.[45] Both have shown to be beneficial, but some evidence suggests that the context-sensitive approach may be more beneficial especially when used in group therapy.[45]

Summary

- Language dysfunction often accompanies survivors of neurologic dysfunction from TBI and nontraumatic causes (stroke, anoxia, infection, brain tumors, dementia, encephalopathy, etc.), often contributing to significant cognitive sensorimotor–behavioral deficits.
- Treatment success depends on accurate diagnosis and determination of the type of speech impairment.
- For those with language dysfunction after a TBI, the accompanying cognitive–sensorimotor–behavioral deficits can be sources of long-term disability.
- Patients may have difficulty with understanding the complexity of language caused by damage to parts of the brain responsible for language production and understanding.
- There are many ongoing studies to gain a better understanding of the pathophysiology, methods/assessments to help with diagnosis, pharmacologic treatment/manipulation/augmentation, or noninvasive brain stimulation to help with the recovery process.
- Studies suggest that patients with aphasia will improve over time, especially if speech therapy is provided, and it

can continue to improve even ten or more years after onset if patients have access to appropriate treatment.

• Researchers are testing new types of speech–language therapy in people with both recent and chronic aphasia, exploring drug therapy, studying advanced imaging methods such as fMRI to explore how language is processed in the normal and injured brain to understand the recovery process, and using noninvasive brain stimulation (TMS, tDCS) to promote recovery. An exciting time to be an aphasia survivor indeed!

Review Questions

1. Which of these is true about aphasia?
   a. A disorder of speech or language that occurs after injury to the right frontal/parietal lobe
   b. A disorder of speech or understanding caused by damage to one or more of the areas of the brain responsible for language
   c. Classified based on oral comprehension, written comprehension, fluency, and repetition
   d. Improvement in language and communication requires intense speech therapies within the first 3 months to take advantage of brain reorganization/plasticity
2. In Broca's aphasia,
   a. patients often have right-sided weakness or paralysis.
   b. patients have fluent jargon speech with normal prosody.
   c. patients have fluent speech with impaired repetition.
   d. the lesion localizes to posterior third of the superior gyrus.
3. In Wernicke's aphasia,
   a. the lesion is located in the posterior third of the inferior temporal gyrus.
   b. patients have halting, effortful speech with imprecise articulation and paraphasia.
   c. Speech is fluent; patients can't understand but can repeat.
   d. Speech is fluent; there is normal prosody but poor repetition.

Answers on page 395.
Access the full list of questions and answers online.
Available on ExpertConsult.com

References

1. NIH National Institute on Deafness and Other Communication Disorders. [website]. 2017. Available at: https://www.nidcd.nih.gov/health/aphasia. accessed on March 27, 2020
2. Balardin JB, Miotto EC. A review of Constraint-Induced Therapy applied to aphasia rehabilitation in stroke patients. *Dement Neuropsychol.* 2009;3(4):275-282.
3. Lam JM, Wodchis WP. The relationship of 60 disease diagnoses and 15 conditions to preference-based health-related quality of life in Ontario hospital-based long-term care residents. *Med Care.* 2010;48(4):380-387.
4. Pujol J, Deus J, Losilla JM, et al. Cerebral lateralization of language in normal left-handed people studied by functional MRI. *Neurology.* 1999;52(5):1038-1038.
5. Ardila A, Bernal B, Rosselli M. How localized are language brain areas? A review of brodmann areas involvement in oral language. *Arch Clin Neuropsychol.* 2016;31(1):112-122.
6. Hickok G. The functional neuroanatomy of language. *Phys Life Rev.* 2009;6(3):121-143.
7. Shewan CM, Kertesz A. Reliability and validity characteristics of the Western Aphasia Battery (WAB). *J Speech Hear Disord.* 1980;45(3):308-324.
8. Fong MWM, Van Patten R, Fucetola RP. The factor structure of the boston diagnostic aphasia examination, 3rd edition. *J Int Neuropsychol Soc.* 2019;00;1-5.
9. Brady MC, Kelly H, Godwin J, et al. Speech and language therapy for aphasia following stroke. *Cochrane Database Syst Rev.* 2016;(6):CD000425.
10. Mattioli F, Ambrosi C, Mascaro L, et al. Early aphasia rehabilitation is associated with functional reactivation of the left inferior frontal gyrus: a pilot study. *Stroke.* 2014;45(2):545-552.
11. Cherney LR, Patterson JP, Raymer A, et al. Evidence-based systematic review: effects of intensity of treatment and constraint-induced language therapy for individuals with stroke-induced aphasia. *J Speech Lang Hear Res.* 2008;51(5):1282-1299.
12. Conklyn D, Novak E, Boissy A, et al. The effects of modified melodic intonation therapy on nonfluent aphasia: a pilot study. *J Speech Lang Hear Res.* 2012;55(5):1463-1471.
13. Russo MJ, Prodan V, Meda NN, et al. High-technology augmentative communication for adults with post-stroke aphasia: a systematic review. *Expert Rev Med Devices.* 2017;14(5):355-370.
14. Saxena S, Hillis AE. An update on medications and noninvasive brain stimulation to augment language rehabilitation in post-stroke aphasia. *Expert Rev Neurother.* 2017;17(11):1091-1107.
15. Berthier ML, Green C, Lara JP, et al. Memantine and constraint-induced aphasia therapy in chronic poststroke aphasia. *Ann Neurol.* 2009;65(5):577-585.
16. Zago S, Ferrucci R, Fregni F, et al. Bartholow, Sciamanna, Alberti: pioneers in the electrical stimulation of the exposed human cerebral cortex. *Neuroscientist.* 2008;14(5):521-528.
17. Priori A. Brain polarization in humans: a reappraisal of an old tool for prolonged non-invasive modulation of brain excitability. *Clin Neurophysiol.* 2003;114(4):589-595.
18. Nitsche MA, Cohen LG, Wassermann EM, et al. Transcranial direct current stimulation: State of the art 2008. *Brain Stimul.* 2008;1(3):206-223.
19. Nitsche MA, Paulus W. Sustained excitability elevations induced by transcranial DC motor cortex stimulation in humans. *Neurology.* 2001;57(10):1899-1901.
20. Sebastian R, Tsapkini K, Tippett DC. Transcranial direct current stimulation in post stroke aphasia and primary progressive aphasia: Current knowledge and future clinical applications. *NeuroRehabilitation.* 2016;39(1):141-152.
21. Rossi S, Hallett M, Rossini PM, et al. Safety, ethical considerations, and application guidelines for the use of transcranial magnetic stimulation in clinical practice and research. *Clin Neurophysiol.* 2009;120(12):2008-2039.

22. Bikson M, Grossman P, Thomas C, et al. Safety of transcranial direct current stimulation: evidence based update 2016. *Brain Stimul.* 2016;9(5):641-661.

23. Biou E, Cassoudesalle H, Cogne M, et al. Transcranial direct current stimulation in post-stroke aphasia rehabilitation: a systematic review. *Ann Phys Rehabil Med.* 2019;62(2):104-121.

24. Dionisio A, Duarte IC, Patricio M, et al. Transcranial magnetic stimulation as an intervention tool to recover from language, swallowing and attentional deficits after stroke: a systematic review. *Cerebrovasc Dis.* 2018;46(3-4):178-185.

25. Demeurisse G, Demol O, Derouck M, et al. Quantitative study of the rate of recovery from aphasia due to ischemic stroke. *Stroke.* 1980;11(5):455-458.

26. Enderby P. Disorders of communication: dysarthria. *Hand Clin Neurol.* 2013;110:273-281.

27. Gurevich N, Scamihorn SL. Speech-language pathologists' use of intelligibility measures in adults with dysarthria. *Am J Speech Lang Pathol.* 2017;26(3):873-892.

28. Barsties B, De Bodt M. Assessment of voice quality: current state-of-the-art. *Auris Nasus Larynx.* 2015;42(3):183-188.

29. Mackenzie C. Dysarthria in stroke: a narrative review of its description and the outcome of intervention. *Int J Speech Lang Pathol.* 2011;13(2):125-136.

30. Alfwaress FS, Bibars AR, Hamasha A, et al. Outcomes of palatal lift prosthesis on dysarthric speech. *J Craniofac Surg.* 2017;28(1):30-35.

31. Mahler LA, Ramig LO, Fox C. Evidence-based treatment of voice and speech disorders in Parkinson disease. *Curr Opin Otolaryngol Head Neck Surg.* 2015;23(3):209-215.

32. Stathopoulos ET, Huber JE, Richardson K, et al. Increased vocal intensity due to the Lombard effect in speakers with Parkinson's disease: simultaneous laryngeal and respiratory strategies. *J Commun Disord.* 2014;48:1-17.

33. Roggeman S, Truyers C, Safin I, et al. Constrained-induced dysarthria therapy: case report. *Ann Rehabil Med.* 2019;43(1):115-117.

34. Sellars C, Hughes T, Langhorne P. Speech and language therapy for dysarthria due to non-progressive brain damage. *Cochrane Database Syst Rev.* 2005;(3):CD002088.

35. Mitchell C, Bowen A, Tyson S, et al. Interventions for dysarthria due to stroke and other adult-acquired, non-progressive brain injury. *Cochrane Database Syst Rev.* 2017;1:CD002088.

36. Hillis AE, Work M, Barker PB, et al. Re-examining the brain regions crucial for orchestrating speech articulation. *Brain.* 2004; 127(Pt 7):1479-1487.

37. Basilakos A. Contemporary approaches to the management of post-stroke apraxia of speech. *Semin Speech Lang.* 2018;39(1):25-36.

38. Ballard KJ, Wambaugh JL, Duffy JR, et al. Treatment for acquired apraxia of speech: a systematic review of intervention research between 2004 and 2012. *Am J Speech Lang Pathol.* 2015;24(2):316-337.

39. Steel J, Ferguson A, Spencer E, et al. Social communication assessment during post-traumatic amnesia and the post-acute period after traumatic brain injury. *Brain Inj.* 2017;31(10): 1320-1330.

40. Xiao H, Jacobsen A, Chen Z, et al. Detecting social-cognitive deficits after traumatic brain injury: an ALE meta-analysis of fMRI studies. *Brain Inj.* 2017;31(10):1331-1339.

41. Association RLAHPS. *Rehabilitation of the Head Injured Adult*: Comprehensive Physical Management. Professional Staff Association of the Rancho Los Amigos Hospital; 1979.

42. Steel J, Ferguson A, Spencer E, et al. Language and cognitive communication during post-traumatic amnesia: a critical synthesis. *NeuroRehabilitation.* 2015;37(2):221-234.

43. Diehl SK, Wallace SE. A modified multimodal communication treatment for individuals with traumatic brain injury. *Augment Altern Commun.* 2018;34(4):323-334.

44. Elbourn E, Togher L, Kenny B, et al. Strengthening the quality of longitudinal research into cognitive-communication recovery after traumatic brain injury: a systematic review. *Int J Speech Lang Pathol.* 2017;19(1):1-16.

45. Finch E, Copley A, Cornwell P, et al. Systematic review of behavioral interventions targeting social communication difficulties after traumatic brain injury. *Arch Phys Med Rehabil.* 2016; 97(8):1352-1365.

46. Fager SK, Brady S, Barlow SM, et al. In: Cifu D, ed. *Braddom's Physical Medicine and Rehabilitation*, Chapter 3: Adult Neurogenic Communication and Swallowing Disorders Table 3-1, Aphasia Types. Philadelphia, PA: Elsevier Health Sciences; 2015:54.

47. Mulheren R, Azola A, et al. *Principles of Rehabilitation Medicine*. 1st ed. New York: McGraw-Hill; 2018.

48. Fager SK, Brady S, Barlow SM, et al. In: Cifu D, ed. *Braddom's Physical Medicine and Rehabilitation*, Chapter 3: Adult Neurogenic Communication and Swallowing Disorders Table 3-3, Dysarthria Types. Philadelphia, PA: Elsevier Health Sciences; 2015:57.

49. National Aphasia Association. Available at: https://www.aphasia.org/. Accessed on March 27, 2020

33

Cognitive Functioning After Traumatic Brain Injury

DOUGLAS B. COOPER, PHD

Cognitive impairments are frequently observed after traumatic brain injury (TBI) and can lead to short-term and long-term disability and poor vocational outcomes. Given the implications of cognitive impairments on postinjury functioning, healthcare providers need to be knowledgeable about the evaluation and management of postinjury cognitive impairments.

Posttraumatic Amnesia and Outcomes

Having problems creating new memories after a TBI is termed *anterograde amnesia* or *posttraumatic amnesia (PTA)*. The duration of PTA increases with TBI severity and is used along with other acute neurologic indicators, such as Glasgow Coma Scale (GCS) scores, and neuroimaging to help determine the severity of injury (mild, moderate, severe). The duration of PTA has been shown to be a good predictor of recovery and long-term cognitive outcomes.

- PTA lasting up to 1 hour is seen with mild TBI (mTBI).

Outcomes: Expectations of full recovery; symptoms dissipate in days/weeks

- PTA between 1 and 24 hours is seen in individuals with moderate TBI.

Outcomes: Expectations of full recovery for most; symptoms dissipate in weeks/months

- PTA over 24 hours is associated with a severe TBI.

PTA between 1 to 14 days

Outcomes: Majority still attain good outcome but may not return to full baseline level of functioning; recovery most dramatic in first 3 to 6 months

PTA between 2 and 4 weeks

Outcomes: Up to 50% may experience moderate disability and protracted recovery

PTA greater than 4 weeks

Outcomes: Most will experience some degree of disability; severe disability for more than one-third of cases

PTA can be evaluated retrospectively by asking a patient about the first clear memory after their injury. More reliable assessment of PTA can be completed prospectively through serial administration of a standardized psychometric instrument.

Prospective Assessment of Posttraumatic Amnesia

1. Galveston Orientation and Amnesia Test (GOAT)
2. Orientation Log (O-Log)

Although behavioral checklists/rating scales of agitation have been developed to assess individuals in PTA, more extensive assessment of cognitive abilities in this stage of recovery is unlikely to yield significant additional meaningful clinical information. *Retrograde amnesia,* loss of memory for the events immediately preceding a TBI, can also occur for some individuals with more severe TBI. Assessment of the duration of PTA and inquiry about potential retrograde amnesia should always be included as part of a clinical history in individuals with TBI.

Recovery of Cognitive Abilities After Traumatic Brain Injury

Recovery of cognitive abilities varies based upon severity of TBI. The Institute of Medicine (IOM) concluded that there is inadequate or insufficient evidence of long-term cognitive impairments after mTBI.[1] Individuals who sustain moderate TBIs demonstrate a slower recovery of cognitive abilities and less uniform cognitive outcomes. Individuals who sustain severe TBIs commonly display a diffuse pattern of cognitive impairments.

- Limited evidence of cognitive impairment beyond days/weeks in mTBI/concussion

TABLE 33.1	Predictors of Positive Cognitive Outcomes after Traumatic Brain Injury
Preinjury intelligence	
Preserved parenchymal volumes	
Less severe traumatic brain injury	
Age (<40 years)	
Absence of medico-legal/disability contexts	

- More protracted recovery in moderate TBI. Primary cognitive domains: information processing speed, declarative memory, and executive functions.
- Long-term cognitive impairments are common in individuals who sustain severe TBI. Longer course of recovery with increased likelihood of residual cognitive impairments.

Table 33.1 summarizes several factors that have been empirically demonstrated to positively affect long-term cognitive outcomes after TBI.[2]

Neuropsychological Evaluation After Traumatic Brain Injury

Objective evaluation of neuropsychological functioning is an important part of assessment and treatment, given the frequency of cognitive difficulties after TBIs. Neuropsychological testing is a standardized set of tests measuring multiple domains of cognitive functioning and other factors that have been shown to influence performance on cognitive tests. Common cognitive domains and neuropsychological tests are summarized in Table 33.2.

Neuropsychological test selection based on:
- The test's reliability or consistency over time
- Validity of the construct being measured
- Degree of measurement error
- Research with known clinical groups demonstrating relationships between the test and specific neural structures or systems.
- Consideration of nonneurologic factors such as
- Age
- Level of education
- Primary language
- Ethnicity
- Physical disability.

Neuropsychological tests are administered in a standardized fashion by either the treating neuropsychologist or a neuropsychological technician sometimes referred to as a *psychometrician*.

Contraindications for neuropsychological testing include:
- Concurrent use of opioid analgesics
- Individuals still in posttraumatic amnesia (PTA)
- Severe expressive/receptive aphasia.

TABLE 33.2	Neuropsychological Assessment After Traumatic Brain Injury
Domain of Functioning	**Neuropsychological Tests**
Serial monitoring after acute traumatic brain injury	JFK Coma Recovery Scale-Revised Orientation Log Galveston Orientation and Amnesia Test Agitated Behavior Scale
General cognitive functioning and full neuropsychological batteries	Wechsler Adult Intelligence Scale –4th Edition Neuropsychological Assessment Battery Repeatable Battery for the Assessment of Neuropsychological Status
Effort/validity	Dot Counting Test Test of Memory Malingering Green Word Memory Test Rey 15-Item Test (with recognition) Word Choice Test Embedded Measures of Performance Validity
Academic achievement	Wide Range Achievement Test–4th edition Woodcock-Johnson Tests of Achievement–4th edition
Sensory-motor functions	Grooved Pegboard Test Manual Finger Tapping Test
Language	Verbal Fluency Tests Multilingual Aphasia Examination Boston Naming Test
Visuospatial–constructional	Clock Drawing Test Rey-Osterrieth Complex Figure Test Judgement of Line Orientation Hooper Visual Organization Test
Learning and memory	California Verbal Learning Test–3rd edition Wechsler Memory Scale–4th Edition Rey Auditory Verbal Learning Test
Attention/Processing Speed	Trail Making Test Continuous Performance Tests Symbol Digit Modalities Test Paced Serial Addition Test Digit Span
Executive functions	Wisconsin Card Sorting Test Booklet Category Test Stroop Test Delis-Kaplan Executive Functions Test
Functional abilities	Texas Functional Living Scale Independent Living Scale
Emotional functioning and personality	Personality Assessment Inventory Minnesota Multiphasic Personality Inventory-2 Restructured Form

Secondary influences on cognitive functioning that can lead to artificially low test scores or variability in task engagement include:
- Somatization
- Adoption of the sick role
- Secondary gain
- Malingering
- Oppositional personalities

To evaluate for secondary influences on testing, neuropsychological evaluation should always include objective measures of both symptom validity (SVT) and performance validity (PVT).

- *Symptom validity* refers to a patient's self-reported symptoms or complaints and evaluates the possibility of overreporting or underreporting symptoms.
- *Performance validity* evaluates the extent to which an individual puts forth optimal effort.

PVTs can either be standalone instruments specifically designed to assess performance validity or embedded validity tests, which are empirically derived scores or patterns of scores within common neuropsychological tests that occur very infrequently in control subjects or known clinical samples. Multiple PVTs should be included to minimize false positive errors.

Neuropsychological test scores are compared with a normative data set, often made up of individuals matched by age, gender, education, and other relevant demographic/background variables. Tests can also be compared with data from individuals with similar TBI severity and/or time since injury.

Common referral questions for neuropsychological evaluation after TBI include:
1. Characterization of cognitive strengths and weaknesses and emotional and behavioral abilities
2. Differential diagnosis (i.e., whether the patient's reported cognitive difficulties are caused by TBI or some other condition or nonneurologic factor such as pain, sleep, psychiatric conditions, preinjury level of functioning)
3. Assist with rehabilitation treatment planning and determination of the presence of cognitive impairments that would be the focus/target of rehabilitation interventions
4. Serial neuropsychological evaluations over time are often conducted to assess recovery or changes in cognition after intervention; sufficient duration between testing should be allowed (e.g., >6 months) to minimize the effects of practice
5. Nonclinical settings (e.g., forensic or administrative contexts) to assist with determination of limitations or functional restrictions such ability to drive, live independently, manage one's money or return to work/fitness for duty

Although computerized neuropsychological test batteries are commercially available that provide reliable and well-standardized assessment of abilities, computerized assessment is highly limited in the interpretation of test results. As a result, caution should be used in relying on computer-test batteries in isolation.

Review Questions

1. Which of these are not associated with positive cognitive outcomes after traumatic brain injury (TBI)?
   a. Absence of medico-legal context
   b. Less severe injury
   c. Gender
   d. Preinjury intelligence
2. Loss of memory for events immediately preceding a TBI is called what?
   a. Preexisting amnesia
   b. Anterograde amnesia
   c. Posttraumatic amnesia (PTA)
   d. Retrograde amnesia
3. Duration of posttraumatic amnesia can be evaluated in the following ways except
   a. prospectively.
   b. using standardized measures such as the Orientation Log (O-Log).
   c. retrospectively.
   d. using computerized test batteries.

Answers on page 395.
Access the full list of questions and answers online. Available on ExpertConsult.com

References

1. Committee on Cognitive Rehabilitation Therapy for Traumatic Brain Injury. *Cognitive Rehabilitation Therapy for Traumatic Brain Injury*: Evaluating the Evidence. Washington DC: Institute of Medicine; 2011.
2. Dikmen SS, Corrigan JD, Levin HS, et al. Cognitive outcome following traumatic brain injury. *J Head Trauma Rehabil.* 2009;24:430-438.

34

Neurosensory Dysfunction

KELLY M. HEATH, MD, FABPMR (BIM)

Neurosensory disorders after traumatic brain injury (TBI) are a complex process, and the pathophysiology is partially understood. TBI can affect all the senses, including hearing, smell, vision, and balance.

Hearing Impairment

Anatomy

The cochlea is the organ of hearing. Sound waves hit the tympanic membrane and transmit via the coordinated movement of the three ossicles (malleus, incus, and stapes) onto the oval window continuing the wave through the perilymph of the scala vestibuli and tympani. This causes the cilia to move within the endolymph, transmitting sound waves to the cochlear nerve.[1]

Hearing Loss

Conductive Hearing Loss

Conductive hearing loss is disruption of the external and middle ear, including the ear canal, tympanic membrane, and ossicles. Causes include hemotympanum, tympanic membrane rupture, and ossicular disruption.[2-5]

Sensorineural Hearing Loss

Sensorineural hearing loss is disruption of the inner ear or auditory nerve. Causes include temporal bone fracture, labyrinthine concussion, and brainstem contusion. This is the most common hearing deficit in TBI and is more prevalent in blast-related TBI because the ear is particularly susceptible to overpressurization during a blast.[2-5]

Mixed Hearing Loss

Mixed hearing loss involves both conductive and sensorineural hearing loss.

Tests: Tuning fork to lateralize lesion, audiometry to assess frequency/type of hearing loss, auditory brainstem response (ABR) to diagnose auditory nerve or pathway disruption

Treatment: Hearing aids, frequency magnification (FM) devices, or cochlear implant for severe bilateral loss[2-5]

Tinnitus

Tinnitus is perceived sound in the absence of external auditory stimulation.[6-7]

Tests: Audiometry, Tinnitus Impact Screening Interview (TISI), Tinnitus Handicap Inventory (THI)

Treatment: Devices (hearing aids, tinnitus masking devices), cognitive behavioral therapy and tinnitus retraining therapy (cognitive-based therapy combining counseling with sound therapy), medication to treat associated anxiety, or sleep

Hyperacusis

Sound that is comfortable to most individuals will be perceived as unbearable to individuals with this condition.[6]
Treatment: Sound therapy

Labyrinthine Concussion

Labyrinthine concussion is a term used to describe hearing loss and vertigo after TBI.[8] This term is used because proposed pathophysiology is damage to the bony labyrinth.

Central Auditory Processing Disorder

Central auditory processing disorder involves damage along the central auditory pathway.[4,7] This damage affects the ability to process auditory input with impaired localization of sound, difficulty hearing in the presence of background noise, or difficulty perceiving temporal speech patterns.
Tests: Audiometry, ABR, temporal processing and pattern testing, dichotic speech test, monaural low-redundancy speech test, binaural interaction test
Treatment: Compensation using hearing aids, amplification systems, auditory training with a qualified audiologist or speech therapist

Acoustic Neuroma

Acoustic neuroma should be ruled out with unilateral hearing loss and disequilibrium.

Anosmia

Anatomy

The olfactory nerve passes through the cribriform plate to the olfactory bulb, passing sensory information of smell from the nose to the entorhinal cortex, hypothalamus, dorsal medial thalamic nucleus, and orbitofrontal cortex.

Anosmia

Anosmia is the lack of smell. The olfactory nerve is the most commonly injured cranial nerve in mild TBI.[9]
Symptoms: Food is tasteless, loss of appetite, difficulty smelling
Tests: University of Pennsylvania Smell Identification Test, electroencephalogram to rule out seizure if parosmia is present

Visual Dysfunction

Anatomy

Primary visual pathway: Visual information from the eye passes to the optic nerve, optic chiasm (partial decussation), optic tract,

lateral geniculate body, and projects to (1) occipital cortex (primary visual cortex), (2) tectum (pupillary function), and (3) superior colliculus (eye movement and multisensory integration)
Secondary visual pathway: Extrastriate visual cortex, inferior temporal area (visual identification and recognition of objects)

Ocular Injury

Damage to tear film, cornea (keratitis or corneal scar), crystalline lens (traumatic cataract or lens dislocation), vitreous (vitreal hemorrhage), and retina (retinal detachment, retinal hemorrhage, retinopathy)[10,11]
Tests: Visual acuity, Snellen eye chart, ocular examination, pupillary testing, spontaneous nystagmus (improved detection with Frenzel lenses), slit lamp biomicroscopy

Oculomotor Dysfunction

Alignment Deficits

Alignment deficits are a deviation of gaze and can be either tropia, a malalignment of one eye when both eyes are uncovered, or a phoria, a latent deviation when binocular vision is broken. Cranial nerve (CN) palsies are the most common cause of alignment deficits. More common in severe TBI.[10,12,13]
Pathophysiology: Damage along the efferent visual pathway. Neural problem is identified much more often in vertical phorias.
Horizontal
    Eso: Eyes turn in
    Exo: Eyes turn out
Vertical
    Hyper: Eye alignment more superior in orbit (up)
    Hypo: Eye alignment more inferior in orbit (down)
Symptoms: Diplopia, impaired depth perception, headaches
    CN 3 (oculomotor): Ptosis, exotropia, lack of mydriasis, lack of accommodation, horizontal diplopia
    CN 4 (trochlear): Compensatory head tilt, hyperphoria and hypertropia, vertical diplopia
    CN 6 (abducens): Esotropia, horizontal diplopia
Tests:
    Hirschberg: Measures alignment with eyes uncovered
    Cover/crossed cover: Looking for deviation between being covered and uncovered
    Maddox rod: Aids in determining deviations in vertical and horizontal planes
    Treatment: Prism lenses: horizontal or vertical depending on deficit, vision therapy

Accommodation Deficits

Accommodation deficits are an inability to maintain clear vision, sustain or change focus on an object. Accommodative insufficiency (most common), accommodative excess, dynamic accommodative infacility[10,13-16]
Pathophysiology: Crystalline lens changes through ciliary control to focus on an object through a complex pathway involving retinal cones, optic nerve, lateral geniculate

nucleus (LGN), occipital lobe, posterior parietal lobe, frontal eye field, oculomotor nucleus, parasympathetic accessory oculomotor nucleus with contribution from the cerebellum

Symptom Blurred vision

Tests:

Accommodative amplitude test: Small accommodative target (20/20–20/30)—distance of the first sustained blur using either the pushup or the minus lens method

Amplitude facility with lens flippers: The patient should be able to clear these lenses monocularly within 11 cycles per minute without evidence of fatigue.

Treatment: Plus powered lenses (insufficiency), vision therapy

Vergence Deficits

Vergence deficits are deficits in disjunctive eye movement—convergence insufficiency, convergence excess, divergence insufficiency. Convergence insufficiency is the most common oculomotor deficit after mild TBI.[12,13,15-19]

Symptoms: Diplopia, eyestrain, vision-related headaches, dizziness, exophoria, intermittent exotropia during near vision and fatigue

Tests:

Near-point convergence (NPC): Small target to measure the break in binocular vision or object doubles

Step vergence: Positive and negative fusional vergence amplitudes measured with a prism rod

Treatment: Oculomotor (vision) therapy, fusional prisms, patching—complete or partial (Table 34.1)

Versional Deficits

Versional deficits are deficits in conjugate eye movement. Smooth pursuits are conjugate eye movements to smoothly and accurately track a slow-moving object. Saccades are rapid eye movements that allow quick and accurate scanning from one object to another.[13,16,20,21]

Pathophysiology: Lesion along pathway from frontal eye fields, paramedian pontine reticular formation, rostral mesencephalon, parietal cortex, basal ganglia, superior colliculus, or cerebellum

Symptoms: Slow reading, loss of place when reading, misreading, floating text, and dizziness

Tests: Northeastern State University College of Optometry Oculomotor Test, Developmental Eye Movement Test, saccadic oculomotor testing, pursuit eye movement testing

Treatment: Large-print text, typoscope, vision therapy

Visual Field Deficits

Visual field deficits are seen with damage to the afferent visual pathway. This is caused by penetrating injuries directly to the optic chiasm or the visual cortex or severe white matter tract damage along the pathway.[22]

Hemianopsia or Quadrantanopsia

Symptoms: Ignoring one-half of an object, bumping into objects on one side, difficulty reading, slow rate of reading

Tests: Confrontation visual fields finger counting, Goldmann perimetry

Treatment: Compensatory, yoked prisms, half-Fresnel prisms, mirrors, visual scanning strategies

Other

Central scotoma: Central area of vision loss

Monocular vision: Complete loss of vision in one eye

Other Visual Disorders

Light Sensitivity

Light sensitivity is ocular discomfort in the presence of light.[11,19]

Pathophysiology: Anomalous dark-light adaptation thresholds caused by disordered thalamic processing. Fluorescent light sensitivity is believed to be caused by anomalous critical flicker fusion frequency threshold.

Treatment: Tints 30% to 40% for indoors, 80% to 85% for outdoor, blue or gray for fluorescent, wear wide-brimmed hat

Color Blindness

Color blindness is damage to the retina, optic nerve, parvocellular pathway of LGN, or visual area V4.

TABLE 34.1 Vergence Deficits

Vergence Deficit	Primary Treatment	Secondary Treatment
Convergence insufficiency	Oculomotor therapy	Prism lenses, surgery
Convergence excess	Plus powered lenses	Oculomotor therapy
Fusional vergence dysfunction	Oculomotor therapy	
Divergence insufficiency	Prism lenses	Oculomotor therapy

Syndromes

Posttrauma Vision Syndrome

Posttrauma vision syndrome is a constellation of binocular visual symptoms that can present after trauma caused by the disruption of visual processing at multiple levels from midbrain and cortex.[10] Symptoms include diplopia (exotropia/esotropia), blurred near vision (accommodative insufficiency), movement of print when reading (convergence insufficiency), asthenopia (oculomotor dysfunction), headaches (increased myopia), and photophobia (low blink rate).

Visual Midline Shift Syndrome

Visual midline shift syndrome is a shift in the perception of the visual midline that occurs with homonymous visual field deficits.[10]

Dual Sensory Deficits/Multisensory Deficits

Visual Vestibular Deficits[12]

Pathophysiology: Deficit along the vestibular ocular pathway from eye to inner ear

Symptoms: Dizziness, vertigo, nausea, photosensitivity to fluorescent lighting, sensitivity to visual motion, especially in visually stimulating environments

Treatment: Assess and treat any visual and vestibular deficits through coordinated oculomotor and vestibular therapy.

Visual Processing Dysfunction

Visual processing dysfunction include visual spatial, visual analysis, and visual motor integration deficits. Ocular exam and acuity are often normal.[12]

Diagnostics for Visual Disorders

Laboratory Tests[10,12,13]

Visual evoked potential: Series of lights mount a recording measured by electrodes on the scalp

Electroretinogram: Measures retina pigment epithelium (activity of rod and cone cells) during photo stimulation by placing electrodes via contact lenses or foil tucked into the conjunctiva

Electrooculogram: Indirectly measures retina pigment epithelium by varying illumination during eye movement; recorded via electrodes on the canthi

Bedside Tests[10,13]

Vestibular/oculomotor screening (VOMS): Assessment of severity of symptoms with visual and ocular provocative maneuvers

King-Devick Test: Timed test to read numbers on three test cards; tests oculomotor function

Subjective visual attention test: Search and cross out a letter or symbol; assess overall visual attention

Imaging

Computed tomography (CT): Detects structural damage—cranial fractures, hematomas

Magnetic resonance imaging (MRI): Detects brain damage in areas of the ocular pathway

Therapeutic Options

Vision Rehabilitation

Oculomotor therapy for accommodation and vergence includes three general phases. The first phase uses large targets with slow change. The second phase increases speed and decreases targets. Target training with monocular vision (patched) first and then progresses to binocular vision tasks. Accommodative flippers are also used in this phase. The third phase trains large jumps between stimuli presented (step vergence training).[13,14,17,18]

Example of exercises:

Accommodation: Small copy of letters/numbers/objects handed to patient, same large copy on wall, and the patient moves between the two, reading line by line

Vergence: Stereograms, Brock string, step vergence amplitude training using prisms, step vergence facility training using prism flippers

Pursuit: Laser light follow, bouncing light, maze follow

Saccades: Identify differences in two pictures, read letters/numbers/objects spaced out on a page

Prisms

Prisms are applied to glasses to bend light to shift an object from its position. Prisms can be placed vertically or horizontally depending on the deficit correcting. They can be unilateral or bilateral. They are most effective in divergence insufficiency, esophoria, and vertical heterophoria.[22]

Yoked prisms: Prism oriented in the same direction on both glasses, shifting visual perception

Homonymous hemianopsia/quadranopsia: Horizontal yoked prism oriented in the direction of visual loss displaces objects from the nonseeing into the seeing hemifield

Visual neglect: Yoked prisms may work but require larger magnitudes

Visual midline shift syndrome: Yoked prisms center the visual midline

Enhanced sector prisms: Bilateral prisms on portions of eyeglasses to improve awareness of the peripheral field; can be effective for homonymous hemianopsia/quadrantopsia, scotoma

Fresnel prisms: Stick-on prisms

Patching

Patching can be used to correct diplopia but renders the patient monocular impairing peripheral vision. Central occlusion patches can decrease diplopia while looking directly at an object but maintains peripheral vision.

Vestibular/Balance

Vestibular Pathway Anatomy

The labyrinth is responsible for vestibular function. It is composed of both the semicircular canals and otolith organs to transmit information regarding motion via the vestibular nerve.[23]

Semicircular canals: Three canals—the superior, posterior, and horizontal. The canals detect rotation through endolymph motion, which displaces the cupula bending the hair cells. The output is to coordinate compensatory eye and head movements through the vestibular ocular reflex (VOR) (Box 34.1).

    Semicircular canal dysfunction: Deficits in gaze stability with lateral head movement (horizontal VOR)

Otolith organs: Utricle and saccule. Otolith organs contain otoconia, small calcium carbonate particles embedded in the gelatinous membrane of the macula that convey the direction of gravity with head tilt. They also coordinate upright posture during movement through the vestibular spinal reflex (VSR) (see Box 34.1).

    Otolith dysfunction: Deficits in postural stability caused by VSR involvement (isolated otolith deficit should be considered in workup of postural instability)[24]

Information travels to the vestibular nerve through two divisions within the vestibular ganglion (Scarpa's ganglion). The superior division receives input from the superior and horizontal semicircular canals and utricle. The inferior division receives input from posterior semicircular canal and saccule. The vestibular nerve combines with the cochlear nerve to form vestibulocochlear nerve. It then travels through the internal auditory canal through the petrous temporal bone to the posterior fossa, entering the brainstem at the pontomedullary junction. Here the vestibular nerve separates from the cochlear nerve. The majority of the fibers go to the ipsilateral vestibular nuclear complex in the pons. The rest go to the flocculonodular lobe of the cerebellum.

The vestibular nuclear complex is made up of four afferent vestibular nuclei located under the fourth ventricle in the pons and extends caudal toward the medulla. The medial column contains the medial vestibular nucleus, which receives afferent input from the lateral semicircular ducts. The lateral column contains the superior (afferents from superior and posterior semicircular ducts), lateral (afferents from both semicircular ducts and otoliths), and inferior vestibular nuclei (afferents from utricle and saccule).

• BOX 34.1   Canals and Otolith Movement

Posterior: left to right along frontal axis (head to ear)
Utricle: linear movement in the horizontal plane
Horizontal: left to right along vertical axis (rotate head)
Saccule: linear movement in the vertical plane
Superior: up down (nod)

Efferent information creates the VOR and the VSR. The cerebellum regulates the VOR and VSR through inhibitory input.

VOR: The superior and medial vestibular nuclei travel via the ascending tract of Dieters to the ipsilateral oculomotor nuclei of the abducens/lateral rectus. The superior and medial vestibular nuclei travel via medial longitudinal fasciculus (MLF) to all other oculomotor nuclei.

VSR: The lateral vestibular nuclei travel via the lateral vestibular tract on the ipsilateral motor neurons in the spinal cord to activate ipsilateral trunk and proximal limb extensors and inhibit contralateral proximal extensors. The medial vestibular nuclei travel via medial vestibulospinal tract to bilateral motor neurons in the cervical spinal cord to coordinate head and neck motion.

Dizziness

Dizziness is a common symptom in TBI.[25,26] It is an initial symptom in up to 75% of TBI and lasting symptom at 5 years in up to 50% in moderate TBI. Dizziness is often a subjective complaint in postconcussion syndrome. Dizziness is a negative predictive factor and strong predictor of failure to return to work 6 months postconcussion. Dizziness is a broad term that can describe any of these:

Vertigo: Hallucination of motion of the body or environment either rotary or linear; cardinal symptom of vestibular dysfunction

Imbalance: Impaired ability to maintain the body in space; symptom of chronic vestibular or neurological disease

Disequilibrium: Feeling of disorientation often described as "drunkenness"; symptom of vestibular, neurological, multisensory, metabolic, or psychogenic disorders

Lightheadedness: Syncope or presyncope; symptom of cardiovascular or cerebrovascular disease

Pathophysiology: Direct or indirect damage to the vestibular end organs, vestibular nerve, or along the pathway to the brainstem, including disruption to visual, motor, and oculomotor pathways.

Vertigo of Central Vestibular System Origin

Vestibular Migraines

Vestibular migraines are also described as migraine-associated dizziness (Box 34.2).[29]

Treatment: Verapamil, amitriptyline, or beta blocker; vestibular therapy

Cerebrovascular

Vertebrobasilar insufficiency, cerebellar or lateral medullary infarction: vertigo +/- neurological signs such as weakness, dysarthria, incoordination. Vertebrobasilar insufficiency may cause drop attacks.[27,28]

Tests: MRI for ischemic changes; Doppler studies may reveal stenosis of the vertebrobasilar circulation

Treatment: Platelet inhibitors

ICHD-3 Criteria

A: At least five episodes fulfilling criteria C and D
B: A current or past history of migraine without aura or migraine with aura
C: Vestibular symptoms of moderate or severe intensity lasting between 5 minutes and 72 hours
D: At least half of the episodes are associated with at least one of the following:
1. Headache with 2 of 4: unilateral, pulsating, moderate or severe intensity, aggravated by routine activity
2. Photophobia or phonophobia
3. Visual aura

Structural

Injury to brain parenchyma or tracts: diffuse axonal injury, contusion/hemorrhage in the brainstem, thalamus, or posterior fossa
Treatment: Vestibular therapy

Vertigo of Peripheral Vestibular System

Posttraumatic Meniere's Syndrome or Endolymphatic Hydrops

This is a disruption in the endolymphatic compartment in the ear; symptoms include episodic vertigo, fluctuating hearing loss, and tinnitus.[27,28]
Test: Audiogram shows sensorineural loss at both low and high frequencies
Treatment: Salt restriction, diuretic
episodic: meclizine

Benign Paroxysmal Positional Vertigo

Benign paroxysmal positional vertigo (BPPV) is the most common inner ear vertigo after head trauma.[30-32]
Presentation: Positional rotary vertigo: otoconia dislodge and get stuck in the semicircular canals.
Test: Dix-Hallpike positive for rotary nystagmus
Treatment: Epley maneuver, canalith repositioning maneuvers, vestibular therapy. TBI-induced BPPV may require more repositioning treatments than idiopathic BPPV. Brandt-Daroff head exercises at home; antiemetic for symptom management

Unilateral Vestibular Hypofunction

Unilateral vestibular hypofunction is the acute onset of continuous vertigo (i.e., vestibular neuritis, fracture of temporal bone, labyrinthine concussion).
Test: Horizontal nystagmus. May require Frenzel glasses or electronystagmography (ENG) to diagnose. Veering gait toward lesion, positive Romberg, past pointing. ENG/video nystagmography: unilateral caloric weakness on affected side; CT for temporal bone fracture
Treatment: Resolves in days to weeks. Symptomatic: Vestibular suppressants, antiemetics; vestibular therapy for incomplete recovery

Bilateral Vestibular Hypofunction

Presentation: Ataxia and oscillopsia (eye bobbing)
Causes: Ototoxic medications, bilateral labyrinthine concussion, basilar skull fracture
Test: Positive dynamic visual acuity test, bilateral impairment on caloric testing, severe decrease gain on rotational chair
Treatment: Vestibular therapy to help reduce symptoms

Superior Semicircular Canal Dehiscence

Superior semicircular canal dehiscence is vertigo with sound or pressure accompanied by disequilibrium/unsteadiness and ear fullness. Dehiscence of the bone over the superior semicircular canal creates a third window for inner ear fluid motion.
Test: High-resolution CT scan of inner ear, reduced threshold on vestibular myogenic evoked response (VEMP) testing
Treatment: Surgical plugging

Perilymphatic Fistula

Perilymphatic fistula is vertigo with head tilt, sound or external ear pressure accompanied by disequilibrium. Disruption of the oval or round window causes leakage of perilymph from the inner ear to the middle ear.
Test: Tragus pressure will cause vertigo and deviation of the eyes, unilateral sensorineural hearing loss
Treatment: Bed rest, head elevation, laxatives; if this fails, surgical patching of the window

Other Causes of Dizziness

Exercised Induced

Autonomic disruption with heart rate elevation. Dizziness is accompanied by increase in heart rate.[28]
Treatment: Guided exercise program

Cervicogenic Dizziness (Whiplash)

Dizziness or disequilibrium with neck pain. Neck injuries can affect the cervical colic reflex, creating dizziness.[24,28,33]
Tests: Diagnosis of exclusion of other vestibular disorders and neck pain; dizziness provoked by body on head movement rather than whole-body movement
Treatment: Physical therapy/treatment of neck disorder

Postural Instability

Postural stability relies on the vestibular, somatosensory, and visual system. Posture control is mediated through the VSR.[24,33]
Diagnosis: Deficits seen in computer dynamic posturography (CDP), especially sensory organization test (SOT), cervical vestibular myogenic evoked response (cVEMP)
Treatment: Vestibular therapy including exercise program

Oculomotor Deficits

See vision section.

Visual Vertigo

Discomfort, postural instability, and symptoms of dizziness, lightheadedness, and/or disorientation in intense visual motion stimulation (watching movies, crowds, driving, etc.)

Psychogenic

Panic disorder, anxiety disorder, depression.
Treatment: anxiety/panic: benzodiazepine; depression: selective serotonin reuptake inhibitors (SSRIs)

Medication Induced

Benzodiazepines, antihypertensives, diuretics, anticonvulsants
Treatment: Stop medications with side effects on vestibular system

Metabolic

Hyponatremia
Treatment: Treat derangement.

Visual-Perceptual Dysfunction

Refer for visual testing.

Diagnostic Tests for Vestibular Disorders

Laboratory Tests[1,3,30,34,35]

Video nystagmography (VNG) measures eye movement/nystagmus while patient is wearing infrared video goggles and eye-tracking software. Tests include gaze testing, oculomotor testing, Dix-Hallpike testing, position testing, and bithermal caloric testing. VNG assesses extraocular muscles, horizontal semicircular canals, superior branch of the vestibular nerve, and vestibular and oculomotor pathways within the CNS.

Gaze testing: Observes for nystagmus with visual fixation and without visual fixation

Peripheral: Horizontal jerk nystagmus in primary gaze, diminished with fixation; unidirectional away from the lesion

Central: Vertical or torsional nystagmus in primary gaze, enhanced with fixation; may be bidirectional or direction changing

Oculomotor testing: Spontaneous gaze, saccade, smooth pursuit, and optokinetic nystagmus (OKN). Indicators of central nervous system dysfunction. Vertical pursuit and vertical saccade most sensitive tests. Can be influenced by comorbid convergence issues, cervical involvement, and migraine.

Dix-Hallpike test: Vertical or horizontal nystagmus with torsional changes on the head

Position testing: Lateral roll test, horizontal head shake test

Bithermal calorics: VOR assessed after irrigating external auditory canal with cold and warm water in each ear. Only test that can isolate one labyrinth (horizontal semicircular canal) from the other. Difference of 20% to 25% between ears suggests abnormal peripheral function. Cold opposite, Warm same (COWS).

Electronystagmography is a battery of tests performed with electrodes around the eyes rather than infrared video goggles in the VNG.

Rotational chair: Measures slow component velocity of true motion VOR. Three values are compared—gain, symmetry, and phase. Assesses horizontal semicircular canals, superior branch of the vestibular nerve. In TBI, low overall gain in rotation attributable to peripheral or central vestibular or oculomotor deficit.

CDP involves static and dynamic postural control tests using computerized platform. It includes the SOT, which is the ability to maintain postural control while changing visual and somatosensory input, and motor control test (MCT), which measures sway, center of gravity, and lower extremity weight symmetry during platform movement. It assesses multisensory input for balance. It is scored 0 to 100, with lower scores being more impaired. Brain-injured patients show abnormal sway, lower composite score, increased reliance on visual input, and poor use of vestibular input. Findings in mild TBI: higher magnitudes of anterior–posterior movement; abnormal composite SOT

Video head impulse testing (vHIT) involves quick movements of the head with goggles to measure VOR; contraindicated with cervical complaints given speed of head movement.

VEMP: Reduced thresholds in semicircular dehiscence; elevated thresholds in most other vestibular dysfunction

cVEMP: Tests saccular and inferior vestibular nerve function

Bedside Tests[24,30,36]

Dix-Hallpike test: Vertical or horizontal nystagmus with torsional changes on the head; assesses for displaced otoconia in the semicircular canals

Horizontal headshake test: Assess nystagmus post head shaking with nystagmus beating toward the neurologically active labyrinth. Horizontal nystagmus on horizontal or vertical head shake seen in peripheral lesions. Vertical nystagmus is seen in brainstem lesions. Nystagmus will last longer in central lesions.

Head thrust test (HTT): Patient fixes on a target while examiner moves head through 5 to 10 degrees of horizontal movement. Tests angular VOR. Corrective saccade with movement to the hypoactive side indicates pathology peripherally and centrally.

Vibration testing: Mastoid bone vibration will elicit nystagmus with peripheral vestibular dysfunction.

Dynamic visual acuity (DVA): Comparison of static acuity to dynamic acuity (patient moves head) measured in Snellen or ETDRS acuity chart. Assesses horizontal semicircular canals and vestibular nerve. Three-line or more difference is considered impaired VOR. Seen in peripheral vestibular hypofunction, central processing, or visual system dysfunction.

Subjective visual vertical test (SVV): Estimation of the physical vertical orientation of a target; assesses utricular function

Dynamic gait index (DGI): Eight-item scale assessing gait with head turns, changes of speed and around obstacles; lower numbers more severe impairment; 22 of 24 indicates balance dysfunction

Modified Clinical Test of Sensory Integration in Balance (mCTSIB): Test of vision, vestibular and somatosensory system; eyes open and eyes closed on firm surface, eyes open and eyes closed on foam surface

Functional gait assessment (FGA): Modification of DGI. 10-item gait test—walk at normal speeds, fast speed, slow speed, with vertical and horizontal head turns, with eyes closed, over obstacles, in tandem, backward and stairs

Balance error scoring system (BESS): Errors counted in 20 seconds with eyes closed in double-leg stance, tandem, and single leg stance on firm surface and foam. Normative data exist.

Dizziness handicap inventory (DHI): 25-item questionnaire most commonly used. Assesses the person's perceived effect of dizziness and unsteadiness on the functional, emotional, and physical aspects of their life. Scored 0 to 100 with higher score more perceived impairment. Can be used as an outcome measure.

Activities-Specific Balance Confidence Scale: 16-item questionnaire rates level of confidence in performing specific activities. Score of 67 or less indicates risk of falling. Can be used as an outcome measure.

Post-Concussion Symptom Scale (PCSS): 22-item questionnaire that assesses severity of broad range of symptoms postconcussion on a 0 to 6 scale

Visual vertigo scale (VVS): 15-item questionnaire that assesses severity of vertigo symptoms during the last month. Higher score more symptom severity up to 60.

Imaging

MRI posterior fossa: Identify structural pathology
CT scan: If basilar skull fracture suspected

Therapy Treatment

Vestibular Therapy

Improve functional balance through retraining using adaptation, substitution, and habituation/desensitization.[26,37-40]

Canalith repositioning maneuver: Diagnostic and therapeutic BPPV if present

Adaptation: Used to treat gaze instability. The goal is central reprogramming by reducing the amount of retinal slip. Progress from seated to standing to walking.

X1 and X2 paradigm:
  X1: Patient rotates head 30 degrees in horizontal (yaw) and vertical (pitch) planes while fixing on a stationary object.
  X2: Patient fixes on a target that they move opposite their head.

Two-target VOR training: Moves eyes between target in hand and on a wall

Substitution: Improve postural stability by using all systems including vestibular, visual, and somatosensory to create alternative strategies for gaze stability.

Cervico-ocular reflex training: X1 exercises, active eye–head movements between two targets, visualization of imaginary targets

Postural control/somatosensory retraining: Balance exercises using various conditions, including eyes open/closed, head turning, changes in surface (foam, floor, etc.). Start

in standing and progress to walking. Use of glasses to vary visual input: foveal glasses, optokinetic glasses, vision-restricted glasses, pinhole glasses, green-red glasses.

Habituation: Reduction in the pathological response to a specific movement by repeated exposure to the provocative movement; treats motion sensitivity

Exercises include performing provoking movement identified from the Motion Sensitivity Quotient or patient identified in incremental steps such as riding an elevator, watching videos, or reading in the car.

Other Therapy Options[33,36,38]

Graded Exertional Exercise

Subthreshold/subsymptom exercise programs help restore normal cerebral homeostasis. Strengthens muscle groups to improve balance reaction times. Also used for return to duty and return to play.

Optokinetic Nystagmus Training

Use of virtual reality, computer programs to treat visual vertigo

Cervical Proprioception Rehabilitation Program

For cervicogenic dizziness; restore cervical range of motion, manual therapy for hypomobility

Psychological Assessment and Treatment

Cognitive behavioral therapy

Pharmacology

Vestibular System Suppression[41]

Antihistamines

Meclizine: Decreases middle ear labyrinth excitability and blocks conduction in the middle ear vestibular-cerebellar pathway. Can interfere with central compensation; discontinue if ineffective within 2 weeks.

Dimenhydrinate/Diphenhydramine: Treats motion sickness

Antiemetics

Ondansetron: Used for symptomatic management of severe vomiting—use with caution; has many side effects

Benzodiazepines

Central suppressants of vestibular system. Use when anticholinergic medication is contraindicated or for psychogenic vertigo.

Adverse effects: Habituation, sedation, memory impairment

Drugs That Cause Dizziness[41]

Ototoxic: Aminoglycosides, loop diuretics, chemotherapeutic agents

Orthostatic hypotension: Antihypertensives, dopaminergic agents when taken with antihypertensives, phenothiazines, tricyclic antidepressants (TCAs), nefazodone, trazodone

Dizziness: SSRIs, anticonvulsants, hypnotics, lidocaine, caffeine

Review Questions

1. A 27-year-old Operation Enduring Freedom veteran presents to your office with a chief complaint of brief episodes of vertigo. He also reports tinnitus and intermittent hearing loss. You order and audiogram. The most likely result will be
   a. conductive hearing loss.
   b. mixed hearing loss.
   c. sensorineural hearing loss.
   d. normal hearing test.

2. A 35-year-old man presents 3 months after traumatic brain injury (TBI) with dizziness. Examination reveals vertical gaze nystagmus, saccadic smooth pursuit, and a normal dynamic visual acuity test. Which of these are on the differential?
   a. Vestibular neuritis
   b. Benign paroxysmal positioning vertigo
   c. Brainstem contusion
   d. Perilymphatic fistula

3. A 32-year-old woman presents to the concussion clinic 3 months postconcussion. She continues to complain of headache, difficulty reading, double vision, and feeling dizzy. She has had 8 weeks of vestibular therapy. You refer her to neuroophthalmology. Testing reveals impaired near-point convergence and negative fusional vergence amplitudes. You recommend to the patient
   a. oculomotor therapy.
   b. prism lenses.
   c. patching for the double vision.
   d. sumatriptan for the headache.

Answers on page 396.
**Access the full list of questions and answers online.
Available on ExpertConsult.com**

References

1. Lei-Rivera L, Sutera J, Galatioto JA, Hujsak BD, Gurley JM. Special tools for the assessment of balance and dizziness in individuals with mild traumatic brain injury. *NeuroRehabilitation.* 2013;32(3):463-472.
2. Shangkuan WC, Lin HC, Shih CP, et al. Increased long-term risk of hearing loss in patients with traumatic brain injury: a nationwide population-based study. *Laryngoscope.* 2017;127(11):2627-2635.
3. Shepard NT, Handelsman JA, Clendaniel RA. Balance and dizziness. In: Zafonte RD, Katz DI, Zasler ND, ed. *Brain Injury Medicine.* 2nd ed. New York, NY: Demos; 2013:779-793.
4. Lew HL, Jerger JF, Guillory SB, Henry JA. Auditory dysfunction in traumatic brain injury. *J Rehabil Res Dev.* 2007;44(7):921-928.
5. Munjal SK, Panda NK, Pathak A. Relationship between severity of traumatic brain injury (TBI) and extent of auditory dysfunction. *Brain Inj.* 2010;24(3):525-532.
6. Coelho DH, Hoffer M. Audiologic impairment. In: Zafonte RD, Katz DI, Zasler ND, eds. *Brain Injury Medicine.* 2nd ed. New York, NY: Demos; 2013:769-778.
7. Fausti SA, Wilmington DJ, Gallun FJ, Myers PJ, Henry JA. Auditory and vestibular dysfunction associated with blast-related traumatic brain injury. *J Rehabil Res Dev.* 2009;46(6):797-810.
8. Chen JX, Lindeborg M, Herman SD, et al. Systematic review of hearing loss after traumatic brain injury without associated temporal bone fracture. *Am J Otolaryngol.* 2018;39(3):338-344.
9. Costanzo RM, Reiter ER, Yelverton JC. Smell and taste. In: Zafonte RD, Katz DI, Zasler ND, eds. *Brain Injury Medicine.* 2nd ed. New York, NY: Demos; 2013:794-808.
10. Padula WV, Singman E, Vicci V, Munitz R, Magrun WM. Evaluating and treating visual dysfunction. In: Zafonte RD, Katz DI, Zasler ND, eds. *Brain Injury Medicine.* 2nd ed. New York, NY: Demos; 2013:750-768.
11. Greenwald BD, Kapoor N, Singh AD. Visual impairments in the first year after traumatic brain injury. *Brain Inj.* 2012;26(11):1338-1359.
12. Fox SM, Koons P, Dang SH. Vision rehabilitation after traumatic brain injury. *Phys Med Rehabil Clin N Am.* 2019;30(1):171-188.
13. Ventura RE, Jancuska JM, Balcer LJ, Galetta SL. Diagnostic tests for concussion: is vision part of the puzzle? *J Neuroophthalmol.* 2015;35(1):73-81.
14. Thiagarajan P, Ciuffreda KJ. Effect of oculomotor rehabilitation on accommodative responsivity in mild traumatic brain injury. *J Rehabil Res Dev.* 2014;51(2):175-191.
15. Gallaway M, Scheiman M, Mitchell GL. Vision therapy for post-concussion vision disorders. *Optom Vis Sci.* 2017;94(1):68-73.
16. Hunt AW, Mah K, Reed N, Engel L, Keightley M. Oculomotor-based vision assessment in mild traumatic brain injury: a systematic review. *J Head Trauma Rehabil.* 2016;31(4):252-261.
17. Alvarez TL, Kim EH, Vicci VR, Dhar SK, Biswal BB, Barrett AM. Concurrent vision dysfunctions in convergence insufficiency with traumatic brain injury. *Optom Vis Sci.* 2012;89(12):1740-1751.
18. Thiagarajan P, Ciuffreda KJ. Effect of oculomotor rehabilitation on vergence responsivity in mild traumatic brain injury. *J Rehabil Res Dev.* 2013;50(9):1223-1240.
19. O'Neil M, Gleitsmann K, Motu'apuaka M, et al. *Visual Dysfunction in Patients with Traumatic Brain Injury: A Systematic Review.* Washington, DC: Department of Veterans Affairs (US); 2014.
20. Shaikh AG, Ghasia FF. Physiology and pathology of saccades and gaze holding. *NeuroRehabilitation.* 2013;32(3):493-505.
21. Mani R, Asper L, Khuu SK. Deficits in saccades and smooth-pursuit eye movements in adults with traumatic brain injury: a systematic review and meta-analysis. *Brain Inj.* 2018;32(11):1315-1336.
22. Bansal S, Han E, Ciuffreda KJ. Use of yoked prisms in patients with acquired brain injury: a retrospective analysis. *Brain Inj.* 2014;28(11):1441-1446.
23. Khan S, Chang R. Anatomy of the vestibular system: a review. *NeuroRehabilitation.* 2013;32(3):437-443.
24. Akin FW, Murnane OD. Head injury and blast exposure: vestibular consequences. *Otolaryngol Clin North Am.* 2011;44(2):323-334
25. Chamelian L, Feinstein A. Outcome after mild to moderate traumatic brain injury: the role of dizziness. *Arch Phys Med Rehabil.* 2004;85(10):1662-1666.
26. Wallace B, Lifshitz J. Traumatic brain injury and vestibulo-ocular function: current challenges and future prospects. *Eye Brain.* 2016 6;8:153-164.
27. Smouha E. Inner ear disorders. *NeuroRehabilitation.* 2013; 32(3):455-462.

28. Maskell F, Chiarelli P, Isles R. Dizziness after traumatic brain injury: overview and measurement in the clinical setting. *Brain Inj.* 2006;20(3):293-305.

29. Furman JM, Marcus DA, Balaban CD. Vestibular migraine: clinical aspects and pathophysiology. *Lancet Neurol.* 2013;12(7):706-715.

30. Chandrasekhar SS. The assessment of balance and dizziness in the TBI patient. *NeuroRehabilitation.* 2013;32(3):445-454.

31. Motin M, Keren O, Groswasser Z, Gordon CR. Benign paroxysmal positional vertigo as the cause of dizziness in patients after severe traumatic brain injury: diagnosis and treatment. *Brain Inj.* 2005 20;19(9):693-697.

32. Suarez H, Alonso R, Arocena M, Suarez A, Geisinger D. Clinical characteristics of positional vertigo after mild head trauma. *Acta Otolaryngol.* 2011;131(4):377-381.

33. Scherer MR, Schubert MC. Traumatic brain injury and vestibular pathology as a comorbidity after blast exposure. *Phys Ther.* 2009;89(9):980-992.

34. Kaufman KR, Brey RH, Chou LS, Rabatin A, Brown AW, Basford JR. Comparison of subjective and objective measurements of balance disorders following traumatic brain injury. *Med Eng Phys.* 2006;28(3):234-239.

35. King JE, Pape MM, Kodosky PN. Vestibular test patterns in the NICoE intensive outpatient program patient population. *Mil Med.* 2018;183(suppl 1):237-244.

36. Weightman MM. Balance and functional abilities assessment and intervention. In: Weightman MM, Radomski MV, Mashima PA, Roth CR, eds. *Mild TBI Rehabilitation Toolkit.* Fort Sam Houston, TX: Borden Institute; 2014:45-95.

37. Aligene K, Lin E. Vestibular and balance treatment of the concussed athlete. *NeuroRehabilitation.* 2013;32(3):543-553.

38. Alsalaheen BA, Mucha A, Morris LO, et al. Vestibular rehabilitation for dizziness and balance disorders after concussion. *J Neurol Phys Ther.* 2010;34(2):87-93.

39. Gurley JM, Hujsak BD, Kelly JL. Vestibular rehabilitation following mild traumatic brain injury. *NeuroRehabilitation.* 2013;32(3):519-528.

40. Balaban CD, Hoffer ME, Gottshall KR. Top-down approach to vestibular compensation: Translational lessons from vestibular rehabilitation. *Brain Res.* 2012;1482:101-111.

41. Lin E, Aligene K. Pharmacology of balance and dizziness. *NeuroRehabilitation.* 2013;32(3):529-542.

35

Emotional Dyscontrol

JUSTIN B. OTIS, MD, AND HAL S. WORTZEL, MD

OUTLINE

Emotional dyscontrol encompasses a spectrum of disorders involving aberrant regulation of emotion on a moment-to-moment basis. These conditions typically involve unpredictable and disproportionately intense (relative to the inciting stimulus) emotional reactions or displays of affect. There is diminished or absent ability to exercise voluntary control over the emotional responses (Arciniegas and Wortzel 2019). The emotional dysregulation manifests with sudden shifts that onset and terminate quickly (i.e., affective dysregulation) as opposed to the more persistent changes in emotion typifying disorders of mood (e.g., depression, mania). Common examples include irritability, affective lability, and pathological laughing and crying (PLC).

At the other end of the spectrum lies apathy, an impairment involving diminished motivation that may manifest with reduced drive relating to cognition, behavior, and emotion. Both dysregulated excess of emotion or the diminished capacity to generate emotion may serve as substantial sources of suffering for persons with brain injury and their families. Clinicians must be both diagnostically and therapeutically attentive to this disabling spectrum of neuropsychiatric conditions to maximize functional recovery after brain injury. This chapter offers definitions for irritability, affective lability, PLC, and apathy along with recommendations regarding the assessment and treatment of these disorders.

Irritability

Irritability is a common experience among healthy individuals. Annoyance, impatience, anger, and loss of temper are manifestations of irritability and may be present in normal day-to-day life. However, these experiences may be exacerbated by brain injury and become sources of distress and functional impairment. Traumatic brain injury (TBI) may increase both the frequency and intensity of irritable episodes.

- Irritability involves both subjective emotional components (e.g., feeling angry or annoyed) and outward manifestations of that feeling (e.g., demonstrating anger) (Alderman 2003).
- Irritability is a common manifestation of posttraumatic emotional dysregulation.
  - In its early form, posttraumatic irritability tends to manifest with "snappiness," typically as a reaction to modest stressors or sources of frustration.
  - Chronic forms of posttraumatic irritability involve recurrent and fleeting outbursts that are experienced as ego dystonic and constitute a change from preinjury patterns of response (Eames 2001).

Reported rates of posttraumatic irritability vary widely, likely as a consequence of the various definitions and methodologies employed across applicable investigations. Nonetheless, irritability is thought to be a common problem in the early recovery period, with most persons enjoying improvement over time (Yang et al. 2013).

Assessment for posttraumatic irritability needs to take into account injury severity and insight. Persons recovering from more severe injuries are often less aware of and able to report on irritability that is readily apparent to families and care providers. Hence, evaluators must consider the degree to which self-awareness is preserved when relying on patient self-report. In the setting of intact self-awareness, the Neurobehavioral Symptom Inventory (NSI) and the Irritability Questionnaire represent useful assessment tools.

When self-awareness is in question, informant-based assessment is preferred and is usefully guided by the Neuropsychiatry Inventory (NPI). Differential diagnosis in the setting of irritability requires recognizing the regularity with which irritability presents among even healthy persons; irritability is not necessarily indicative or a consequence of brain injury. Preexisting emotionality, various psychiatric disorders (especially depression, irritable mania, anxiety disorders, or posttraumatic stress disorder), substance use, pain, and medications may cause or contribute to irritability (Arciniegas and Wortzel 2014). These conditions, when identified, serve as appropriate initial targets for treatment rather than more direct management of irritability itself.

The treatment of irritability involves consideration of the severity of symptoms and cognitive status:
- For mild to moderate irritability with intact cognition:
  - Counseling and psychotherapy (Rees and Bellon 2007)
  - Group therapy and manualized anger self-management training (Hart et al 2012)
- For severe irritability and/or cognitive or behavioral impairment:
  - Case reports describe sertraline, valproate, methylphenidate, carbamazepine, quetiapine, aripiprazole, buspirone, and propranolol as beneficial treatments (Arciniegas and Wortzel 2014).
  - Selective serotonin reuptake inhibitors (SSRIs) are beneficial across a range of affective dysregulation disorders (except apathy), with modest side effect profiles, ease of use, and efficacy on comorbid conditions. They are considered first-line pharmacotherapy for posttraumatic irritability.
  - Sertraline, citalopram, and escitalopram are preferred because of short half-lives, modest drug and CYP450 interactions, and modest side effect profiles.
  - Amantadine has a relatively robust evidence base, including randomized controlled trials for posttraumatic irritability (Hammond et al. 2014, 2015, 2018), but caution is advised in the setting of cooccurring cognitive impairment.
  - An open-label trial of quetiapine suggests that low doses may reduce posttraumatic irritability and aggression and improve cognition (Kim and Biljani 2006).

Affective Lability

Affective (or emotional) lability involves:
- Contextually congruent, albeit exaggerated, emotional reactions to personally meaningful stimuli
- Episodes are provoked, variable in intensity, and only partially susceptible to voluntary control or distraction (Arciniegas and Wortzel 2014)
- Episodes may involve partially stereotyped outbursts of anger, anxiety, crying, elation, irritability, or laughing

Affective lability by definition occurs periodically and involves relatively brief emotional shifts that are independent of any underlying persisting depressive, bipolar, or anxiety disorders, which are also common after traumatic brain injury and add to diagnostic complexity (Ponsford et al 2018). Determinations regarding prevalence after brain injury are complicated by various definitions and assessment methods employed across investigations (Arciniegas and Wortzel 2014).

That said, one investigation reports rates for mild TBI (mTBI) as high as 28% in the 1-week to 3-month postinjury period (Villemure et al 2011). Higher rates and the propensity for persistent problems occur with injuries of greater severity. In the setting of moderate to severe TBI, prevalence rates may range from 33% to 46% in the early postinjury period and from 14% to 62% more chronically (Arciniegas and Wortzel 2019).

Once again, evaluation necessitates consideration for cognitive deficits—more specifically, the capacity for self-awareness. Accordingly, evaluation for affective lability may be facilitated via either clinician-administered scales, such as the Neuropsychiatric Inventory-Clinician (NPI-C) or the Neurobehavioral Rating Scale-Revised (NRS-R), or via self-assessment tools such as the Affective Lability Scale or the Center for Neurologic Study-Lability Scale (CNS-LS) (Arciniegas and Wortzel 2019).

Affective lability is a feature shared across many neuropsychiatric conditions and thus is not necessarily indicative of or referable to brain injury. Considerations regarding differential diagnosis should involve a broad range of conditions spanning medicine and psychiatry, including depression, mania, substance abuse, and personality disorder.

The treatment of affective lability involves:
- Behavioral interventions such as counseling, patient and family education, and/or psychotherapy
- First-line pharmacotherapy options for severe or persisting symptoms include sertraline, citalopram, or escitalopram (Arciniegas and Wortzel 2014)
- Second-line interventions are typically guided by comorbidities:
  - With inattention and/or slow processing speed: methylphenidate
  - With comorbid irritability and/or aggression: amantadine
  - With irritability/anger or aggression (at self or others): valproate or carbamazepine
  - With a comorbid seizure disorder: lamotrigine

Pathological Laughing and Crying

PLC is the prototypical disorder of emotional dyscontrol. The clinical manifestations may involve numerous disconnects between stimuli and emotional response in terms of both valance and intensity and disparity between demonstrated affect verses internal emotional experience. Other terms encountered in the medical literature to describe PLC include *pseudobulbar affect, emotional incontinence,* and *involuntary emotional expression disorder.*
- PLC is characterized by frequent and brief episodes of stereotyped, intense, and uncontrollable laughing or crying that are exaggerated in comparison with the stimulus and may be contextually inappropriate (e.g., laughing induced by somber circumstances) (Wortzel et al 2008).
- The internal emotional experience may bear little resemblance to the associated affective display (e.g., crying may occur absent associated sadness).

PLC is a relatively uncommon neuropsychiatric manifestation of TBI, especially compared with irritability and affective lability. Unlike these latter two forms of emotional dyscontrol, which frequently present in the setting of psychiatric illness and may even occur in healthy persons, PLC occurs in the setting of an underlying neurological condition (e.g., multiple sclerosis, stroke, and various neurodegenerative conditions). In essence, neurologic insults compromise the networks that integrate internal emotional states with affective displays and that instill elements of volitional control.

TBI is among the neurologic insults that may yield PLC. Prevalence of pathological laughter and crying ranges in the literature from 5% to 21% in the first year postinjury, with more severe injuries carrying greater risk of PLC. Pathological crying is four times more prevalent than pathological laughing after severe TBI (Roy et al 2015).

PLC is often apparent based on clinical interview, collateral information from caregivers, and direct observation. That said, various measures may aid in diagnosis and provide a means for quantifying symptom severity and to monitor progress with treatment. When self-awareness is preserved, the Pathological Laughter and Crying Scale is a good option (Arciniegas and Wortzel 2019). When insight is limited, a clinician-administered approach using the NPI-C is more useful (Arciniegas and Wortzel 2019). PLC frequently cooccurs with depressive disorders, anxiety disorders, posttraumatic stress disorder (PTSD), and behavioral dyscontrol (i.e., aggression) after TBI (Roy et al. 2015; Tateno et al. 2004).

PLC should be distinguished from normal emotionality, essential crying (Green et al. 1987), and personality disorders (e.g., borderline and/or histrionic personality disorder). Importantly, seizures may yield episodes of ictal laughing (gelastic seizures) or crying (dacrystic or quiritarian seizure). Altered consciousness and postictal confusion (which do not feature in PLC) are clues suggestive of seizures (Chahine and Chemali 2006).

Treatment of pathological laughter and crying includes:
- Education regarding the nature and underlying causes of PLC for patients and families, to reduce distress and embarrassment
- First-line medication options include SSRIs such as citalopram, escitalopram, or sertraline (Wortzel et al 2008)
- Augmentation options, when results are insufficient, include amantadine, carbamazepine, lamotrigine, methylphenidate, or valproate (Arciniegas and Wortzel 2014)
- Although approved by the US Food and Drug Administration (FDA) for pseudobulbar affect, dextromethorphan/quinidine (Nuedexta) is more appropriate when SSRIs prove ineffective, as combination therapy or augmentation (Hammond et al 2018).

Apathy

Apathy is appropriately regarded as a syndrome involving diminished goal-directed cognition, emotion, and behavior as a consequence of insult or injury to the brain that is not better accounted for by another cognitive or emotional condition.

Apathy manifests as a loss of motivation causing diminished ability to respond to stimuli (both internal and external) with goal-directed responses (Reekum and Reekum 2013). Apathy may affect cognition, behavior, and emotion (i.e., the capacity to think, do, or feel).

Apathy complicates a number of neuropsychiatric conditions, including TBI, and is associated with poor response to rehabilitation and other therapies along with increased caregiver burden. A variety of terms are used to describe apathy across a spectrum of severity, with the term *akinetic mutism* used to denote the near-complete loss of voluntary responses to stimuli in the setting of intact sensorimotor functions and arousal. The medical literature presents a wide range of prevalence estimations for apathy in the setting of TBI, from 20% to 71% (Worthington and Wood 2018).

Diminished motivation features across a wide variety of neuropsychiatric conditions, many of which may occur after TBI. Clinicians must be particularly vigilant to differentiate apathy from depression, because pharmacologic therapies typically used for depression (e.g., SSRIs) may exacerbate apathy. Unlike depression, apathy features diminished or blunted emotions as opposed to dysphoric emotional states (e.g., persistent sadness, hopelessness, helplessness).

Given the nature of apathy and diminished drive to act, patients struggling with apathy frequently lack the ability or drive to offer complaints in relation to this experience. Hence, informant-based interview is often necessary and should seek information regarding motivational behaviors, flattened affect, lack of initiation, and diminished interest or participation in activities (Reekum and Reekum 2013). Diagnostic assessment may be facilitated by the Apathy Assessment Scale (Marin 1991) or the NPI.

The treatment of posttraumatic apathy involves:
- Nonpharmacologic interventions, such as verbal cueing, task checklists, computer retraining, cognitive interventions, music therapies, structured activity kits, multisensory stimulation environments
- Medications that target dopamine systems:
  - Methylphenidate or dextroamphetamine is an appropriate first-line options for TBI-related apathy.
  - Bromocriptine and amantadine have been reported to be beneficial for apathy in the setting of TBI.
- Medications that augment the cholinergic system:
  - Acetylcholinesterase inhibitors such as donepezil, rivastigmine, or galantamine
- Medications that target other neurotransmitters systems with stimulating effect, such as modafinil, carbidopa-levodopa, bupropion, venlafaxine, protriptyline, and selegiline
- Treatment with antidepressants, such as SSRIs, may exacerbate apathy (Reekum and Reekum 2013).

Review Questions

1. A 46-year-old male building contractor with a history of posttraumatic epilepsy presents for evaluation 12 weeks after a traumatic brain injury (TBI) with loss of consciousness (LOC) for 40 minutes when he was struck with an iron beam during a residential construction project. His wife accompanies him and reports that he has lost interest in their favorite TV shows, and she has a much harder time getting him to help around the house. When he is asked about this, he reports a general disinterest in his usual activities. He and his spouse deny any apparent dysphoric emotions but instead report he is emotionally muted, consistent with his affectively blunted presentation. The most appropriate first-line intervention for this patient's condition would be
   a. methylphenidate.
   b. paroxetine.
   c. carbamazepine.
   d. bupropion.

2. A 23-year-old woman with a history of migraine headaches presents with her boyfriend for worsened headaches and increased emotionality after a low-velocity motor vehicle collision in which she was a restrained driver with no loss of consciousness. During evaluation, she is very talkative and superficial with history and details, hushes her boyfriend when he attempts to provide any history, has very expressive nonverbal communication, and portrays congruent but exaggerated emotional expressivity across a full range of emotional states and topics. Her affect is most consistent with:
   a. apathy.
   b. affective lability.
   c. histrionic personality disorder.
   d. pathological laughing and crying.

3. The son of a 52-year-old man accompanying his father to clinic requests an evaluation for his father's mood changes. He has noted over the past few months, his father has inappropriate outbursts of childlike laughter during sad movies and serious conversations. These outbursts have caused conflict in his family, leading to increased tension between the patient and his wife. The patient reports he is unable to control it and wants to regain control of his emotions and repair his relationship with his wife. A US Food and Drug Administration (FDA)–approved treatment for his condition is
   a. clonidine.
   b. dextromethorphan/quinidine.
   c. topiramate.
   d. escitalopram.

Answers on page 396.
Access the full list of questions and answers online. Available on ExpertConsult.com

References

1. Alderman N. Contemporary approaches to the management of irritability and aggression following traumatic brain injury. *Neuropsychol Rehabil.* 2003;13(1-2):211-240.
2. Arciniegas DB, Wortzel HS. Emotional and behavioral dyscontrol after traumatic brain injury. *Psychiatr Clin North Am.* 2014;37(1): 31-53.
3. Arciniegas DB, Wortzel HS. Emotional dyscontrol. In: Silver JM, McAllister TW, Yudofsky SC, eds. *Textbook of Traumatic Brain Injury.* 3rd ed. Washington DC: American Psychiatric Publishing; 2019:329-344.
4. Chahine LM, Chemali Z. Du rire aux larmes: pathological laughing and crying in patients with traumatic brain injury and treatment with lamotrigine. *Epilepsy Behav.* 2006;8(3):610-615.
5. Eames PG. Distinguishing the neuropsychiatric, psychiatric, and psychological consequences of acquired brain injury. In: Wood RL, McMillan TH, eds. *Neurobehavioral Disability and Social Handicap Following Traumatic Brain Injury.* UK:Psychology Press; 2001: 29-64.
6. Green RL, McAllister TW, Bernat JL. A study of crying in medically and surgically hospitalized patients. *Am J Psychiatry.* 1987;144(4):442-447.
7. Hammond FM, Bickett AK, Norton JH, et al. Effectiveness of amantadine hydrochloride in the reduction of chronic traumatic brain injury irritability and aggression. *J Head Trauma Rehabil.* 2014;29(5):391-399.
8. Hammond FM, Sherer M, Malec JF, et al. Amantadine effect on perceptions of irritability after traumatic brain injury: results of the amantadine irritability multisite study. *J Neurotrauma.* 2015;32(16):1230-1238.
9. Hammond FM, Sauve W, Ledon F, Davis C, Formella AE. Safety, tolerability, and effectiveness of dextromethorphan/quinidine for pseudobulbar affect among study participants with traumatic brain injury: results from the PRISM-II open label study. *PM R.* 2018;10(10):993-1003.
10. Hart T, Vaccaro MJ, Hays C, Majuro RD. Anger self-management training for people with traumatic brain injury: a preliminary investigation. *J Head Trauma Rehabil.* 2012;27(2): 113-122.
11. Kim E, Bijlani M. A pilot study of quetiapine treatment of aggression due to traumatic brain injury. *J Neuropsychiatry Clin Neurosci.* 2006;18(4):547-549.
12. Marin RS, Biedrzycki RC, Firinciogullari S. Reliability and validity of the Apathy Evaluation Scale. *Psychiatry Res.* 1991;38(2): 143-162.
13. Ponsford J, Always Y, Gould KR. Epidemiology and natural history of psychiatric disorders after TBI. *J Neuropsychiatry Clin Neurosci.* 2018:262-270.
14. Reekum R, Reekum E. Apathy. In: Arciniegas DB, Nasler ND, Vanderploeg RD, Jaffee MS, eds. *Management of Adults with Traumatic Brain Injury.* Washington, DC: American Psychiatric Publishing; 2013:283-302.
15. Rees RJ, Bellon ML. Post concussion syndrome ebb and flow: longitudinal effects and management. *NeuroRehabilitation.* 2007;22(3): 229-242.
16. Roy D, McCann U, Han D, et al. Pathological laughter and crying and psychiatric comorbidity after traumatic brain injury. *J Neuropsychiatry Clin Neurosci.* 2015;27(4):299-303.
17. Tateno A, Jorge RE, Robinson RG. Pathological laughing and crying following traumatic brain injury. *J Neuropsychiatry Clin Neurosci.* 2004;16(4):426-434.

18. Villemure R, Nolin P, Le Sage N. Self-reported symptoms during post-mild traumatic brain injury in acute phase: influence of interviewing method. *Brain Inj.* 2011;25(1):53-64.

19. Worthington A, Wood RL. Apathy following traumatic brain injury: a review. *Neuropsychologia.* 2018;118(Pt B):40-47.

20. Wortzel HS, Oster TJ, Anderson CA, et al. Pathological laughing and crying: epidemiology, pathophysiology and treatment. *CNS Drugs.* 2008;22(7):531-545.

21. Yang CC, Huang SJ, Lin WC, et al. Divergent manifestations of irritability in patients with mild and moderate-to-severe traumatic brain injury: perspectives of awareness and neurocognitive correlates. *Brain Inj.* 2013;27(9):1008-1015.

36

Agitation and Restlessness

LINDSAY MOHNEY, DO, BRUNO S. SUBBARAO, DO, AND BLESSEN C. EAPEN, MD

Agitation after traumatic brain injury (TBI) is a clinical manifestation of the natural recovery process and is often associated with posttraumatic amnesia (PTA).[1] Most definitions denote an excess of behaviors (motor or verbal) that interfere with patient care, pose a risk to persons or property, or require action from staff.[1,2] These include some combination of aggression, restlessness, disinhibition, akathisia, inappropriate vocalizing, and emotional liability. These behaviors must be present in the absence of other physical, medical, or psychiatric causes.[1]

The incidence among patients varies widely, between 11% and 70%. Studies have shown agitation duration varies from a few days to several weeks, although it typically resolves within 4 weeks.[2] The most consistent predictors of agitation are impaired cognition, ongoing PTA, and lower functional status. Other variables associated with worse agitation behaviors include more severe injury, premorbid history of substance abuse, and presence of infection.[3] The pathology underlying posttraumatic agitation is likely multifactorial, involving a complicated combination of cerebral structural lesions, biochemical abnormalities, and external factors including damage to the frontal and temporal lobes, injury to the prefrontal cortex, damage to the thalamus and limbic system, and impaired regulation of serotonin, norepinephrine, and dopamine.[1,4]

Diagnosis

A detailed history of present illness and medical comorbidities and an in-depth social history should be obtained. A comprehensive physical examination should be performed next, including vital signs, neurological examination, cardiopulmonary evaluation, and musculoskeletal examination. Evaluation should include assessment for secondary conditions common in TBI that may contribute to agitation, such as expressive aphasia leading to behavioral outbursts as the individual becomes frustrated with the inability to communicate.

Agitation is a diagnosis of exclusion after other conditions have been ruled out.[1,4]

- Medical
  - Medication side effects: Many drugs may exacerbate agitation including: opioids, benzodiazepines, dopamine agonists (e.g., metoclopramide), H_2-receptor antagonists (e.g., omeprazole), and anticholinergic medications (e.g., oxybutynin)
  - Pain (headache, polytrauma, postop, heterotopic ossification, spasticity, shoulder subluxation, occult fracture, skin lesion, etc.)
  - Infection
  - Metabolic disturbance (electrolytes, thyroid, hypoglycemia)
  - Hypoxemia (pulmonary embolism)
  - Urinary retention/incontinence
  - Nausea, constipation
  - Neurological
    - Hydrocephalus
    - Seizures
    - Intracranial mass lesions
  - Psychiatric
    - Personality disorders/psychosis/anxiety/mood disorders
    - Sundowning in patients with dementia
    - Substance use/acute intoxication
- Workup/laboratory tests
  - Complete blood count with differential
  - Complete metabolic panel
  - Thyroid function tests
  - Urinalysis with urine culture
  - Urine toxicology screen
  - Cerebrospinal fluid analysis
  - Computed tomography head/magnetic resonance imaging brain
  - Electroencephalogram
  - X-ray

Assessment

In practice, agitation is typically assessed clinically. In fact, one study showed fewer than half the brain injury specialists use objective measures of agitation in their practice.[1] Objective measures of agitation can be used to determine the effectiveness of treatment.

- Agitated Behavior Scale (ABS)[1,5,6]
  - Only measure of agitation developed specifically for and validated in the TBI population
  - Helpful for monitoring patient's recovery progression and assessing effectiveness of interventions
  - High interrater reliability
  - Can be completed in 5 to 10 minutes of observation
  - See Table 36.1
- Overt Aggression Scale (OAS)[1,6]
  - Observational scale that requires training to administer
  - Can be completed in 3 to 5 minutes

- Allows recording of type, severity, and frequency of different aggressive behaviors such as verbal, physical against objects, physical against self, and physical against others
- There are additional items that register the intervention applied by the staff

Management and Treatment Recommendations

Agitated behavior has been associated with longer lengths of stay in both hospital and acute rehabilitation settings, increased cost of care, and increased amount of support needed after hospitalization. Agitation can also impede community reintegration, including alienation from family, loss of employment, and potential legal issues.[1] Thus, management is essential to ensure safety, ease caregiver burden, and maximize cooperation in therapies.

TABLE 36.1 Agitated Behavior Scale[5]

1 = Absent: The behavior is not present.

2 = Present to a slight degree: The behavior is present but does not disrupt appropriate behavior. The individual may redirect spontaneously.

3 = Present to a moderate degree: The individual needs to be redirected from an agitated to an appropriate behavior but benefits from such cueing.

4 = Present to an extreme degree: The individual is not able to engage in appropriate behavior because of the interference of the agitated behavior, even when external cueing or redirection is provided.

1. Short attention span, easy distractibility, inability to concentrate
2. Impulsive, impatient, low tolerance for pain or frustration
3. Uncooperative, resistant to care, demanding
4. Violent and/or threatening violence toward people or property
5. Explosive and/or unpredictable anger
6. Rocking, rubbing, moaning, or other self-stimulating behavior
7. Pulling at tubes, restraints, etc.
8. Wandering from treatment areas
9. Restlessness, pacing, excessive movement
10. Repetitive behaviors—motor and/or verbal
11. Rapid, loud, or excessive talking
12. Sudden changes of mood
13. Easily initiated or excessive crying and/or laughter
14. Self-abusiveness—physical and/or verbal

Total Score

<21	Normal
22–28	Low agitation
29–35	Moderate agitation
>35	Severe agitation

- First line: Environmental modification[1,4,7]
  - Reduce stimuli:
    - Minimize light, noise, and distractions—low-level lighting, draw curtains, turn off television, etc.
    - Limit number of visitors at one time
    - Staff and family should speak in low volume, slowly, one at a time
    - Implement rest periods throughout the day to minimize impact of fatigue.
  - Avoid/minimize restraints: Use noncontact restraints if able (e.g., safety net beds), padded hand mittens, one-to-one staff supervision
  - Minimize tubes and lines: Cover them if essential for patient care (e.g., place abdominal binder)
  - Frequent reorientation by staff and family
  - Consistent schedule and staff
  - Timed toileting
  - Create a familiar environment: Allow family to bring in personal possessions
  - Ensure good sleep cycle regulation and sleep quality
    - Encourage good sleep hygiene
    - Consider use of trazodone, melatonin
- Behavior modification[1,4]
  - Allow patient to express feelings of restlessness by allowing them to pace (if safe) or be walked/wheeled around by staff

- Mobile patients may require a closed unit or sensors for safety
- Deescalation techniques
- Structured behavioral programs
  - May have limited application given cognitive and impaired safety awareness. Anosognosia (lack of awareness of deficits) is also a challenge.

Pharmacological Management

For patients who exhibit agitated behaviors despite environmental and behavioral modification, addition of a pharmacological agent may be considered. Every TBI is different, thus the choice of therapy should be based on clinical presentation and medical comorbidities. The ideal agent is nonsedating, would not affect cognitive recovery, and has a low side effect profile. Agents that slow cognition may prolong/exacerbate agitation. As with most medications, the general principle for administration is "start low, go slow," beginning with the lowest dose available and slowly increasing for effectiveness. Frequent reassessment is essential to determine the need for continuation of the pharmacological agents (Table 36.2).

TABLE 36.2 Summary of Pharmacological Management Options for Agitation in Traumatic Brain Injury

Medication	Dosing	Benefits	Important Side Effects	Comments
Beta Blockers[4,7,8]				
Propranolol	Starting dose: 20–60 mg/day, divided into twice a day (BID) or four times a day (QID) Maximum dose up to 420 mg/day has been used	• Best evidence for efficacy • Also treats dysautonomia, anxiety, tremor, and migraines • Improves restlessness and disinhibition	• Hypotension • Bradycardia • Lethargy	No adverse effect on motor or cognitive recovery
Antiepileptic Drugs (AEDs)[1,4,7,8,9]				

Carbamazepine	Aggression-limiting effects seen with dosing 300–900 mg/day, divided BID or three times a day (TID)	• Mood-stabilizing AEDs reduce agitation with aggression, irritability, and disinhibition.
		• Consider treatment if agitation associated with epilepsy or bipolar disorder.
			• Hyponatremia
			• Sedation
			• Nausea
			• Rare but serious:
			  • Aplastic anemia
			  • Agranulocytosis
			  • Stevens-Johnson syndrome
				Improvement in behavior seen within 4 days
				Need to monitor serum levels for toxicity
				Potential to negatively affect psychomotor speed

Valproic acid	Starting dose: 250 mg BID May be titrated up 250 mg every 2–3 days to maximum of 1000–2500 mg/day	• Less likely than carbamazepine to have negative impact on cognition and has safer side effect profile	• Sedation • Nausea/emesis • Weight gain • Hepatotoxicity	Potential for rapid efficacy

TABLE 36.2 Summary of Pharmacological Management Options for Agitation in Traumatic Brain Injury—cont'd

Medication	Dosing	Benefits	Important Side Effects	Comments
Antidepressants[1,4,7]				
Selective serotonin reuptake inhibitors (SSRIs, e.g., sertraline)	Starting dose: 25–50 mg/day Dosing titrated every 3–7 days up to 200 mg/day	• Helpful for agitation with depressive or behavioral component • Can improve symptoms of Kluver-Bucy syndrome and pseudobulbar affect	• Decreased libido • Serotonin syndrome • QTc prolongation	Antidepressant effect noted in 2 or more weeks' quicker time to effect for behavioral disorders
Tricyclic antidepressants (TCAs, e.g., amitriptyline)	Starting dose: 10 mg/day Maximum dose: 250 mg/day	• May be recommended as a second-line agent	• Sedation • QTc prolongation • May lower seizure threshold • Anticholinergic effects	May increase confusion
Trazodone	Starting dose: 50–100 mg Increased sleep usually seen by 150 mg	• Shown to decrease agitation and aggressive behaviors • Can also be used for sleep cycle regulation	• Anticholinergic effects • Priapism • Sedation	Can precipitate serotonin syndrome if used with an SSRI
Lithium[1,9]	Starting dose: 300 mg BID Titrate by serum drug levels and side effects: 0.5–1.2 mEq/L is therapeutic and >1.4 mEq/L is toxic level	• Can help in patients with mania and cyclic mood disorders	• Increased thirst • Polyuria • Sedation • Movement disorders • Seizures • QTc prolongation • Renal impairment	May cause decreased cognition and lethargy
Antipsychotics[4,7]				
Typical antipsychotics (e.g., haloperidol)	Starting dose: 0.5mg May repeat every 15-30 minutes as needed until symptoms are controlled.	• Typically reserved for severe agitation or aggressive crisis	• Extrapyramidal effects • Neuroleptic malignant syndrome • QTc prolongation • Sedation	Can be given intramuscularly (IM) or intravenously May have deleterious effects on cognition and motor recovery Associated with longer time in posttraumatic amnesia Not recommended for long-term use
Atypical antipsychotics (e.g., quetiapine, ziprasidone, olanzapine)	Dosing dependent on agent selected. Use lowest efficacious dose.	• Better side effect profile compared with typical agents	• Sedation • Extrapyramidal symptoms • Dizziness	Can be given IM Not recommended for long-term use unless concomitant psychiatric disease
Neurostimulants[3,4,7,10]				
Amantadine	Starting dose: 50 mg per day in divided doses, typically morning and noon 200–400 mg/day used for improving wakefulness and cognition	• Effective for acute and chronic agitation after traumatic brain injury (TBI) • Also improves wakefulness, apathy	• Irritability • Tachycardia • Elevated blood pressure • Lowered seizure threshold	Effects seen within several days Must be weaned when discontinuing because of risk for neuroleptic malignant syndrome with abrupt withdrawal

Continued

| TABLE 36.2 | Summary of Pharmacological Management Options for Agitation in Traumatic Brain Injury—cont'd | | | |

Medication	Dosing	Benefits	Important Side Effects	Comments
Methylpheni-date	Dose: 10–60 mg/day in divided doses, usually at 8:00 a.m. and noon	• Effective for acute and chronic agitation after TBI • Can also improve attention/concentration	• Insomnia • Decreased appetite • Elevated blood pressure	Quick onset of action
Anxiolytics[1,3,4,7]				
Buspirone	Usual dose of 5–20 mg TID Maximum dosing recommended 60 mg/day, but as high as 180/day seen	• Can be considered a second-line agent for agitation in the absence of anxiety • No significant adverse neurological or cognitive effects; not a respiratory depressant; nonsedating, nonaddictive	• Light headedness • Headache • Risk of serotonin syndrome with concomitant use of antidepressants	2–3 week delay in therapeutic action
Benzodiaze-pines (e.g., lorazepam, diazepam)	Dosing dependent on agent selected. Use lowest efficacious dose.	• Useful for rapid resolution of agitation crisis	• Paradoxical agitation • Anterograde amnesia • Disinhibition • Sedation • Impaired coordination • Respiratory depression	Recommend starting long-acting agents concurrently Discontinue as soon as possible to minimize chances of delaying cognitive recovery Risk of dependence and addiction

Review Questions

1. What is the only measure of agitation developed for and validated in the traumatic brain injury (TBI) population?
   a. Overt Aggression Scale (OAS)
   b. Agitated Behavior Scale (ABS)
   c. Galveston Orientation and Amnesia Test (GOAT)
   d. Ranchos Los Amigos Scale (RLAS)
2. What is the recommended first-line management of agitated behavior?
   a. Metoprolol
   b. Haloperidol
   c. Bilateral wrist restraints
   d. Limit the number of visitors to one at a time.

3. Which medication should be considered in an agitated patient with paranoia and delusions?
   a. Beta blocker
   b. Atypical antipsychotic
   c. Selective serotonin reuptake inhibitor (SSRI)
   d. Benzodiazepine

Answers on page 396.
Access the full list of questions and answers online.
Available on ExpertConsult.com

References

1. Lombard LA, Zafonte RD. Agitation after traumatic brain injury: Considerations and Treatment Options. *Am J Phys Med Rehabil.* 2005;84:797-812.
2. Brooke M, Questad K, Patterson D, Bashak K. Agitation and Restlessness after Closed Head Injury: A Prospective study of 100 consecutive admissions. *Arch Phys Med Rehabil.* 1992;73:320-323.
3. Bogner J, Barrett R, Hammond F, et al. Predictors of agitated behavior during inpatient rehabilitation for traumatic brain injury. *Arch Phys Med Rehabil.* 2015;96(8 suppl 3):S274-S281.
4. Luaute J, Plantier D, Wiart L, Tell L, et al. Care management of the agitation or aggressiveness crisis in patient with TBI. Systematic review of the literature and practice recommendations. *Ann Phys Rehabil Med.* 2016;56:58-67.
5. Bogner J, Corrigan J, Stange M, Rabold D. Reliability of the Agitated Behavior Scale. *J Head Trauma Rehabil.* 1999;14(1):91-96.
6. Castaño Monsalve B, Laxe S, Bernabeu Guitart M, Bulbena Vilarrasa A. Behavioral scales used in severe and moderate traumatic brain injury. *Neurorehabilitation.* 2014;35:67-76.

7. Bhatnagar S, Iaccarino MA, Zafonte R. Pharmacotherapy in rehabilitation of post-acute traumatic brain injury. *Brain Res.* 2016;1640:164-179.

8. Brooke M, Patterson D, Questad K, Cardenas D, Farrel-Roberts L. The Treatment of Agitation during initial hospitalization after traumatic brain injury. *Arch Phys Med Rehabil.* 1992;73:917-921.

9. Kalra I, Watanabe T. Mood stabilizers for traumatic brain injury-related agitation. *J Head Trauma Rehabil.* 2017;32(6):E61-E64.

10. Hammond F, Malec J, Zafonte R, Sherer M, et al. Potential Impact of Amantadine on aggression in chronic traumatic brain injury. *J Head Trauma Rehabil.* 2017;32(5):308-318.

37

Sleep Dysfunction and Fatigue

DMITRY ESTEROV, DO, AND BILLIE SCHULTZ, MD

Evaluation of Posttraumatic Fatigue

Introduction

- Fatigue is one of the most commonly reported symptoms after brain injury (BI); reported rate of fatigue varies.
  - One study reported fatigue in 53% of those studied.[1]
  - Other studies have suggested 21% to 70% of individuals with traumatic brain injury (TBI) experience fatigue, greater than estimates for the general population of 3% to 22%.[2]

Definition

- No standardized uniform definition exists. It has been described as an awareness of a negative balance between available energy and the mental and physical requirements of activities.[2]
- Distinction between central fatigue and peripheral fatigue[3]:
  - Central fatigue: Dysfunction of supratentorial structures involved in mentation

- Peripheral fatigue: Of physical, metabolic, or muscular origin
- Often both are involved after TBI.
- Fatigue versus excessive daytime sleepiness (EDS): Although they are similar, there is a difference in that sleepiness typically responds to appropriate amount of rest. Sleepiness is more defined by difficulty maintaining wakefulness, whereas fatigue is multidimensional.

Etiology

- The exact etiology is unknown and is likely multifactorial.
- There are associations with conditions that are frequently reported after TBI, such as depression, pain, and disturbed sleep.[1]
- Chronic pain can lead to symptoms of fatigue.[1]
- It has been reported with neuroendocrine abnormalities.
- Coping hypothesis is a theory that fatigue after BI is caused by an increase in mental effort needed to overcome impaired attention and processing speed, thus the brain compensates to overcome these cognitive deficits.

Scales/Metrics Used

- There is no one universally applied scale, although a number of scales have been used to measure fatigue after BI (Table 37.1).
- "Measurement overlap" is important to keep in mind, in that measures of depression, pain, and other health problems often pertain to fatigue and thus are likely to correlate with fatigue measures.

General Medical Workup

- Initial testing can include erythrocyte sedimentation rate (ESR), complete blood count, chemistry panel, liver panel, and fasting blood glucose.[4]
- Cardiopulmonary
  - Obstructive sleep apnea, chronic obstructive pulmonary disease (COPD), heart failure

TABLE 37.1	Measures of Assessing Fatigue	
Measure	**Key Features**	
Global Fatigue Index (GFI)	One of the most widely used measures of fatigue, used with a variety of populations with chronic conditions, including human immunodeficiency virus, multiple sclerosis, and cancer	
Epworth Sleepiness Scale	Measures daytime sleepiness rather than fatigue but has been used in studies in those with traumatic brain injury (TBI). There are eight items, each of which rates a routine daytime situation on a 4-point scale from 0 (would never doze) to 3 (high chance of dozing). Subjects who score 10 or more are considered to have excessive daytime sleepiness.	
Fatigue Severity Scale (FSS)	A one-dimensional fatigue scale composed of nine items each ranging from 1 (no impairment) to 7 (severe impairment), with higher scores indicating more severe fatigue. Has been used in trials of individuals with TBI and used in trials of modafinil for fatigue after TBI.[6]	
Modified Fatigue Impact Scale	A multidimensional fatigue measure found to be reliable and has been used in studies in individuals with TBI. A 21-item self-report instrument in which subjects rate the extent to which fatigue has caused problems for them from 0 (no problem) to 4 (extreme problem), with higher scores indicating a greater impact of fatigue. Subscales for cognitive, physical, and psychosocial functioning can also be calculated.[6]	
Barrow Neurological Institute Fatigue Scale	Designed for use in early stages of measuring fatigue, such as on acute rehabilitation.	

- Metabolic
- Anemia/iron deficiency
- Endocrine
  - Anterior pituitary dysfunction
  - Thyroid/growth hormone/testosterone/cortisol
- Psychiatric
- Alcohol or drug dependence
- Infectious
- Neoplastic
- Medication induced
  - Assessing necessity of medications that increase fatigue:
    - Antiepileptics
    - Antihistamines
    - Antipsychotics
    - Antihypertensives (propranolol, verapamil)
    - Antiemetics (Phenergan, Zofran)
- Sleep disorders (see later)

Management

- Home exercise program
- Rehabilitation approach
  - Compensatory strategies with energy conservation
  - Instructions to pace oneself/brain breaks
- Dietary counseling and weight reduction
- Psychiatric counseling or referral to mental health specialists as indicated
  - Cognitive behavioral therapy (CBT) has been shown to help with fatigue in other conditions but is not proven to help with fatigue specifically after TBI[5]
- Pharmacological treatments of fatigue
  - Modafinil is US Food and Drug Administration (FDA) approved for treatment of EDS associated with narcolepsy, obstructive sleep apnea, and shift work sleep disorder.[6]
  - Modafinil has been shown to help with Excessive Daytime Sleepiness (EDS) but not with measures of fatigue.[5]

- Methylphenidate has been shown to benefit in one class III crossover study of 24 patients.[5]
- Hormone replacement can be considered for endocrine abnormalities, but more research is needed.

Evaluation of Sleep Dysfunction

Introduction

- Sleep disorders are common after a TBI, with one study finding incidence to be three times higher compared with the general population.[7]
- Prevalence is higher in those with severe TBI compared with mild TBI.[8]
- Sleep dysfunction is a component of fatigue but not necessarily the primary cause of fatigue.

Overview of Normal Sleep

- Sleep stages divided into nonrapid eye movement (NREM) and rapid eye movement (REM)
  - Five stages overall: wake (W), N1, N2, N3, and R
  - N1–N3 are considered NREM
- Characteristics of each stage[9]
  - W: As individuals become drowsy and the eyes close, the alpha rhythm is the predominant pattern. An epoch is considered stage W if it contains greater than 50% alpha waves
  - N1: Very short duration, considered light sleep
  - N2: Presence of sleep spindles and K complexes
  - N3: Considered the deepest stage of sleep and characterized by delta waves
  - REM sleep: electroencephalogram (EEG) is the same as in awake state but characterized by muscle atonia and episodic bursts REMs; stage when dreams occur

- Slow-wave/deep NREM sleep is more prominent in the first third of the night, and REM sleep is more prominent in the last part of the night or morning hours.

Pathophysiology/Changes to Sleep After Traumatic Brain Injury

- A metaanalysis of polysomnography data after TBI showed that TBI patients had poorer sleep efficiency, shorter total sleep duration, and greater wake after sleep onset time. Although sleep architecture was similar between the groups, a trend suggested that TBI patients may spend less time in REM sleep. TBI patients reported greater subjective sleepiness and poorer perceived sleep quality.[9]
- Biochemical substrates have been found to be altered after TBI.
  - Lower levels of cerebrospinal fluid of a neuropeptide called *hypocretin-1* (orexin) are associated with excessive daytime sleepiness in TBI in acute phase but return to baseline in chronic phase.[12] Low cerebrospinal fluid (CSF) orexin is initially found to be low in narcolepsy.
  - Lowered melatonin is found to be associated with altered REM sleep post TBI.
- Damage to the hypothalamus, brainstem, and reticular activating system can disrupt arousal and the sleep–wake cycle.[10]
- Coup-contrecoup injury most frequently damages inferior frontal and anterior temporal regions, including the basal forebrain, which is an area involved in sleep initiation.[10]

Etiology

- Types of sleep disorders most commonly reported after TBI (Table 37.2)
- In a meta-analysis, the most common sleep disturbance after TBI was insomnia, followed by difficulty maintaining sleep and poor sleep efficiency on polysomnography.[11]
- Other factors that can cause insomnia:
  - Medication: neurostimulant use
  - Pain can present in the form of headaches and joint, neck, shoulder, and back pain and can lead to insomnia if untreated
  - Concurrent posttraumatic stress disorder (PTSD): Diagnosis of PTSD also involves sleep disturbances.
    - PTSD-related nightmares can be treated effectively with prazosin and/or image-rehearsal therapy with or without CBT for insomnia.[10]
  - Anxiety and depression are strongly associated with sleep disturbance, and both are common symptoms after TBI.[10]
- Environmental/life habits

Evaluation of Sleep Disorders

- Sleep diary
- Polysomnography (PSG)
  - PSG provides comprehensive data on sleep-onset latency, time in different stages, and monitoring of heart rate and blood oxygenation.
  - Multiple sleep latency testing (MSLT) is often helpful in diagnosing narcolepsy and EDS
- Actigraphy
  - A watchlike device worn on a limb that records patient data to give objective parameters

TABLE 37.2	Common Disorders after Traumatic Brain Injury
Disorder	**Key Features**
Insomnia	Most common sleep disorder after traumatic brain injury (TBI), characterized by poor sleep quantity or quality in the forms of delayed sleep onset, nocturnal awakenings with difficulty returning to sleep, waking too early, and not feeling rested despite adequate sleep hours. Cognitive behavioral therapy (CBT) may be effective.
Obstructive Sleep Apnea	Obstructive sleep apnea and central sleep apnea are reported more frequently in individuals after TBI than in the general population.[13] Treatment includes continuous (CPAP) or bilevel positive airway pressure (BiPAP), mandibular advancement devices, surgical approaches to the proximal airway, and conservative treatments such as weight loss and body positioning during sleep.
Narcolepsy	Involves daytime sleepiness, cataplexy (episodic loss of muscle function), hypnagogic hallucinations (dreamlike experiences while falling asleep, dozing, or awakening), and sleep paralysis (inability to move on awakening). Multiple sleep latency test (MSLT) can show sleep latency sooner than normal subjects and presence of naps containing rapid eye movement (REM) sleep.
Hypersomnia (aka Pleiosomnia)	Increased need for sleep. TBI patients often require more sleep than healthy controls, correlating with TBI severity.
Circadian Rhythm Sleep Disorders	Disruption of normal 24-hour cycle of body patterns such as body temperature and melatonin secretion.
Excessive Daytime Sleepiness (EDS)	Daily episodes of irrepressible need to sleep or unintentional lapses into sleep at potentially inappropriate times, including during sedentary activities.[13] Often accompanied by a shorter period to fall asleep on the MSLT.

Management

- Pharmacological interventions for insomnia
  - Melatonin and melatonin agonists (ramelteon)
  - Tricyclic antidepressants: Can treat neuropathic pain; also used for posttraumatic headaches and may help with insomnia caused by sedating effect
  - Hypnotics including zolpidem, zopiclone, eszopiclone, zaleplon
  - Benzodiazepines: Rarely used secondary to dependency; shown to reduce REM sleep percentage[10]
  - Trazodone
  - Mirtazapine
- Caution in older adults with all sedating medications, which can increase risk of falls at night
- Neurostimulants
  - Modafinil is recommended for use in patients with narcolepsy and those with obstructive sleep apnea.

- Bright light therapy
  - Exposing a person to a source of bright light (>10,000 lux) for greater than 20 minutes daily to help promote improved circadian rhythm and decreased daytime sleepiness
- Psychological interventions
  - CBT – Studies in patients with insomnia show it can improve both nocturnal sleep quality and reduce daytime fatigue.[10] Includes:
  - Stimulus control: reassociating the bed with rest and relaxation rather than anxiety
  - Sleep restriction: limiting the time spent in bed to the actual time spent sleeping versus the time spent trying to fall asleep – assessed by sleep diary
  - Cognitive restructuring of thoughts about sleep
    - Sleep hygiene education: improving lifestyle factors and environmental factors

Review Questions

1. Which of these sleep stages is associated with sleep spindles and K complexes on electroencephalogram (EEG)?
   a. N1
   b. N2
   c. N3
   d. REM
2. Which of these is correct regarding the Barrow Neurologic Institute Fatigue Scale (BNI Fatigue Scale)?
   a. It is a 27-point scale measuring fatigue.
   b. It is primarily designed for use early after injury and in acute rehabilitation.

   c. It is used commonly in the outpatient setting.
   d. It is used during evaluation for a sleep study.
3. Which of these medications has been shown to help treat fatigue specifically after traumatic brain injury (TBI)?
   a. Methylphenidate
   b. Modafinil
   c. Amantadine
   d. Atomoxetine

Answers on page 397.
Access the full list of questions and answers online.
Available on ExpertConsult.com

References

1. Englander J, Bushnik T, Oggins J, Katznelson L. Fatigue after traumatic brain injury: association with neuroendocrine, sleep, depression and other factors. *Brain Inj.* 2010;24(12):1379-1388.
2. Cantor JB, Ashman T, Gordon W, et al. Fatigue after traumatic brain injury and its impact on participation and quality of life. *J Head Trauma Rehabil.* 2008;23(1):41-51.
3. Mollayeva T. A systematic review of fatigue in patients with traumatic brain injury: the course, predictors and consequences. *Neurosci Biobehav Rev.* 2014;47:684-716.
4. Zasler ND, Katz DI, Zafonte RD. *Brain Injury Medicine: Principles and Practice.* 2nd ed. New York, NY: Demos Medical Publishing; 2013.
5. Cantor JB, Ashman T, Bushnik T, et al. Systematic review of interventions for fatigue after traumatic brain injury: a NIDRR traumatic brain injury model systems study. *J Head Trauma Rehabil.* 2014;29(6):490-497.
6. Jha A, Weintraub A, Allshouse A, et al. A randomized trial of modafinil for the treatment of fatigue and excessive daytime sleepiness in individuals with chronic traumatic brain injury. *J Head Trauma Rehabil.* 2008;23(1):52-63.
7. Theadom A, Cropley M, Parmar P, et al. Sleep difficulties one year following mild traumatic brain injury in a population-based study. *Sleep Med.* 2015;16:926.
8. Nakase-Richardson R, Sherer M, Barnett SD, et al. Prospective evaluation of the nature, course, and impact of acute sleep abnormality after traumatic brain injury. *Arch Phys Med Rehabil.* 2013;94:875.
9. Patel AK, Araujo JF. Physiology, sleep stages. [Updated 2018 Oct 27]. In: *StatPearls* [Internet]. Treasure Island, FL: StatPearls Publishing; 2018. https://www.ncbi.nlm.nih.gov/books/NBK526132/ Date of Access: 04/01/2020
10. Viola-Saltzman M, Watson NF. Traumatic brain injury and sleep disorders. *Neurol Clin.* 2012;30(4):1299-1312. doi:10.1016/j.ncl.2012.08.008.
11. Mathias JL, Alvaro PK. Prevalence of sleep disturbances, disorders, and problems following traumatic brain injury: a meta-analysis. *Sleep Med.* 2012;13:898.
12. Baumann CR, Bassetti CL, Valko PO, et al. Loss of hypocretin (orexin) neurons with traumatic brain injury. *Ann Neurol.* 2009;66:555.
13. Sandsmark DK. Sleep-wake disturbances after traumatic brain injury: synthesis of human and animal studies. *Sleep.* 2017;40(5). doi:10.1093/sleep/zsx044.

38

Mood and Anxiety Disorders

NAZANIN BAHRAINI, PHD, SUZANNE MCGARITY, PHD, AND HAL S. WORTZEL, MD

OUTLINE

Epidemiology

Etiology

Evaluation

    Diagnostic Criteria

    Differential Diagnosis

    Screening and Assessment

Intervention

    Pharmacological Interventions

    Psychological Interventions

Traumatic brain injury (TBI) results in an increased risk for psychiatric illness, including mood and anxiety disorders, substance abuse, sleep disorders, and psychosis.[1-4] As in the general population, mood disorders are most common, with depression being the most prevalent psychiatric disorder after TBI. Risk for depression spans the range of TBI severity. Anxiety disorders are also common and frequently coexist with depression.[2,5] Studies show that individuals with TBI experience all variants of anxiety disorders, including generalized anxiety disorder (GAD), panic disorder, specific phobias, and obsessive–compulsive disorder, with GAD being the most commonly reported anxiety disorder after TBI.[6-7]

Depression and anxiety are associated with greater cognitive and functional impairment and can complicate recovery and increase TBI-related disability.[7-10] Thus, timely identification and treatment of these disorders after TBI is critical to improving outcomes and psychosocial functioning.

In this chapter, we review prevalence, etiology, evaluation, and treatment of posttraumatic depression (PTD) and GAD, the two most common psychiatric disorders after TBI. Posttraumatic stress disorder (PTSD) is no longer classified as an anxiety disorder according to the *Diagnostic and Statistical Manual of Mental Disorders, fifth edition* (DSM-5),[11] and is covered separately in Chapter 39.

Epidemiology

Previous studies on psychiatric outcomes after TBI feature considerable variability in prevalence of depression and anxiety disorders in the months and years postinjury, with prevalence rates of anxiety as high as 70% and rates of depressive disorders ranging from 25% to 50%.[1-3] Methodological differences (e.g., study design, measures, injury severity classification, follow-up period) have contributed to variable findings regarding the prevalence of depression and anxiety after TBI. Longitudinal or prospective studies of depression and anxiety after TBI have mostly been limited to the first year postinjury but are generally methodologically more rigorous and valid, particularly when structured diagnostic interviews are employed. Some studies with longer follow-up periods have shown elevated rates of mood and anxiety disorders that increase in the first year postinjury and gradually decline over the next few years.[4] Other investigations suggest that psychiatric disorders may continue to emerge after the first year postinjury.[2-3,12]

Preinjury anxiety, depression, and substance abuse represent the most robust risk factors for postinjury depression and anxiety.[1-2,4] Unemployment and unstable employment are also risk factors for depression.[13,14] Some research suggests that a history of TBI may increase the risk of depression and anxiety, perhaps as a consequence of cumulative damage from multiple TBIs.[15-17]

Etiology

There are numerous mechanisms whereby depression and anxiety may develop after TBI. Biological mechanisms and psychosocial and adjustment-related mechanisms may all play a role. Psychosocial factors may serve as stronger determinants of depression, especially as time since injury progresses.[18-20] Biological or organic changes associated with TBI may also contribute to increased risk of mood and anxiety disorders. Focal and diffuse injuries to prefrontal and limbic circuits that regulate emotions may cause or contribute to increased risk for depression and anxiety.[21]

TABLE 38.1	*Diagnostic and Statistical Manual of Mental Disorders*, Fifth Edition (DSM-5) Symptom Criteria for Major Depression[11]	
Symptom Criterion (Symptoms most helpful in differentiating depressed and nondepressed persons with traumatic brain injury [TBI] are noted with a checkmark)		
1. **Depressed mood** most of the day, nearly every day. In persons with TBI, this may manifest as irritability, frustration, anger, and aggression versus sadness, feeling blue, or tearfulness		✓
2. **Decreased interest or pleasure** in most activities, most of the day, nearly every day		✓
3. **Significant weight change or change in appetite** nearly every day.		
4. **Sleep disturbance** (insomnia or hypersomnia)		
5. **Psychomotor retardation or agitation** (observable by others, not merely subjective feelings of restlessness or being slowed down)		
6. **Fatigue** or loss of energy nearly every day		
7. **Feelings of worthlessness** or excessive or inappropriate guilt nearly every day		✓
8. **Diminished ability to think or concentrate**, or indecisiveness, nearly every day		
9. **Recurrent thoughts of death**, recurrent suicidal ideation without a specific plan, or a suicide attempt or a specific plan for committing suicide		✓

Evaluation

Diagnostic Criteria

The DSM-5[11] provides the current criteria for diagnosing major depression and GAD. For a diagnosis of major depression, the individual must be experiencing five or more symptoms listed in Table 38.1 during the same 2-week period, and at least one of the symptoms should be either depressed mood or loss of interest or pleasure. GAD shares some features and symptoms with depression but is largely characterized by excessive anxiety and worry about a number of events or activities, occurring more days than not for at least 6 months. The individual finds it difficult to control worry and anxiety that is associated with at least three of the symptoms listed in Table 38.2. In addition, for a diagnosis of major depression and GAD, the symptoms must cause the individual clinically significant distress or impairment in important areas of functioning, and they must also not be a result of substance abuse or another medical condition.

Differential Diagnosis

Depression, anxiety, and other TBI-related sequelae share many common symptoms, including fatigue, irritability, poor concentration, and sleep disturbance, making differential diagnosis difficult. Current evidence indicates that organic TBI-related sequelae that overlap with depressive symptoms do not contribute to significant false-positive diagnoses of depression among those with TBI.[22] As shown in Table 38.2, symptoms such as feelings of hopelessness and worthlessness and difficulty enjoying activities may be most helpful in differentiating those who are depressed

TABLE 38.2	Diagnostic and Statistical Manual of Mental Disorders, Fifth Edition (DSM-5) Symptom Criteria for Generalized Anxiety Disorder[11]
Symptom Criterion	

1. **Excessive anxiety or worry** about a number of events or activities occurring more days than not
2. **Difficulty controlling the worry**
3. **Anxiety or worry associated with three or more of these symptoms:**
   - Restlessness, feeling keyed up or on edge
   - Easily fatigued
   - Difficulty concentrating or mind going blank
   - Irritability
   - Muscle tension
   - Sleep disturbance (difficulty falling or staying asleep)

from those who may be experiencing other affective and somatic sequelae after TBI.[22-23]

Other psychiatric conditions commonly associated with TBI, such as apathy, anxiety, emotional lability, and dysregulation, also require careful clinical consideration when making a differential diagnosis. As outlined in Table 38.3, Seel et al.[22] highlighted overlapping and differentiating features of depression and other common neuropsychiatric sequelae of TBI (e.g., anxiety, apathy, and emotional dysregulation) that may be helpful to keep in mind when evaluating individuals with TBI for these conditions.

Screening and Assessment

Depression and anxiety—and psychiatric disorders in general—are frequently underdiagnosed and undertreated in persons with TBI, making early identification and management of these conditions paramount. Screening and

TABLE 38.3	Overlapping and Differential Features of Common Neuropsychiatric Sequelae of Traumatic Brain Injury			
Feature	Depression	Anxiety	Apathy	Emotional Dysregulation
Mood	Sad, irritable, frustrated	Worried, distressed	Flat, lacks emotion	Frustrated, angry, tense
Activity Level	Low energy and activity	Restless, edgy	Lack of energy, initiative, activity	Impulsive
Physiological	Underaroused	Hyperaroused	Underaroused	Fluctuating arousal
Attitude	Loss of interest, pleasure	Overconcerned	Loss of interest, goals	Argumentative
Awareness	Overestimates problems	Overestimates problems	Underestimates problems	Underestimates problems
Cognitions	Rumination, focuses on loss, failure	Rumination, focuses on harm, danger	Lack concern about failure	Rumination
Coping Style	Active avoidance, social withdrawal	Active avoidance	Dependent, compliant	Uncontrolled outbursts

Adapted from Seel et al.[22]

TABLE 38.4	Recommended Measures for Screening and Assessment of Depression and Anxiety in Persons with Traumatic Brain Injury	
Measure	Purpose	Description
Structured Clinical Interview for Diagnostic and Statistical Manual of Mental Disorders, Fifth Edition (DSM-5) Disorders (SCID–5)[28-29]	Diagnostic	Semistructured interview guide for making major DSM-5 diagnoses; administered by a clinician or trained mental health professional who is familiar with the DSM-5 classification and diagnostic criteria
Patient Health Questionnaire-9 (PHQ-9)[30-31]	Screening; symptom monitoring	Nine-item self-report measure of depression severity based on DSM-5 symptom criteria for depression; completed in 5 minutes; minimal training required
Beck Depression Inventory-II (BDI-II)[32-33]	Screening; symptom monitoring	21-item self-report measure of depression severity based on the DSM-5 symptom criteria for depression; completed in 5–10 minutes; minimal training required
Neurobehavioral Functioning Inventory (NFI) Depression Scale[34-35]	Screening; symptom monitoring	13-item self-report measure of frequency of depressive symptoms; completed in 5–10 minutes; minimal training required
Generalized Anxiety Disorder-7 (GAD-7)[36]	Screening; symptom monitoring	7-item self-report measure of anxiety severity based on DSM-5 symptom criteria for GAD; completed in 5 minutes; minimal training required
Brief Symptom Inventory-18 Item (BSI-18)[37-38]	Screening; symptom monitoring	18-item screen of psychological distress with a Global Severity Index (GSI), and three clinical subscales: somatization, anxiety, and depression; completed in 5 minutes; interpretation requires doctoral-level training in psychology

assessment of depression and anxiety can be enhanced by using psychometrically sound measures. Suggested measures for these purposes are listed in Table 38.4. Screening for these conditions should be a standard component of TBI assessment. Among those who screen positive, structured diagnostic interviews are the gold standard for diagnosis.

Self-report measures of symptoms should not be used as standalone tools for diagnostic purposes because they have limited usefulness in terms of differential diagnosis and may contribute to symptom misattribution. But when used as screening measures or in concert with diagnostic interviews or other clinician-administered assessments, self-report measures of symptoms may offer further insight into areas that patients perceive as most problematic. Individuals with depression and anxiety may overestimate the level of impairment and difficulties.[24] Thus it is prudent to take both self-report and objective measures of functioning into account when evaluating persons with anxiety and depression. Gathering information from reliable collateral sources (e.g., family members or caregivers) may provide for a more accurate depiction of the patient's functional status. Last, given the increased risk of suicide among those with TBI, screening for suicidal ideation may also be warranted.[25-27]

Intervention

There is no single gold standard for treating depression or anxiety after TBI. There is, however, growing recognition that identifying subgroups of patients who share similar risk factors, symptom clusters, and symptom trajectories may allow for more tailored and effective treatment. In the next sections are pharmacological and psychotherapeutic approaches that enjoy the best evidentiary support. More research is needed to identify specific patient subgroups who may have differential responses to these treatments, however.

Pharmacological Interventions

Antidepressant medications have shown mixed results for treating post-TBI depression.
- Selective serotonin reuptake inhibitors (SSRIs: sertraline, fluoxetine, and citalopram) remain one of the most evidence-based approaches to treating posttraumatic depression and anxiety.[39-40]
  - SSRIs are first-line pharmaceutical treatment because of their broad impact on mood, irritability and anger; anxiolytic properties; and generally favorable tolerability.
  - Sertraline has shown favorable results on both depressive and anxiety symptoms and quality of life[41-43] and has low potential for significant drug interactions. Moreover, there is some evidence indicating that sertraline may be effective in preventing posttraumatic depression.[44]
- Other classes of medications, including serotonin-norepinephrine reuptake inhibitors (SNRIs) and tricyclic antidepressants (TCAs), are less well studied.
  - Although these other classes of medications have shown some favorable outcomes in treating depression and may also have a positive impact on pain and anxiety, the tolerability and safety of these medications is less certain, leading most experts to regard them as second-line pharmacotherapies for depression after TBI.[21]

Like most pharmacological options, patients with TBI may experience side effects with antidepressants, including nausea, headaches, sedation, and insomnia.
- Cognitive deficits associated with TBI can also be exacerbated by anticholinergic effects of some SSRIs (e.g., paroxetine).
- Other antidepressants (e.g., bupropion) may lower the seizure threshold and thereby increase risk of seizures after TBI.

- Benzodiazepines, although widely used in the community to treat anxiety disorders, tend to exacerbate common problems caused by TBI (e.g., cognitive impairment, fatigue) and are generally best avoided.

Especially for patients with more severe TBI, careful titration (start low, go slow) and monitoring effects of medication (including treatment response and side effects) are recommended. Other general pharmacological considerations for individuals with TBI are found in Chapter 59. Electroconvulsive therapy may be considered to treat depression among individuals with TBI who fail to respond adequately to other interventions.[21,45]

Psychological Interventions

Cognitive behavioral therapy (CBT) approaches are the first line of treatment for persons with depression and anxiety disorders with or without TBI. There is a growing body of evidence supporting the efficacy of CBT-based interventions for treating depression,[40,46-48] anxiety,[47,49] and hopelessness[50-51] in those with TBI. Problem-solving therapy (PST), especially when paired with goal attainment, may be particularly helpful in those with TBI given that impairment in problem solving is a core aspect of executive dysfunction (ED), and deficits in ED and psychiatric disorders are often mutually exacerbating.

Other behavioral interventions, such as behavioral activation training (BAT), even in simple forms such as activity scheduling and overcoming avoidance, have also shown favorable outcomes for treating depression among those with TBI. Behavioral activation may be especially helpful for improving mood and anxiety in individuals with significant cognitive impairments, which may preclude the effective use of cognitive techniques such as identifying and challenging negative thoughts.[48,52] Third-wave CBT therapies, such as mindfulness-based cognitive therapy (MBCT), are also showing potential for treatment of depression in those with moderate to severe TBI, but more research is needed.[53] Most of these interventions have focused primarily on depressive symptoms, and there is generally less research to guide psychological interventions for GAD and other anxiety disorders after TBI.

TBI-related cognitive impairments in domains such as memory, verbal communication, attention, abstract thinking, and self-awareness can impose significant barriers to the effective delivery of psychotherapeutic interventions. Modifications to psychotherapeutic interventions under such circumstances are necessary and appropriate. Common accommodations include writing down key points from the session, speaking slowly in short sentences, repetition, breaking down content into shorter segments, and appropriate pacing to prevent fatigue.

Overall, decisions about which therapeutic approach to use (e.g., CBT, PST, BAT) largely depends on patient presentation, and therapists should tailor therapy approaches to the cognitive and physical limitations of patients.

Review Questions

1. Which of these factors is most strongly associated with increased risk for posttraumatic brain injury (TBI) depression and anxiety?
   a. Age
   b. Injury severity
   c. Preinjury psychiatric history
   d. Education level

2. Determinants of depression and anxiety may include all of these *except*
   a. focal injuries to prefrontal regions.
   b. diffuse axonal injuries to prefrontal or limbic circuits.
   c. difficulty adjusting to disability.
   d. age at injury.

3. For a diagnosis of major depression, the individual must be experiencing five or more symptoms during the same 2-week period and at least one of the symptoms should be either depressed mood or
   a. sleep disturbance.
   b. decreased interest or pleasure in most activities.
   c. fatigue.
   d. recurrent thoughts of death.

Answers on page 397.
Access the full list of questions and answers online. Available on ExpertConsult.com

References

1. Fann JR, Burington B, Leonetti A, Jaffe K, Katon WJ, Thompson RS. Psychiatric illness following traumatic brain injury in an adult health maintenance organization population. *Arch Gen Psychiatry.* 2004;61(1):53.

2. Gould KR, Ponsford JL, Johnston L, Schönberger M. The nature, frequency and course of psychiatric disorders in the first year after traumatic brain injury: a prospective study. *Psychol Med.* 2011;41(10):2099-2109.

3. Scholten AC, Haagsma JA, Cnossen MC, Olff M, Beeck EFV, Polinder S. Prevalence of and risk factors for anxiety and depressive disorders after traumatic brain injury: a systematic review. *J Neurotrauma.* 2016;33(22):1969-1994.

4. Alway Y, Gould KR, Johnston L, Mckenzie D, Ponsford J. A prospective examination of Axis I psychiatric disorders in the first 5 years following moderate to severe traumatic brain injury. *Psychol Med.* 2016;46(06):1331-1341.

5. Jorge RE, Robinson RG, Moser D, Tateno A, Crespo-Facorro B, Arndt S. Major depression following traumatic brain injury. *Arch Gen Psychiatry.* 2004;61(1):42. doi:10.1001/archpsyc.61.1.42.

6. Whelan-Goodinson R, Ponsford J, Johnston L, Grant F. Psychiatric disorders following traumatic brain injury: their nature and frequency. *J Head Trauma Rehabil.* 2009;24(5):324-332.

7. Diaz AP, Schwarzbold ML, Thais ME, et al. Psychiatric disorders and health-related quality of life after severe traumatic brain injury: a prospective study. *J Neurotrauma.* 2012;29(6):1029-1037.

8. Hibbard MR, Ashman TA, Spielman LA, Chun D, Charatz HJ, Melvin S. Relationship between depression and psychosocial functioning after traumatic brain injury. *Arch Phys Med Rehabil.* 2004;4(2).

9. Hart T, Brenner L, Clark A, et al. Major and minor depression after traumatic brain injury. *Arch Phys Med Rehabil.* 2011;92:1211-1219.

10. Haagsma JA, Scholten AC, Andriessen TM, Vos PE, Beeck EFV, Polinder S. Impact of depression and post-traumatic stress disorder on functional outcome and health-related quality of life of patients with mild traumatic brain injury. *J Neurotrauma.* 2015;32(11):853-862.

11. *Diagnostic and Statistical Manual of Mental Disorders: DSM-5.* Arlington, VA: American Psychiatric Association; 2013.

12. Hart T, Hoffman JM, Pretz C, Kennedy R, Clark AN, Brenner LA. A longitudinal study of major and minor depression following traumatic brain injury. *Arch Phys Med Rehabil.* 2012;93(8):1343-1349.

13. Seel RT, Kreutzer JS, Rosenthal M, et al. Depression after traumatic brain injury: A NIDRR model systems multi-center investigation. *Neurorehabilitation.* 2010;27(1):73-81.

14. Dikmen SS, Bombardier CH, Machamer JE, Fann JR, Temkin NR. Natural history of depression in traumatic brain injury. *Arch Phys Med Rehabi.* 2004;85(9).

15. Kerr ZY, Marshall SW, Harding HP, Guskiewicz KM. Nine-year risk of depression diagnosis increases with increasing self-reported concussions in retired professional football players. *Am J Sports Med.* 2012;40(10):2206-2212.

16. Dams-Oconnor K, Spielman L, Singh A, et al. The impact of previous traumatic brain injury on health and functioning: a TRACK-TBI study. *J Neurotrauma.* 2013;30(24):2014-2020.

17. Corrigan JD, Bogner J, Mellick D, et al. Prior history of traumatic brain injury among persons in the traumatic brain injury model systems national database. *Arch Phys Med Rehabil.* 2013;94(10):1940-1950.

18. Gomez-Hernandez R, Max JE, Kosier T, Paradiso S, Robinson RG. Social impairment and depression after traumatic brain injury. *Arch Phys Med Rehabil.* 1997;78(12):1321-1326.

19. Hoofien D, Gilboa A, Vaki E. Traumatic brain injury (TBI) 10-20 years later: a comprehensive outcome study of psychiatric symptomatology, cognitive abilities and psychosocial functioning. *Brain Inj.* 2001;15(3):189-209.

20. Jorge RE, Robinson RG, Arndt SV, Forrester AW, Geisler F, Starkstein SE. Comparison between acute- and delayed-onset depression following traumatic brain injury. *J Neuropsychiatry Clin Neurosci.* 1993;5(1):43-49.

21. Jorge RE, Arciniegas DB. Mood disorders after TBI. *Psychiatr Clin North Am.* 2014;37(1):13-29.

22. Seel RT, Macciocchi S, Kreutzer JS. Clinical considerations for the diagnosis of major depression after moderate to severe TBI. *J Head Trauma Rehabil.* 2010;25(2):99-112.

23. Kaelin D, Katz D, Kreutzer J, Macciocchi S, Seel R. Diagnosing major depression following moderate to severe traumatic brain injury—evidence-based recommendations for clinicians. *US Neurology.* 2010;06(02):41-47.

24. Fann J, Katon W, Uomoto J, Esselman P. Psychiatric disorders and functional disability in outpatients with traumatic brain injuries. *Am J Psychiatry.* 1995;152(10):1493-1499. doi:10.1176/ajp.152.10.1493.

25. Bahraini NH, Simpson GK, Brenner LA, Hoffberg AS, Schneider AL. Suicidal ideation and behaviours after traumatic brain injury: a systematic review. *Brain Impairment.* 2013;14(01):92-112.

26. Fralick M, Sy E, Hassan A, Burke MJ, Mostofsky E, Karsies T. Association of concussion with the risk of suicide. *JAMA Neurology.* 2019;76(2):144-151.

27. Brenner LA, Bahraini NH. Concussion and risk of suicide: who, when and under what circumstances? *Nat Rev Neurol* 15, 132–133 (2019).

28. First MB, Williams JBW, Karg RS, Spitzer RL. *Structured Clinical Interview for DSM-5 Disorders, Clinician Version (SCID-5-CV)*. Arlington, VA: American Psychiatric Association; 2016.

29. Kennedy RE, Livingston L, Riddick A, Marwitz JH, Kreutzer JS, Zasler ND. Evaluation of the neurobehavioral functioning inventory as a depression screening tool after traumatic brain injury. *J Head Trauma Rehabil.* 2005;20(6):512-526.

30. Kroenke K, Spitzer RL, Williams JB. The PHQ-9: validity of a brief depression severity measure. *J Gen Intern Med.* 2001;16(9):606-613.

31. Fann JR, Bombardier CH, Dikmen S, et al. validity of the patient health questionnaire-9 in assessing depression following traumatic brain injury. *J Head Trauma Rehabil.* 2005;20(6):501-511.

32. Beck AT, Steer RA, Brown GK. *Manual for the Beck Depression Inventory-II*. San Antonio, TX: Psychological Corporation; 1996.

33. Homaifar BY, Brenner LA, Gutierrez PM, et al. Sensitivity and specificity of the beck depression inventory-II in persons with traumatic brain injury. *Arch Phys Med Rehabil.* 2009;90(4):652-656.

34. Seel RT, Kreutzer JS. Depression assessment after traumatic brain injury: an empirically based classification method. *Arch Phys Med Rehabil.* 2003;84(11):1621-1628.

35. Czuba KJ, Kersten P, Kayes NM, et al. Measuring neurobehavioral functioning in people with traumatic brain injury: Rasch analysis of neurobehavioral functioning inventory. *J Head Trauma Rehabil.* 2016;31(4):E59-E68.

36. Hart T, Fann JR, Chervoneva I, et al. Prevalence, risk factors, and correlates of anxiety at 1 year after moderate to severe traumatic brain injury. *Arch Phys Med Rehabil.* 2016;97(5):701-707.

37. Lancaster MA, Mccrea MA, Nelson LD. Psychometric properties and normative data for the Brief Symptom Inventory-18 (BSI-18) in high school and collegiate athletes. *Clin Neuropsychol.* 2016;30(2):338-350.

38. Meachen S-J, Hanks RA, Millis SR, Rapport LJ. The reliability and validity of the brief symptom inventory−18 in persons with traumatic brain injury. *Arch Phys Med Rehabil.* 2008;89(5):958-965.

39. Salter KL, Andrew MJ, Foley NC, Sequeira K, Teasell RW. Pharmacotherapy for depression posttraumatic brain injury: a meta-analysis. *J Head Trauma Rehabil.* 2016;31(4): E21-E32.

40. Fann JR, Hart T, Schomer KG. Treatment for depression after traumatic brain injury: a systematic review. *J Neurotrauma.* 2009;26(12):2383-2402.

41. Vattakatuchery J, Lathif N, Joy J, Cavanna A, Rickards H. Pharmacological interventions for depression in people with traumatic brain injury: systematic review. *J Neurol Neurosurg Psychiatry.* 2014;85:e3.

42. Ashman TA, Cantor JB, Gordon WA, et al. A randomized controlled trial of sertraline for the treatment of depression in persons with traumatic brain injury. *Arch Phys Med Rehabil.* 2009;90(5):733-740.

43. Turner-Stokes L, Hassan N, Pierce K, Clegg F. Managing depression in brain injury rehabilitation: the use of an integrated care pathway and preliminary report of response to sertraline. *Clin Rehabil.* 2002;16(3):261-268.

44. Jorge RE, Acion L, Burin DI, Robinson RG. Sertraline for preventing mood disorders following traumatic brain injury. *JAMA Psychiatry.* 2016;73(10):1041-1047.

45. Martino C, Krysko M, Petrides G, Tobias KG, Kellner CH. Cognitive tolerability of electroconvulsive therapy in a patient with a history of traumatic brain injury. *J ECT.* 2008;24(1):92-95.

46. Ashman T, Cantor JB, Tsaousides T, Spielman L, Gordon W. Comparison of cognitive behavioral therapy and supportive psychotherapy for the treatment of depression following traumatic brain injury: a randomized controlled trial. *J Head Trauma Rehabil.* 2014;29(6):467-478.

47. Ponsford J, Lee NK, Wong D, et al. Efficacy of motivational interviewing and cognitive behavioral therapy for anxiety and depression symptoms following traumatic brain injury. *Psychol Med.* 2016;46(05):1079-1090.

48. Fann JR, Bombardier CH, Vannoy S, et al. Telephone and in-person cognitive behavioral therapy for major depression after traumatic brain injury: a randomized controlled trial. *J Neurotrauma.* 2015;32(1):45-57.

49. Soo C, Tate RL. Psychological treatment for anxiety in people with traumatic brain injury. *Cochrane Database Syst Rev.* 2007 Issue 3. Art. No.: CD005239. DOI: 10.1002/14651858.CD005239.pub2.

50. Brenner LA, Forster JE, Hoffberg AS, et al. Window to hope: a randomized controlled trial of a psychological intervention for the treatment of hopelessness among veterans with moderate to severe traumatic brain injury. *J Head Trauma Rehabil.* 2018;33(2):E64-E73.

51. Simpson GK, Tate RL, Whiting DL, Cotter RE. Suicide prevention after traumatic brain injury: a randomized controlled trial of a program for the psychological treatment of hopelessness. *J Head Trauma Rehabil.* 2011;26(4):290-300.

52. Juengst SB, Kumar RG, Wagner AK. A narrative literature review of depression following traumatic brain injury: prevalence, impact, and management challenges. *Psychol Res Behav Manag.* 2017;10:175-186.

53. Bedard M, Felteau M, Marshall S, et al. Mindfulness-based cognitive therapy: benefits in reducing depression following a traumatic brain injury. *Adv Mind-Body Med.* 2012;26(1):14-20.

39

Posttraumatic Stress Disorder

DOUGLAS B. COOPER, PHD, CHRISTOPHER TICKNOR, MD, AND JAN KENNEDY, PHD

Posttraumatic stress disorder (PTSD) is a psychiatric disorder that occurs in individuals who have experienced or witnessed a traumatic event, such as a:

- Serious accident
- Sexual assault
- Combat/war experience
- Natural disaster
- Terrorism act

It is a frequent psychiatric comorbidity in individuals with traumatic brain injuries (TBIs), especially in combat-exposed service members and veterans. It has received considerable attention after the conflicts in Iraq (Operation Iraqi Freedom [OIF]) and Afghanistan (Operation Enduring Freedom [OEF]), and together, PTSD and TBI have been termed the *signature wounds* of these conflicts. PTSD appears to be an important mediator of poor outcomes and negative sequalae after TBI. Diagnosis and treatment of PTSD after TBI can be challenging because of the overlap of core symptoms of these two conditions.

History of Posttraumatic Stress Disorder

Extreme emotional reactions to traumatic events involving bodily harm or death have been noted throughout recorded history. Battle trauma and flashback-like dreams were described by Hippocrates (460–377 BCE). During World War I, the term *shell shock* was used to describe symptoms believed to be caused by the effects of direct cerebral trauma. However, many soldiers without evidence of head trauma presented with shell shock symptoms, leading to a controversy as to whether symptoms were neurogenic or psychogenic.

Up to as recently as World War II and the Vietnam War, understanding of this phenomenon was lacking, and stigma associated with PTSD continued. Although the most recognized setting for this reaction was in combat, similar reactions were noted among individuals exposed to other types of trauma. This realization lead to the current conceptualization of PTSD as a human response to psychologically overwhelming trauma. PTSD was first officially recognized as a disorder in 1980 in the third edition of the *Diagnostic and Statistical Manual of Mental Disorders* (DSM-III). It was classified as an anxiety disorder in DSM-III and DSM-IV and moved to a new category, trauma and stressor related disorders, with the release of DSM-5 in 2013.

Posttraumatic Stress Disorder Prevalence

The lifetime prevalence of PTSD is around 6.8% among adults in the United States. Women's lifetime risk for PTSD is twice that of men. Although exposure to significant stressors such as motor vehicle accidents, natural disasters, rape, and assault is common in civilian populations—with more than 75% reporting a lifetime exposure—only a small percentage of individuals develop PTSD. Risk factors for the development of PTSD include preexisting psychiatric conditions, poor social support, family history of psychiatric conditions, low IQ, and female gender.

Development of PTSD varies significantly based on the type of traumatic experience and individuals are most likely to develop PTSD after exposure to assaultive violence (including sexual assault) and combat. Prevalence rates of PTSD among Vietnam-era veterans range considerably, because most epidemiological data were collected well after the end of the war. Studies of veterans serving in the conflicts in Afghanistan and Iraq have shown a prevalence of PTSD ranging from 10% to 20% in combat-deployed individuals, more than twice the rate in civilian populations.

Comorbidities of Posttraumatic Stress Disorder and Other Psychiatric Disorders

PTSD is highly comorbid with other psychiatric conditions. Approximately 80% of individuals with PTSD have also been diagnosed with one or more additional psychiatric disorders (lifetime rates). Approximately half of people with PTSD also have major depressive disorder (MDD); 40% of those with PTSD have been diagnosed with generalized anxiety disorder. Over 20% of those with PTSD also have a substance use disorder, developed either as a consequence of PTSD or serving as a risk factor for the development of PTSD. Studies have found that 11% to 39% of bipolar patients also meet criteria for PTSD. PTSD is associated with an increased risk for suicide. Among people who have been diagnosed with PTSD at some point in their lifetime, approximately 27% have attempted suicide.

Prevalence of Posttraumatic Stress Disorder in Individuals with Traumatic Brain Injury

Prevalence of PTSD varies depending on the severity of TBI. In a large, multisite prospective study of trauma patients,[1] rates of PTSD at 12 months postinjury were highest for individuals with:
- No TBI (24%)
- Mild TBI (22%)
- Moderate TBI (19%)
- Severe TBI (17%)

It has been argued that rates of PTSD are lower in individuals with moderate to severe TBI because loss of consciousness and/or posttraumatic amnesia interfere with the process of encoding trauma-related memories. In contrast, among those with mild TBI (mTBI), combat-deployed samples[2] have shown an increase in PTSD in service members who experienced mTBI with loss of consciousness (44% with PTSD) versus mTBI with alteration of consciousness (27%) or a nonbrain injury (16%). This finding, which has been replicated in other independent samples, suggests some type of neurochemical or neurobiological change may make an individual with mTBI more susceptible to the subsequent development of PTSD. This finding has also been shown in civilian samples.

Diagnosis of Posttraumatic Stress Disorder

There is no biomarker or laboratory procedure used to diagnose PTSD. A semistructured, clinical interview of specific trauma-related symptoms remains the gold standard. Several self-report measures have been developed and validated for use with individuals who have experienced psychological trauma, although most are best used as screening tools. The diagnostic criteria for posttraumatic stress disorder[3] are detailed in Table 39.1.

Overlap of Posttraumatic Stress Disorder and Traumatic Brain Injury Symptoms

There is a significant overlap of symptoms of PTSD and mTBI, especially in individuals reporting persistent postconcussive symptoms after mTBI. Studies have attempted to identify symptoms that are specific only to

TABLE 39.1 Diagnostic Criteria For Posttraumatic Stress Disorder[3]

Criteria	Description of Symptoms
Severe stressor	Person was exposed to death, threatened death, serious injury, actual or threatened sexual assault/violence through direct exposure, witnessing, indirectly (though a close friend or family member) or repeated indirect exposures in the course of professional duties (e.g., first responders)
Intrusion symptoms (one symptom required)	Recurrent, involuntary, and intrusive memories related to the stressor, including nightmares, flashbacks, and prolonged distress after exposure to trauma-related stimuli
Avoidance behaviors (one symptom required)	Avoidance of situations, external reminders, or thoughts associated with the traumatic experience
Negative alterations in cognition and mood (two symptoms required)	Feelings of guilt, persistent/distorted negative beliefs and expectations about oneself and/or the world, inability to recall key features of a traumatic event, persistent distorted blame of self/others for the event or its consequences, feeling emotionally alienated from others, constricted affect (inability to experience positive emotions), or markedly diminished interest in previously enjoyable activities
Alterations in arousal and Reactivity (two symptoms required)	Experiencing irritability, aggression, self-destructive behaviors, hypervigilance, exaggerated startle response, sleep disturbance, or problems with concentration
Duration	Persistence of symptoms for more than a month (note: delayed onset can occur)
Functional impact	Symptoms must be of sufficient severity to cause functional impairment in social and/or occupational functioning

TABLE 39.2	Overlapping Symptoms of Posttraumatic Stress Disorder (PTSD) and Persistent Postconcussive Symptoms (PCS)		
PTSD	**Both PTSD and PCS**	**PCS**
	Depression	
	Anxiety	
Nightmares/ reexperiencing	Insomnia	Headache[a]
Guilt	Irritability/anger	Sensitivity to light
Shame	Cognitive difficulties	Dizziness[a]
	Fatigue	
	Avoidance	

[a]In highly distressed individuals with PTSD, headaches and dizziness are also frequently reported.

one condition but not the other. However, nearly all symptoms have been shown to occur in individuals with high psychological distress. Table 39.2 should serve as a heuristic only.

Posttraumatic Stress Disorder Interventions

General treatment principles of PTSD suggest that cure is obtainable, but realistically, diminishing symptoms may be a more practical goal. Although primary care providers are often the first to evaluate patients with PTSD, a referral to a mental health professional or therapist is often indicated. Persistent sleep abnormalities are present in more than 60% of people who develop the chronic form of PTSD. Rapid eye movement (REM) sleep has been shown to play a role in maintenance of disturbing, fear-based memories. Nightmares, often considered a hallmark of PTSD, may require a sleep study to evaluate physiological measures of autonomic activity during sleep.

Specific psychotherapy modalities are first-line treatment to help patients with PTSD. Exposure therapy (ET) is thought by many to be the foundation for psychotherapy counseling and the treatment of PTSD. Repeated exposure to processing memories of a traumatic event can desensitize patients to the physiological and behavioral manifestations of PTSD.

Prolonged exposure (PE) therapy teaches patients with PTSD how to gain control over symptoms by facing negative feelings. PE involves talking about trauma with a therapist in confronting and challenging avoidance and other persistent negative behaviors. Cognitive processing therapy (CPT) assists patients in correcting overgeneralizations that danger is ever present and allows patients to establish more control and predictability in routine activities.

Trauma-focused cognitive behavior therapy (TFCBT) assists the patient in reexperiencing a traumatic event through engaging with memories, referred to as *imaginal exposure*. Managing everyday reminders in a therapeutic approach helps patients avoid triggers. Specific modalities to accomplish this are Eye Movement Desensitization and Reprocessing Therapy (EMDR), a process that involves recalling distressing images of the trauma while receiving neurosensory inputs.

Non-TFCBT therapy includes present-centered therapy (PCT) which focuses on real-world relationships and employment challenges rather than the trauma itself.

There is a growing body of literature in OEF/OIF populations that has demonstrated efficacy of ET, CPT, and TFCBT in reducing PTSD symptoms in veterans diagnosed with cooccurring PTSD and mTBI. Less is known about the effectiveness of these treatments with individuals with moderate or severe TBI, although severe memory/cognitive impairments can negatively affect psychotherapeutic treatments.

Pharmacotherapy for Posttraumatic Stress Disorder

The combination of pharmacotherapy with psychotherapeutic intervention is generally more effective for treating PTSD than either intervention alone. Pharmacotherapy research supports the use of short-term and long-term medications, primarily consisting of selective serotonin reuptake inhibitors (SSRIs). Sertraline and paroxetine are approved by the US Food and Drug Administration (FDA) for treating adults with PTSD. Venlafaxine, duloxetine, and atypical antipsychotics such as quetiapine, aripiprazole, and risperidone may assist patients with disorganized thinking and hyperreactivity.

The use of benzodiazepines is generally discouraged because of a lack of scientific evidence supporting their use amid concerns about dependency and withdrawal. Prazosin, an alpha-1 adrenergic antagonist, has demonstrated efficacy for some patients in treating nightmares. Use of trazodone is preferable to benzodiazepines for insomnia. The

TABLE 39.3	Medications and Target Doses Used to Treat Posttraumatic Stress Disorder (PTSD)

Selective Serotonin Reuptake Inhibitors (SSRIs)

Sertraline 100–200 mg daily

Citalopram 20–40 mg daily

Paroxetine 20–40 mg daily

Medications for Nightmares

Prazosin 1–2 mg each night at bedtime

Medications for PTSD-Related Insomnia

Trazodone 50–200 mg each night at bedtime

beta-adrenergic antagonist propranolol can reduce an increased arousal of defensive threat responses that often accompanies the CNS adrenergic overdrive of PTSD symptoms. Propranolol likely reduces traumatic recall in PTSD by indirectly decreasing the memory-enhancing influence of stress hormones such as cortisol and adrenaline.

Patients with PTSD should be screened for comorbid depression, panic disorder, and substance use disorders, including alcohol use disorder. Naltrexone and disulfiram may assist patients in achieving sobriety if alcohol use disorder is a complicating factor. Patients with PTSD should be regularly screened for the development of self-destructive behaviors and/or suicidal ideation. If self-destructive behaviors or suicidal thinking is present, urgent referral to an emergency room or a mental health professional is indicated.

Review Questions

1. What is the estimated prevalence of posttraumatic stress disorder (PTSD) among adults in the United States?
   a. 1%–2%
   b. 2%–4%
   c. 6%–8%
   d. 10%–12%
2. Which factors confer risk for development of PTSD?
   a. Preexisting psychiatric conditions, less than high school education
   b. Age during the trauma, poor social support
   c. Unemployment, family history of psychiatric conditions
   d. Family history of psychiatric conditions, female gender

3. Which comorbid condition is most frequently associated with PTSD?
   a. Bipolar disorder
   b. Major depressive disorder
   c. Generalized anxiety disorder
   d. Substance use disorder

Answers on page 397.
Access the full list of questions and answers online. Available on ExpertConsult.com

References

1. Zatzick DF, Rivara FP, Jurkovich GJ, et al. Multisite investigation of traumatic brain injuries, posttraumatic stress disorder, and self-reported health and cognitive impairments. *Arch Gen Psychiatry*. 2010;67(12):1291-1300.
2. Hoge CW, McGurk D, Thomas JL, Cox AL, Engel CC, Castro CA. Mild traumatic brain injury in U.S. soldiers returning from Iraq. *N Engl J Med*. 2008;358(5):453-463.
3. American Psychiatric Association. *Diagnostic and Statistical Manual of Mental Disorders*. 5th ed. Washington, DC: APA Press; 2013.

40

Behavioral Dyscontrol

SUZANNE MCGARITY, PHD, NAZANIN BAHRAINI, PHD, AND HAL WORTZEL, MD

The term *behavioral dyscontrol* broadly refers to impairment in one's ability to self-regulate behavior in response to either internal or external stimuli, typically yielding actions that are impulsive and contextually inappropriate. Posttraumatic dyscontrol of this type often manifests as disinhibition and aggression. Self-directed violence, including suicidal behavior, may also be considered a form of behavior dyscontrol and is included in the discussion herein. Behavioral dyscontrol may complicate the acute period after traumatic brain injury (TBI) of any severity, although as a chronic sequala, it is more common after moderate to severe TBI. Behavioral dyscontrol creates substantial challenges for patients, providers, and caregivers, often interfering with the provision of optimal treatment and potentially placing patients, providers, and families in harm's way.

In this chapter, we:
1. Review definitions for disinhibition, aggression, and self-directed harm.
2. Provide data on incidence rates.
3. Present key factors in assessment and diagnosis.
4. Review best practices for treatment and management in medical or rehabilitation settings.

Disinhibition

Disinhibition refers to:
- Nonaggressive behavior that is socially inappropriate
- The behavior can be verbal, physical, or sexual behavior
Patients who exhibit disinhibition demonstrate poor ability to:
- Exercise patience
- Contain impulses

- Conform to societal standards and expectations
- Manage frustration effectively

Disinhibited behavior may occur in the context of emotional dysregulation, in which common observable signs may include labile affect, exaggerated emotional responses, or pathological laughing and crying (please refer to Chapter 35 for more information on emotional dyscontrol after brain injury).

The frequency with which various forms of behavioral dyscontrol occur after brain injury is not well established. The applicable literature is complicated by a challenging nosology wherein many terms are used to capture various behaviors. That said, clinical experience indicates that disinhibition is fairly common in the early recovery stages of moderate to severe TBI. The prevalence of disinhibition after moderate to severe TBI has been reported to range from 12% to 32%.[1]

Assessment of disinhibition must account for:
- Cultural considerations
- Presence of painful conditions and associated pain behaviors
- Premorbid personality characteristics
- Other conditions such as mania, psychosis, medications, or substances of abuse that may result in similar types of behaviors

The underlying cause of disinhibited behavior will heavily influence decisions about treatment and management. Assessment of disinhibited behavior can include self-report measures and/or clinician-observation tools. The patient's level of self-awareness and reliable reporting will often determine the best methods for assessment. Assessment may be facilitated with use of the Neuropsychiatric Inventory (NPI) or its clinician administered version (NPI-C), with both versions capturing applicable data in a disinhibition subscale.[2,3]

Treatment and management of posttraumatic disinhibition may include pharmacological, behavioral, and environmental management strategies.

Pharmacotherapy for posttraumatic disinhibition includes:
- First-line agents as selective serotonin reuptake inhibitors (SSRIs)[4]
- Alternative pharmacotherapy options include anticonvulsants, such as valproate, carbamazepine, and lamotrigine[4]

- Antiandrogenic agents have been reported to be effective for reducing disinhibited sexual behavior.[5]
- Atypical antipsychotics warrant consideration when patients do not respond to other approaches.

Environmental safety measures and behavioral strategies commonly incorporate the use of a behavior modification plan.

Behavior modification plans:
- Serve to modify or eliminate the specific dysfunctional behaviors observed in the patient
- Identify internal and external precipitants of the problematic behavior to better inform the use of appropriate behavior modification strategies, such as:
  - Reinforcement of desired behavior (i.e., not engaging in the disinhibited behavior or replacing it with more socially acceptable behavior)
  - Adverse consequences (e.g., not receiving attention) for the undesired behavior
- Are most successful when formulated using patient, clinician, and caregiver feedback
- Require consistency across settings and care providers to ensure successful implementation

Aggression

Once again, epidemiology is complicated by a difficult nosology. The term *aggression* historically has been applied to a broad host of emotional and behavioral problems (e.g., irritability, agitation). More precisely applied, the term *aggression* refers to verbal or behavioral outbursts or physical violence directed either at objects or people in the environment.

Aggression is a fairly common complication during recovery from moderate to severe TBI. Agitation and aggression within the context of the early posttraumatic confusional state may occur in 30% to 80% of patients.[1] During the late postinjury period after nonpenetrating severe TBI, rates of aggression have been reported to range from 15% to 51%.[1] Studies using the NPI to identify agitation/aggression report frequency of chronic posttraumatic aggression at approximately 20%.[1]

Assessment and management of aggression involves carefully attending to:
- Severity of the behavior and impact on others
- Frequency of the behavior
- Differentiation between purposeful and instrumental behavior (i.e., directed at a specific person with effort to obtain a desired outcome) versus reactive and explosive behavior (i.e., involving impulsive actions with no discernable target or identifiable purpose)
- Premorbid psychological factors, such as mood, psychosis, substance use, and personality disorders, which can contribute to an increased incidence of posttraumatic aggression or even be the cause of such behaviors[1]
- Consideration that virtually all behaviors, including aggressive and sexual behaviors, are relevant and adaptive in specific situations, although obviously inappropriate in other contexts

Aggression that occurs in the context of brain injury tends to manifest as impulsive reactions in response to a perceived threat or other unpleasant environmental stimuli (e.g., pain upon dressing change, a stranger assisting with toileting). Aggressive behaviors involving clear targets and discernable objectives should prompt careful consideration in relation to the differential diagnosis and alternative etiologies (i.e., not traumatic injury) for such behaviors.

Anatomically speaking, posttraumatic aggression is most closely associated with injury to the frontal lobes, more specifically the lateral orbitofrontal subcortical circuit (LOFC).[4]

The LOFC:
- Supports social comportment and intelligence, including the ability to determine the contextual appropriateness of any given behavior
- Imparts constraints dictated by social norms and consequences on these impulses, facilitating inhibition of aggression and sexual behaviors when circumstances mandate restraint
- When injured, increases the likelihood of misplaced aggression in response to relatively trivial stimuli[4]

Aggressive behaviors are among the most challenging types of posttraumatic conditions to manage. They pose barriers to effective care and treatment because they often result in disruption of supportive relationships with both providers and caregivers and can pose safety threats for the patient, caregivers, and treatment team. Understanding the etiology of the aggression is of utmost importance in determining how best to manage this type of behavioral dyscontrol. There is no one strategy that will effectively manage aggression for all individuals.

The best approach to managing posttraumatic aggression involves:
- A multidisciplinary and collaborative effort involving both nonpharmacological and pharmacological strategies
- Early response to behavior when first observed so providers and caregivers can work quickly to develop a management plan before social and legal consequences interfere with access to care[6]
- Thoughtful, front-end assessment that describes the nature, frequency, and severity of the behavior to establish a baseline against which subsequent gains (or losses) may be measured
- Once a baseline has been established, a combination of environmental and behavioral techniques are appropriate first-line interventions
- Behavioral analysis and management, including positive and negative reinforcement, self-controlled time outs, and assertiveness training, should be implemented[4]
- Realistic goal setting that aims to reduce the frequency and severity of undesired behaviors is typically more practical than complete elimination, especially in early periods of recovery and rehabilitation after brain injury

Understandable emotional reactions to aggressive behavior may precipitate reactive responses from caretakers and prescribers. This sometimes results in otherwise helpful treatment strategies being abandoned or altered in response to behaviors that are consistent with (or perhaps even relatively improved from) baseline. Systematic collection of quantifiable data can help avoid such countertherapeutic responses and is facilitated by structured assessment such as the Overt Aggression Scale.[7]

The medication management of aggression typically requires discerning between acute and chronic aggression.

- Acute aggression often requires more aggressive interventions to rapidly restore behavioral control and ensure safety.
- Acute aggression may also warrant use of antipsychotics, although these medications are ideally avoided for the purposes of long-term management of persons with TBI.
  - When antipsychotics are warranted, atypical antipsychotics such as quetiapine, olanzapine, and aripiprazole are preferred because of their more favorable side effect profiles, particularly in relation to cognitive and motoric functioning.[4]
  - If atypical agents fail to afford sufficient benefit, haloperidol becomes a reasonable alternative, although it requires monitoring for akathisia and extrapyramidal side effects.
- Benzodiazepines may also be indicated to help control acute aggression. Agents with short- or moderate-duration half-lives and no active metabolites are preferred (e.g., lorazepam).
- When using antipsychotics and benzodiazepines, low and frequent dosing rapidly titrated to effectiveness and/ or sedation is suggested. Agents should be promptly down titrated and discontinued on restoration of behavioral control.[4]

When aggression manifests as a more chronic sequalae of TBI, initial treatment choices are typically directed by comorbid neuropsychiatric conditions. Common target examples include depression, mood lability, psychosis, anxiety, seizures, or pain.

- Aggression cooccurring with depression calls for an antidepressant acting on the serotonin system (e.g. sertraline, escitalopram, or citalopram).
- SSRIs are also the treatment of choice for emotional lability or pathological laughing or crying and anxiety, but buspirone is another reasonable initial option in the setting of anxiety and aggression.[4]
- Anticonvulsants (e.g., carbamazepine and valproic acid) are first-line treatments for aggression that cooccurs with seizures.
- Aggression associated with mania should be managed with mood stabilizers (e.g., valproic acid, carbamazepine, lithium). Lithium does require special consideration because persons with brain injury may have increased susceptibility to neurotoxic side effects. Atypical antipsychotics also may prove helpful in these cases.
- Aggression cooccurring with psychosis calls for an atypical antipsychotic (e.g., quetiapine, olanzapine, or aripiprazole).
- When aggression lacks a clear cooccurring target or other treatments have already been optimized, evidence-based options to target aggression more directly include SSRIs,

amantadine, tricyclic antidepressants, buspirone, methylphenidate, valproate, lithium, and the beta-adrenergic receptor antagonists.[4]

Suicide

Suicide is defined as death because of deliberate, self-directed behavior. *Self-directed violence* (SDV) is a broader term used to encapsulate death by suicide, suicidal behaviors such as preparatory behaviors, suicide attempts, and nonsuicidal self-injurious behaviors such as cutting or burning oneself without the intent to die. Persons with brain injury are at increased risk for self-directed harm, particularly death by suicide, even many years after injury.[8-13]

There are several possible reasons underlying this association:

- The previously described anatomy of aggression is once again applicable, increasing the risk for aggression whether directed outwardly or toward oneself.
- Death by suicide and brain injury share common risk factors such as premorbid psychiatric history and/or substance use disorders, along with demographic factors such as male gender, age, and current or past military service.[8,14,15]
- Persons with brain injury commonly encounter psychosocial stressors such as interpersonal, financial, and legal problems that may increase risk for suicide.[16]

Persons with TBI should be screened for suicide risk during the acute recovery phase, if they are able to engage in the screening process, and as part of ongoing rehabilitative care.

- Screening can include brief standardized instruments that include asking directly about suicidal ideation, such as the Patient Health Questionnaire (PHQ-9), in which Item 9 asks, "Over the last 2 weeks, how often have you been bothered by thoughts that you would be better off dead or of hurting yourself in some way?"[17] Studies have demonstrated predictive utility of Item 9 in determining elevated risk for suicide.[18]
- If patients screen positive for suicide risk, a comprehensive evaluation should follow (i.e., past suicidal behavior, characteristics of current ideation, and intent and relevant risk factors and protective factors).
- Risk should be stratified by temporality and severity (i.e., level of acute risk and chronic risk).[19]
- A management plan for mitigating risk in the current care setting must follow. Examples of management strategies for moderate to high acute risk include transfer to an inpatient psychiatric unit or adjustments to the current care environment such as line-of-site observation and removing sharp objects.

After immediate safety concerns are addressed, providers may consider approaching suicidal thinking and behavior with a combination of both pharmacological and therapeutic interventions. If evidence of thoughts or behavior related to SDV is observed or reported in the context of a diagnosed psychiatric condition, for example, a mood or psychotic disorder, pharmacological management of the underlying condition may be an appropriate first-line approach. Behavioral interventions can help mitigate risk of self-directed harm after brain injury.

Safety planning is an essential component of suicide prevention when working with individuals at increased risk for suicide. The safety plan is developed collaboratively with the patient to identify warning signs that occur at the onset of a crisis and highly personal, individualized coping skills and resources to use both to prevent crises and manage to crises more effectively when they occur.[20] Such plans are especially important for persons with TBI because they often struggle with cognitive deficits that compromise the ability to remember and implement coping strategies in a timely or effective fashion.

Several evidence-based treatments may be effective in reducing risk of death by suicide for persons with TBI.

Evidence-based therapies that have demonstrated reduction of suicide risk include:
- Cognitive therapy for suicide prevention (CT-SP)
- Cognitive behavioral therapy (CBT)

- Dialectical behavioral therapy (DBT)
- Problem-solving therapy (PST)[21]

There are also more recently developed treatments that demonstrate empirical support for reducing suicide risk specifically in brain injury populations.

Examples include:
- Window to Hope (WtoH), an approach that incorporates behavioral activation, cognitive restructuring, problem solving, and relapse prevention
- Problem-Solving Therapy for Suicide Prevention (PST-SP), a brief intervention that focuses on using problem-solving skills and coping strategies to enhance safety planning[24]

Both approaches target hopelessness associated with distress in persons with brain injury. It is recommended that any therapeutic intervention for suicide prevention after brain injury aims to address the common key presenting problems that lead to distress and result in elevated risk: ineffective coping, poor problem solving, social isolation, and a lack of pleasant or rewarding activities.

Review Questions

1. When assessing and diagnosing posttraumatic disinhibition, providers must consider premorbid personality characteristics, pain conditions and pain behaviors, and
   a. Age
   b. Cultural factors
   c. Blood type
   d. Length of posttraumatic amnesia
2. A patient presents with disinhibited behavior involving inappropriate comments to members of the care team about their physical appearance. An appropriate behavior modification plan would include
   a. rewarding a day without such comments with a movie selected by the patient.
   b. designating one provider as the individual who will respond to such comments.

   c. eliminating breaks or free time until the patient no longer makes inappropriate comments.
   d. administering a benzodiazepine whenever comments are observed.
3. Which of these is an appropriate first-line pharmacological treatment for posttraumatic disinhibition?
   a. Carbamazepine
   b. Quetiapine
   c. Electroconvulsive therapy
   d. Sertraline

Answers on page 398.
Access the full list of questions and answers online.
Available on ExpertConsult.com

References

1. Arcinegas DB, Wortzel HS. Emotional and behavioral dyscontrol after TBI. *Psychiatr Clin North Am*. 2014;37:31-53.
2. Cummings JL, Mega M, Gray K, Rosenberg-Thompson S, Carusi DA, Gornbein J. Neuropsychiatric Inventory: comprehensive assessment of psychopathology in dementia. *Neurology*. 1994;44(12):2308-2314.
3. Kaufer DI, Cummings JL, Ketchel P, et al. Validation of the NPI-Q, a brief clinical form of the Neuropsychiatric Inventory. *J Neuropsychiatry Clin Neurosci*. 2000;12(2):233-239.
4. Wortzel HS, Silver JS. Behavioral dyscontrol. In: Silver JM, McAllister TW, Arcinegas DB, eds. *Textbook of Traumatic Brain Injury*. 3rd ed. Washington, DC: American Psychiatric Association Publishing; 2019:395-411.
5. Guay DR. Drug treatment of paraphilic and nonparaphilic sexual disorders. *Clin Ther*. 2009;31(1):1-31.
6. Wortzel HS, Arciniegas DB. A forensic neuropsychiatric approach to traumatic brain injury, aggression, and suicide. *J Am Acad Psychiatry Law*. 2013;41(2):274-286.

7. Yudofsky SC, Silver JM, Jackson W, Endicott J, Williams D. The Overt Aggression Scale for the objective rating of verbal and physical aggression. *Am J Psychiatry*. 1986;143(1):35-39.
8. Brenner LA, Ignacio RV, Blow FC. Suicide and traumatic brain injury among individuals seeking Veterans Health Administration Services. *J Head Trauma Rehabil*. 2011;26(4):257-264.
9. Bahraini NH, Simpson G, Brenner LA, et al. Suicidal ideation and behaviors after traumatic brain injury: a systematic review. *Brain Impair*. 2013;14(suppl 1):92-112.
10. Simpson G, Tate R. Suicidality in people surviving a traumatic brain injury: prevalence, risk factors and implications for clinical management. *Brain Inj*. 2007;21(13-14):1335-1351.
11. Tsaousides T, Cantor JB, Gordon WA. Suicidal ideation following traumatic brain injury: prevalence rates and correlates in adults living in the community. *J Head Trauma Rehabil*. 2011;26(4):265-275.
12. Fisher LB, Pedrelli P, Iverson GL, et al. Prevalence of suicidal behaviour following traumatic brain injury: longitudinal follow-up

data from the NIDRR Traumatic Brain Injury Model Systems. *Brain Inj*. 2016;30(11):1311-1318.

13. Mackelprang JL, Bombardier CH, Fann JR, et al. Rates and predictors of suicidal ideation during the first year after traumatic brain injury. *Am J Public Health*. 2014;104(7):e100-e107.

14. Fazel S, Wolf A, Pillas D, et al. Suicide, fatal injuries, and other causes of premature mortality in patients with traumatic brain injury: a 41-year Swedish population study. *JAMA Psychiatry*. 2014;71(3):326-333.

15. Kaplan MS, Huguet N, McFarland BH, et al. Suicide among male veterans: a prospective population-based study. *J Epidemiol Community Health*. 2007;61(7):619-624.

16. Centers of Disease Control. *Suicide Prevention*. Atlanta, GA: Centers for Disease Control and Prevention; 2018. Available from https://www.cdc.gov/vitalsigns/pdf/vs-0618-suicide-H.pdf. Accessed January 9, 2019.

17. Kroenke K, Spitzer RL, Williams JB. The PHQ-9: validity of a brief depression severity measure. *J Gen Intern Med*. 2001;16(9):606-613.

18. Simon GE, Rutter CM, Peterson D, et al. Does response on the PHQ-9 Depression Questionnaire predict subsequent suicide attempt or suicide death? *Psychiatr Serv*. 2013;64:1195-1202. doi:10.1176/appi.ps.2012005.

19. Wortzel HS, Homaifar B, Matarazzo B, Brenner LA. Therapeutic risk management of the suicidal patient: stratifying risk in terms of severity and temporality. *J Psychiatr Pract*. 2014;20(1):63-67. doi:10.1097/01.pra.0000442940.46328.63.

20. Stanley B, Brown GK. *The Safety Planning Intervention Manual*: Veteran Version. Washington, DC: US Department of Veterans Affairs; 2018.

21. Brown GK, Jager-Hyman S. Evidence-based psychotherapies for suicide prevention: Future directions. *Am J Prev Med*. 2014;47(3 suppl 2):S186-S194.

22. Brenner LA, Forster JE, Hoffberg AS, et al. Window to hope: a randomized controlled trial of a psychological intervention for the treatment of hopelessness among veterans with moderate to severe traumatic brain injury. *J Head Trauma Rehabil*. 2018; 33(2):E64-E73. doi:10.1097/HTR.0000000000000351.

23. Simpson GK, Tate RL, Whiting DL, Cotter RE. Suicide prevention after traumatic brain injury: a randomized controlled trial of a program for the psychological treatment of hopelessness. *J Head Trauma Rehabil*. 2011;26(4):290-300. doi:10.1097/HTR.0b013e3182225250.

24. Barnes SM, Monteith LL, Gerard GR, Hoffberg AS, Homaifar BY, Brenner LA. Problem-solving therapy for suicide prevention in veterans with moderate-to-severe traumatic brain injury. *Rehabil Psychol*. 2017;62(4):600-608. doi:10.1037/rep0000154.

41

Substance Abuse

ALPHONSA THOMAS, DO, AND CHRISTINE GREISS, DO

Substance abuse disorders are a relatively common occurrence in the traumatic brain injury (TBI) population. Premorbid rates of substance use are around the same or may even exceed those of the general population. Whether it is associated with the mechanism of injury or post injury behavior, clinicians must be astute in managing these conditions.

Epidemiology

- 36% to 51% are intoxicated during injury.
- 22% to 29% drink hazardously between 1 to 3 years postinjury. Alcohol use peaks 2 years postinjury and stabilizes afterward.
- Alcohol is the most commonly abused substance in TBI.
- 37% to 66% of TBI patients abuse alcohol, whereas 10% to 44% abuse illicit drugs.
- Daily cigarette use is prominent in TBI patients.

Risk Factors

- Young age
- Male gender
- Unmarried
- Greater TBI severity
- Repetitive injury
- History of substance abuse
- Psychiatric disorders
- Damage to specific neural circuits: prefrontal cortex (PFC), nucleus accumbens, and the ventral tegmental area. These areas are thought to mediate substance abuse behavior.

Definitions

- Unhealthy (or risky) consumption constitutes a substance use disorder (SUD)
- "Risky" drinking:
  - 15+ drinks/week, 5+ drinks/day for men
  - 8+ drinks/week, 4+ drinks/day for women
- Abuse (older term from *Diagnostic and Statistical Manual of Mental Disorders, Fourth Edition* [DSM-IV])[6]
  - Continued use despite imminent consequence
  - Behavior centers around acquisition, consumption, and recovery
- DSM-V combines the DSM-IVs categories of substance abuse and substance dependence into a single group called substance use disorder.[1,7]

Screening

The goals of screening individuals are to identify those with histories of substance misuse and to treat accordingly. Screening also helps to identify issues earlier to manage and treat these individuals effectively. All patients should be intermittently screened for substance misuse. Individuals with TBI often have associated cognitive and neurobehavioral impairments that can limit or confound testing results.

- These standardized measures are self-report questionnaires.
- Alcohol abuse and dependence:
  - Alcohol Use Disorder Identification Test (AUDIT): Currently recommended for use in TBI research. Most sensitive to low levels of hazardous alcohol use and can detect episodes of binge drinking. Can detect problems drinking earlier than other screening measures.[5]
  - Cut-down, Annoyed, Guilty, Eye-Opener (CAGE) questionnaire
  - Brief Michigan Alcohol Screen Test
- Illicit drug use:
  - A screening standard for drug use in TBI has not been recommended.
  - Drug Abuse Screening Test (DAST): Most commonly used self-report measure for detecting drug abuse[5]
  - Simple Screening Instrument (SSI)

Effect on Recovery/Long-Term Consequences[1,2]

- Increased extent of brain damage (greater brain atrophy, diminished white matter integrity)
- Exacerbation of existing neurological sequela (physical, cognitive, psychological)
- Lowers seizure threshold
- Increased risk of mood/psychiatric impairments, suicide attempts
- Increased risk for additional TBIs
- Impaired vocational outcome

Interventions

There is no cure or definitive treatment for substance abuse disorders. The unique challenges in treating the brain injury population are the cognitive impairments limiting learning and the efficacy of brief interventions/didactic lesson-based strategies. It is important to educate families also on the consequences of substance misuse on TBI recovery and risks of developing a substance use disorder after TBI.

Behavioral Interventions

- Cognitive behavioral therapy (CBT)
  - Helps patients modify construed thought processes and alter behaviors that may promote substance use

- Mindfulness-based relapse-prevention therapies
  - Includes the use of meditation to increase awareness of thoughts, feelings, and the environment to manage drug cravings/use
- Counseling
  - Includes 12-step programs such as Alcoholic Anonymous
- Referral to community resources is an integral part of disposition planning in rehabilitation
  - The Substance Abuse and Mental Health Services Administration (SAMHSA)'s Behavioral Health Treatment Services Locator is an electronic database of thousands of treatment programs for different addictions, ages, and settings.
  - When referring to programs, be cognizant of the patient's cultural background and socioeconomic status.
- Financial incentives and addressing barriers have resulted in better patient compliance than motivational interviewing.
- A community-based model using intensive case management has been shown to improve outcomes.

Pharmacological Management

Pharmacological management of SUD is recommended in moderate to severe cases. These agents reduce alcohol consumption, prevent relapse, and promote abstinence. No one agent has been deemed superior to the others in the TBI population.

- US Food and Drug Administration (FDA)–approved pharmacological interventions exist for the management of alcohol and opiate dependence (Table 41.1).

TABLE 41.1 **US Food & Drug Administration (FDA)–Approved Pharmacological Interventions for Alcohol and Opioid Dependence**

Drug	FDA Indication	Mechanism of Action	Dosing	Clinical Benefit	Monitoring
Naltrexone	Opioid or alcohol dependence	Opioid antagonist	380 mg IM q4 week; 50–100 mg QD	Decreases craving	Depression, LFTs
Methadone	Opioid dependence	Opioid receptor agonist	15–30 mg for first dose; max. 40 mg in a day	Decreases craving	Depression, creatinine level, respiratory status
Buprenorphine	Opioid dependence	Nonselective, mixed agonist–antagonist opioid receptor modulator	Restricted distribution	Decreases craving	Respiratory status, LFTs
Disulfiram	Alcohol dependence	Inhibits the enzyme acetyl dehydrogenase	125–500 mg qAM	Aversion therapy	LFTs, CBC, electrolytes
Acamprosate	Alcohol dependence	NMDA receptor antagonist and modulates GABA A receptors	666 mg TID	Decreases craving	Depression, creatinine level

CBC, Complete blood count; *IM,* intramuscular; *LFT,* liver function test; max., maximum; *qAM,* every morning; *QD,* daily; *TID,* three times a day. (From Zasler ND, Katz DI, Zafonte RD. *Brain Injury Medicine: Principles and Practice.* 2nd ed. New York, NY: Demos Medical Pub.; 2013.)

- Questionable efficacy in TBI
  - Alcohol dependence: disulfiram, acamprosate, and naltrexone
  - Opioid dependence: naltrexone, buprenorphine, and methadone
- Topiramate (not FDA approved) is often used.
- These treatments are typically administered after 7 to 10 days of abstinence to help patient avoid withdrawal.
- Baseline liver and kidney function should be assessed. Naltrexone has a risk of hepatotoxicity.
- This is best used in conjunction with behavioral interventions or when an individual has failed management with behavioral techniques alone.
- Consider multiple agents if monotherapy is ineffective.

Four-Quadrant Model

A four-quadrant model for TBI was derived from a similar method used for patients with mental illness and substance abuse (Fig. 41.1). Corrigan et al. developed a model for TBI to help direct treatment of TBI and SUD based on condition severity (low or high). This is useful in identifying the settings where individuals with specific TBI characteristics can likely be found and which methods of intervention are commonly used.[5]

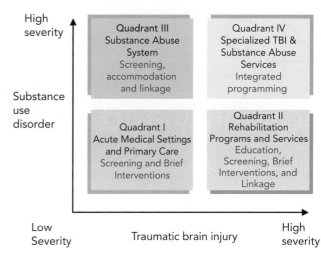

• **Fig. 41.1** Four-quadrant model.[1] (From Zasler ND, Katz DI, Zafonte RD. *Brain Injury Medicine: Principles and Practice.* 2nd ed. New York, NY: Demos Medical Pub.; 2013.)

How Much Is Safe?

There are many risk factors associated with alcohol use and TBI, and therefore it is difficult to answer this question. The benefit of abstaining from alcohol is clear in that it does not pose any detriment to recovery.

Review Questions

1. Prior history of substance misuse is the strongest independent predictor of
   a. substance use after traumatic brain injury (TBI).
   b. life satisfaction.
   c. social reintegration.
   d. employment.
2. How long after a TBI does alcohol use peak?
   a. 1 year
   b. 2 years
   c. 5 years
   d. 10 years

3. The use of naltrexone has been associated with
   a. nephrotoxicity.
   b. neuropathy.
   c. hepatotoxicity.
   d. suicide.

Answers on page 398.
Access the full list of questions and answers online.
Available on ExpertConsult.com

References

1. Zasler ND, Katz DI, Zafonte RD. *Brain Injury Medicine: Principles and Practice.* 2nd ed. New York, NY: Demos Medical Pub.; 2013.
2. Bjork JM, Grant SJ. Does traumatic brain injury increase risk for substance abuse? J Neurotrauma. 2009;26:1077-1082.
3. Merkel SF, Cannella LA, Razmpour R, et al. Factors affecting increased risk for substance use disorders following traumatic brain injury: what we can learn from animal models. *Neurosci Biobehav Rev.* 2017;77:209-218.
4. Bryce S, Spitz G, Ponsford J. Screening for substance use disorders following traumatic brain injury: examining the validity of the AUDIT and the DAST. *J Head Trauma Rehabil.* 2015;30(5): E40-E48.

5. Corrigan JD, Bogner J, Hungerford DW, Schomer K. Screening and brief intervention for substance misuse among patients with traumatic brain injury. *J Trauma.* 2010;69(3):722-726.
6. American Psychiatric Association. *Diagnostic and Statistical Manual of Mental Disorders,* fourth edition text revision *(DSM-IV-TR).* Washington DC: American Psychiatric Association; 2000.
7. American Psychiatric Association. *Diagnostic and Statistical Manual of Mental Disorders,* Fifth Edition Text Revision *(DSM-V-TR).* Washington DC: American Psychiatric Association; 2013.

42

Sexuality and Intimacy

PAUL KI YOO, DO, AND KIRK LERCHER, MD, MBS

Sexual dysfunction is a well-known, yet seldom discussed, complication in individuals who have sustained a traumatic brain injury (TBI). This is likely because it can be uncomfortable for the patient, significant other, and healthcare professional to address these issues. This can cause issues with intimacy, which can lead to relationship problems and emotional distress in both the patient and their partner or spouse.[1]

Common problems documented in men are:
- Decreased desire or drive for sexual activity[1,3,6,8]
- Difficulty maintaining an erection[1,3,6]
- Decreased arousal[1,3,6]
- Difficulty achieving orgasm[1,5]
- Ejaculatory dysfunction[1,5]
Similar problems are documented in women, such as:
- Decreased desire for sexual activity[2,3,5]
- Difficulty achieving orgasm[2,3,5]
- Decreased vaginal lubrication and pain during sex[1-5]

There are many factors that contribute to sexual dysfunction after a brain injury. Structural damage to the brain is the primary contributor,[9] However, there are social, emotional, physical, and cognitive factors that also play a significant role in sexual dysfunction.

Contributing Factors to Sexual Dysfunction

Anatomical Factors

There are many areas in the brain that contribute to sexual function.
- The frontal lobes, limbic, and paralimbic regions are associated with sexual drive, assertiveness, initiation, and sexual preference.[3]

- Injury to the orbitofrontal region can lead to:
  - Disinhibition[3,5]
  - Hypersexual responses such as inappropriate sexual talk, self-exposure, and genital touching[3,5]
- Injuries involving the dorsolateral frontal injury can lead to:
  - Apathy[1,5,6]
  - Attention deficits[5-7]
  - Initiation impairments[5,6]
- Temporal lobe injuries can also lead to hypersexual behaviors.
  - Kluver bucy syndrome is a rare complication caused by damage to the bilateral anterior temporal lobes, and can present with hypersexuality, hyperorality, and exploratory behaviors.[1,3,6]
  - Seizures in the temporal lobes can manifest with hypersexual or hyposexual behaviors.[6]
- Brainstem lesions:
  - Brainstem lesions can affect both sensory input and motor output to the body.[5]
  - Damage to areas such as the reticular activating system in the midbrain and pons can affect arousal and alertness.[6]
  - The brainstem connects the limbic and paralimbic structures such as the hippocampus, amygdala, hypothalamus, and cingulate gyrus. These areas are involved in producing erections and other sexually related behaviors.[6]
- The neuroendocrine system:
  - The hypothalamus and pituitary gland is commonly affected in traumatic brain injuries.[1]
  - Can lead to alterations in hormone levels such as testosterone, progesterone, and estrogen, which can then cause changes in menstrual cycle and fertility in women and decreased sperm production and infertility in men.[2,5]
  - Subcortical structures such as the thalamus are thought to play a role in penile erection.[7]
- Neurotransmitters:
  - Dopamine and serotonin can affect sexual desire.[8]
  - Damage to these neurotransmitter pathways can lead to changes in sexual function.[2,7]

Physical and Functional Factors

Patients can have physical and functional limitations that can make intimacy with their partners difficult.

- Hemiparesis or spasticity can make positioning and movement difficult and can also cause pain.[7]
- Visuospatial deficits or hemineglect from right hemispheric lesions can also interfere with intimacy.[7]
- Fatigue has also been reported to be a contributing factor in the importance and frequency of sex in brain injury patients.[5,7]
- Oral–motor dysfunction have reported in difficulty kissing and expressing romantic vocalizations.[2,7]
- Headaches, visual impairments, and auditory impairments were also reported to interfere with intimacy.[2]
- Neurogenic bowel and bladder can lead to decreased sexual activity due to fear, anxiety, and embarrassment about having an accident.[2]
- Sensory impairments to certain areas of the body can lead to decreased arousal and difficulty achieving an orgasm. Difficulties with personal hygiene and physical appearance may also affect a patient's sexual life.[5,10]

Cognitive Factors

Individuals with brain injuries will often present with cognitive deficits that will interfere with their independence and activities of daily living, as well as sexual dysfunction.

Common cognitive deficits include:
- Attention and concentration difficulties
  - Can lead to difficulties with sexual arousal and ability to focus on sexual activities[5]
  - Partners can feel neglected or disinterested due to lack of attention.[2]
- Short-term memory deficits[6]
  - May lead to difficulty remembering important events or dates[5]
  - Patients may miss opportunities that can lead to intimacy.[1,5]
- Impaired initiation
  - Can lead to decreased frequency of sexual encounters[5,10]
  - Poor initiation can give the impression of disinterest in their significant other.[5]
- Difficulty with abstract thinking
  - Can limit patient's ability to fantasize, leading to decreased sexual drive and/or arousal[1,5]
- Impaired goal-directed behaviors and planning[5]

Emotional and Psychiatric Factors

Many emotional and psychiatric factors can contribute to sexual dysfunction[1-3,5,7,10]:
- Depression
- Adjustment disorder
- Anxiety
- Poor self-esteem and/or body image
- Fear of intimacy

These are common sequalae of TBI caused by sudden changes in function, quality of life, and independence. This can lead to apathy, decreased sexual drive, and arousal.[5,7] Patients may distance themselves emotionally from their significant others, which can cause relationship difficulties, avoidance of intimacy, and separation or divorce.[2,3]

Partners and spouses of TBI patients may experience a change in dynamics in their relationship from an intimate partner to one of a caregiver or parent–child.[2,3] Some may be unable to overcome the idea of being intimate with a disabled partner.[7] In some cases, the significant other may feel that they are now living with a stranger and feel intimacy is incompatible.[1,2]

Fear itself may lead to an avoidance of intimate activity. Especially in patients who have had a stroke, there can be a fear that sexual activity may lead to another stroke.[7]

Medications

Medications that may contribute to sexual dysfunction may include:
- Antidepressants
- Antiepileptics
- Antipsychotics
- Antihypertensives

TBI patients typically are started on antidepressants due to mood difficulties and to help with neuro-recovery.[7,8] Many are also started on antiepileptic and/or antipsychotic medications due to seizures, agitation, and irritability.[3]

Dopamine has been shown to have an excitatory effect on sexual desire. Serotonin, on the other hand, has been shown to inhibit sexual function. Medications that have antidopaminergic or serotonergic may further alter sexual function.[2]

Antihypertensive can also cause difficulty with erections by lowering the cavernosal artery pressure and can lead to erectile dysfunction.[7]

Treatment

The topic of sexual dysfunction can be uncomfortable to approach by both the patient and their significant other and the healthcare professional.[10] However, it is a common problem that occurs after a brain injury and should be addressed because it can cause negative changes in a patient's marriage or relationship.[6]

A comprehensive approach should be made to treat sexual dysfunction after a brain injury.
- The PLISSIT model is comprised of four steps: Permission to address sexuality, provide Limited Information about sexual functioning and disability, give Specific Suggestions about particular complaint, and Intensive Therapy.[3,10]
- The BETTER model follows similar principles as the PLISSIT model, but includes a record keeping step. The steps include: Bring up the topic, Explain concerns, Tell about resources, Time the discussion to patient's preference, Educate patient about disability and treatments, and Record discussion and information shared in patient's medical record.[3,10]

- The ALLOW model includes these steps: Ask about sexual function, Legitimize concerns, identify Limitations in evaluation of dysfunction, Open up the discussion, and Work together to develop goals and treatment plans.[3]
- Create an open and comfortable environment to discuss and address issues of sexual dysfunction.[3,5,10]
- A comprehensive medical examination is important to rule out any underlying medical issues that may contribute to decreased sexual function.[2,3,5,10]
  - Screening for medical comorbidities such as diabetes, heart disease, endocrine function, or hormone levels
  - Urological or obstetric/gynecological examination
  - Rule out inhibiting factors such as pain or other focal neurological deficits.
- Interdisciplinary approach to address sexual dysfunction[2,5,10]:
  - Physical and occupational therapy can help with education and optimization of comfortable positioning

along with adaptive aids and equipment that can assist with intimacy.
- Speech therapy can assist with cognitive and communicative barriers to sexuality.
- Counseling through a sexual health educator, sex therapist, or marital therapist can help with the emotional and social issues that may be present.
- Medications such as performance-enhancing medications and lubrication for women can also help with sexual activity.

Summary

Sexual dysfunction is a common and multifactorial complication that can occur after TBI. Different components such as structural, functional, social, emotional, and medical factors can contribute significantly to sexual dysfunction. This is a complication that should be addressed by the healthcare professional and the patient and partner. Treatment should be comprehensive and involve an interdisciplinary approach.

Review Questions

1. Kluver-Bucy syndrome is a condition caused by damage to the
   a. Left frontal lobe injury
   b. Bilateral anterior temporal lobes
   c. Right parietal lobe
   d. Brainstem
2. What cognitive factors can contribute to sexual dysfunction?
   a. Fatigue
   b. Attention/concentration deficits
   c. Spasticity
   d. Depression

3. Which area in the brainstem is involved with alertness and can contribute to decreased sexual arousal?
   a. Reticular activating system
   b. Hippocampus
   c. Amygdala
   d. Hypothalamus

Answers on page 398.
Access the full list of questions and answers online. Available on ExpertConsult.com

References

1. Latella D, Maggio MG, De Luca R, et al. Changes in sexual functioning following traumatic brain injury: an overview on a neglected issue. *J Clin Neurosci.* 2018;58:1-6.
2. Blessen CE, Cifu DX. *Rehabilitation after Traumatic Brain Injury.* St. Louis, MO: Elsevier; 2018.
3. Cifu DX, Kaelin DL, Kowalske KJ, et al. *Braddom's Physical Medicine and Rehabilitation.* 5th ed. St. Louis, MO: Elsevier; 2016.
4. Sander AM, Maestas KL, Pappadis MR, Hammond FM, Hanks RA. multicenter study of sexual functioning in spouses/partners of persons with traumatic brain injury. *Arch Phys Med Rehabil.* 2016;97(5):753-759.
5. Zollman FS. *Manual of Traumatic Brain Injury.* 2nd ed. New York, NY: Demos Medical Publishing; 2016.
6. Zasler ND, Katz DI, Zafonte RD. *Brain Injury Medicine.* New York, NY: Demos Medical Publishing; 2007.
7. Park JH, Ovbiagele B, Feng W. Stroke and sexual dysfunction—a narrative review. *J Neurol Sci.* 2015;350(1-2):7-13.
8. Chollet F, Tardy J, Albucher JF, et al. Fluoxetine for Motor Recovery after Acute Ischaemic Stroke (FLAME): a randomised placebo-controlled trial. *Lancet Neurol.* 2011;10(2):123-130.
9. Goldin Y, Cantor JB, Tsaousides T, Spielman L, Gordon W. Sexual functioning and the effect of fatigue in traumatic brain injury. *J Head Trauma Rehabil.* 2014;29(5):418-426.
10. Grenier-Genest A, Gerard M, Courtois F. Stroke and sexual functioning: a literature review. *Neurorehabilitation.* 2017;41(2):293-315.

Rehabilitation Concepts

43

Therapeutic Exercise/Rehabilitation

KIMBERLY BENSON PT, DPT, JOEL DAN SCHOLTEN, MD, AND
KATHARINE STOUT, PT, DPT, MBA

Rehabilitation post brain injury occurs in a variety of setting with multiple team members. Regardless of timing, goal-directed care is important. Each individual sustaining brain injury presents with unique mobility and cognitive challenges; therefore, no single intervention is recommended for everyone. Periodic reevaluation of functional status is required to align goals and the plan of care to maximize the patient's return to independence. It is critical to incorporate the entire interdisciplinary team, including the patient and family, in developing the rehabilitation plan.

The entire rehabilitation team should work toward common patient-centered goals in a transdisciplinary approach[1] that benefits the patient by providing the most comprehensive approach to rehabilitation. Open communication assists with identifying possible complications such as normal pressure hydrocephalous (NPH), seizures, infections, and neuroendocrine dysfunction.

Individuals post brain injury recover at different rates and to different extents. Rehabilitation interventions should include efforts to prevent sequalae that may impair future function and recovery, such as periarticular calcification resulting from prolonged immobilization.[2] In survivors of traumatic brain injury (TBI), time of posttraumatic amnesia—along with several other factors time factors, such as inflammation, timing of neurotoxic events, and neurorestorative events—may affect recovery timelines.[2,3] For survivors of acquired/nontraumatic brain injuries (such as stroke and anoxic injuries), initial severity of motor deficits followed by early return of motor function tend to be the best predictor of functional return.[4] In this chapter, we explore current trends and highlight key concepts in rehabilitation and therapeutic exercises post brain injury.

Motor Control

Literature based on animal studies reveals timing, intensity, and frequency of rehabilitation post brain injury are important factors to consider with recovery.[5] Rehabilitation can both promote and inhibit neural plasticity based on timing, frequency, and intensity. Animal model findings suggest that the window of opportunity to start symptom-specific, skilled rehabilitative training is early (within days) but not immediately (within hours).[5,6] There is a dearth of human studies on this subject; therefore, best practice continues to evolve, but current literature supports early intervention to promote mobility and decrease sequelae of immobility.[7]

Longitudinal studies suggest that recovery from hemiparesis proceeds through a series of fairly stereotypical stages over the first 6 months poststroke, irrespective of the kind of therapeutic intervention.[8] Biernaskie and colleagues found that rehabilitative training was more effective in improving functional outcomes when initiated at 5 days rather than 30 days after stroke.[9]

Therapeutic interventions to promote motor recovery are derived from different therapeutic approaches, such as exercise and functional-based activities, proprioceptive neuromuscular facilitation (PNF), and neurodevelopmental therapy (NDT). The Brunnstrom approach is another philosophy that breaks down motor recovery into six phases: flaccidity, spasticity and synergies emerge, increased spasticity, decreased spasticity and synergies, able to move freely through complex movement combinations, spasticity is no longer apparent, and normal motor function returns.[10] Based on current literature, no one approach is best, and often the mixed approach is needed to maximize function.[11,12]

Therapeutic concepts such as task-oriented training, progressive practice to increase movement speed and precision, compensatory adaptations, strengthening, and cardiovascular fitness are ingrained in the rehabilitation goals for patients with most neurological diseases.[13-15] The frequency, timing, intensity, and environmental conditions of practice are critical to consider when developing plans of care for patients with brain injuries. Following TBI, use of the Rancho Los Amigo Scale-Revised (RLAS-R) can guide the progression of therapeutic interventions according to phases of recovery.

For example, in cognitive level III, the family should be speaking with the patient in a normal tone and performing passive range of motion (PROM). In contrast, at cognitive level VI RLAS-R, the family and providers shift focus toward patient-initiated movements with assistance to complete task as needed. Sessions may include route finding, task-specific training, and higher-level balance retraining. The ability to layer physical, cognitive, and behavioral expectations changes as a person progresses through the stages of recovery, and the team can adapt rehabilitation strategies to maximize recovery.

- Consider frequency, intensity, and timing when prescribing activities.
- A mixed approach to therapeutic intervention offers the best recovery. Knowing how and when to layer on cognitive and behavioral expectations with physical activity can help the team formulate the strategy to maximize recovery.

Mobility and Range of Motion

Mobility is important to recovery no matter the severity or type of brain injury. Key considerations are medical stability, impaired balance, range of motion (ROM), muscle weakness, and premorbid motor skills.[16] Providing early intervention can reduce complications such as contractures, pressure sores, heterotrophic ossification, and deconditioning. Inclusion of therapy services early after injury can assist with initiating family education on PROM and positioning and promote multiple benefits, including early participation in therapeutic exercise. Functional mobility tasks such as transfers and standing can double as therapeutic exercise in the early stages of recovery. Therapy can assist with maintaining functional strength and improving cardiovascular function, which may decrease consequences of immobility.

Spasticity and tone changes can occur over time after a brain insult and must be monitored and used to adjust the treatment plan accordingly. A limb that at one time was flaccid may progress to hypertonicity, and incorporating therapeutic exercise as tone changes throughout recovery is assessment dependent.[17]

Mobility changes throughout recovery. It is imperative to assess and update treatment plans periodically to align with the patient's abilities.

Strength and Endurance

Strength and endurance training is vital to the prevention of secondary complications and promotion of a healthy lifestyle. Most physical therapy interventions focus on physical impairments that are a direct result of the injury, such as gait kinematics, spasticity, flexibility, muscle performance, balance, and functional skills. However, not all brain injuries result in primary physical impairments. Adapting strategies to accommodate other impairments, including cognitive, behavioral, and motivational deficits, is important to focus on and plays a key role in strength and endurance training. Physical capacity and endurance are key components to focus on during recovery for not only the health benefits but also the reduction of secondary complications.[18,19]

The promotion of a healthy lifestyle is critical to reduce secondary complications. Addressing cognitive, behavioral, and motivational factors that may inhibit strength and endurance training should be considered.

Exercise and Activity

Based on physical activity guidelines recommended by the US Department of Health and Human Services, adults should participate in at least 150 to 300 minutes a week of moderate-intensity or 75 to 150 minutes a week of vigorous-intensity aerobic physical activity—or an equivalent combination of moderate- and vigorous-intensity aerobic activity, preferably spread throughout the week. Adults with disability and chronic conditions should also strive for the 150 minutes of moderate to vigorous activity per week, incorporating an exercise plan that accommodates their abilities.[20]

Prescribing exercise to meet the recommend intensity, frequency, and duration is important in survivor's overall health. Educating patients on exercise and its benefits is an important role of the rehabilitation team. Monitoring progression using the modified Borg scale—reported as rate of perceived exertion (RPE)—is a simple way to monitor exercise intensity. Combining aerobic, muscle strengthening, bone strength, flexibility, and balance activities is needed to maximize the health benefits.

Rehabilitation specialists have multiple therapeutic modalities available to achieve the recommended guidelines. The timing and progression of activities are important to overall recovery.[21] Access to therapeutic exercises, technology (for example, exoskeletons, functional e-stim, virtual reality equipment), and knowledge in promoting mobility despite impairments allows patients to remain active. Providers need to set the expectation that exercise is possible after brain injury and to assist survivors of a brain injury to identify a mode of exercise that accommodates their level of function.

Adults with disability and chronic conditions should strive for the 150 minutes of moderate to vigorous activity per week. Prescribing an exercise plan that accommodates their abilities and incorporates intensity, duration, and frequency is most beneficial.

Mobility Aids, Orthoses, Casting, and Splinting

In many cases, mobility aids may enhance mobility after brain injury. More options become available as technology advances; understanding the device function and the needs of your patient is vital to prescribe the appropriate device

(Table 43.1).[22] Early orthosis use may improve kinematics but must be monitored to maximize functional mobility outcomes and prevent complications.[23] Frequent evaluation of impact and benefit of technology is required in the absence of technology gold standards after brain injury.[23]

Multiple devices are available to assist with positioning, mobility, and function. Having a multidisciplinary team will maximize utilization and progression of needed devices.

Measurement of Therapeutic Exercise Benefit

Tracking the impact of rehabilitation intervention is critical through the incorporation of objective measures. Objective measures of physical functional after brain injury fall into several categories (Table 43.2). Given the heterogenic nature of brain injury and patient presentation, no single measure is suitable for all patients.

Additional rehabilitation measures can be found online. The National Institutes of Health has developed a rehabilitation tests and measures database, currently managed by the Shirly Ryan AbilityLab. It is a free online resource of many tests and measures applicable across domains for the brain injury population and available at https://www.sralab.org/rehabilitation-measures.[24]

The emergence of a global measure of progress called the goal attainment scale (GAS) is a valid way to incorporate multiple aspects of rehabilitation and work toward a specific goal of the patient.[25] Goal attainment scaling allows multiple providers on the rehabilitation team to interview the patient, capture meaningful daily activities, and break down those activities to task level. Goals are then determined and included in the rehabilitation plan. This method allows

TABLE 43.1 Rehabilitation Devices

Types of Aids	Examples
Aids to support independent living	Kitchen adaptations, bathroom adaptations, ramps, stairlifts, handrails, lift chairs
Seating and positioning aids	Wheelchair: power base or manual base
Transfer aids	Hoyer lift, sliding board, gait belts
Mobility aids	Cane, crutches, walker, rollator, scooter
Orthotics	Spinal, ankle-foot orthotics, knee-ankle-foot orthotic, dynamic splints, functional e-stim
Rehabilitation tools	Exoskeletons, body weight support devices, robotics, standing frames
Casting and splitting	Dynamic splints, serial casting

TABLE 43.2 Objective Measures for Mobility and Function[a]

Area of Function	Tests
Muscle tone	• Ashworth Scale/Modified Ashworth Scale (AS/MAS) • Spinal Cord Assessment Tool for Spastic Reflexes • Motor Evaluation Scale for Upper Extremity in Stroke (MESUPES)
Gait	• 10 Meter Walk Test (10MWT) • Times up and Go (TUG) • 2 minute Walk Test (2MWT) • 6 minute Walk Test (6MWT)
Balance/functional mobility measures	• Berg Balance Score (BBS) • Tinetti Falls Efficacy Scale (Tinetti FES) • Dynamic Gait Index (DGI) • Rivermead Motor Assessment (RMA) • Functional Gait Assessment (FGA) • Activities-Specific Balance Confidence Scale • High-Level Mobility Assessment Tool (HiMAT)
Activities of daily living	• Barthel Index (BI) • Functional Independence Measure (FIM) • Modified Rankin Handicap Scale (MRS) • Medical Outcomes Study Short Form 36 (SF–36) • Community Integration Questionnaire (CIQ) • Four Step Square Test (FSST) • Fugl-Myer Assessment of Motor Recovery After Stroke (FMA) • Orpington Prognostic Score (OPS)

[a]Table is not meant to be all inclusive; instead it is a sampling from each area of function.

objective tracking of individual progress toward clearly defined goals in a very heterogenic population.

Establishing patient-centered goals and using objective measures to track progress allows for multiple providers to work together to maximize function is a very heterogenic population.

Summary

Rehabilitation is based on a team approach, with ongoing evaluation through the acute, subacute, and chronic phases.[26] As Hammod et al have described, individuals post brain injury are at a higher risk for developing comorbidities during the course of recovery.[27] Rehabilitation takes place in a multitude of environments based on a person's abilities and goals. Providers must adjust the plan of care based on periodic assessments of the intervention effectiveness using objective measures. Engaging the entire care team, caregivers, and the patient throughout the recovery process promotes the best outcome.

Review Questions

1. A 25-year-old man status post aneurysm rupture 4 months earlier presents with hemiparesis. The patient would like to return to independent ambulation but is limited by lacking full dorsiflexion during swing phase of gait. The patient would benefit most from what type of intervention?
   a. Therapeutic exercise and device evaluation
   b. Device evaluation
   c. Therapeutic exercise
   d. Botox

2. A 53-year-old man status post ischemic stroke 2 months ago is presenting with moderate dysmetria, severe dysdiadochokinesia, and weakness. Based on his impairments, he is most likely to have what level of mobility after 1 year?
   a. Independent with mobility and self-care
   b. Assistance with mobility and self-care
   c. Dependent for mobility and self-care
   d. Modified independent with mobility and self-care

3. A physical therapist (PT) calls you to report a sudden change in presentation in a traumatic brain injury (TBI) patient, noting increased tone, increased agitation, ataxic gait pattern, and urinary incontinence. The most likely explanation would be
   a. normal brain injury recovery.
   b. normal pressure hydrocephalous.
   c. electrolyte imbalance.
   d. fatigue from increased activity.

Answers on page 399.
Access the full list of questions and answers online. Available on ExpertConsult.com

References

1. Choi BCK, Pak AWP. Multidisciplinarity, interdisciplinarity and transdisciplinarity in health research, services, education and policy: 1. Definitions, objectives, and evidence of effectiveness. *Clin Invest Med*. 2006;29(6):351-364.
2. Stocchetti N, Zanier ER. Chronic impact of traumatic brain injury on outcome and quality of life: a narrative review. *Crit Care*. 2016;20(1):148.
3. Brown AW, Malec JF, McClelland RL, Diehl NN, Englander J, Cifu DX. Clinical elements that predict outcome after traumatic brain injury: a prospective multicenter recursive partitioning (decision-tree) analysis. *J Neurotrauma*. 2005;22(10):1040-1051.
4. Coupar F, Pollock A, Rowe P, Weir C, Langhorne P. Predictors of upper limb recovery after stroke: a systematic review and meta-analysis. *Clin Rehabil*. 2012;26(4):291-313.
5. Hylin MJ, Kerr AL, Holden R. Understanding the Mechanisms of recovery and/or compensation following injury. *Neural Plast*. 2017;2017:7125057.
6. Humm JL, Kozlowski DA, James DC, Gotts JE, Schallert T. Use-dependent exacerbation of brain damage occurs during an early post-lesion vulnerable period. *Brain Res*. 1998;783(2):286-292.
7. Königs M, Beurskens EA, Snoep L, Scherder EJ, Oosterlaan J. Effects of timing and intensity of neurorehabilitation on functional outcome after traumatic brain injury: a systematic review and meta-analysis. *Arch Phys Med Rehabil*. 2018;99(6):1149-1159.e1.
8. Kwakkel G, Kollen B, Lindeman E. Understanding the pattern of functional recovery after stroke: facts and theories. *Restor Neurol Neurosci*. 2004;22(3-5):281-299.
9. Biernaskie J, Chernenko G, Corbett D. Efficacy of rehabilitative experience declines with time after focal ischemic brain injury. *J Neurosci*. 2004;24(5):1245-1254.
10. Brunnstrom S. Motor testing procedures in hemiplegia: based on sequential recovery stages. *Phys Ther*. 1966;46(4):357-375.
11. Bland DC, Zampieri C, Damiano DL. Effectiveness of physical therapy for improving gait and balance in individuals with traumatic brain injury: a systematic review. *Brain Inj*. 2011;25(7-8):664-679.
12. Kawahira K, Shimodozono M, Etoh S, Kamada K, Noma T, Tanaka N. Effects of intensive repetition of a new facilitation technique on motor functional recovery of the hemiplegic upper limb and hand. *Brain Inj*. 2010;24(10):1202-1213.
13. Dobkin BH. Confounders in rehabilitation trials of task-oriented training: lessons from the designs of the EXCITE and SCILT multicenter trials. *Neurorehabil Neural Repair*. 2007;21(1):3-13.
14. Dobkin BH. Training and exercise to drive poststroke recovery. *Nat Clin Pract Neurol*. 2008;4(2):76-85.
15. Dobkin BH. Motor rehabilitation after stroke, traumatic brain, and spinal cord injury: common denominators within recent clinical trials. *Curr Opin Neurol*. 2009;22(6):563-569.
16. Williams GP, Schache AG, Morris ME. Mobility after traumatic brain injury: relationships with ankle joint power generation and motor skill level. *J Head Trauma Rehabil*. 2013;28(5):371-378.
17. Aloraini SM, Gäverth J, Yeung E, MacKay-Lyons M. Assessment of spasticity after stroke using clinical measures: a systematic review. *Disabil Rehabil*. 2015;37(25):2313-2323.
18. Bushnik T, Englander J, Wright J. Patterns of fatigue and its correlates over the first 2 years after traumatic brain injury. *J Head Trauma Rehabil*. 2008;23(1):25-32.

19. Mossberg KA, Amonette WE, Masel BE. Endurance training and cardiorespiratory conditioning after traumatic brain injury. *J Head Trauma Rehabil.* 2010;25(3):173-183.

20. U.S. Department of Health and Human Services. *Physical Activity Guidelines for Americans.* 2nd ed. Washington, DC: U.S. Department of Health and Human Services; 2018.

21. Griesbach GS. Exercise after traumatic brain injury: is it a double-edged sword? *PM R.* 2011;3(6 suppl 1):S64-S72.

22. Lannin NA, Herbert RD. Is hand splinting effective for adults following stroke? A systematic review and methodologic critique of published research. *Clin Rehabil.* 2003;17(8):807-816.

23. Rogozinski BM, Schwab SE, Kesar TM. Effects of an articulated ankle foot orthosis on gait biomechanics in adolescents with traumatic brain injury: a case-series report. *Phys Med Rehabil Int.* 2018;5(2): 1144.

24. Shirley Ryan AbilityLab. *Rehabilitation Measure Database.* Available from: https://www.sralab.org/rehabilitation-measures.

25. Turner-Stokes L. Goal attainment scaling (GAS) in rehabilitation: a practical guide. *Clin Rehabil..* 2009;23(4):362-370.

26. Hammond FM, Malec JF. Rethinking brain injury. *Brain Inj Pro.* 2013;10(N1):6-10.

27. Hammond FM, Corrigan JD, Ketchum JM, et al. Prevalence of medical and psychiatric comorbidities following traumatic brain injury. *J Head Trauma Rehabil.* 2019;34(4):E1-E10.

44

Assistive Technology

SHEITAL BAVISHI, DO

As defined by Public Law 100-407[1]

*Assistive technology means any item, piece of equipment or
product system, whether acquired commercially off the shelf,
modified, or customized, that is used to increase, maintain,
or improve the functional capabilities of children with disabilities. (Federal Register, August 19, 1991, p. 41272)*[2]

History and Legislation

Technology-Related Assistance for Individuals
With Disabilities Act (The Tech Act)

- Signed into law in 1988 and amended in 1994
- All states have to develop systems for providing a variety
  of technology assistance to children and adults with disabilities and their parents and guardians.

- The purpose of PL 100-407 is to provide financial assistance to the states to enable them to conduct needs
  assessments, identify technology resources, provide assistive technology (AT) services, and conduct public
  awareness programs, among others.[2]

The federal regulations go on to state that an array of
services is included when considering applications for
AT. Such services include activities such as evaluation of a
person's needs for AT devices, purchasing or leasing AT
devices for people, designing and fabricating devices, coordinating services offered by those who provide AT services,
providing training or technical assistance to a person who
uses AT, and training and technical assistance to those who
work with people who use AT devices, such as teachers or
employers.[2]

Individuals With Disabilities Education Act, Public Law 105-17

- Guarantees the right of all children with disabilities to a
  free and appropriate public education in the least restrictive environment passed in 1997
- Most important is the development of an Individualized
  Education Program (IEP) for every student who is enrolled in special education, which are now extended to
  preschool programs for students who are entitled to an
  Individualized Family Services Plan (IFSP) and to those
  who are eligible for rehabilitation services through the
  development of an Individualized Written Rehabilitation
  Plan (IWRP)
- Requires the development of an Individualized Transition Plan (ITP) for all special education students of
  14 years of age or older to prepare the student for post-
  school environments
- As part of the IEP planning process, IDEA mandates that
  the AT needs of all students be considered [P.L. 105-17,
  Section 1414 (d)(3)(B)(v)]. This provision applies equally
  to students with learning disabilities who may require the
  use of a device, such as a spelling checker, to assist them
  with written communication.[2]

Reauthorization of the Rehabilitation Act (2003)

- Recognized role of employment in enabling individuals with disabilities to become economically self-sufficient and integrated into communities
- Mandates that AT devices and services are considered and provided as a means to acquire vocational training and to enter into and maintain employment
- Vocational rehabilitation (VR) has become an important source of funding for AT devices.

Augmentative and Alternative Communication

Definition

- Tools, systems, and strategies that are used specifically to assist or support communication
- Multimodal
- Supplement deficient oral communication or limited oral communication skills
- Low-technology (do not use electronics) or high-technology (use electronics) devices

Information and Communication Technologies

Definition

- Any device or application used for communication
- Includes technology such as email, internet, and mobile phones that enable users to access, store, transmit, and manipulate information[3]

Switches

Switches are devices that can be connected to other devices to control them.
- Can be simple or more complex and can be activated in different ways (pushing, pulling, sipping and puffing, pressing, blinking)
- Can be generic, able to connect to various devices with adapter cords, or designed with a specific functionality for a specific device
- Single switches are less physically demanding but are slower when there are more options to scan.
- Multiswitch scanning is more cognitively and physically complicated but allows the options to be organized in such ways that choices can be made faster.
  Choosing the most appropriate switch depends on multiple variables:
  - Consideration must be made to the patient's cognitive and physical abilities
  - Complexity of what is being controlled
  - Cost

- Mounting options
- Necessary to try multiple switches before settling on the best option

Environmental Control

Environmental control (EC) devices allow a person to interact with their environment and assist in maintaining independence with daily living.
- Control home devices: lights, locks, security system, television, music players, robotic vacuums
- Vehicle controls: remote start, doors, ramps
- Communication: telephone, video phone, computers
Electronic devices are now sold as smart devices and can be remotely controlled by a single device. Apps have been developed that allow users to use their smartphones, electronic tablets, and computers to remotely control devices throughout their homes, including lights, alarm systems, thermostats, televisions, etc. Devices that are not designed to be remotely controlled can be plugged into electronic switches that can be controlled remotely, essentially making them into smart devices.

Voice-activated devices are becoming more available commercially. Multiple products that can connect to multiple smart devices throughout a home environment allow people to speak commands to activate them. This gives patients with significant physical impairments the ability to manage their environment around them without the assistance of others.

Considerations for Environmental Controls

- Physical impairments
- Cognitive deficits
- Verbal communication impairments

Electronic Memory Aids

Cognitive deficits after traumatic brain injury (TBI) are quite common. Problems with memory, attention, and executive function are common and can significantly limit an individual's independence. More and more, technology is being used to compensate. Some devices have been adapted to help, whereas others have been designed to fill a specific need. These devices come in various styles (see Table 44.1 and 44.2). Some have a single purpose and others, such as smartphones, are more complex and have multiple functions.

Types of Electronic Memory Aids (Table 44.1)

- Watches with alarms
- Mobile phones and tablets: notes, calendars, alarms, applications
- Electronic pill boxes with alarms
- Digital recorders
  To help with memory, devices such as smartphones, tablets, and personal digital assistants (PDAs) can be

TABLE 44.1	Types of Devices
Assistive technology	Low tech: • Planners/organizers • Calendars • Journals • Switches High tech: • Personal digital assistant • Digital voice recorders • Computers • Cameras • Smartphones • Environmental control devices (Table 44.2)
Augmentative and alternative communication	Low tech: • Communication boards (picture or letter) • Yes/no buttons • Notepads High tech: • Text to talk • Eye gaze systems • Electronic communication device
Information and communication technologies	• Tablets • Computers • Internet • Mobile apps • Telerehabilitation

TABLE 44.2	Environmental Control Devices
Smart devices • Phones • Tablets • Voice-controlled intelligent personal assistant	
Applications	
Voice-activated controls	
Electronic switches	

used to create lists and take notes. Some can even transcribe, eliminating the need to manually type in the information. There is good evidence that devices such as PDAs and smartphones, when used as cognitive aids, improve independence and confidence for individuals who have had TBIs.[4,7] Studies have shown that use of devices can achieve higher memory goals[5] and increase completion of tasks.[6]

Brain–Computer Interfaces

Brain–computer interface (BCI) systems (Box 44.1) are made up of electrodes that stimulate or record neural

• BOX 44.1	Brain–Computer Interface (BCI)
BCI	Neuroprosthetic device that replaces biological motor output pathways from the brain, sensory input pathways to the brain, or cognitive processes mediated by connections within the central nervous system, allowing the user to interact freely with his or her environment. Different BCI systems may bypass, replace, or compensate for lost sensorimotor, visual, auditory, cognitive, affective, or volitional functions of an individual.

activity, a signal processing and decoding module, and an environmental interface to capture or produce changes in physical states that are also experienced by others. BCI facilitates communication of thoughts, social interaction, and reaction to and control over the physical world. BCI has the advantage of being completely hands free, allowing it to be used by severely disabled users, and BCI control does not rely on voice control, as many who are severely disabled have problems with voice production.[8,9]

Considerations for Assistive Technology, Augmentative and Alternative Communication, and Information and Communication Technologies

Use of AT, augmentative and alternative communication (AAC), and information and communication technologies (ICT) devices requires evaluation of factors that influence successful use of the devices. Evaluations should be completed by trained speech language pathologists, physical therapists, and/or occupational therapists to evaluate barriers. Facilitators, preferred features, and desirable functions need to be assessed before recommending or using an AT or AAC device.

Common barriers:
- Physical factors (vision, fine motor skills etc.)
- Cognitive factors (memory, executive function etc.)
- Psychosocial
- Access to device
- Funding
- Support team
- Reliability
- Speed of internet connection or device

Facilitators to successful use include motivation, training, support team, consumer involvement about choice of device, individualized approach (goals and needs), funding, ongoing assessment, and reevaluation. Features that need to be considered are ease of use, capacity for storage, and congruence with needs. Therefore, proper assessment with an AAC-trained therapist is recommended, and ongoing training, repetition, and visits are recommended for both the person and caregiver/support team for the brain-injured person.[3]

Review Questions

1. Assistive technology (AT) as defined by public law is
   a. a device that is used to decrease the functional capabilities of individuals with disabilities.
   b. a device that is customized for an individual with a disability.
   c. a device that can be off the shelf, modified, or customized to increase the functional capabilities of individuals with disabilities.
   d. a device that is obtained commercially off the shelf for an individual with a disability.
2. Federal regulations state which of these services must be included when considering applications of AT?
   a. Purchasing or leasing devices
   b. Designing and fabricating devices
   c. Coordinating services offered by providers of AT services
   d. All of the above
3. Individualized Education Program (IEP) was developed under the provision of which act?
   a. The Tech Act
   b. Individuals With Disabilities Education Act (IDEA)
   c. Reauthorization of Rehabilitation Act
   d. Americans With Disabilities Act

Answers on page 399.
Access the full list of questions and answers online. Available on ExpertConsult.com

References

1. Braddom R. *Physical Medicine and Rehabilitation*. 3rd ed. 2007: 523-539.
2. http://natri.uky.edu/resources/fundamentals/laws.html
3. Brunner M, Hemsley B, Togher L, Palmer, S. Technology and its role in rehabilitation for people with cognitive-communication disability following a traumatic brain injury. *Brain Inj*. 2017;4:1-16.
4. Ferguson S, Friedland D, Woodberry E. Smartphone technology: gentle reminders of everyday tasks for difficulties post-brain injury. *Brain Inj*. 2015;29(5):583-591.
5. Lannin N, Carr B, Allaous J, et al. A randomized controlled trial of effectiveness of handheld computers for improving everyday memory functioning in patients with memory impairments after acquired brain injury. *Clin Rehabil*. 2014;28(5):470-481.
6. Dowd MM, Lee PH, Sheer JB, et al. Electronic reminding technology following traumatic brain injury: effects on timely task completion. *J Head Trauma Rehabil*. 2011;26(5):339-347.
7. Evald L. Prospective memory rehabilitation using smartphones in patients with TBI: what do participants report? *Neuropsychol Rehabil*. 2015;25(2):283-297.
8. Craig A, Tran Y, McIsaac P, Boord P. The efficacy and benefits of environmental control systems for the severely disabled. *Med Sci Monit*. 2004;11(1):RA32-39.
9. Pfurtscheller G, Allison BZ, Brunner C, et al. The hybrid BCI. *Front Neurosci*. 2010;4:42.

45

Community Reentry

ERIC T. SPIER, MD

OUTLINE

- Defining the Problem
- Population Considerations
- Settings in the Continuum of Care
- Special Problems

The goal of this chapter is to define the meaning of community reentry in patients with a brain injury (BI) diagnosis. Patients who benefit from this service have had an alteration in their independence and ability to live in a community setting. Because challenges include premorbid factors, injury characteristics, and patient expectations, the services are best provided in a specialty setting.

Community reentry services include:

- Productive activity
- Return to school or habilitation services
- Vocational needs
- For most brain injury survivors, transportation issues and driving

Agency is the primary goal for people seeking reentry rehabilitation services. This is defined by a level of 6 to 8 on the Glasgow Outcome Scale-Extended (GOS-E) or a score of 4 to 5 on the Glasgow Outcome Scale (GOS). Patients who are expected to achieve a recovery of high-moderate disability to good recovery are usually the targets of reentry. Limitations to achieving these goals range from a high-level expressive aphasia preventing a person's return to a communications job to severe mental and physical fatigue preventing full-time work from being possible at all. Sixteen model systems projects contribute to a common longitudinal data system that tracks patients from emergency care through postacute rehabilitation to postinjury outcomes, including return to work (RTW). In a data review of 20 years of traumatic brain injury model systems data, the most clinically predictive indicator of a good GOS or GOS-E is duration of posttraumatic amnesia (PTA) or injury severity.

Variables that add predictive power were:

- Premorbid education
- Productivity
- Occupational category[1]

For those who are not able to achieve competitive employment after discharge, supportive employment may be an intermediate goal. Competitive employment is in a real job, not with a group of others with disabilities, and not for subminimal wages in the community. This is contrasted with supported employment, a service used to progress someone to competitive employment. Supportive employment includes resource facilitation with services like job coaching and was developed in the late 1980s by Wehman and colleagues at Virginia Commonwealth University. Resource facilitation is an evidence-based partnership that helps survivors identify and retain services to help them meet employment goals.[2]

These services are mentored by therapists with special training and degrees. These providers are referred to as *vocational rehabilitation* (VR) *specialists*. They usually fall into two categories: certified rehabilitation counselor (CRC) or occupational therapists (OTs) with specialty training.

VR services are poorly supported, but the degree to which they do exist has been in part because of the Rehabilitation Act of 1973 (amended in 1998), which created the Department of Vocational Rehabilitation (DVR). The DVR provides federal grants to provide VR services for persons with disabilities. VR services are time limited and expected to be comprehensive and individualized.

Successful programming includes:

- Assessment
- Job placement
- Job training and support
- Rehabilitation counseling
- Long-term follow along
  RTW services may include:
- Situational assessment
- Followed by work site assessment
- Driving evaluation
- Job coaching
  Various accommodations can help a person be successful once returning to work. Examples of work accommodations include:
- Temporarily limited hours
- Oversight and feedback from coemployees

- Additional time to review work
- Compensatory strategies
- Structured rest breaks
- Option to work from home

Defining the Problem

The goals of an acute rehabilitation stay are to address acute medical needs, therapy needs, and basic activities of daily living (ADLs). Inpatient rehab is not typically to achieve complete independence but does include anything that would allow a person to be independent for more than 24 hours at a time.

This may also include:

- RTW
- School
- Managing a household
- Engaging independently in productive activity outside a home
- Transportation

Goals of higher-level independence are not funded in an inpatient rehabilitation facility (IRF) based on the logic that regaining higher level skills can be achieved without medical oversight. However, the complexity of safely reentering the community needs a coordinated interdisciplinary system of providers and specialists who individualize the care for each acquired brain injury (ABI) patient. One can imagine the difference in skills needed between a nuclear reactor operator and an air traffic controller.

The patient's primary rehabilitation team works with involved parties to recommend accommodations. Leaving complex executive decision making to the patient in whom these skills (and insight into them) may be lacking is a faulty strategy. Services geared toward higher level independence are difficult to find because they don't reimburse well enough to be profitable in a for-profit system. These services are either creatively delivered in a well-funded minority or subsidized in nonprofit settings. In either case, only a minority of patients have access to the resource, whether it is because of society's value on agency or poor funding. Discharging patients before addressing reentry goals is the unfortunate but most common outcome.

Driving laws vary from state to state, but the safety and legality of driving again after brain injury is clearly important. A patient's safety awareness and deficits should be reviewed in an inpatient setting to determine whether driving is a realistic goal.

Then the therapy team can look at driving readiness from a discipline-specific perspective to include:

- Safety awareness
- Vision
- Reaction time
- Ability to interpret and see signage

This is followed by an on-the-road assessment, the gold standard of driving readiness testing. At this point, the patient can present to the department of motor vehicles for licensure. The laws regarding how these steps are carried out vary slightly between programs and states.

Some community reentry programs have a teacher or other representative on the rehab team who serves as a liaison between the patient and the school to determine the best course of action. This may include completing coursework in parallel to being in rehab therapy or a return to school program that begins at home if medical complications make school attendance impossible.

Schools can create accommodations such as:

- Limited classroom time
- A live scribe or iPad
- Additional time for assignments
- Preferential seating
- Early access to lecture material
- Adjustment to attendance policies
- Extended test time
- The option to test in a separate environment

Population Considerations

Reentry services are most critical for working and school-age individuals where lifetime dollars lost by not returning to the workforce have the biggest societal consequence, to say nothing of impact to patient and family. The Centers for Medicare and Medicaid Services (CMS) leads the industry in what services should be provided. CMS, by design, is only responsible for retirees over age 65 and permanently disabled individuals who are not returning to work. Most private insurances follow basic CMS guidelines, so the expectation to provide reentry services is also largely absent with private funding sources.

Workers' compensation (WC) and the Department of Defense (DoD) avert that complication by design but have a secondary set of pitfalls associated with secondary gain. We know, for example, that the relationship between employer and employee does not always set the best intentions, with RTW rates plummeting the more time an employee is out of work. Employees are afraid to lose their benefit by RTW too early and not being successful, whereas WC is guarding against malingering and other abuses to the payment model. The ongoing responsibility WC has for its benefactors affords some of the best long-term outcomes, but it can also lead to unnecessary and expensive medical costs and/or litigation.

A review of the literature demonstrates a dearth of evidence that outcomes after TBI can be predicted or improved.[3,4] Additionally, there is not agreement on what is meant by *community integration* for research and treatment planning.[5] Recent data from the past 5 years are more optimistic. Return to employment long term after TBI, 6 to 10 years, is more likely with patients who are young or have had milder injury.[6] The more time that passes postinjury, the more difficult it is to have a successful return to work, suggesting a benefit to early rehabilitative efforts, but more research is needed.[7] Developing ways that help differentiate those who will most benefit from resources is important.

There is a complicated network of providers involved in rehabilitative care who all share the onus of developing a successful reentry plan. A study assessing the benefit of VR services in the United Kingdom showed inpatients with moderate to severe TBI who received VR services were 27% more likely to be employed 1 year after discharge with a negligible difference in healthcare costs.[8] Identifying who is most likely to benefit from services may be helpful in determining resource allocation. In patients who sustained an TBI, 53% of participants had returned to work 1 year postinjury. Probabilities of being employed were 95% lower for those who had been unemployed before injury and 74% lower for those with a more severe injury.[9]

Settings in the Continuum of Care

High comorbidities exist for the population of people recovering from moderate to severe ABI. Hospital readmission rates and secondary medical costs are high for patients with disorders of consciousness (DOC), and they are frequently passed into lower levels of care too soon. It is imperative for a person's rights and agency to be considered and to be cared for in the appropriate location for their injury type and severity. These patients often continue to improve, and this allows for a rehabilitation team specializing in brain injury medicine (BIM) to identify when to begin reentry specific goals.

The following are settings in which goals may be addressed and some of the strategies that should be employed.

In an IRF, the treatment is a balance between medical necessity and rehabilitation needs—often referred to as the *Goldilocks rule*. Initiating a community reentry plan is not often a realistic option in most settings. When these goals can be initiated and the resources are in place to begin community reintegration, there are some clear advantages to beginning treatment in an acute rehabilitation setting.

- First, the inpatient rehabilitation team services are more intensive and communication is more robust, so it is easier to set a plan in motion.
- Second, setting expectations early can be beneficial to the patient and family. Opportunities for helping with short-term disability, financial planning, and for more protracted cases stress inoculation or other forms of psychological support are helpful.
- Last is identifying the next setting for care for successful reentry. Early intervention equates to better job retention. Resources fade away more rapidly than most families and patients anticipate, so aligning expectations for future care can decrease the shock of discharging.

Postacute residential brain injury settings vary significantly in design and funding. Because this setting is not paid for by CMS and the private insurance industry varies extensively on payer models, there is inconsistent access to the service. These services are designed to help people RTW and gain independence. Settings where reentry services are available can be a critical link between an IRF level of care and reentry goals critical to community independence.

- In the postacute setting, length of stays for brain injury patients tend to be longer because goals include regaining lost function and new skill acquisition. There is little to no medical training in BIM fellowships and residency training

programs about these services. There is opportunity for research and advocacy in this area to potentially increase access to a larger population of people who could benefit from this care. These settings are additionally beneficial because they create structured safe environments where maladaptive behaviors are common and can be addressed more effectively.
- Day program services are intensive comprehensive settings for care that can offer many of the benefits of IRFs without the same medical necessity requirements. They are also hard to find because the resource to funding ratio that makes creating successful programs possible is difficult without philanthropy and community support.
- Outpatient rehabilitation can vary extensively in design and may approach day program intensity in some settings. When timed well in the recovery course with clear setting of expectations, this can be a powerful part of the treatment spectrum in ABI community reentry. It is a good setting to begin handing off more responsibility to the patient and family/support structure. There is still access to resources with opportunities to test independence, build insight, and identify unexpected areas of need.

Special Problems

Injury characteristics are as varied as there are patients. Some injury patterns are encountered frequently enough and present enough challenges that they deserve special discussion.

- Anticipating difficulties presented by some of these deficits can be used to facilitate a successful reentry or at least identify where caution should be taken before proceeding. For example, a patient who has worked as a librarian for many years may be more successful than anticipated because of their old knowledge and skills, and an on-the-job evaluation may be warranted. A counter example is a former air traffic controller with anosognosia who is sure they can return to work in spite of clear deficits.
- Patients with low premorbid level of function and low social support are the poorest outcome predictors for independence after injury. As a result, longer periods of rehabilitation and social work support are often needed. Resilience counseling and psychological support with a focus on the support structure and strategies to build interdependence are needed for success.
- Anosognosia is when a patient has complete unawareness of a lost neurological and/or neuropsychological function. It can be better understood as a complete impairment in self-awareness. Many patients will improve with time and build insight progressing to various levels of impaired self-awareness (ISA). This partial syndrome is the area where treatment is targeted. It is important to develop a consistent strategy with the rehabilitation team that includes clear boundaries, maintenance of rapport, and a focus on building awareness. Studies of anosognosia after TBI demonstrate that 33% of severely injured patients resume a reasonably productive lifestyle 2 to

4 years after injury, but when the follow-up is 10 to 15 years, it is less than 10%.[10] Predictors of outcome post TBI for both work and school after 1 year were shown to be more sensitive to self-centeredness and initiation (aka behavioral difficulties) than for neurological symptoms, physical injuries, cognitive difficulties, and emotional difficulties. Only severity of injury or duration of PTA were as predictive of poor outcome.[11] In another prospective study out of the Netherlands, both psychiatric symptoms postinjury and impaired cognition were considered to be the highest risk factors at 3 years of follow-up for unemployment.[12] These findings are consistent with other more recent prospective studies.[13]

- Aphasia constitutes a large range of deficits and depending on the presentation can have no impact on reentry goals in some patients and be devastating to independence with others. Communication ability relates significantly to psychosocial functioning at 1 year post TBI, and continued speech therapy can prove beneficial.[14] A delivery driver with expressive deficits or speech apraxia may have specific scripts that he can carry with him and have minimal impact on performance, whereas a waiter may benefit from habilitation and move to working in the kitchen where language skills are not an essential function. Patients with fluent receptive Wernicke's aphasia are extremely challenging to reintegrate into life and work after injury. This fact is made more challenging given the frequent copresentation of anosognosia with this deficit.

- Mood disorders are best treated with neuropsychiatry, neuropsychology, and/or other specialists knowledgeable in the treatment of ABI. The need to tease out depression, anxiety, and manic symptoms from affective dysfunction is important. Pseudobulbar affect, deficits in prosody, abulia, alexithymia, and fatigue can complicate the clinical picture with very different treatments needed for similar clinical presentations. Communicating these findings with the patient, social support structure, and treatment team will help develop effective strategies for treatment. Something as simple as explaining deficits in prosody or loss of the ability to interpret a loved one's facial expressions can save a marriage or job.

Review Questions

1. Large clinical studies show definitively that
   a. aphasia is the largest barrier to return to work (RTW).
   b. frontal and temporal injuries associated with anosognosia are the largest barrier to short-term RTW.
   c. time to follow commands (TTFC) is the most significant limitation to RTW .
   d. psychiatric illness postinjury is most correlated barrier for RTW .

2. Goals of community reentry
   a. include school, RTW, vocational, and retirement goals.
   b. are covered through Centers for Medicare and Medicaid Services (CMS) reimbursements.
   c. are covered by Department of Vocational Rehabilitation (DVR) support though state and federal funds.
   d. include support in all inpatient rehabilitation facilities (IRFs).

3. A variable that adds the most predictive power for RTW includes
   a. years since injury.
   b. intellectual quotient.
   c. premorbid education.
   d. medical comorbidities.

Answers on page 399.
Access the full list of questions and answers online. Available on ExpertConsult.com

References

1. Walker WC, Stomberg KA, Marwitz JK,et al. Predicting long-term global outcome after traumatic brain injury: development of a practical prognostic tool using the traumatic brain injury model system national database. *J Neurotrauma*. 2018;35: 1587-1595.
2. Trexler LE, Parrott DR. Models of brain injury vocational rehabilitation: the evidence for resource facilitation from efficacy to effectiveness. *J Vocat Rehabil*. 2018;49:195-203.
3. Saltychev M, Eskola M, Tenovuo O, Laimi K. Return to work after traumatic injury: systematic review. *Brain Inj*. 2013;27 (13-14):1516-1527.
4. Fadyl JK, McPherson KM. Approaches to vocational rehabilitation after traumatic brain injury: a systematic review of the evidence. *J Head Trauma Rehabil*. 2009;24(3):195-212.
5. Sander AM, Clark A, Pappadis MR. What is community integration anyway? Defining meaning following traumatic brain injury. *J Head Trauma Rehabil*. 2010;25(2):121-127.
6. Lexell J, Whilney AK, Jacobson LJ. Vocational outcome 6-15 years after a traumatic brain injury. *Brain Inj*. 2016;30(8):969-974.
7. Cuthbert JP, Pretz CR, Bushnik T, et al. Ten-year employment patterns of working age individuals after moderate to severe traumatic brain injury: a national institute on disability and rehabilitation research traumatic brain injury model systems study. *Am Cong Rehabil Med, Arch Phys Med Rehabil*. 2015;96: 2128-2136.
8. Radford K, Phillips J, Drummond A, et al. Return to work after traumatic brain injury: cohort comparison and economic evaluation. *Brain Inj*. 2013;27(5):507-520.

9. Andelic N, Stevens LF, Sigurdardottir S, Arango-Lasprilla JC, Roe C. Associations between disability and employment 1 year after traumatic brain injury in a working age population. *Brain Inj*. 2012;26(3):261-269.

10. Prigatano GP, Schacter DL, eds. *Awareness of Deficit After Brain Injury*: Clinical and Theoretical Issues. New York, NY: Oxford University Press; 1991.

11. Willmott C, Spitz G, Ponsford JL. Predictors of productivity outcomes for secondary and tertiary students following traumatic brain injury. *Brain Inj*. 2015;29(7-8):929-936.

12. Grauwmwijer E, Heijenbrok-Kal MH, Haitsma IK, Ribbers GM. A prospective study on employment outcome 3 years after moderate to severe traumatic brain injury. *Arch Phys Med Rehabil*. 2012;93:993-999.

13. Benedictus MR, Spikman JM, van der Naalt J. Cognitive and behavioral impairment in traumatic brain injury related to outcome and return to work. *Arch Phys Med Rehabil*. 2010;91:1436-1441.

14. Tran S, Kenny B, Power E, et al. Cognitive-communication and psychological functioning 12 months after severe traumatic brain injury. *Brain Inj*. 2018;32(13-14):1700-1711.

46

Involving Family in Rehabilitation: Role of Physiatry

LILLIAN FLORES STEVENS, PHD, AND ANGELLE SANDER, PHD, FACRM

Why Should Physiatrists Involve Family in Treatment?

- Family members are the primary source of support for persons with traumatic brain injury (TBI) regarding:
  - Physical assistance (e.g., transfers, basic and instrumental activities of daily living)
  - Ongoing monitoring and supervision of impact of cognitive deficits on activities (e.g., medication management, medical appointment tracking, decision-making accuracy)
  - Monitoring emotional status (e.g., symptoms of depression and anxiety)
  - Assistance with implementing treatment team recommendations (e.g., physical and occupational therapy exercises, safety precautions)
  - Helping with integration into the community and social and leisure activities
- There is a bidirectional relationship between caregiver and patient health.[1-3]
  - Patients' psychosocial functioning and well-being affect family caregivers' health.
  - Caregivers' psychosocial functioning and well-being affect patient rehabilitation outcomes and community participation.

How Does Traumatic Brain Injury Affect Family Members?

Although there is variability in individual response to caring for a person with TBI, research has documented frequent negative impacts, including[4,5]:
- Decreased physical health
- Increased and often long-lasting emotional distress, including depression and anxiety
- Increased financial strain and higher likelihood of leaving the labor force
- Increased family strain (e.g., decreased communication, increased marital strain)
- Disruption of family roles
- Inattention to their own physical and mental health needs

What Do Family Caregivers Need?

- Clear, honest information about the medical status and needs of the person with injury in language they can understand[6]
- Education on physical, cognitive, emotional, and behavioral changes anticipated in the person with injury
- Information on resources to help with daily needs (e.g., obtaining needed outpatient treatment, getting financial assistance)
- Information on how to get emotional support (e.g., caregiver support groups, Brain Injury Association of America)
- Referrals for services to help them adjust to the caregiving role and their own emotions, if needed (e.g., individual counseling/psychotherapy, family therapy)

What Can Physiatrists Do to Help Family Members?

- Involve them in treatment planning, goal setting, and decision making.

TABLE 46.1 **Recommendations for Family Interventions Based on Distress Level[4]**

Nature of Family Distress	General Level of Intervention
Family functioning well before injury but experiencing normal distress related to injury.	• Education about traumatic brain injury (TBI) • Assistance in beginning to consider the longer term consequences • Reinforcement of existing coping strategies
Mild preexisting disturbances in family dynamics appear to be exacerbating normal reaction to TBI-related stress.	• Education about TBI • Assistance in developing longer term contingency plans • Intensive counseling and assistance in developing mutually supportive coping skills
Long-standing and pathological family dysfunction is an obstacle to coping with injury and to the rehabilitation process.	• Standard TBI education, support, and long-term planning • Additional intensive family therapy

TABLE 46.2 **Family Intervention Considerations Based on Treatment Setting[5]**

Treatment Setting	Typical Family Member Experience	Intervention Considerations
Inpatient/acute trauma	• Emotionally overwhelmed and confused • Difficulty processing and recalling what health professionals tell them	• Brief education and normalization of traumatic brain injury (TBI)–related sequalae (e.g., agitation, posttraumatic amnesia) that can be confusing to family members • Emotional support to family members experiencing grief and/or distress
Inpatient rehabilitation	• Hope and joy, because patients often show rapid improvement • May have unrealistic expectations of the pace of future recovery and unawareness of long-term problems	• Regular updates on progress, facilitate realistic hope and discharge plans • Neuropsychological assessment to identify remaining deficits and areas of strength and provide family members with education and training on strategies to manage remaining deficits • Case management to facilitate access to resources
Postacute rehabilitation	• Increased emotional distress as they adjust to life at home and become aware of injury-related limitations	• Work with family members to set functional goals for activities at home and in the community • Cognitive rehabilitation as needed to develop and implement compensatory strategies • Neuropsychological assessment to help identify remaining impairments and areas of strength and provide family members with education and training on strategies to manage remaining deficits • Individual or family psychotherapy as needed to assist family members in coping with injury-related changes

• Explain things to them in clear language—avoid medical jargon.
• Be familiar with referral sources that can help them adjust, such as psychologists/neuropsychologists, social workers, and nurse educators.

• Be familiar with differing intervention needs based on different levels of family distress (Table 46.1).
• Be familiar with family reactions and needs depending on the stage of brain injury recovery and treatment setting (Table 46.2).

Review Questions

1. When considering the impact on rehabilitation, what is the best way to characterize the relationship between patient and caregiver?
   a. Unidirectional: The caregiver's psychosocial functioning affects the injured individual's rehabilitation outcomes.
   b. Unidirectional: The patient's rehabilitation outcome affects their caregiver's psychosocial functioning.
   c. Bidirectional: The psychosocial functioning of patients affects their family caregiver's health, and the psychosocial functioning of caregivers affects patient rehabilitation outcomes.
   d. None: The patient-caregiver relationship does not affect rehabilitation outcomes.

2. Which is the need considered most important by family caregivers?
   a. The need for emotional support.
   b. The need for medical information and education.
   c. The need for instrumental support.
   d. The need for financial relief.

3. What factor would be most important to consider when addressing the needs of family members during the acute rehabilitation phase of recovery?
   a. Family members may experience hope and joy in witnessing improvements and may have unrealistic expectations about the future.
   b. Family members may experience increased emotional distress as they become more aware of how the limitations of the person with injury affect their daily lives.
   c. Family members may be emotionally overwhelmed and confused and have difficulty processing and recalling detailed information.
   d. Family members may be processing grief and distress related to the injury.

Answers on page 399.
Access the full list of questions and answers online. Available on ExpertConsult.com

References

1. Winstanley J, Simpson G, Tate R, Myles B. Early indicators and contributors to psychological distress in relatives during rehabilitation following severe traumatic brain injury: findings from the Brain Injury Outcomes Study. *J Head Trauma Rehab*. 2006; 21:453-466.
2. Sady MD, Sander AM, Clark AN, Sherer M, Nakase-Richardson R, Malec JF. Relationship of pre-injury caregiver and family functioning to community integration in adults with traumatic brain injury. *Arch Phys Med Rehab*. 2010;91: 1542-1550.
3. Sander AM, Maestas KL, Sherer M, Malec JF, Nakase-Richardson R. Relationship of caregiver and family functioning to participation outcomes after postacute rehabilitation for traumatic brain injury: a multicenter investigation. *Arch Phys Med Rehab*. 2012; 93:842-848.
4. Malec JF, Van Houtven CH, Tanielian T, Atizado A, Dorn MC. Impact of TBI on caregivers of Veterans with TBI: burden and interventions. *Brain Inj*. 2017;31(9):1235-1245.
5. Sander AM. Treating and collaborating with family caregivers in the rehabilitation of persons with traumatic brain injury. In: Sherer M, Sander AM, eds. *Handbook on the Neuropsychology of Traumatic Brain Injury, Clinical Handbooks in Neuropsychology*. New York, NY: Springer; 2014:271-282.
6. Kreutzer JS, Marwitz JH, Klyce DW, et al. Family needs on an inpatient brain injury rehabilitation unit: a quantitative assessment. *Brain Inj*. 2018;33(4):228-236.

Special Topics

47

Pediatric Traumatic Brain Injury

DAVID CANCEL, MD, JD, RUTH E. ALEJANDRO, MD, FAAPMR AND DARA D. JONES, MD

OUTLINE

Traumatic brain injury is (TBI) is defined as "an alteration in brain function, or other evidence of brain pathology, caused by an external force."[1] In children, a pediatric TBI disrupts the normal stages of growth required for full maturation of the developing brain. This is further complicated by different stages of growth and development throughout a child's life. This chapter highlights features of pediatric TBI that distinguish it from that of adult TBI.

Epidemiology

Epidemiological features of pediatric TBI include age, gender, premorbid developmental and environmental history, and mechanisms of injury.
- TBI is leading cause of death and disability in pediatric trauma.[2]
- Under age 10, 50% of TBIs are from transport-related accidents, falls, and assaults.
- In older children, the most common cause is from motor vehicle crashes.[3]

- The largest affected pediatric groups are infants and adolescents. The most common cause of TBI under age 4 is falls.[4]

Morbidity and Mortality

Morbidity and mortality rates often reflect the severity of injury, presence of additional injuries, and the age of the child. There is greater morbidity with the presence of serious concomitant injuries—longer hospitalization, increased infections, fewer ventilator-free days, and higher level of care required on discharge from the hospital.[5]
- Morbidity in survivor rates are 75% to 95% with good recovery, 10% with moderate disability, 1% to 3% severe disability.
- "Abusive head trauma is most common TBI-related cause of death under 4 years of age."[4]
- Children younger than age 2 have a mortality rate of 50% and worse outcomes compared with older children.
- In severe TBI, mortality rates vary from 12% to 62%, in moderate TBI 4%, in mild TBI (mTBI) less than 1%.[6]

Age and Gender

Age and gender-related factors play a role in the location, mechanism, and severity of injury.
- Relative risk for TBI is equal between both genders before age 2.[3]
- Cognitive and academic outcomes are worse in the younger age group.[7]
- By age 10, 16% will sustain at least one head injury necessitating medical care.[8]
- TBI mortality increased between 2013-2017 due to increase in suicide mortality despite decrease in motor vehicle crashes in previous years.[9]
- Boys, rural children, and children ages 15-19 had higher mortality rates between 1999-2017 than girls, urban, and younger children[9]
- The majority of sports-recreation related concussions occur in children under 18 years of age.[10]
- Male:female ratio in school-aged children is 2:1.[11]
- In adolescence, this mortality risk increases to a ratio of 4:1.[12]

- Anatomical and physiological factors include head and neck strength differences; with women having less head–neck mass and neck girth to absorb impact and acceleration forces.[13]

Preinjury history can serve as a risk factor for injury. This can include home settings and premorbid conditions.

In very young victims, these can be homes with poor coping skills,[14] limited financial means,[15] psychiatric/psychological difficulties, fewer family resources,[16] and a single-parent household.[17] In older children, hyperactivity and attention deficit may be a risk factor.[18] There has been an association with Hispanic ethnicity and mTBI.[19] Mild TBI can be associated with 50% rate of premorbid learning disabilities or poor academic performance,[20] and 17% of children with persistent deficits after mTBI had previous head injury; hyperactivity; learning, behavioral, psychiatric/neurological conditions; and family difficulties.[21]

As with adults, injury characteristics were predictive of outcomes. In pediatric TBI, additional predictive value was seen in neuroimaging findings that showed bilateral brain edema, multiple and/or diffuse brain lesions, decreased brain volumes, and increased ventricular size.[22,23]

Measurement, Pathophysiology, and Classification of Traumatic Brain Injury

The classification of pediatric TBI severity involves the integration of acute injury measurement scales and understanding the pathophysiology and mechanisms of injury. Pediatric versions of widely used assessment scales are used to help address limitations in testing. These are because of the differences in the developmental level of the pediatric population being tested. These can be used to classify injury severity, which in turn can predict outcomes. Description of these scales will focus on the differences when used in children.

Measurement Scales

- For children 3-15 years of age, the Children's Orientation and Amnesia Test (COAT). This test incorporates the developmental level when assessing patients[26]
- Glasgow Coma Scale (GCS): Used frequently; appears best for ages 5 years and above; therefore age-appropriate cognitive–linguistic pediatric coma scales are used[24]
- Loss of Consciousness (LOC): As in adults, describes the time frame of consciousness/coma[25]
- Post-Traumatic Amnesia (PTA) can be assessed via the Children's Orientation and Amnesia Test (COAT). Duration used to predict short and long term outcome after pediatric TBI.[26]
- As in adults, the classification system for grading TBI severity often incorporates GCS, LOC and PLA[27]

Pathophysiological Differences

Complex, multifactorial contributions to brain injury can result from pathophysiological differences. These include developmental responses postinjury that distinguish pediatric from adult TBI.

Brain Development

- Increased cerebral water content and blood volume[28]
- Larger head:body ratio
- Immature nerve cell myelination
- Weaker neck musculature and ligamentous connections
- Increased blood-brain permeability
- Decreased skull absorption of mechanical forces[29]

Post–Brain Injury Development

- Brain atrophy
- Impaired brain autoregulation[29]
- Increased diffusion of excitotoxic neurotransmitters[30]

Classification of Pediatric Traumatic Brain Injury

The mechanical properties of pediatric brain tissue and the immature skull play an important role in defining the underlying injury. Infant brain tissue is mostly composed of axons. Increased myelination of astrocytes and oligodendrocytes decrease the "stiffness" of the brain tissue.[31] Age-dependent variances in skull thickness and infant cranial suture fusions should also be considered.[32] Because of this, most pediatric brain injuries result in generalized brain injury.[33]

The developing brains of the pediatric group respond differently to trauma than adults, with more susceptibility to hypoxic–ischemic insults, hypotension, posttraumatic swelling, and diffuse injuries.[33] Despite the similarities in brain injury mechanisms reviewed, individual differences with varying complex patterns of neuromuscular and neuropsychological impairments are evident in all patients with TBI.[34]

Abusive Head Trauma

AHT, also known as *shaken baby syndrome*, is a unique feature of pediatric TBI. Child abuse is the major cause of AHT in the youngest subgroups. Pathological mechanisms of inertial forces alone are associated with an increased likelihood of diffuse injury, traumatic axonal injury, and subdural hematoma.[35] Anatomical factors include open fontanelles, softer skulls with poorer impact absorption, and weaker neck musculature with relatively large heads. These factors making infants likely to sustain a diffuse TBI.[36]

Concussion and Mild Traumatic Brain Injury

A distinct subset of pediatric TBI involves concussion, considered a form of mTBI. *Concussion* is defined as "a traumatically induced transient disturbance of brain function."[37]

TABLE 47.1	"Types of Head injury"	
Penetrating Head Injury (PHI)	**Closed Head Injury (CHI)**	
• Damages skull, dura • Leads to focal lesion[32] • Lower incidence of PHI compared with adults[33]	• Generalized injury[34] • Diffuse damage • Majority of pediatric traumatic brain injuries occur via CHI[35]	

TABLE 47.2	"Primary versus Secondary Injuries"
Primary Injury	**Secondary Injury**
• Damage at the initial time of injury • Via direct and/or indirect contact acceleration-deceleration forces[40] • Presence or lack of skull fracture[41] • Most likely from motor vehicle accidents involving high-velocity acceleration–deceleration forces[42]*	• From hours after injury up to weeks or longer • Via altered regulatory mechanisms • Children more likely to have indirect brain trauma than from intracranial hemorrhages[43] • Secondary brain damage (from treatable causes)
• Contusions • Coup–contrecoup injuries • Cranial nerve injuries • Diffuse axonal injuries (DAI)[42]	• Increased intracranial pressure and cerebral edema: most common complications in children[43] • Hydrocephalus: can occur in rehab settings or remotely postinjury[44]

*Acceleration–deceleration forces: combination of translational and rotational acceleration is the most damaging mechanism of inertial forces; correlated more with subdural hematoma and DAI (the latter correlated with long-term functional disabilities)

TABLE 47.3	Assessment of Abusive Head Trauma
Risk factors	Male gender, young mother (under 21 years of age), and multiparity[47]
Presenting symptoms	Nonspecific (i.e., altered state of consciousness, seizures, vomiting, breathing difficulty, apnea, increasing head circumference, failure to thrive, and delayed development), and the traumatic event is not easily disclosed[48]
Unique features of abusive head trauma	Subdural hematoma (diffuse, inter-hemispheric, or posterior fossa locations) and retinal hemorrhage (most common findings)[49] with multiple fractures of varying ages, irritability, poor feeding, vomiting, observed periods of apnea, and skin lesions[50]

Although concussion and mTBI are not unique to pediatric TBI and the topic is reviewed elsewhere in this textbook, it is worth noting certain aspects of concussion in children:

- From 2001 - 2012, 70% of ED visits for sports related concussions were among children.[38]
- In males, higher rates in contact sports—American Football, Basketball, Soccer and Baseball[39]
- In females—Soccer, Basketball and Hockey[39]
- Second-impact syndrome is a controversial and rare but serious complication seen with children who have reinjury during the initial postinjury period.[40]

Total rest is no longer recommended. Current guidelines recommend symptom-limited cognitive and physical rest in the immediate postinjury period (up to 48 hours), followed by a gradual or graded increase in physical activity. In children, there is also a gradual return to learn protocol to allow the transition back to academic activity. This should precede the return to sport protocol, with resolution of concussion-related symptoms before a return to play.[41]

Rehabilitation Strategies in Pediatric Traumatic Brain Injury

Sections after this address common issues pertaining to the treatment of pediatric brain injury in the rehabilitation setting. These include pharmacological management for cognition and arousal, dysautonomia, and spasticity. This is followed by selected medical complications in children with TBI.

Medications for Cognition, Arousal, and Dysautonomia

- **Amantadine:** N-methyl-D-aspartate receptor antagonist used to improve arousal and attention in children[42]
- **Melatonin:** Postulated to help reset the sleep–wake cycle[43] with possible neuroprotective role in TBI[44]; children may secrete more, not less, melatonin in the acute stages of brain injury[45]
- **Bromocriptine:** Dopamine D2 agonist cited in multiple case reports for treatment-resistant central hyperthermia[46-48]
- **Morphine:** Centrally acting opioid analgesic used in children with autonomic instability[49,50]
- **Beta-adrenergic receptor antagonists:** Used in autonomic instability; slows cerebral metabolism and catecholamine-induced catabolic state[51]
- **Clonidine:** Used for sympathetic hyperactivity in combination with beta blockers[52]
- **Gabapentin:** Effective for dysautonomia in which standard treatments were ineffective[53]

Medications for Spasticity

Treatment goals for spasticity in the child with a brain injury not only include goals for improving gross and fine motor function but also seek to improve positioning, comfort, ease of care, and decreased need for surgical intervention in a growing child.[54] Unlike in adults, spasticity management in pediatric patients must also incorporate future physical and developmental stages.

Oral Medications

- **Baclofen:** Gamma aminobutyric acid (GABA B) receptor agonist at the level of the spinal cord; adverse effects include sedation and fatigue; abrupt discontinuation may cause withdrawal-increased spasticity, seizures, hyperthermia, altered mental status; most severe withdrawal complication is rhabdomyolysis and multiorgan failure[55]; treatment of withdrawal usually involves reinstitution of oral baclofen[56]

- **Tizanidine:** Centrally acting alpha-2 adrenergic agonist that increases presynaptic inhibition of motor neurons; adverse effects include sedation, drowsiness, hypotension, dizziness, and dry mouth; contraindicated in patients taking antihypertensives[57]

- **Benzodiazepines:** Act at spinal cord and supraspinal levels by mediating GABA A receptors; adverse effects include ataxia, urinary retention, constipation, and hypersalivation[58]

- **Dantrolene:** Inhibits release of calcium at the level of the sarcoplasmic reticulum; adverse effects of weakness, gastrointestinal symptoms, hepatoxicity with features of acute hepatitis[59]; no cases of hepatotoxicity have been reported in children[60]

- **Clonidine:** Centrally acting alpha-2 adrenergic agonist that increases presynaptic inhibition of motor neurons; common effects include hypotension, sedation, and dry mouth; contraindicated in patients taking antihypertensives; has additional benefit of use in treatment of sympathetic hyperactivity[61]

- **Gabapentin:** Inhibits presynaptic glutamate release by modulating calcium channels; has the adverse effects of sedation, dizziness, and ataxia[62]

Interventional Medications

- **Botulinum toxin:** For treatment of focal spasticity; blocks transmission of acetylcholine from the presynaptic nerve terminal at the neuromuscular junction; adverse events include localized pain and excessive weakness; more severe adverse events can include respiratory failure and systemic weakness[63]

- **Intrathecal baclofen:** GABA B receptor agonist, blocking polysynaptic and monosynaptic afferent neuronal transmission; used for generalized spasticity; contraindications include hypersensitivity to oral baclofen[64]
  - Complications include dose-related causes (overdose or withdrawal) and implant malfunction[65]; symptoms of baclofen withdrawal can include itching, rebound spasticity, hallucinations, seizures, and eventual rhabdomyolysis; treatment of withdrawal can include restarting oral baclofen, administering diazepam, or dantrolene[66]
  - For intrathecal baclofen withdrawal can also give cyproheptadine, a serotonin agonist[67]

- **Neurolysis with alcohol/phenol:** Alcohol and phenol effect neurolysis through the destruction of peripheral nerves; adverse events include injection site pain, dysesthesia, and hypotension[68]

Medical Complications in Pediatric Traumatic Brain Injury

These are selected medical complications with differences in their frequency, management, and outcomes.

- **Heterotopic ossification:** Lower frequency compared with adults[69]; risk factors include severity of injury,[70] autonomic instability,[71] and persistent vegetative state[69]; concerns over bisphosphonates because of long half-life, unknown teratogenic effect, and impact on growing bone[72]

- **Venous thromboembolism** Incidence significantly lower than adults[73]; associated with older age, surgery, transfusion, ventilation, injury severity and lower GCS score[74]

- **Epilepsy and prophylaxis:** 5% to 21% of children experience posttraumatic seizures; 32% to 40% develop a recurrence[75]; posttraumatic seizures most associated with younger age, severity of injury, and nonaccidental trauma[76]; prophylaxis in first week advised but none afterward unless posttraumatic seizures occur[77]

- **Attention deficit hyperactivity disorder (ADHD):** Commonly seen after TBI; often associated with both premorbid and postinjury ADHD[78]

- **Depression:** Occurs less frequently in children than in adults[79]; serotonergic antidepressants, cognitive behavioral interventions show best preliminary evidence for treatment[80]

- **Endocrine dysfunction:** Most common is growth hormone deficiency (varies from 2%–57% of cases); second most common is gonadotropin-releasing hormone (GnRH) deficiency (4%–37%)[81]; unique to children; precocious puberty, requiring GnRH agonist therapy[81,82]

- **Olfactory dysfunction:** May affect children because of role of olfaction in diet,[83] resulting in decreased feeding and ability to thrive

Functional Outcomes in Pediatric Brain Injury

Functional domains most sensitive to TBI are intellectual functioning, processing speed, attention, and verbal memory. Most recovery include intellectual functioning and processing speed.[84] On the other hand, children with a significant premorbid history are more likely to have negative lasting impact from their injury.[85]

- **Glasgow Outcome Scale Extended Peds (GOS-E Peds):** Designed to predict outcome measures from infancy to adulthood; modeled after the Glasgow Outcome Scale (GOS)[86]

- **Children's Orientation and Amnesia Test (COAT):** Derived from the Galveston Orientation and Amnesia Test (GOAT); measures PTA and cognitive functioning in children and adolescents from 3 to 15 years; made up of 16 items that assess general orientation, temporal orientation, and memory[87]

- **Time to Follow Commands (TFC):** Interval in days from injury until individual followed simple verbal commands twice within 24 hr interval[87]; TFC and PTA both added statistically significant predictive power above and beyond the GCS[88]
- **Functional Independence Measure for Children (WeeFIM):** Adaptation of the Functional Independence Measure (FIM) used in adults; for children from 6 months to 7 years without disabilities and older children with developmental disabilities; three domains: self-care (eight items), mobility (five items), and cognition (five items); has been further expanded to include children up to 18 years, allowing interface with the adult FIM[89]
- **Pediatric Evaluation of Disability Inventory (PEDI):** Assesses self-care (73 items), mobility (59 items), social function (65 items), caregiver assistance (20 items); for children ages 6 months to 7.5 years with physical limitations, combination of physical and cognitive limitations; also used in older children with developmental disabilities[90]

Review Questions

1. A 13-year-old boy is tackled during a football game. He does not lose consciousness but was disoriented for 20 seconds and cannot recall his injury. His headache is improving, but during sideline evaluation he is unsteady and has difficulty with single-leg stance during balance testing.

   The next best step is
   a. home rest for 1 week, then graded return to learn/play.
   b. home monitoring with family, then graded return to learn/play.
   c. computed tomography (CT) scan, then graded return to learn/play.
   d. magnetic resonance imaging (MRI), then graded return to learn/play.

2. You are at a long-term care facility seeing a 7-year-old girl with severe traumatic brain injury (TBI). The child has been noted to have weight gain, onset of menses, and signs of breast development. What is the most likely treatment option?
   a. Gonadotropin-releasing hormone (GnRH) agonist
   b. GnRH antagonist
   c. Estrogen
   d. Testosterone

3. You are following a child with TBI in the outpatient clinic. His mother notes that the child is "different" since the injury. He has behavioral issues in school. He keeps getting up in the middle of class to wander about, disrupting lessons. Teachers report that he is unable to focus on schoolwork. At home he takes longer to fall asleep. What is the most likely cause of the changes in behavior?
   a. Depression
   b. Anxiety
   c. Attention deficit hyperactivity disorder (ADHD)
   d. Oppositional defiant disorder

Answers on page 400.
Access the full list of questions and answers online. Available on ExpertConsult.com

Reference

1. Menon DK, Schwab K, Wright DW, et al. Position statement: definition of traumatic brain injury. *Arch Phys Med Rehabil.* 2010;91:1637-1640.
2. Rutland-Brown W, Langlois JA, Thomas KE, Xi YL. Incidence of traumatic brain injury in the United States, 2003. *J Head Trauma Rehabil.* 2006;21:544-548.
3. Summers CR, Ivins B, Schwab KA. Traumatic brain injury in the United States: an epidemiological overview. *Mt Sinai J Med.* 2009;76:105-110.
4. National Center for Injury Prevention and Control. Traumatic brain injury-related emergency department visits, hospitalizations, and deaths – United States, 2007 and 2013. Atlanta, GA: Department of Health and Human Services, Centers for Disease Control and Prevention. *MMWR Surveill Summ.* 2017;66(9):1-16. doi:10.15585 /mmwr.ss6609a1.
5. Stewart TC, Alharfi IM, Fraser DD. The role of serious concomitant injuries in the treatment and outcome of pediatric severe traumatic brain injury. *J Trauma Acute Care Surg.* 2013;75(5): 836-842.
6. Kraus JF. Epidemiological features in brain injury in children: occurrence, children at risk, causes and manner of injury, severity and outcomes. In: Broman SH, Michels ME, eds, *Traumatic Head Injury in Children.* New York, NY: Oxford University Press; 1995:22-39.
7. Prasad MR, Swank PR, Ewing-Cobbs L. Long-Term School Outcomes of Children and Adolescents With Traumatic Brain Injury. *J Head Trauma Rehabil.* 2017;32(1):E24–E32.
8. Barlow KM, Crawford S, Stevenson A, Sandhu SS, Belanger F, Dewey D. Epidemiology of postconcussion syndrome in pediatric mild traumatic brain injury. *Pediatrics.* 2010;126(2):e374-e381.
9. Cheng P, Li R, Schwebel DC, et al. Traumatic brain injury mortality among U.S. children and adolescents ages 0-19 years, 1999-2017. *J Safety Research.* 2020; 72:93-100.
10. Halstead MD, Walter KD, Council of Sports Medicine and Fitness. Sport-related concussion in children and adolescents. *Pediatrics,* 2018; 142(6):e20183074
11. Sosin DM, Sniezek JE, Thurman DJ. Incidence of mild and moderate brain injury in the United States, 1991. *Brain Inj.* 1996;10:47-54.
12. Annegers JF. The epidemiology of head trauma in children. In: Shapiro K, ed. *Pediatric Head Trauma.* Mount Kisco, NY: Futura; 1983:1-10.

13. Tierney RT, Sitler MR, Swanik CB, Swanik KA, Higgins M, Torg J. Gender differences in head-neck segment dynamic stabilization during head acceleration. *Med Sci Sports Exerc.* 2005; 37(2):272-279.

14. Anderson VA, Morse S, Klugg G, et al. Predicting recovery from head injury in young children: a prospective analysis. *J Int Neuropsychol Soc.* 1997;3:568-580.

15. Parslow RC, Morris KP, Tasker RC, Forsyth RJ, Hawley CA. Epidemiology of traumatic brain injury in children receiving intensive care in the U.K. *Arch Dis Child.* 2005;90:1182-1187.

16. Taylor HG, Drotar D, Wade SL, Yeates KO, Stancin T, Klein S. Recovery from traumatic brain injury in children: the importance of the family. In: Broman SH, Michel ME, eds. *Traumatic Head Injury in Children.* New York, NY: Oxford University Press; 1995; 188-218.

17. Rivara JB, Jaffe KM, Fay GC, et al. Family functioning and injury severity as predictors of child functioning one year following traumatic brain injury. *Arch Phys Med Rehabil.* 1993;74:1047-1055.

18. Max JE, Lansing AE, Koele SL, et al. Attention deficit hyperactivity disorder in children and adolescents following traumatic brain injury. *Dev Neuropsych.* 2004;25(1-2):159-177.

19. Lumba-Brown A, Yeates KO, Sarmiento K, et al. Centers for Disease Control and Prevention Guideline on the diagnosis and management of mild traumatic brain injury among children. *JAMA Pediatr.* 2018;172(11):e182853.

20. Dicker BG. Profile of those at risk for minor head injury. *J Head Trauma Rehabil.* 1992;7:83-91.

21. Ponsford J, Willmott C, Rothwell A, et al. Cognitive and behavioral outcome following mild traumatic head injury in children. *J Head Trauma Rehabil.* 1999;14(4):360-372.

22. Ewing-Cobbs L, Prasad MR, Kramer L, et al. Late intellectual and academic outcomes following traumatic brain injury sustained during early childhood. *J Neurosurg.* 2006;105:2887-2896.

23. Bonnier C, Marique P, Van Hout A, Potelle D. Neurodevelopmental outcome after severe traumatic brain injury in very young children: role for subcortical lesions. *J Child Neurol.* 2007;22:519-529.

24. Kirkham FJ, Newton CRJC, Whitehouse W. Pediatric coma scales. *Dev Med Child Neurol.* 2008;50:267-274.

25. Wagner AK, Arenth PM, Kwasnica CK, Rogers EH. Traumatic Brain Injury. In: Braddom RL, ed. *Physical Medicine and Rehabilitation.* 4th ed. Philadelphia, PA: Elsevier Health Sciences; 2011:1133-1175.

26. Ewing-Cobbs L, Levin HS, Fletcher JM, Miner ME, Eisenberg HM. The children's orientation and amnesia test: relationship to severity of acute head injury and to recovery of memory. *Neurosurgery.* 1990;27(5):683-691; discussion 691.

27. Brasure M, Lamberty GJ, Sayer NA, et al. (2012). Multidisciplinary *Postacute Rehabilitation for Moderate to Severe Traumatic Brain Injury in Adults.* Rockville (MD): Agency for Healthcare Research and Quality (US); Jun. (Comparative Effectiveness Reviews, No. 72.) https://www.ncbi.nlm.nih.gov/books/NBK99000/. Accessed August 26, 2017.

28. Muizelaar J, Marmarou A, DeSalles A, et al. Cerebral blood flow and metabolism in severely head injured children.1. Relationship with GCS, outcome, ICPA and PVI. *J Neurosurg.* 1989;71:63-71.

29. Araki T, Yokota H, Morita A. Pediatric traumatic brain injury: characteristic features, diagnosis, and management. *Neurol Med Chir* (Tokyo). 2017;57(2):82-93.

30. Himwich HE. Early studies of the developing brain. In: Himwich W, ed. *Biochemistry of the Developing Brain.* Vol 1. New York, NY: Marcel Dekker; 1973:2-20.

31. Yamada H. *Strength of Biological Materials.* Baltimore, MD: Williams and Wilkins; 1970.

32. Marr, A.L., & Coronado, V.G. (Eds.) (2004). Central nervous system injury surveillance data submission standards - 2002. Atlanta, GA: Centers for Disease Control and Prevention, National Center for Injury Prevention and Control.

33. Levin, H.S., Culhane, K.A., Mendelsohn, D., Lilly, M.A., Bruce, D., Fletcher, J.M., Chapman, S.B., Harward, H., Eisenberg, H.M. (1993). Cognition in relation to magnetic resonance imaging in head-injured children and adolescents. *Arch Neurol,* Sep; 50(9): 897–905.

34. Graham, D.I., Gennarelli, T.A.: Pathology of brain damage after head injury. In: Head Injury. Copper, P.R., Golfinos, J.G. (Eds.): New York, McGraw-Hill, 2000. pp.133-153.

35. Gennarelli, T., and Thibault, L. (1982). Biomechanics of acute subdural hematoma. *Journal of Trauma,* 22, 680–686.

36. Hahn YS, Chyung C, Barthel MJ, Bailes J, Flannery AM, McLone DG. Head injuries in children under 36 months of age. Demography and outcome. *Childs Nervous System.* 1988a;4:34-40.

37. Harmon KG, Clugston JR, Dec K, et al. American Medical Society for Sports Medicine Position Statement on Concussion in Sport. *Clin J Sport Med.* 2019;29(2):87-100.

38. Coronado VG, Haileyesus T, Cheng TA, et al. Trends in Sports- and Recreation-Related Traumatic Brain Injuries Treated in US Emergency Departments: The National Electronic Injury Surveillance System-All Injury Program (NEISS-AIP) 2001-2012. *J Head Trauma Rehabil.* 2015;30(3):185-197.

39. Sarmiento K, Thomas KE, Daugherty J, et al. Emergency Department Visits for Sports- and Recreation-Related Traumatic Brain Injuries Among Children - United States, 2010-2016. MMWR Morb Mortal Wkly Rep. 2019;68(10):237-242.

40. Gaetz, M. (2004). The neurophysiology of brain injury. *Clinical Neurophysiology,* 115, 4-18.

41. Feng, Y., Abney, T., Okamoto, R., Pless, R., Genin, G., & Bayly, P. (2010). Relative brain displacement and deformation during constrained mild frontal head impact. *J R Soc Interface,* 6; 7(53), 1677-1688.

42. Andriessen, T., Jacobs, B., & Vos, E. (2010). Clinical characteristics and pathophysiological mechanisms of focal and diffuse traumatic brain injury. *J Cell Mol Med,* 14 (10), 2381-2392.

43. Kochanek, P.M., Clark, R.S.B., Ruppel, R.A., Adelson, P.D., Bell, M.J., Whalen, M.J., Robertson, C.L., Satchell, M.A., Seidberg, N.A., Marion, D.W., Jenkins, L.W. (2000). Biochemical, cellular, and molecular mechanisms in the evolution of secondary damage after severe traumatic brain injury in infants and children: lessons learned from the bedside. *Pediatr Crit Care Med,* 1; 4-19.

44. Rumalla K, Letchuman V, Smith KA, Arnold PM. Hydrocephalus in Pediatric Traumatic Brain Injury: National Incidence, Risk Factors, and Outcomes in 124,444 Hospitalized Patients. *Pediatr Neurol.* 2018 Mar;80:70-76.

45. Marseglia L, D'Angelo G, Manti S, et al. Melatonin secretion is increased in children with severe traumatic brain injury. *Int J Mol Sci.* 2017;18(5):1053. doi:10.3390/ijms18051053.

46. Natteru P, George P, Bell R, Nattanmai P, Newey CR. Central hyperthermia treated with bromocriptine. *Case Rep Neurol Med.* 2017;2017:1712083. doi:10.1155/2017/1712083.

47. Parks, S., Sugerman, D., Xu, L., Coronado, V. (2012). Characteristics of non-fatal abusive head trauma among children in the USA, 2003-2008: application of the CDC operational case definition to national hospital inpatient data. *Inj Prev,*18: 392-398.

48. Christian CW, Committee on Child Abuse and Neglect, American Academy of Pediatrics. (2015). The evaluation of suspected child physical abuse. *Pediatrics,* 135(5):e1337-e1354

49. Keenan HT, Runyan DK, Marshall SW, Nocera MA, Merten DF. A population-based comparison of clinical and outcome characteristics of young children with serious inflicted and noninflicted traumatic brain injury. *Pediatrics.* 2004;114(3):633-9.

50. Geddes, J.F., Vowles, G.H., Hacksaw, A.K., et al. (2001). Neuropathology of inflicted head injury in children. II. Microscopic brain injury in infants. *Brain,* 2001 Jul; 124(Pt7):1299-1306

51. Tran TY, Dunne IE, German JW. Beta blockers exposure and traumatic brain injury: a literature review. *Neurosurg Focus.* 2008;25(4):E8. doi:10.3171/FOC.2008.25.10.E8.

52. National Institutes of Health, National Heart, Lung, and Blood Institute. Expert panel on integrated guidelines for cardiovascular health and risk reduction in children and adolescents. *Clinical Practice Guidelines.* 2011. http://www.nhlbi.nih.gov/guidelines/cvd_ped/peds_guidelines_full.pdf. Accessed June 30, 2017.

53. Baguley IJ, Heriseanu RE, Gurka JA, Nordenbo A, Cameron ID. Gabapentin in the management of dysautonomia following severe traumatic brain injury: a case series. *J Neurol Neurosurg Psychiatry.* 2007;78:539-541. doi:10.1136/jnnp.2006.096388.

54. Hansel DE, Hansel CR, Shindle MK, et al. Oral baclofen in cerebral palsy: possible seizure potentiation? *Pediatr Neurol.* 2003;29(3): 203-206.

55. Pérez-Arredondo A, Cázares-Ramírez E, Carrillo-Mora P, et al. Baclofen in the therapeutic of sequel of traumatic brain injury: spasticity. *Clin Neuropharmacol.* 2016;39(6):311-319.

56. Dario A, Tomei G. A benefit-risk assessment of baclofen in severe spinal spasticity. *Drug Saf.* 2004;27(11):799-818.

57. Chang E, Ghosh N, Yanni D, Lee S, Alexandru D, Mozaffar T. A review of spasticity treatments: pharmacological and interventional approaches. *Crit Rev Phys Rehabil Med.* 2013;25(1-2):11-22.

58. Chung CY, Chen CL, Wong AM. Pharmacotherapy of spasticity in children with cerebral palsy. *J Formos Med Assoc.* 2011;110(4): 215-222. doi:10.1016/S0929-6646(11)60033-8.

59. Wilkinson SP, Portmann B, Williams R. Hepatitis from dantrolene sodium. *Gut.* 1979;20(1):33-36.

60. Delgado MR, Hirtz D, Aisen M, et al. Practice Parameter: Pharmacologic treatment of spasticity in children and adolescents with cerebral palsy (an evidence-based review): Report of the Quality Standards Subcommittee of the American Academy of Neurology and the Practice Committee of the Child Neurology Society. *Neurology.* 2010;74(4):336-343. doi:10.1212/WNL. 0b013e3181cbcd2f.

61. Patel MB, McKenna JW, Alvarez JM, et al. Decreasing adrenergic or sympathetic hyperactivity after severe traumatic brain injury using propranolol and clonidine (DASH After TBI Study): study protocol for a randomized controlled trial. *Trials.* 2012; 13:177. doi:10.1186/1745-6215-13-177.

62. Rabchevsky AG, Kitzman PH. Latest approaches for the treatment of spasticity and autonomic dysreflexia in chronic spinal cord injury. *Neurotherapeutics.* 2011;8(2):274-282. doi:10.1007/s13311-011-0025-5.

63. Crowner BE, Torres-Russotto D, Carter AR, Racette BA. Systemic weakness after therapeutic injections of botulinum toxin a: a case series and review of the literature. *Clin Neuropharmacol.* 2010;33(5):243-247. doi:10.1097/WNF.0b013e3181f5329e.

64. Saulino M, Ivanhoe CB, McGuire JR, Ridley B, Shilt JS, Boster AL. Best practices for intrathecal baclofen therapy: patient selection. *Neuromodulation.* 2016;19(6):607-615. doi:10.1111/ner.12447.

65. Awaad Y, Rizk T, Siddiqui I, Roosen N, McIntosh K, Waines GM. Complications of intrathecal baclofen pump: prevention and cure. *ISRN Neurol.* 2012;2012:575168. doi:10.5402/2012/575168.

66. Yeh RN, Nypaver MM, Deegan TJ, Ayyangar R. Baclofen toxicity in an 8-year-old with an intrathecal baclofen pump. *J Emerg Med.* 2004;26(2):163-167.

67. Saulino M, Anderson DJ, Doble J, et al. Best practices for intrathecal baclofen therapy: troubleshooting. *Neuromodulation.* 2016;19(6):632-641. doi:10.1111/ner.12467.

68. Karri J, Mas MF, Francisco GE, Li S. Practice patterns for spasticity management with phenol neurolysis. *J Rehabil Med.* 2017;49(6):482-488. doi:10.2340/16501977-2239.

69. Kluger G, Kochs A, Holthausen H. Heterotopic ossification in childhood and adolescence. *J Child Neurol.* 2000;15(6): 406-413.

70. Simonsen LL, Sonne-Holm S, Krasheninnikoff M, Engberg AW. Symptomatic heterotopic ossification after very severe traumatic brain injury in 114 patients: incidence and risk factors. *Injury.* 2007;38(10):1146-50.

71. Hendricks HT, Geurts AC, van Ginneken BC, Heeren AJ, Vos PE. Brain injury severity and autonomic dysregulation accurately predict heterotopic ossification in patients with traumatic brain injury. *Clin Rehabil.* 2007;21(6):545-553.

72. Boyce AM, Tosi LL, Paul SM. Bisphosphonate treatment for children with disabling conditions. *PM R.* 2014;6(5):427-436. doi:10.1016/j.pmrj.2013.10.009.

73. Leeper CM, Vissa M, Cooper JD, Malec LM, Gaines BA. Venous thromboembolism in pediatric trauma patients: ten-year experience and long-term follow-up in a tertiary care center. *Pediatr Blood Cancer.* 2017;64(8). doi:10.1002/pbc.26415.

74. Yen J, Van Arendonk KJ, Streiff MB, et al. Risk factors for venous thromboembolism in pediatric trauma patients and validation of a novel scoring system: the risk of clots in kids with trauma (ROCKIT score). *Pediatr Crit Care Med.* 2016;17(5): 391-399. doi:10.1097/PCC.0000000000000699.

75. Keret A, Bennett-Back O, Rosenthal G, et al. Posttraumatic epilepsy: long-term follow-up of children with mild traumatic brain injury. *J Neurosurg Pediatr.* 2017;20(1):64-70. doi:10.3171/2017.2. PEDS16585.

76. Liesemer K, Bratton SL, Zebrack CM, Brockmeyer D, Statler KD. Early post-traumatic seizures in moderate to severe pediatric traumatic brain injury: rates, risk factors, and clinical features. *J Neurotrauma.* 2011;28(5):755-762. doi:10.1089/neu.2010.1518.

77. Keret A, Shweiki M, Bennett-Back O, et al. The clinical characteristics of posttraumatic epilepsy following moderate-to-severe traumatic brain injury in children. *Seizure.* 2018;58:29-34.

78. Adeyemo BO, Biederman J, Zafonte R, et al. Mild traumatic brain injury and ADHD: a systematic review of the literature and meta-analysis. *J Atten Disord.* 2014;18(7):576-584.

79. Poggi G, Liscio M, Adduci A, et al. Psychological and adjustment problems due to acquired brain lesions in childhood: a comparison between post-traumatic patients and brain tumour survivors. *Brain Inj.* 2005;19(10):777-785.

80. Fann JR, Hart T, Schomer KG. Treatment for depression after traumatic brain injury: a systematic review. *J Neurotrauma.* 2009;26(12):2383-2402. doi:10.1089/neu.2009.1091.

81. Reifschneider K, Auble BA, Rose SR. Update of endocrine dysfunction following pediatric traumatic brain injury. *J Clin Med.* 2015;4(8):1536-1560. doi:10.3390/jcm4081536.

82. Kaulfers AM, Backeljauw PF, Reifschneider K, et al. Endocrine dysfunction following traumatic brain injury in children. *J Pediatr.* 2010;157(6):894-899.

83. Bakker K, Catroppa C, Anderson V. Olfactory dysfunction in pediatric traumatic brain injury: a systematic review. *J Neurotrauma.* 2014;31(4):308-314. doi:10.1089/neu.2013.3045.

84. Babikian T, Asarnow R. Neurocognitive outcomes and recovery after pediatric TBI: meta-analytic review of the literature. *Neuropsychology.* 2009;23(3):283-296. doi:10.1037/a0015268.

85. Fay TB, Yeates KO, Wade SL, Drotar D, Stancin T, Taylor HG. Predicting longitudinal patterns of functional deficits in children with traumatic brain injury. *Neuropsychology.* 2009;23(3):271-282. doi:10.1037/a0014936.

86. Suskauer SJ, Slomine BS, Inscore AB, Lewelt AJ, Kirk JW, Salorio CF. Injury severity variables as predictors of WeeFIM scores in pediatric TBI: time to follow commands is best. *J Pediatr Rehabil Med.* 2009;2(4):297-307.

87. Iverson GL, Iverson AM, Barton EA. The Children's Orientation and Amnesia Test: educational status is a moderator variable in tracking recovery from TBI. *Brain Inj.* 1994;8(8): 685-688.

88. Davis KC, Slomine BS, Salorio CF, Suskauer SJ. Time to Follow Commands and duration of post-traumatic amnesia predict GOS-E Peds scores 1–2 years after TBI in children requiring inpatient rehabilitation. *J Head Trauma Rehabil.* 2016;31(2): E39-E47. doi:10.1097/HTR.0000000000000159.

89. Ziviani J, Ottenbacher KJ, Shephard K, Foreman S, Astbury W, Ireland P. Concurrent validity of the Functional Independence Measure for Children (WeeFIM) and the Pediatric Evaluation of Disabilities Inventory in children with developmental disabilities and acquired brain injuries. *Phys Occup Ther Pediatr.* 2001; 21(2-3):91-101.

90. Dumas HM, Fragala-Pinkham MA, Haley SM, et al. Item bank development for a revised pediatric evaluation of disability inventory (PEDI). *Phys Occup Ther Pediatr.* 2010;30(3):168-184. doi:10.3109/01942631003640493.

48

Geriatric Traumatic Brain Injury

EKUA GILBERT-BAFFOE, MD, and JAIME M. LEVINE, DO

Population Dynamics

- The population of people in the United States over 64 in 1990 was 29.9 million, versus 40 million in 2010 and 47 million in 2015. This number is expected to project to 88.5 million by 2050 (Census Bureau, n.d).

Epidemiology of Traumatic Brain Injury (TBI) in the United States[8,20]

- Incidence in the general population: 1.7 million
- Prevalence in the general population: 3.17 million
- The elderly account for more than 80,000 TBI-related emergency department visits each year in the United States
- The TBI-related hospitalization rate is 85.1 per 100,000 for people ages 65 to 74 and rises with age. Improvements in initial medical management have led to an increase in the number of elderly living with TBI.

Leading Causes of TBI in the Elderly [8,20,21]

1. Unintentional falls
   - Advancing age increases the risk of falls leading to TBI related to many causes, including coexisting medical problems diabetes, visual and sensory dysfunction, neurological diseases (e.g., Parkinson's disease), muscle weakness, impaired cognition, and polypharmacy.
   - Risk of falls increases dramatically with advancing age above 65.
   - Risk of falling for those older than 85 years old is six times greater than those ages 65 to 74.
2. Traffic-related accidents
   - This includes motor vehicle accidents and pedestrians struck by motor vehicles; these are the second most common cause of TBI in the elderly population.

Sensory Abnormalities of Aging[7]

- Changes in sensorium, which can occur in the aging population, present a unique challenge in the management of the elderly population with TBI.
  - Presbycusis: 60% of older adults experience some degree of presbycusis or sensorineural hearing loss by age 65. It is important not to mistake hearing loss for another cognitive or linguistic deficit after TBI.
  - Assessment of presbycusis should include:
    - Hearing evaluation by speech language pathologist (SLP)
    - Audiology evaluation for more in-depth analysis of any significant deficits
    - Use of hearing aids/noise amplification devices when indicated (but it is important to monitor for overstimulation in the TBI population, who may be more sensitive to noise after their injuries)

Visual Changes with Normal Aging[7]

- This includes decline in extraocular muscle motion, changes in visual acuity, and increases in intraocular pressure. This should be evaluated in this population by:
  - Performing a visual screen if cognitive status appropriate

- Use of visual aids such as corrective lenses when appropriate
- Use of strategic visual aids when appropriate (e.g., patches, partial occlusion glasses, blackout tape depending on the visual impairment).
- Evaluation by a neuroophthalmologist may be required for in-depth assessment of visual impairments.

Orthostasis

- This often occurs after prolonged immobility and subsequently impairs optimization of time spent in therapies. It may also present as a unique challenge in the elderly population, who may have underlying cardiac and vascular disease. Vital signs should be monitored closely as a patient progresses through therapies. These factors should be considered in management (Haring et al., 2015; Levine & Flanagan, 2013):
  - Assess medications: Initial antihypertensives may not be needed, and/or dosing adjustments may be indicated as the patient progresses through rehabilitation. (e.g., because of resolution of posttraumatic hypertension).
  - Use of abdominal binders and lower extremity pressure stockings may be helpful in supporting blood pressure. Slower transitions from supine to sitting and to standing may also decrease the occurrence of symptomatic orthostatic hypotension.
  - Pharmacological agents may be needed to increase or support blood pressure if the aforementioned nonpharmacological supportive strategies are insufficient.

Hydrocephalus[15]

- It is important to monitor for signs and symptoms of hydrocephalus to allow for prompt diagnosis and management.
- The classic triad of the clinical signs—worsening cognition, alterations in gait, and urinary incontinence—may be a rare presentation or difficult to classify in TBI patients because these symptoms may be attributed to the TBI itself.
- Clinical indication of hydrocephalus in this population will be increased fatigue or a change or lack of improvement in functional status (e.g., a change from minimal assistance to maximum assistance for transfers in patient).
- Many of the symptoms of hydrocephalus also overlap with complications after TBI, such as infection. Therefore hydrocephalus should be included in the differential for workup of these symptoms, especially in TBI patients who have suffered subarachnoid hemorrhages that can affect the absorption of cerebrospinal fluid.

Cognition[15]

- Age-related cognitive changes are an expected component of normal aging.

- Most people experience gradual decline in cognitive performance over their life span, particularly in memory.
- It is usually minor and doesn't affect function, termed *mild cognitive impairment* (MCI).
  - MCI increases risk of TBI, because it decreases functional problem-solving skills and increases risk of mechanical fall
  - Slows recovery
  - Increases rehabilitation lengths of stay
- It is critical to establish preinjury cognitive baseline when goal setting in rehabilitation.

Affective

- Emotional changes are common post-TBI
  - Often depression and anxiety (Albrecht et al., 2015; van Reekum et al., 1996)
  - Depression among most prevalent mental health problems in the elderly (Fann et al., 1995; Hibbard et al., 1998)
    - Associated with considerable mortality, including risk of suicide
    - Must differentiate from normal grieving, fatigue, or sleep dysfunction
  - Hard to diagnose
    - Many patients may have cognitive or linguistic deficits, making it difficult to get an accurate verbal report of symptoms
    - Sometimes must rely on behavioral indicators
  - Elderly tend to underreport depressive symptoms.
  - Many sequelae of TBI are similar to depression.
    - Fatigue, cognitive slowing, apathy, somatic complaints, disrupted sleep
  - Treatment for post-TBI depression in the elderly
    - Combination of psychotherapeutic support and medication
    - Medications: Start low and go slow.
    - Select agent carefully.
    - Consider agents to treat more than one condition to minimize polypharmacy.

Behavior[7]

- Behavioral dysregulation after TBI in the elderly is common.
  - Restlessness, agitation, aggression, irritability pose safety challenges and add stress to the environment of care.
  - Treatment: Nonpharmacological approach is first line.
    - Lower the level of stimulus
    - Avoid busy, high-traffic spaces
    - Limit number of visitors
    - Lower the noise level
  - Supportive counseling
  - Eliminate or treat sources of noxious stimulation: pain, constipation, urinary retention, spasticity, infection, stressful contacts.

- Pharmacological approach is reasonable next step.
  - Atypical antipsychotics, antiepileptics, beta blockers
  - Caution with use of centrally acting medications and ensure benefits outweigh risks

Sleep Disturbance[15]

- The combination of age-related sleep changes and altered sleep patterns in people with TBI creates challenges.
  - Sleep hygiene is first-line therapy.
    - Eliminate technology from the bedroom.
    - Retire and awaken at the same time each day.
    - Avoid emotional content in the evenings.
    - Eliminate alcohol and caffeine.
  - Cautious use of pharmacological agents may be considered in refractory cases.
    - Melatonin or melatonin analogs are safe and avoid unwanted side effects.
    - Consider benign agents that have drowsiness as a side effect, such as trazadone.
    - Avoid sedatives and hypnotics because of unwanted side effects.

Outcomes for older individuals with TBI are worse than their younger counterparts when controlling for injury severity (LeBlanc et al., 2006; Mosenthal et al., 2002).

- Older individuals with TBI are more likely to die of their injury, be more dependent for mobility and activities of daily living (ADLs), and be discharged to long-term care facilities than younger people with similar injuries.
- More likely to have medical comorbidities that complicate recovery
- More likely to have less premorbid physical and cognitive reserve

Mortality acutely after TBI is the highest among the elderly than any other age group (Haring et al., 2015; Harrison-Felix et al., 2015; Ivascu et al., 2008; LeBlanc et al., 2006).

- Age at time of injury is an independent predictor of mortality regardless of injury severity (Mosenthal et al., 2002).
- Thought to be caused by a combination of slowed healing because of age, presence of other comorbidities, and the treatment thereof

- Presence of anticoagulants increases risk of hemorrhage or expansion of hemorrhage but also decreases risk of venous thromboembolism.
- Cardiovascular disease may impair compensatory responses to hypotension and hypoxemia acutely, resulting in greater secondary injury after trauma.
- Age-related increase in subdural space may allow further hemorrhage to occur before clinical signs of neurological impairment are noticed ("silent bleeding").
  - May also lead to higher initial Glasgow Coma Scale (GCS) scores, which is misleading

Functional Outcomes[2,9,16-17,19]

- Elderly people with TBI are more likely to have poorer functional outcomes than their younger counterparts.
  - More often require residential settings at time of hospital discharge
  - More often require skilled assistance if discharged to home
  - Only about one-third of elderly people with TBI are discharged home without skilled assistance
  - Reasons for poor outcomes are multifactorial:
    - Aging central nervous system less able to handle stress
    - Cerebral plasticity likely less effective
    - Poorer premorbid cognitive and physical abilities
    - May be on more cognitive-impairing medications

Prevention[3,18]

- Falls are the leading cause of TBI in the elderly
  - Approximately one-third of people age 65 or older fall each year.
  - Screening for falls is a huge part of primary prevention.
  - Interventions for those at risk: home modifications, correction of visual/cardiac abnormalities, therapeutic exercises, reduction/elimination of psychoactive medications, treatment of postural hypotension, assistive devices

Review Questions

1. What is the leading cause traumatic brain injury (TBI) in the elderly?
   a. Motor vehicle collisions
   b. Falls
   c. Violence
   d. Suicide attempts
2. Potential reasons for poor outcomes after TBI in include all of these except
   a. poorer premorbid cognitive and physical functioning.
   b. polypharmacy.
   c. cerebral plasticity likely less effective.
   d. the aging central nervous system is better able to handle stress.

3. Environmental approaches used to treat behavioral dysregulation in an elderly patient after TBI should include
   a. raising the noise level on the rehabilitation unit.
   b. elimination of causes of noxious stimulation such as constipation or pain.
   c. bringing the patient into a busy common area to eat meals.
   d. encouraging large numbers of visitors to enter the patient's room at a time.

Answers on page 400.
Access the full list of questions and answers online.
Available on ExpertConsult.com

References

1. Albrecht JS, Kiptanui Z, Tsang Y, et al. Depression among older adults after traumatic brain injury: a national analysis. *Am J Geriatr Psychiatry*. 2015;23(6):607-614.
2. Albrecht JS, Slejko JF, Stein DM, Smith GS. Treatment charges for traumatic brain injury among older adults at a trauma center. *J Head Trauma Rehabil*. 2017;32(6):E45-E53.
3. Campbell AJ, Spears GF, Borrie MJ. Examination by logistic regression modelling of the variables which increase the relative risk of elderly women falling compared to elderly men. *J Clin Epidemiol*. 1990;43(12):1415-1420.
4. Census Bureau, U. *Statistical Abstract of the United States*: 2011. 2011. Avaliable at: https://www.census.gov/library/publications/2010/compendia/statab/130ed.html
5. Coronado VG, Thomas KE, Sattin RW, Johnson RL. The CDC traumatic brain injury surveillance system: characteristics of persons aged 65 years and older hospitalized with a TBI. *J Head Trauma Rehabil*. 2005;20(3):215-228.
6. Fann JR, Katon WJ, Uomoto JM, Esselman PC. Psychiatric disorders and functional disability in outpatients with traumatic brain injuries. *Am J Psychiatry*. 1995;152(10):1493-1499. doi:10.1176/ajp.152.10.1493.
7. Flanagan SR, Hibbard MR, Riordan B, Gordon WA. Traumatic brain injury in the elderly: diagnostic and treatment challenges. *Clin Geriatr Med*. 2006;22(2):449-468. doi:10.1016/j.cger.2005.12.011.
8. Frieden TR, Houry D, Baldwin G. Centers for Disease Control and Prevention. *Report to Congress on Traumatic Brain Injury In the United States*: Epidemiology and Rehabilitation. Atlanta, GA; 2015. https://www.cdc.gov/traumaticbraininjury/pdf/TBI_Report_to_Congress_Epi_and_Rehab-a.pdf. Accessed February 10, 2019.
9. Gan BK, Lim JHG, Ng IHB. Outcome of moderate and severe traumatic brain injury amongst the elderly in Singapore. *Ann Acad Med Singapore*. 2004;33(1):63-67.
10. Haring RS, Narang K, Canner JK, et al. Traumatic brain injury in the elderly: morbidity and mortality trends and risk factors. *J Surg Res*. 2015;195(1):1-9.
11. Harrison-Felix, C., Pretz, C., Hammond, F. M., Cuthbert, J. P., Bell, J., Corrigan, J., Miller, A. C., & Haarbauer-Krupa, J. Life expectancy after inpatient rehabilitation for traumatic brain injury in the United States. *Journal of Neurotrauma*. 2015;32(23):1893–1901.
12. Hibbard MR, Uysal S, Kepler K, Bogdany J, Silver J. Axis I psychopathology in individuals with traumatic brain injury. *J Head Trauma Rehabil*. 1998;13(4):24-39.
13. Ivascu FA, Howells GA, Junn FS, Bair HA, Bendick PJ, Janczyk RJ. Predictors of mortality in trauma patients with intracranial hemorrhage on preinjury aspirin or clopidogrel. *J Trauma Inj Infect Crit Care*. 2008;65(4):785-788.
14. LeBlanc J, Guise E de, Gosselin N, Feyz M. Comparison of functional outcome following acute care in young, middle-aged and elderly patients with traumatic brain injury. *Brain Inj*. 2006;20(8):779-790.
15. Levine J, Flanagan SR. Traumatic Brain Injury in the Eldery. In: Nathan RDZ, Zasler D, Katz DI, eds. *Zasler Brain Injury Medicine*. 2nd ed. Demos Medical Publishing, LLC; 2013:420-433.
16. McIntyre A, Mehta S, Janzen S, Aubut J, Teasell RW. A meta-analysis of functional outcome among older adults with traumatic brain injury. *NeuroRehabilitation*. 2013;32(2):409-414.
17. Mosenthal AC, Lavery RF, Addis M, et al. Isolated traumatic brain injury: age is an independent predictor of mortality and early outcome. *J Trauma*. 2002;52(5):907-911.
18. Panel on Prevention of Falls in Older Persons AGS and BGS. Summary of the Updated American Geriatrics Society/British Geriatrics Society Clinical Practice Guideline for Prevention of Falls in Older Persons. *J Am Geriatr Soc*. 2011;59(1):148-157.
19. Susman M, DiRusso SM, Sullivan T, et al. Traumatic brain injury in the elderly: increased mortality and worse functional outcome at discharge despite lower injury severity. *J Trauma*. 2002;53(2):219-223; discussion 223-224.
20. Taylor MD, Tracy JK, Meyer W, Pasquale M, Napolitano LM. Trauma in the elderly: intensive care unit resource use and outcome. *J Trauma*. 2002;53(3):407-414.
21. Tinetti ME, Speechley M, Ginter SF. Risk factors for falls among elderly persons living in the community. *N Engl J Med*. 1988;319(26):1701-1707.
22. van Reekum R, Bolago I, Finlayson MA, Garner S, Links PS. Psychiatric disorders after traumatic brain injury. *Brain Inj*. 1996;10(5):319-327.

49

Military Traumatic Brain Injury

AMY O. BOWLES, MD, AND MEGHAN J. MCHENRY, MD

OUTLINE

Traumatic brain injury (TBI) in the military rose to prominence in the early 2000s and was called the signature injury of the wars in Iraq and Afghanistan. Although generally adhering to commonly used academic definitions, the Department of Defense (DoD) differs in the use of imaging findings in the determination of TBI severity; any computed tomography (CT) abnormalities raise the severity level to at least moderate (Table 49.1).[2] Using these definitions, the US military reported about 380,000 TBI among military servicemembers between 2000 and 2018[10]; current incidence rates are about 17,000 per year. Over 80% of brain injuries in active duty personnel are classified as mild. Prevalence studies estimated that approximately 20% of those who deployed to Iraq or Afghanistan sustained a TBI.[9]

A disproportionate fraction of combat-related military TBIs are associated with high-energy explosions.[5] Blast-related injures can be primary (overpressurization), secondary (penetrating trauma or fragmentation injuries), tertiary (injury from being thrown by the blast or structural collapse caused by the blast), or quaternary (burns or toxic exposures after the blast).[6] Blast mechanism of injury is often associated with polytrauma, or injuries to multiple body regions and/or systems, in addition to TBI.[3] Nevertheless, many TBIs in the military occur in garrison (i.e., not in war zones) and are caused by falls, sports and recreational activities, and military training exercises.

- Approximately 20% of those who deployed to Iraq or Afghanistan sustained a TBI.
- Over 80% of brain injuries in active duty military personnel are classified as mild.
- Combat-related military TBIs are often the result of a blast or high-energy explosion.

Screening

Medics and corpsmen serve as the first responders for military medicine, and they perform a Military Acute Concussion Examination (MACE) when servicemembers present with suspected acute TBI.[8] This tool is derived from the Sideline Assessment of Concussion (SAC) and shares many similarities. It includes red flags denoting when patients should be elevated to the next level of care. If TBI is not immediately identified or reported in theater, screening for TBI injury events and historical or current postconcussive symptoms is performed routinely after deployment as part of the DoD's Post-Deployment Health Assessment (PDHA) and Reassessment (PDHRA) programs. These are completed within 30 days and within 3 to 6 months after return from deployment, respectively.[3]

- Medics and Corpsmen are the military's first responders.
- The MACE is performed when servicemembers present with suspected acute TBI.

Management

The US military has resources around the world to manage all levels of trauma and TBI, including a robust medical evacuation system and partnerships with local healthcare organizations and trauma centers. For active duty servicemembers who require inpatient rehabilitation for TBI, the military often partners with the Department of Veterans Affairs (VA) Polytrauma System of Care. For the most part, TBI in military populations is managed the same way as it's managed in civilian settings, particularly when it comes to trauma resuscitation. As in the civilian population, clinicians must be vigilant for cooccurring behavioral health conditions because these can alter management and the trajectory of recovery.

A specific concern in the military population is posttraumatic stress disorder (PTSD) (Table 49.2). Rates of comorbid PTSD among veterans with TBI are as high as 44%.[11] This presents a particular challenge because PTSD shares many symptoms with concussion, including sleep disturbance, neurocognitive symptoms, and mood/behavior changes.[14] In the majority of mild TBI (mTBI) cases, neurocognitive dysfunction resolves over time,[15] typically within 3 months.[4] There is a growing body of literature that suggests that postconcussion

TABLE 49.1 Department of Defense Criteria for Determining Traumatic Brain Injury Severity[a] (Reference: Assistant Secretary of Defense)[2]

Criterion	Mild	Moderate	Severe
Structural imaging	Normal	Normal or abnormal	Normal or abnormal
Loss of consciousness	0–30 min	30 min to 24 hours	>24 h
Alteration of consciousness	Up to 24 h	>24 h; severity based on other criteria	>24 h; severity based on other criteria
Posttraumatic amnesia	0–1 day	1–7 days	>7 days
Glasgow Coma Scale score (best in first 24 hours)	13–15	9–12	3–8

[a]If the patient meets criteria in more than one category, the higher severity level is selected.

From Traumatic brain injury: Updated definition and reporting. Washington, DC: Department of Defense; 2015.

TABLE 49.2 *Diagnostic and Statistical Manual of Mental Disorders*, 5th Edition, Criteria for Diagnosing Posttraumatic Stress Disorder[1]

- Exposure to actual or threatened death, serious injury, or sexual violence
- Intrusion symptoms
- Avoidance symptoms
- Negative alterations in cognition and mood
- Alterations in arousal and reactivity
- Duration more than 1 month
- Causes clinically significant distress or impairment in social, occupational, or other important areas of functioning
- Not attributable to the physiological effects of a substance or another medical condition

From American Psychiatric Association. (2013). Diagnostic and statistical manual of mental disorders (5th ed.). Arlington, VA: American Psychiatric Publishing.

symptoms are more strongly correlated with measures of PTSD and depression than TBI, and veterans with psychiatric disorders more frequently meet diagnostic criteria for postconcussive syndrome than those with mTBI alone.[13] PTSD requires specific treatment, and thus its diagnosis is critically important to the patient's long-term recovery.

Unfortunately, the stigma in military culture associated with seeking behavioral healthcare frequently contributes to misattribution of symptoms, because servicemembers are often reluctant to attribute difficulties to a mental health problem as opposed to a physical one. Treatment of PTSD often leads to an improvement in symptoms attributed to concussion.

- Rates of cooccurring PTSD in veterans with a history of TBI are as high as 44%.
- Treatment of PTSD often leads to improvement in symptoms attributed to concussion.

Return to Duty or Activity

Return to duty guidelines in the military generally parallel those for return to sport, with a similar emphasis on evaluation for exertion-based symptoms.[12] Military specific return-to-activity guidelines, patient education materials, and additional provider tools can be found at https://dvbic. dcoe.mil. Additional resources that can be helpful in the management of military and veteran patients including clinical practice guidelines addressing mTBI and PTSD can be found at https://www.healthquality.va.gov.[7]

- The military has specific return-to-activity guidelines that emphasize evaluation for exertion-based symptoms.

Review Questions

1. Who are the first responders in military medicine?
   a. Flight surgeons
   b. Nurses
   c. Medics and corpsmen
   d. Infantry specialists
2. What tool do military first responders use for the initial acute assessment of servicemembers with known or suspected traumatic brain injury (TBI)?
   a. Sideline Assessment of Concussion (SAC)
   b. Military Acute Concussion Examination (MACE)
   c. Electroencephalogram (EEG)
   d. Automated Neuropsychological Assessment Metrics (ANAM)

3. SPC Smith was thrown by the blast wind when an IED detonated. This is an example of what kind of blast injury?
   a. Primary
   b. Secondary
   c. Tertiary
   d. Quaternary

Answers on page 400.
Access the full list of questions and answers online.
Available on ExpertConsult.com

References

1. American Psychiatric Association. *Diagnostic and Statistical Manual of Mental Disorders*. 5th ed. Arlington, VA: American Psychiatric Publishing; 2013.

2. Assistant Secretary of Defense. *Traumatic Brain Injury: Updated Definition and Reporting*. Washington, DC: Department of Defense; 2015.

3. Armistead-Jehle P, Soble JR, Cooper DB, Belanger HG. Unique aspects of traumatic brain injury in military and veteran populations. *Phys Med Rehabil Clin N Am*. 2017;28:323-337.

4. Carroll LJ, Cassidy JD, Peloso PM, et al. Prognosis for mild traumatic brain injury: results of the WHO Collaborating Centre Task Force on Mild Traumatic Brain Injury. *J Rehabil Med*. 2004;36(433):84-1055.

5. Chapman JC, Diaz-Arrastia R. Military traumatic brain injury: a review. *Alzheimer's & Dementia*. 2014;10:S97-S104.

6. DePalma RG, Burris DG, Champion HR, Hodgson MJ. Blast injuries. *N Engl J Med*. 2005;352:1335-1342.

7. Department of Veterans Affairs, & Department of Defense. *VA/DoD Clinical Practice Guideline for Management of Concussion/Mild Traumatic Brain Injury. Version 2.0—2016*. Available at: https://www.healthquality.va.gov/guidelines/Rehab/mtbi/mTBICPGFullCPG50821816.pdf. Accessed Feburary 12, 2019.

8. French LM, Mccrea M. The military acute concussion evaluation (MACE). *J Spec Oper Med*. 2008;8(1):68-77.9.

9. Helmick KM, Spells CA, Malik SZ, Davies CA, Marion DW, Hinds SR. Traumatic brain injury in the US military: epidemiology and key clinical and research programs. *Brain Imaging Behav*. 2015;9:358-366.

10. Defense and Veterans Brain Injury Center. Available at https://dvbic.dcoe.mil/dod-worldwide-numbers-tbi. Accessed January 9, 2019.

11. Hoge CW, McGurk D, Thomas JL, Cox AL, Engel CC, Castro CA. Mild traumatic brain injury in U.S. soldiers returning from Iraq. *N Engl J Med*. 2008;358:453-463.

12. Ling GSF, Ecklund JM. Traumatic brain injury in modern war. *Curr Opin Anesthesiol*. 2011;24:124-130.

13. Storzbach D, O'Neil ME, Roost SM, et al. Comparing the neuropsychological test performance of operation enduring freedom/operation Iraqi freedom (OEF/OIF) veterans with and without blast exposure, mild traumatic brain injury, and posttraumatic stress symptoms. *J Int Neuropsychol Soc*. 2015;21:353-363.

14. Tanev KS, Pentel KZ, Kredlow MA, Charney ME. PTSD and TBI co-morbidity: Scope, clinical presentation and treatment options. *Brain Inj*. 2014;28:261-270.

15. Vasterling JJ, Jacob SN, Rassmusson A. Traumatic brain injury and posttraumatic stress disorder: conceptual, diagnostic, and therapeutic considerations in the context of co-occurrence. *J Neuropsychiatry Clin Neurosci*. 2018;30:91-100.

50

Sport Concussion

ROSANNA C. SABINI, DO

According to the most recent Consensus Statement of the International Conference on Concussion in Sport, held in 2016, a sport-related concussion is a traumatic brain injury (TBI) induced by biomechanical forces.[1] A concussion may be caused by a direct or indirect force transmitted to the brain resulting in rapid yet short-lived neurological impairments. Loss of consciousness (LOC) does not need to occur to diagnose a concussion, because it does not occur the majority of the time. LOC occurs in less than 10% of concussions, whereas confusion and amnesia (retrograde and/or anterograde) are more common.[2]

Symptoms of a concussion may develop over hours, and resolution typically follows a sequential course. In some instances, the symptoms may be prolonged, lasting days to sometimes weeks. The brain-related pathological changes are mostly caused by a functional rather than a structural injury, which is why imaging via computed tomography (CT) or magnetic resonance imaging (MRI) is often negative. The Fifth International Conference on Concussion in Sport also specified that concussion symptoms cannot be explained by illicit drugs, including alcohol or medications; psychosocial impairments; coexisting medical conditions; injuries to the cervical area; or peripheral vestibular system impairments.[1]

Pathophysiology[3]

A concussion is the result of a complex cellular dysfunction predominantly caused by neurotransmitters that are released after an injury. The consequential response is a cascade of events that ultimately leads to cellular death.

The cascade of damage is thought to begin with the release of glutamate[3]:

Glutamate → efflux of K^+ → stabilized by influx of Ca^{2+} → hyperglycolysis of cell → release of free radicals and enzymes (proteases, lipases, nitrogen oxide) → cytoskeleton damage → glucose overutilization or adenosine triphosphate (ATP) to repair → energy crisis → mitochondrial failure → lactate production → increased membrane permeability → apoptosis or necrosis

During this energy crisis, symptoms may develop and even worsen when physical or cognitive activities are performed.

On-Field Assessment

On-field assessment of a sport-related concussion requires the recognition of the signs and symptoms of a concussion. It is imperative that coaches, athletic trainers, parents, and athletes themselves be educated on the signs and symptoms of a concussion.

If there is any suspicion of a concussion, an athlete should be:
- Immediately removed from the game
- Medically evaluated onsite by a healthcare provider (to rule out more serious injury)
- Administered a sideline evaluation with the Sport Concussion Assessment Tool 5th Edition (SCAT5) assessment tool[4]
- Routinely monitored for deterioration over the initial few hours
- Not allowed to return to play the same day

Concussion grading scales should never be used to determine the severity of a concussion.

Physician Evaluation

After an athlete has been removed from play, they should seek a medical evaluation by a physician expert who is knowledgeable in the management and treatment of concussion.

Assessment of a concussion requires a thorough history and physical examination that includes:
- Injury details (how it occurred, immediate symptoms and evolution, presence of LOC or amnesia)

TABLE 50.1	Post-Concussion Symptom Scale						
	None	Mild		Moderate		Severe	
Headache	0	1	2	3	4	5	6
Nausea	0	1	2	3	4	5	6
Vomiting	0	1	2	3	4	5	6
Dizziness	0	1	2	3	4	5	6
Balance problems	0	1	2	3	4	5	6
Trouble falling asleep	0	1	2	3	4	5	6
Sleeping more than usual	0	1	2	3	4	5	6
Drowsiness	0	1	2	3	4	5	6
Sensitivity to light	0	1	2	3	4	5	6
Sensitivity to noise	0	1	2	3	4	5	6
More emotional than usual	0	1	2	3	4	5	6
Irritability	0	1	2	3	4	5	6
Sadness	0	1	2	3	4	5	6
Nervousness	0	1	2	3	4	5	6
Numbness or tingling	0	1	2	3	4	5	6
Feeling slowed down	0	1	2	3	4	5	6
Feeling like in a fog	0	1	2	3	4	5	6
Difficulty with concentrating	0	1	2	3	4	5	6
Difficulty with remembering	0	1	2	3	4	5	6

- Current symptom description, guided by the 22-item Post-Concussion Symptom Scale (PCSS) (Table 50.1)
- Determine how the symptoms are affected, such as what makes them better or worse
- Discuss how symptoms may interfere with physical activities, work, school, computer/phone use, etc.
- Identify management received thus far such as being left out of school, testing received, or if medication has been taken to assist with the symptoms

When assessing concussion symptoms, it is relevant to group them into four symptom domains:

1. Somatic: headache, nausea, vomiting, light and noise sensitivity, dizziness, poor balance, tinnitus, blurry vision, numbness, or tingling
2. Cognitive: fogginess, difficulty concentrating or remembering, feeling slowed down
3. Sleep: difficulty falling asleep, staying asleep, sleeping more than usual, fatigue, drowsiness
4. Emotional: sadness, irritability, anxiety

Viewing concussion symptoms as domains can assist in understanding how symptoms interrelate with other symptoms; for example, insomnia may lead to daytime fatigue, headaches, and/or irritability. It is important to note that symptoms can be interpreted differently based on the athlete's age or gender. Understanding the athlete's motivations and goals can further assist in the assessment and overall management. Some athletes may confound their symptoms for earlier return to play, whereas others may not understand that the symptoms experienced are related to a concussion nor the importance of immediate treatment.

Prior comorbid history may guide the management of the current concussion. Other relevant medical history to obtain includes a history of:

- Headaches or migraines in self or family members
- Eye or vision problems
- Dizziness
- Anxiety and/or depression
- Sleep difficulties
- Learning disabilities
- The number of prior concussions and recovery time of each injury

The physical examination of a sport-related concussion should at a minimum include a:

- Neurological examination
- Balance assessment using the Balance Error Scoring System (BESS). The BESS tests balance with eyes closed, on firm and soft surfaces, in three stances—feet together, tandem, and on only the nondominant foot

- Visuomotor examination to determine presence of nystagmus and saccades and to test the convergence and vestibular–ocular reflex

If needed, the SCAT5 can also be performed (Child-SCAT5 for those ages 5–12).[5] Computerized testing is not recommended. It is important to note that early in the recovery, cognitive and emotional complaints are likely a result of the somatic symptoms experienced, which need to be prioritized for treatment.

A head CT or brain MRI is usually not recommended initially, because the majority are negative, and their use is limited to high suspicion for structural intracerebral injury, including intracranial hemorrhage, prolonged LOC, post-traumatic amnesia (PTA), persistently altered mental status (Glasgow Coma Scale [GCS] score <15), focal neurological deficit, evidence of skull fracture on examination, or signs of clinical deterioration.[6]

Management and Treatment

General Guidelines

1. Concussion management is always individualized.
2. Protocols available can guide the management and treatment.
3. Goal of recovery should focus on return to play, sports, work, and daily life activities.
4. "When in doubt, sit them out." No athlete should be allowed to return to play until they have been assessed for the presence of a concussion. Risk of reinjury is high when one experiences symptoms of a concussion, and reinjury during unresolved concussion symptoms can lead to worsened symptoms and a prolonged recovery.
5. Provide education and reassurance about recovery, as it can be the most important step! Inform the athlete on the natural course of recovery and the importance of following the treatment recommendations so that symptoms improve in a timely fashion, while maintaining a healthy lifestyle—such as timely and nutritious meals, adequate hydration, reducing stress, and sleeping well.

General Recommendations

1. After 1 or 2 days of relative rest, reintegration of physical and cognitive activity should begin, as tolerated by the symptoms. No complete rest should be recommended because it leads to prolonged symptoms and unnecessary anxiety. In addition, inactivity can lead to iatrogenic symptoms, similar to a concussion.
2. As a general rule, if one feels well performing an activity, they should be allowed to continue that activity. If one feels worse performing an activity, the individual should take a break and try again later. This can include electronics use and interactive video games to test tolerance. Such activities can provide relevant information for clinician guidance of the management. For instance, if a child can tolerate screen time but is not able to read a book in school, this may hint to an underlying psychosocial aspect of the injury that needs to be addressed.
   a. Physical activities performed in the early stages should be limited to those that are noncontact in nature. For example, recommend slow or brisk walks and modify the intensity based on exacerbation of symptoms. The goal is to allow some form of activity because complete rest is not conducive to improving return to previous level of activity.
   b. Cognitive activities should be limited to activities as tolerated by the symptoms. Students should not be removed from school unless there are significant symptoms. Trial of school with rest breaks and modifications is initially recommended. Normalizing previous activities is important for maintaining social interactions with friends while limiting the unnecessary anxiety related to schoolwork missed.
3. Once an athlete is making progress with their symptoms and able to tolerate day-to-day activities, it is important to begin the return to sport strategy as recommended by the Consensus Statement in Sports (Table 50.2). The

TABLE 50.2 Graduated Return to Sport Strategy[1]

Rehabilitation Stage	Functional Exercise	Objective
1. Symptom-limited activity	Daily activities that do not provoke symptoms	Gradual reintroduction of work/school activities
2. Light aerobic exercise	Walking or stationary cycling at slow to medium pace; no resistance training	Increase heart rate
3. Sport-specific exercise	Running or skating drills; no head-impact activities	Add movement
4. Noncontact training drills	Harder training drills, e.g., passing drills; may start progressive resistance training	Exercise, coordination, and increased thinking
5. Full-contact practice	Following medical clearance, participate in normal training activities	Restore confidence and assess functional skills by coaching staff
6. Return to sport	Normal game play	—

athlete is progressed through each of the six stages of activity, with at least 24 hours between each stage of progression. If symptoms worsen at any stage, the athlete is downgraded to the previous stage and reassessed after at least 24 hours at the previous stage. The return to sport strategy should take a minimum of a week and should not be performed any faster to ensure that recovery is occurring. Return to school must successfully precede return to contact sports.

Symptom-Specific Management

Headache

Headache is the most common symptom after a concussion and can present in many forms. It is important to classify the headache because this will assist in the guidance of treatment. In addition to ascertaining the quality and frequency of the headache, it should be noted that association with nausea and light sensitivity is consistent with a posttraumatic migraine. Use of over-the-counter medications, such as acetaminophen or a nonspecific antiinflammatory as needed, can assist with the pain experienced. Personal or familial history of migraines may increase susceptibility to such types of headaches.

If headaches are associated with neck pain, then the treatment is geared toward cervicogenic headache treatments with heat, ice, and neck-stretching exercises. A short course of physical therapy can further assist in the improvement of the pain and decreased prolonged symptoms.

Dizziness

It is important to distinguish the difference between lightheadedness and vertiginous dizziness, because they connotate different management strategies. Lightheadedness can occur in a setting of dehydration and inactivity. However, vertiginous dizziness needs to be further evaluated for the presence of concomitant oculomotor dysfunctions, such as saccades and nystagmus, or an abnormal vestibular-ocular reflex. In these instances, physiological impairments of balance with anterior-posterior sway at the ankles or abnormal dynamic gait with head turns demonstrates a vestibular disorder. Vestibular therapy should be recommended for further evaluation and treatment.

Sleep Disorders

Sleep is a complex, yet essential, aspect of maintaining a healthy mind and body and restoring the energy one needs to be active during the day. Sleep can be affected by pain, stress, mood, and other factors. If sleep is not optimized, it can worsen fatigue, mood, and day-to-day functioning. Therefore it is imperative that optimizing sleep is integral to maximizing recovery. Management begins with good sleep hygiene habits as dictated by cognitive behavioral therapy. Short-term use of melatonin could also be considered.

Mood and Cognitive Complaints

Experiencing the symptoms of a concussion—especially with the presence of pain and poor sleep—can lead to emotional distress and certainly will affect how one performs their day-to-day tasks. Early on, somatic symptoms need to be addressed first, because if they improve, so do the emotional and cognitive complaints. Specific management of these symptoms should be addressed further when recovery does not follow the natural course and becomes prolonged. If recovery is prolonged, neuropsychologist involvement for an interview, counseling, and paper–pencil neurocognitive testing is recommended.

Recovery

The expected time frames for recovery are about 10 to 14 days in adults and about 4 weeks in children.[1] In the setting of recovery beyond this time frame, an athlete should be referred to a physician who is an expert in concussion management (if not already working with one). Common risk factors related to prolonged symptoms are presence of migrainous symptoms, fogginess, or amnesia; being younger in age, female, or an overexerter; or having a history of multiple concussions, psychiatric disturbances, or learning disability.[7] In addition, a higher PCSS score at the initial evaluation has been shown to consistently be a factor in prolonged recovery.

Further evaluation into underlying an cause must be sought out when concussion symptoms last greater than 2 months. For optimal management of concussion, especially when faced with complex cases, it is important to have a multidisciplinary team approach. Appropriate management requires acknowledgment of the symptoms experienced by the patient along with emotional support and reassurance. Sometimes, a thorough history and physical examination can reveal undiagnosed vestibular or ocular dysfunctions that can be treated with a vestibular referral and significantly improve outcomes.

The term *postconcussion syndrome* should not be used, because it is a nonspecific psychiatric diagnosis that is not reflective of persistent ongoing symptoms related to a nonprogressive injury. The likely cause for prolonged symptoms is considered a constellation of symptoms that can be related to premorbid psychosocial aspects of the individual—such as premorbid anxiety, depression, and family dynamics—which can limit the recovery resilience in times of stress.

Prevention

Although helmets are often thought to protect the brain, they are unable to prevent the concussive force that is transmitted to the brain and hitting against the skull. New technologies with accelerometers on helmets may provide information regarding force sustained but do not reflect the impact that the brain ultimately sustains.[1] Helmets of such nature should not be used a method for diagnosing a concussion. Despite their limitations, helmets should be worn for contact sports and high-impact activities such as skiing or bicycling, because they can protect the face and prevent skull fractures.

Review Questions

1. A 12-year-old girl presents a few days after she fell off the couch at home while playing with her sister. She had a headache and felt dizzy afterward. Today she reports that she is doing better but had difficulty concentrating on the board at school because of the headaches. What should the management recommendations be for this child?
   a. Home schooling until headaches are resolved
   b. Removal from school until headaches have completely resolved
   c. Perform neurocognitive testing to determine fitness for return to school
   d. Full days at school with as-needed pain medications and schoolwork modifications

2. The same patient returns at your follow up 2 weeks later and notes that she is significantly worse. Now she complains not only of headaches but also dizziness, nausea, anxiety, and cognitive inefficiencies. The child's mother states she had to stay home a few days because she was not feeling well. What should the next course of management be?
   a. Child has worsened concussion symptoms and should be removed from school until symptoms have resolved.

   b. Determine whether a new concussion has been sustained while trying to recover from the original.
   c. Speak with the child about stressors encountered to identify alternate cause of why the symptoms are worse.
   d. Child should be continued on previous recommendations with full reintegration back to school.

3. Which symptom should be prioritized in the management of an acute concussion?
   a. Sleep difficulties
   b. Cognitive complaints
   c. Headache
   d. Dizziness

Answers on page 400.
Access the full list of questions and answers online. Available on ExpertConsult.com

References

1. McCrory P, Meeuwisse W, Dvorak J, et al. Consensus statement on concussion in sport—the 5(th) International Conference on Concussion in Sport held in Berlin, October 2016. *Br J Sports Med*. 2017;51(11):838-847.
2. Lovell M, Collins M, Bradley J. Return to play following sports-related concussion. *Clin Sports Med*. 2004;23(3):421-441, ix.
3. Giza CC, Hovda DA. The new neurometabolic cascade of concussion. *Neurosurgery*. 2014;75 (suppl 4):S24-S33.
4. Sport Concussion Assessment Tool—5th edition. *Br J Sports Med*. 2017;51(11):851-858.
5. Davis GA, Purcell L, Schneider KJ, et al. The child sport concussion assessment tool 5th edition (Child SCAT5): background and rationale. *Br J Sports Med*. 2017;51(11):859-861.
6. Giza CC, Kutcher JS, Ashwal S, et al. Summary of evidence-based guideline update: evaluation and management of concussion in sports: report of the Guideline Development Subcommittee of the American Academy of Neurology. *Neurology*. 2013;80(24):2250-2257.
7. Sabini RC, Nutini DN, Nutini M. Return-to-play guidelines in concussion: revisiting the literature. *Phys Sports Med*. 2014;42(3): 10-19.

51

Gender-Specific Issues in Traumatic Brain Injury

MONICA VERDUZCO-GUTIERREZ, MD, AND JASON EDWARDS, DO

OUTLINE

Epidemiology

Outcomes

Sports-Related Concussion

Intimate Partner Violence

Although sex-based differences regarding the incidence of traumatic brain injury (TBI) have been well documented, there is a dearth of literature examining sex and gender effects on TBI-related outcomes and related gender-specific issues. Of note, much of the existing literature discusses gender and sex interchangeably. The National Institutes of Health (NIH) defines *sex* as "biological differences between females and males, including chromosomes, sex organs, and endogenous hormonal profiles," whereas *gender* is defined as "socially constructed and enacted roles and behaviors which occur in a historical and cultural context and vary across societies and over time."[1] Perhaps the complex interplay between sex and gender can help explain some of the inconsistencies found in sex and gender-based TBI research. There is a need for future studies specifically examining sex and gender differences in TBI to help elucidate the full extent of their effects.

Epidemiology

The international incidence of TBI is reported to be 349 per 100,0000 person-years.[2] When analyzed by sex, the annual incidence of TBI among females is 195 per 100,000 compared with 388 per 100,000 for males.[2] In the United States, rates of TBI-related emergency department visits by sex in 2010 showed an average of 800 per 100,000 visits for males versus 633.7 per 100,000 for females.[3] When examining the rates of TBI-related deaths, men had over twice the rate of deaths compared with

women between the years of 2001 and 2010.[3] Additionally, men had nearly double the rate of TBI-related hospitalizations compared with women between 2001 and 2010, suggesting men may be at higher risk of suffering a more severe brain injury.[3]

The relative risk of sustaining a TBI is near equal for males and females below the age of 2 and over the age of 65.[4,5] The largest discrepancy is found between the ages of 10 and 14, with males having the highest risk for TBI.[5,6]

Outcomes

Studies on gender-related outcomes after TBI have explored the effects of hormonal influences, including the potential neuroprotective effects of the steroid sex hormones estrogen and progesterone. Animal studies have shown neuroprotective effects of both, but attempts to replicate these findings in clinical studies have yielded conflicting results.[7-9] A shorter duration of amenorrhea after TBI has been found to be associated with improved outcomes, with subjects experiencing a longer durations of amenorrhea found to have worse global outcome ratings when controlling for severity of injury.[10,11] These findings could be attributed to protective effects of female sex hormones.[10,11] However, other studies have shown evidence of higher mortality and worse functional outcomes in women after moderate to severe TBI.[12,13] Additional research has shown peri- and postmenopausal women as having reduced mortality and fewer complications after moderate to severe TBI, whereas premenopausal women exhibit similar mortality rates as men.[14,15] More research is needed to further explore the effects of sex hormones in relation to TBI outcomes.

Sports-Related Concussion

Gender differences have also been reported regarding sports-related concussion incidence, clinical presentation, and recovery. Data indicate an overall higher incidence of concussion among women compared with that of men in sports

324

played with the same rules.[16-18] Although controversial, some studies suggest the increased incidence of sports-related concussion in females is related to reporter bias, because males were found to have less intent to report future concussions than their female counterparts.[19,20] This may be because of differences in gender norms as opposed to biologically determined sex, because female athletes with greater conformity to the norms of risk-taking behavior were more likely to return to play while symptomatic, and intent to report future concussions was greater among athletes who conformed less to traditional masculine gender norms of self-reliance and winning.[20]

One proposed explanation for the increased incidence relates to the biomechanical differences between men and women, specifically head-to-neck ratio, neck strength, and dynamic stability.[21-23] Weaker neck strength was found to correlate with athletes who had sustained a concussion.[22]

In terms of outcome and recovery, females appear to take longer to recover than their male counterparts and experience more severe and longer lasting neuropsychological deficits relative to baseline than do males.[24-27]

Intimate Partner Violence

Whereas consequences of mild TBIs (mTBI)—in particular sports-related mTBIs—have gained increased international attention, TBI related to intimate partner violence (IPV) has garnered relatively little recognition in comparison. The paucity of research on IPV-related TBI is confounded by hesitancy of victims to disclose abuse or seek medical treatment

and the lack of uniform screening guidelines.[28] IPV is highly gendered and is a common cause of TBI because head, face, and neck injuries are among the most common IPV-related injuries reported.[29] Per the Centers for Disease Control and Prevention, IPV refers to "physical, sexual, or psychological harm by a current or former partner or spouse."[30] The National Intimate Partner and Sexual Violence Survey indicates that 1 in 4 women in the United States experienced contact sexual violence or physical violence compared with 1 in 10 men.[31]

Brain injuries sustained by women experiencing IPV are unique in that these women are more likely to sustain repetitive injuries—most often caused by blows to the head, neck, or face, with 29% to 39% of women also reporting attempted strangulation, a potential cause of hypoxic-ischemic brain injury.[29,32-35]

One poorly studied population that appears to be at increased risk for IPV—and thus for IPV-related TBI—is the lesbian, gay, bisexual, and transgender (LGBT) population.[36] Data are currently lacking, but beyond being at increased risk, research has shown that LGBT individuals face additional barriers to seeking treatment that are unique to their sexual orientation or gender identity including fear of outing oneself when seeking help, the lack of LGBT-friendly resources, and potential homophobia from service providers.[36,37]

Sex and gender-based differences regarding IPV-related TBI add complexity to an already understudied topic. Further research is needed to define and address barriers that discourage victims from reporting events and seeking treatment.

Review Questions

1. Strengthening of which muscles may decrease incidence of concussion in young athletes?
   a. Neck
   b. Temporalis and frontalis
   c. Deltoids
   d. Abdominal
2. When comparing the sexes, which statement is true regarding the incidence of traumatic brain injured (TBI)-related hospitalizations and TBI-related deaths?
   a. Women have higher rates of TBI-related hospitalizations but a lower incidence of TBI-related deaths.
   b. Women have lower rates of TBI-related hospitalizations but a higher incidence of TBI-related deaths.
   c. Women have higher rates of TBI-related hospitalizations but a lower incidence of TBI-related deaths.
   d. Women have lower rates of TBI-related hospitalizations and a lower incidence of TBI-related deaths.
3. Administration of progesterone in clinical studies on TBI has consistently shown what effect on outcomes?
   a. Reduced mortality
   b. Decreased disability
   c. Conflicting results
   d. More adverse events

Answers on page 401.
Access the full list of questions and answers online.
Available on ExpertConsult.com

References

1. National Institutes of Health. *Sex & Gender*. Office of Research on Women's Health [Internet]. National Institutes of Health. [cited 2019 Jan 16]. Available at: https://orwh.od.nih.gov/sex-gender.
2. Nguyen R, Fiest KM, McChesney J, et al. The international incidence of traumatic brain injury: a systematic review and meta-analysis. *Can J Neurol Sci*. 2016;43(6):774-785.
3. Centers for Disease Control and Prevention. *TBI Data and Statistics. Concussion. Traumatic Brain Injury*. CDC Injury Center [Internet]. [cited 2019 Jan 16]. Available at: https://www.cdc.gov/traumaticbraininjury/data/index.html.
4. Crowe L, Babl F, Anderson V, Catroppa C. The epidemiology of paediatric head injuries: data from a referral centre in Victoria, Australia. *J Paediatr Child Health*. 2009;45(6):346-350.

5. Mushkudiani NA, Engel DC, Steyerberg EW, et al. Prognostic value of demographic characteristics in traumatic brain injury: results from The IMPACT Study. *J Neurotrauma.* 2007;24(2):259-269.

6. Faul M, Xu L, Wald MM, Coronado VG. Traumatic brain injury in the United States: emergency department visits, hospitalizations and deaths 2002-2006. Centers for Disease Control and Prevention, National Center for Injury Prevention and Control; 2010. [cited 2019 Feb 9]. Available at: https://www.cdc.gov/traumaticbraininjury/pdf/blue_book.pdf.

7. Herson P, Koerner I, Hurn P. Sex, sex steroids, and brain injury. *Semin Reprod Med.* 2009;27(3):229-239.

8. Stein DG, Cekic MM. Progesterone and vitamin D hormone as a biologic treatment of traumatic brain injury in the aged. *PM&R.* 2011;3:S100-S110.

9. Skolnick BE, Maas AI, Narayan RK, van der Hoop RG, MacAllister T, Ward JD, et al. A clinical trial of progesterone for severe traumatic brain injury. *N Engl J Med.* 2014;371(26):2467-2476.

10. Ripley DL, Harrison-Felix C, Sendroy-Terrill M, Cusick CP, Dannels-McClure A, Morey C. The impact of female reproductive function on outcomes after traumatic brain injury. *Arch Phys Med Rehabil.* 2008;89(6):1090-1096.

11. Colantonio A, Mar W, Escobar M, et al. Women's health outcomes after traumatic brain injury. *J Womens Health.* 2010;19(6):1109-1116.

12. Slewa-Younan S, van den Berg S, Baguley IJ, Nott M, Cameron ID. Towards an understanding of sex differences in functional outcome following moderate to severe traumatic brain injury: a systematic review. *J Neurol Neurosurg Psychiatry.* 2008;79(11):1197-1201.

13. Munivenkatappa A, Agrawal A, Shukla D, Kumaraswamy D, Devi B. Traumatic brain injury: does gender influence outcomes? *Int J Crit Illn Inj Sci.* 2016;6(2):70.

14. Berry C, Ley EJ, Tillou A, Cryer G, Margulies DR, Salim A. The effect of gender on patients with moderate to severe head injuries. *J Trauma.* 2009;67(5):950-953.

15. Davis DP, Douglas DJ, Smith W, et al. Traumatic brain injury outcomes in pre- and post- menopausal females versus age-matched males. *J Neurotrauma.* 2006;23(2):140-148.

16. NCAA Sports Medicine Handbook [Internet]. 25th ed. The National Collegiate Athletic Association; 2014. [cited 2019 Feb 9]. Available at: http://www.ncaapublications.com/p-4374-2014-15-ncaa-sports-medicine-handbook.aspx.

17. Rosenthal JA, Foraker RE, Collins CL, Comstock RD. National high school athlete concussion rates from 2005-2006 to 2011-2012. *Am J Sports Med.* 2014;42(7):1710-1715.

18. Marar M, McIlvain NM, Fields SK, Comstock RD. Epidemiology of concussions among united states high school athletes in 20 sports. *Am J Sports Med.* 2012;40(4):747-755.

19. Miyashita TL, Diakogeorgiou E, VanderVegt C. Gender differences in concussion reporting among high school athletes. *Sports Health.* 2016;8(4):359-363.

20. Kroshus E, Baugh CM, Stein CJ, Austin SB, Calzo JP. Concussion reporting, sex, and conformity to traditional gender norms in young adults. *J Adolesc.* 2017;54:110-119.

21. Tierney RT, Sitler MR, Swanik CB, Swanik KA, Higgins M, Torg J. Gender differences in head-neck segment dynamic stabilization during head acceleration. *Med Sci Sports Exerc.* 2005;37(2):272-279.

22. Collins CL, Fletcher EN, Fields SK, et al. Neck strength: a protective factor reducing risk for concussion in high school sports. *J Prim Prev.* 2014;35(5):309-319.

23. Viano DC, Casson IR, Pellman EJ. Concussion in professional football. *Neurosurgery.* 2007;61(2):313-328.

24. Benedict PA, Baner NV, Harrold GK, et al. Gender and age predict outcomes of cognitive, balance and vision testing in a multidisciplinary concussion center. *J Neurol Sci.* 2015;353(1-2):111-115.

25. Covassin T, Elbin RJ, Harris W, Parker T, Kontos A. The role of age and sex in symptoms, neurocognitive performance, and postural stability in athletes after concussion. *Am J Sports Med.* 2012;40(6):1303-1312.

26. Berz K, Divine J, Foss KB, Heyl R, Ford KR, Myer GD. Sex-specific differences in the severity of symptoms and recovery rate following sports-related concussion in young athletes. *Phys Sports Med.* 2013;41(2):58-63.

27. Brooks BL, Iverson GL, Atkins JE, Zafonte R, Berkner PD. Sex differences and self-reported attention problems during baseline concussion testing. *Appl Neuropsychol Child.* 2016;5(2):119-126.

28. Goldin Y, Haag HL, Trott CT. Screening for history of traumatic brain injury among women exposed to intimate partner violence. *PM&R.* 2016;8(11):1104-1110.

29. Kwako LE, Glass N, Campbell J, Melvin KC, Barr T, Gill JM. Traumatic brain injury in intimate partner violence: a critical review of outcomes and mechanisms. *Trauma Violence Abuse.* 2011;12(3):115-126.

30. 2015 NISVS Data Brief Violence Prevention Injury Center CDC [Internet]. 2019 [cited 2019 Feb 2]. Available at: https://www.cdc.gov/violenceprevention/datasources/nisvs/2015NISVSdatabrief.html.

31. Smith SG, Zhang X, Basile KC, et al. *The National Intimate Partner and Sexual Violence Survey (NISVS)*: 2015 Data Brief—updated release [Internet]. Atlanta, GA: National Center for Injury Prevention and Control, Centers for Disease Control and Prevention; 2018. [cited 2019 Feb 2]. Available at: https://www.cdc.gov/violenceprevention/datasources/nisvs/2015NISVSdatabrief.html?CDC_AA_refVal=https%3A%2F%2Fwww.cdc.gov%2Fviolenceprevention%2Fnisvs%2F2015NISVSdatabrief.html.

32. Campbell JC, Webster D, Koziol-McLain J, et al. Risk factors for femicide in abusive relationships: results from a multisite case control study. *Am J Public Health.* 2003;93(7):1089-1097.

33. Sutherland CA, Bybee DI, Sullivan CM. Beyond bruises and broken bones: the joint effects of stress and injuries on battered women's health. *Am J Community Psychol.* 2002;30(5):609-636.

34. Wilbur L, Higley M, Hatfield J, et al. Survey results of women who have been strangled while in an abusive relationship. *J Emerg Med.* 2001;21(3):297-302.

35. Mcquown C, Frey J, Steer S, et al. Prevalence of strangulation in survivors of sexual assault and domestic violence. *Am J Emerg Med.* 2016;34(7):1281-1285.

36. Rothman EF, Exner D, Baughman AL. The prevalence of sexual assault against people who identify as gay, lesbian, or bisexual in the United States: a systematic review. *Trauma Violence Abuse.* 2011;12(2):55-66.

37. Brown TNT, Herman JL. *Intimate Partner Violence and Sexual Abuse Among LGBT People: A Review of Existing Research.* Los Angeles, CA: The Williams Institute; 2015.

52

Postconcussion Syndrome Assessment, Management, and Treatment

ABANA AZARIAH, MD, AND THOMAS WATANABE, MD

OUTLINE

Mild traumatic brain injury (mTBI) makes up 85% to 90% of all traumatic brain injury (TBI) cases. Based on clinical outcomes and formal research, most people with an mTBI will have self-limiting symptoms (<3 months) and follow a predictable course toward good recovery. A small number (<5%) of mTBI patients, however, will go on to have persistent symptoms, placing them in a category described as postconcussion syndrome (PCS). PCS implies both chronicity and a group of signs and symptoms and is a possible sequela of mTBI. Patients with PCS present with slow and/or incomplete recovery, associating them with higher levels of disability and frequent healthcare service utilization.

The etiology of PCS has never been agreed on. It has been well documented that in the early stages after a mTBI, symptoms are largely a result of numerous organic factors occurring within the brain. These can occur at the macroscopic and microscopic levels.[1] Prolongation of symptoms however, such as those seen in patients with PCS, are thought to be perpetuated by early psychological distress, preexisting mental health disorders, and mental health.[2,3] Several studies have suggested early psychological factors play an important etiological role in PCS also.[4-7] Adequately addressing these psychological elements can help toward symptomatic and functional recovery. Premorbid factors, such as biopsychosocial stability of the individual and the complexity of the initial injury, also have been suggested to play a role in etiology.[8-10] Knowledge regarding etiologies of

PCS also provides a basis for the development of a treatment plan.

Diagnostic Criteria

There is no universally accepted definition of PCS. It is loosely described as a constellation of symptoms occurring in individuals with mTBI. The onset and duration of symptoms remain vague, although many have suggested symptom duration of at least 3 months. Objective findings including physical examination, radiological evidence, and laboratory findings are largely absent, leaving the diagnosis of PCS based almost entirely on subjective symptoms, which may be problematic.

Currently, two criteria exist for PCS:
1. *Diagnostic and Statistical Manual of Mental Disorders*, Fourth Edition (DSM-IV, Table 52.1)
2. International Classification of Diseases 10th edition (ICD-10, Table 52.2).

The advantage of employing formal criteria is that it provides a basic framework for healthcare providers who may have minimal clinical experience in managing patients with a history of remote mTBI. It also provides a list of commonly reported symptoms that can guide clinicians during the initial history intake and gathering of objective evidence (i.e., physical and neurological examination). It can also provide a working definition for research. The DSM-IV criteria require that "reported disturbances cause significant impairment in social or occupational functioning and represent a significant decline from a previous level of functioning." The focus on functional *decline* implies a more recent event. Its presence can help clinicians disentangle chronic premorbid symptoms versus recent symptoms resulting from a new mTBI.[11]

Having mentioned these utilities, limitations when using these criteria exist, and strict adherence to these guidelines is not recommended. The most obvious limitation seen is the emphasis on subjective symptoms over objective findings (e.g., neuropsychological tests). The ICD-10 criteria, for example, do not require objective evidence of cognitive complaints.[12] Tables 52.1 and 52.2 list symptoms that are vague and can be present in patients with a multitude of medical and psychological diagnoses. In fact, the psychological measures used in several studies that looked at PCS, the Hospital Anxiety and Depression Scale or the Impact of Events Scale, were developed to address

emotional distress in medical patients and are not specific to mTBI.[13]

On the contrary, the DSM-IV criteria do require a neuropsychological assessment as a measure of cognitive function. They do not, however, provide rigid guidelines regarding when the assessment should be administered. We believe this degree of freedom is in fact appropriate and allows testing to be individualized as opposed to simply being a protocol-driven decision. Furthermore, the cutoff of 3 months for symptom reporting may not always apply to each individual case. The rigid guideline of waiting 3 months before diagnosis of PCS should be reconsidered because of such high variability of patient presentation, risk factor associations, and related lack of relevance to treatment decision making.

As discussed earlier, the ICD-10 and DMS-IV criteria have some major discrepancies between them. Studies comparing prevalence rates using the different criteria show a three to six times higher rate using the DSM-IV.[14] Higher prevalence rates using DMS-IV is likely because of the additional requirements of documented objective evidence of cognitive impairment and impairment in functioning required by the ICD-10.

Clinical Assessment

Clinical assessment should include a detailed history and physical, including an evaluation of concomitant medical conditions, injury-related diagnoses, and psychosocial issues.

Fig. 52.1 lists common medical and psychosocial conditions that may influence the reporting of symptoms after most recent mTBI. Diagnosis of depression, posttraumatic stress, anxiety, and certain personality types (high achievers,

---

TABLE 52.1 Postconcussional Syndrome (Research Criteria from the DSM-IV)

These criteria must be met for the diagnosis of postconcussional disorder:
A. Requires history of head trauma causing significant cerebral concussion
B. Objective evidence on neuropsychological testing of decline in some of his or her cognitive abilities, e.g., attention, concentration, learning, or memory
C. The person must report three or more subjective symptoms, and these symptoms must be present for at least 3 months:
1. Easily fatigued
2. Disordered sleep
3. Headache
4. Vertigo or dizziness
5. Irritability or aggression on little or no provocation
6. Anxiety, depression, or affective lability
7. Changes in personality (social or sexual inappropriateness)
8. Apathy or lack of spontaneity

Disturbance causes significant impairment in social or occupational functioning and represents a significant decline from a previous level of functioning.

DSM-IV, Diagnostic and Statistical Manual of Mental Disorders, Fourth Edition.

TABLE 52.2 Postconcussional Syndrome (Research Criteria from the ICD-10)

For those undertaking research into this condition, these criteria are recommended:
A. The general criteria of F07 must be met. The general criteria for F07, personality and behavioral disorders caused by brain disease, damage, and dysfunction, are as follows: G1. Objective evidence (from physical and neurological examination and laboratory tests) and/or history of cerebral disease, damage, or dysfunction. G2. Absence of clouding of consciousness and of significant memory deficit. G3. Absence of sufficient or suggestive evidence for an alternative causation of the personality or behavior disorder that would justify its placement in section F6 (other mental disorders caused by brain damage and dysfunction and to physical disease).
B. History of head trauma with loss of consciousness, preceding the onset of symptoms by a period of up to 4 weeks (objective electroencephalography [EEG], brain imaging, or oculonystagmographic evidence for brain damage may be lacking).
C. At least three of these:
1. Complaints of unpleasant sensations and pains, such as headache, dizziness (usually lacking the features of true vertigo), general malaise and excessive fatigue, or noise intolerance
2. Emotional changes, such as irritability, emotional lability—both easily provoked or exacerbated by emotional excitement or stress, or some degree of depression and/or anxiety
3. Subjective complaints of difficulty in concentration and in performing mental tasks and of memory complaints without clear objective evidence (e.g., psychological tests) of marked impairment
4. Insomnia
5. Reduced tolerance to alcohol
6. Preoccupation with aforementioned symptoms and fear of permanent brain damage to the extent of hypochondriacal overvalued ideas and adoption of a sick role

ICD-10, International Classification of Diseases 10th Edition

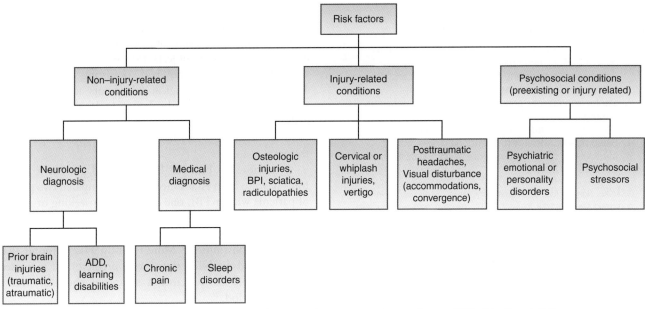

• **Fig. 52.1** Risk factors for the development of postconcussive syndrome. *ADD,* Attention deficit disorder; *BPI,* brachial plexus injuries;

dependent, or insecure) should be carefully reviewed because they have shown to be predictive of development of PCS.[6,15,16] Other risk factors that have also been identified are higher symptoms scores acutely,[17] early manifestation of emotional symptoms,[18] migraine headaches,[19] and within a military population history of TBI, both predeployment and deployment psychological distress and loss of consciousness (LOC) with the injury.[20]

After a detailed history is obtained, a focused physical examination should be completed. The chronicity of symptoms being observed could have resulted from missed findings on prior examinations resulting in an inadequate assessment and management of symptoms. Complaints of chronic pain, for example limb, back, neck, shoulder pain or posttraumatic headaches, may be the result of associated injuries and should be treated adequately and the patient reassessed before diagnosis of PCS.[13,21] For review of common physical examination findings in mTBI, refer to earlier chapters in this book.

Management and Treatment

As mentioned earlier, a complete and thorough history and examination is essential in developing a treatment plan. Additionally, a good understanding of the patient's psychosocial status and stressors can help the treatment team develop strategies that they can then use in their therapy or counseling sessions. A holistic approach is often recommended when considering management and treatment of PCS. Fig. 52.2 addresses some of the physical, cognitive, and psychosocial problems commonly seen in PCS. Note that the interventions are broadly categorized into pharmacological (Table 52.3), rehabilitation, and psychological, but they have a significant degree of overlap and often occur simultaneously.

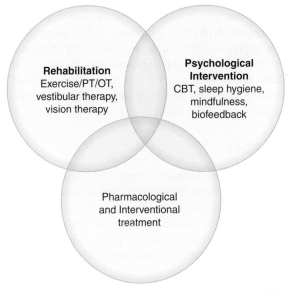

• **Fig. 52.2** Holistic treatment of postconcussion syndrome. *CBT,* Cognitive behavioral therapy; *PT,* physical therapy; *OT,* occupational therapy.

Because many of the risk factors for the development of PCS can be conceptualized in a biopsychosocial model, it is reasonable to employ cognitive and behavioral interventions as part of a treatment plan. When cognitive deficits persist, patients may develop a loss of confidence, leading to anxiety and avoidant behavior.[16] These problems may worsen cognitive decline.

Cognitive behavioral therapy (CBT) may help address the anxiety and other maladaptations such as symptom misattribution.[22] A systematic review found support for CBT in the treatment of PCS.[23] Early, brief psychological

TABLE 52.3	Pharmacological Treatment for Postconcussional Syndrome

1. Pain syndromes/headaches: analgesics (acetamino-phen, NSAIDs), neuropathic pain medications (e.g., gabapentin, pregabalin), nerve blocks anmv, and other interventional procedures
2. Depression/anxiety: antidepressants, mood stabilizers, anxiolytics
3. Posttraumatic stress disorder: prazosin, SSRIs, SNRIs
4. Sleep agents: melatonin, trazodone, TCAs, others
5. Medications for specific neurobehavioral deficits: meth-ylphenidate, others

NSAIDS, Nonsteroidal antiinflammatory drugs; *SNRI,* serotonin and norepinephrine reuptake inhibitor; *SSRI,* selective serotonin reuptake inhibitor; *TCAs,* tricyclic antidepressants.

treatment has been demonstrated to decrease the likelihood of prolonged PCS. Education, reassurance, and a gradual resumption of "normal" activities were identified as important parts of this treatment.[24] Lange demonstrated a strong relationship between depression and postconcussion symptoms, supporting the need for efforts to minimize the development of depression and address it when it is established.[5] Although activity is often considered part of the management of physical symptoms and in resumption of return to play for athletes, the role of activity in enhancing cognitive and behavioral function should not be overlooked. Supervised activity has been demonstrated to decrease anxiety and may help reduce fear of reinjury, assisting in reactivation after concussion.[25]

Outcomes

Studies that have addressed outcomes after mTBI in a longitudinal fashion fairly consistently demonstrate that as duration of symptoms lengthens, the rate and extent of recovery lessen. Barker-Collo found that whereas 50% of subjects had symptom improvement between 1 and 6 months, only 4.2% demonstrated significant improvement between 6 and

12 months.[26] Additionally, several studies support the concept that prolonged symptoms have more of a psychological basis, whereas early symptoms are more biological. Losoi evaluated a group of subjects with mTBI over 1 year and showed that those who had persisting symptoms at 12 months had psychological risk factors acutely and had more symptoms at 6 months. Interestingly, all subjects in an orthopedic control group who had concussion-like symptoms at 12 months also had identifiable psychological risk factors.[27]

A relationship between litigation and persistent symptoms has also been established. Paniak compared two groups of patients with mTBI, one of which was seeking or receiving financial compensation. That group was found to have an increase in symptom severity and incidence at both 3 and 12 months postinjury.[28] More recently, Hanks found that litigation and disability status were predictors of increased symptoms on the concussion symptom checklist over a 6-month period.[29]

Clinicians treating patients with mTBI should be cognizant of early symptoms of anxiety, depression, and/or irritability given their relationship to persistence of symptoms after injury and overall outcome.

Summary

- Lack of consensus regarding definition/conceptual framework of PCS makes evaluation of risk factors and natural history difficult.
- Identification of risk factors and presenting symptoms may lead to earlier identification of at-risk individuals, which may decrease the likelihood of evolution to PCS.
- When evaluating patients with prolonged symptoms it is important to review the clinical history and conduct a thorough examination to identify reasons for lack of symptom resolution.
- Psychological factors play a prominent etiological role for PCS and predominate as symptoms become more chronic.
- A holistic approach is recommended for management and treatment of PCS.

Review Questions

1. According to *Diagnostic and Statistical Manual of Mental Disorders,* fourth edition (DSM-IV) criteria, symptoms related to concussion need to have persisted for at least how many month before making the diagnosis of postconcussion syndrome (PCS)?
   a. 3 weeks
   b. 6 weeks
   c. 9 weeks
   d. 12 weeks
2. What is greatest limitation in the current criteria for PCS?
   a. Duration of symptom reporting
   b. Recommendation to obtain neuroimaging
   c. Overreliance on pain symptoms
   d. Emphasis on subjective symptoms

3. Compared with acute symptoms, more prolonged symptoms seen in PCS are based more on which of these factors?
   a. Headaches
   b. Psychological factors
   c. Visual disturbance
   d. Sleep disturbance

Answers on page 401.
Access the full list of questions and answers online.
Available on ExpertConsult.com

References

1. Lishman WA. Physiogenesis and psychogenesis in the 'post-concussional syndrome'. *Br J Psychiatry*. 1988;153(4):460-469.

2. Silverberg ND, Iverson GL. Etiology of the post-concussion syndrome: physiogenesis and psychogenesis revisited. *Neuro Rehabilitation*. 2011;29(4):317-329.

3. Stein MB, Jain S, Giacino JT, et al. Risk of posttraumatic stress disorder and major depression in civilian patients after mild traumatic brain injury: a TRACK-TBI study. *JAMA Psychiatry*. 2019;76(3):249-258.

4. King NS, Wenden FJ, Caldwell FE, Wade DT. Early prediction of persisting post‚Äêconcussion symptoms following mild and moderate head injuries. *Br J Clin Psychol*. 1999;38(1):15-25.

5. Lange RT, Iverson GL, Rose A. Depression strongly influences postconcussion symptom reporting following mild traumatic brain injury. *J Head Trauma Rehabil*. 2011;26(2):127-137.

6. Meares S, Shores EA, Taylor AJ, et al. The prospective course of postconcussion syndrome: The role of mild traumatic brain injury. *Neuropsychology*. 2011;25(4):454.

7. Snell DL, Siegert RJ, Hay-Smith EJ, Surgenor LJ. Associations between illness perceptions, coping styles and outcome after mild traumatic brain injury: preliminary results from a cohort study. *Brain Inj*. 2011;25(11):1126-1138.

8. Ponsford J, Willmott C, Rothwell A, et al. Factors influencing outcome following mild traumatic brain injury in adults. *J Int Neuropsychol Soc*. 2000;6(5):568-579.

9. Jacobs B, Beems T, Stulemeijer M, et al. Outcome prediction in mild traumatic brain injury: age and clinical variables are stronger predictors than CT abnormalities. *J Neurotrauma*. 2010;27(4):655-668.

10. Stulemeijer M, Werf SP, Jacobs B, et al. Impact of additional extracranial injuries on outcome after mild traumatic brain injury. *J Neurotrauma*. 2006;23(10):1561-1569.

11. Castillo RJ, Carlat DJ, Millon T, et al. *Diagnostic and Statistical Manual of Mental Disorders*. Washington, DC: American Psychiatric Association Press; 2007.

12. World Health Organization. *The ICD-10 Classification of Mental and Behavioural Disorders: Diagnostic Criteria for Research*. Geneva: World Health Organization; 1993.

13. Stalnacke BM. Postconcussion symptoms in patients with injury-related chronic pain. *Rehabil Res Practice*, 2012, 528265.

14. McCauley SR, Boake C, Pedroza C, et al. Postconcussional disorder: Are the DSM-IV criteria an improvement over the ICD-10? *J Nerv Ment Dis*. 2005;193(8);540-550.

15. Ponsford J, Cameron P, Fitzgerald M, Grant M, Mikocka-Walus A, Schönberger M. Predictors of postconcussive symptoms 3 months after mild traumatic brain injury. *Neuropsychology*. 2012;26(3):304.

16. Kay T, Newman B, Cavallo M, Ezrachi O, Resnick M. Toward a neuropsychological model of functional disability after mild traumatic brain injury. *Neuropsychology*. 1992;6(4):371.

17. Heyer GL, Schaffer CE, Rose SC, Young JA, McNally KA, Fischer AN. Specific factors influence postconcussion symptom duration among youth referred to a sports concussion clinic. *J Pediatr*. 2016 ;174:33-38.

18. Dischinger PC, Ryb GE, Kufera JA, Auman KM. Early predictors of postconcussive syndrome in a population of trauma patients with mild traumatic brain injury. *J Trauma*. 2009;66(2):289-297.

19. Iverson GL, Gardner AJ, Terry DP, et al. Predictors of clinical recovery from concussion: a systematic review. *Br J Sports Med*. 2017;51(12):941-948.

20. Stein MB, Ursano RJ, Campbell-Sills L, et al. Prognostic indicators of persistent post-concussive symptoms after deployment-related mild traumatic brain injury: a prospective longitudinal study in US Army soldiers. *J Neurotrauma*. 2016;33(23):2125-2132.

21. Iverson GL, McCracken LM. 'Postconcussive' symptoms in persons with chronic pain. *Brain Inj*. 1997;11(11):783-790.

22. Broshek DK, De Marco AP, Freeman JR. A review of postconcussion syndrome and psychological factors associated with concussion. *Brain Inj*. 2015;29(2):228-237.

23. Al Sayegh A, Sandford D, Carson AJ. Psychological approaches to treatment of postconcussion syndrome: a systematic review. *J Neurol Neurosurg Psychiatry*. 2010;81(10):1128-1134.

24. Mittenberg W, Canyock EM, Condit D, Patton C. Treatment of post-concussion syndrome following mild head injury. *J Clin Exp Neuropsychol*. 2001;23(6):829-836.

25. Sandel N, Reynolds E, Cohen PE, Gillie BL, Kontos AP. Anxiety and mood clinical profile following sport-related concussion: From risk factors to treatment. *Sport Exerc Perform Psychol*. 2017;6(3):304.

26. Barker-Collo S, Theadom A, Jones K, et al. Reliable individual change in post concussive symptoms in the year following mild traumatic brain injury: data from the longitudinal, population-based brain injury incidence and outcomes New Zealand in the community (Bionic) study. *JSM Burns Trauma*. 2016;1(1):1006.

27. Losoi H, Silverberg ND, Wäljas M, et al. Recovery from mild traumatic brain injury in previously healthy adults. *J Neurotrauma*. 2016;33(8):766-776.

28. Paniak C, Reynolds S, Toller-Lobe G, Melnyk A, Nagy J, Schmidt D. A longitudinal study of the relationship between financial compensation and symptoms after treated mild traumatic brain injury. *J Clin Exp Neuropsychol*. 2002;24(2):187-193.

29. Hanks RA, Rapport LJ, Seagly K, Millis SR, Scott C, Pearson C. Outcomes after concussion recovery education: effects of litigation and disability status on maintenance of symptoms. *J Neurotrauma*. 2019;36(4):554-558.

53

Nontraumatic Brain Injury

RANI HALEY LINDBERG, MD

OUTLINE

Ischemia

Infection

Tumors

Autoimmune Brain Disorders

Nontraumatic brain injury (NTBI) is a broad category of brain disorders not resulting from traumatic forces. Included in this category are acquired brain injuries resulting from ischemic cerebrovascular disease, infection, neoplasm, and autoimmune disorders (Table 53.1). These pathologies result in impairments of physical function, cognition, language, and behavior. Evaluation for these disorders includes comprehensive history and physicals with symptomatology dependent on location of lesion and degree of injury/inflammation (Table 53.2). Treatment involves supportive care, rehabilitation, and education in addition to addressing specific brain issues (Table 53.3). In general, the NTBI population is an older demographic with more comorbidities that those with traumatic brain injury (TBI). Functional recovery after TBI tends to be better than after NTBI.[12]

Ischemia

- Focal ischemia is the most common stroke and is categorized into three types (Table 53.4). Symptoms lasting less than 24 hours are transient ischemic attacks (TIAs) and greater than 24 hours qualify as a stroke.[1-3]
- Ischemia is the leading cause of long-term disability in the United States.[1]
- Greater than 795,0000 individuals experience a new or recurrent stroke in the United States yearly.[1]
- Approximately 12% of stokes are preceded by a TIA.
- Incidence of recurrent stroke is 12% to 15%.
- Modifiable and nonmodifiable risk factors serve as targets for prevention. Hypertension is the greatest modifiable risk factor, and age is the most important nonmodifiable factor (Table 53.5).[1-3]

- Those presenting within 4.5 hours of initial symptoms may be eligible for intravenous thrombolysis with tissue plasminogen activator (tPA) and/or thrombectomy/embolectomy by a neurointerventionalist.[2]
- Most recovery occurs within 3 months. Lower limb function recovers before upper limb in most. Indicators of poor functional recovery include complete paralysis of the upper limb, prolonged flaccidity, severe proximal spasticity, and late return of proprioceptive facilitation of proximal traction response of the arm. Return of hand function within 4 weeks is an indicator of good functional return.[13]
- Multidisciplinary programs can reduce mortality rates, support recovery, and decrease the need for long-term care and disability.[13]

TABLE 53.1	Pathophysiology
Ischemia[1-3]	• Insufficient blood flow to brain causing cell death—this can be systemic hypoperfusion (see Chapter 55) or focal ischemia • Injury includes an inner core of severe necrosis with an outer layer of less severe injury (penumbra) • Penumbra reperfusion stops cell injury and decreases infarction size
Infection[4-6]	• Meningitis: infection and inflammation of the meninges from bacterial or viral pathogens • Encephalitis: inflammation of the brain tissue from viral pathogens • Meningoencephalitis: process affecting both the meninges and brain tissue and can be bacterial or viral
Tumors[7,8]	• Primary or metastatic lesions resulting from abnormal proliferation of malignant or benign cells • Cancers that can metastasize to brain: lung, colon, breast, kidney, and skin
Autoimmune[9-11]	• Immune-mediated inflammatory responses to tissues in the CNS

CNS, Central nervous system.

TABLE 53.2	Clinical Evaluation		
	History and Physical Items	**Labs and Tests**	**Imaging**
Ischemia[1-3]	• Emphasis on cardiovascular and neurological history, physical examination, and review of systems • Time of onset is important for early intervention • Delineate stroke risk factors (see Table 53.3)	• Complete blood counts (CBC) • Basic Metabolic Panel (BMP) • Lipid panels • Liver function tests • Hemoglobin A1c • Hypercoagulability panel (antiphospholipid antibody panel, protein C and S, factor V Leiden) • Echocardiogram • Electrocardiogram	• Preferred initial: computerized tomography (CT) of the brain without contrast • CT can be negative in the first 24 h and helps rule out hemorrhage to direct use of thrombolytic therapy. • Magnetic resonance imaging (MRI) is used to confirm and/or identify subtle strokes • Angiography is an adjunct to CT and MRI and identifies areas of vascular abnormality and voids in blood flow
Infection[4-6]	• Signs/symptoms: fever, headache, nausea, vomiting, vision changes, drowsiness, photosensitivity, and stiff neck • Behavioral changes and confusion can be seen. • Initially presents with flulike syndrome • Rash may be seen in bacterial meningitis	• CBC • BMP • Blood cultures • Cerebrospinal fluid (CSF) analysis and culture • Viral serology	• MRI with contrast is preferred • Imaging may be negative in meningitis and encephalitis • Meningitis: imaging detects potential entry point of infection • Abscess: MRI with contrast may show an encapsulated mass with necrotic center
Tumors[7,8]	• Signs/symptoms: headache, confusion, nausea, vomiting, weakness, balance impairment, cranial nerve palsies, fever, weight loss • Headache is the most common symptom • Seizure is a common presenting sign	• CBC • BMP • CSF analysis • Serum tumor markers • Biopsy	• CT and MRI of brain and body • MRI with gadolinium contrast is preferred modality (look for enhancement with central necrosis and surrounding edema)
Autoimmune[9-11]	• Fatigue, headache, seizures, stroke, and cranial nerve palsies are common • Relapsing, remitting, and progressive • Past medical and family history of autoimmune disease • Examination findings can include skin findings such as rash, purpura	• CBC • BMP • Blood cultures • CSF analysis and culture • Autoantibodies N-methyl-D-aspartate (NMDA) receptor • Brain biopsy	• CT and MRI • CT angiography is helpful in cerebral vasculitis and can show alternating areas of stenosis causing a beading-type appearance of the blood vessel

TABLE 53.3	Treatment
Disorder	**Treatment**
Ischemia[1-3]	• Thrombolysis with tissue plasminogen activator • Thrombectomy/embolectomy • Oral Antiplatelet • HMG-CoA reductase inhibitor • Addressing modifiable risk factors
Infection[4-6]	• Oral or intravenous (IV) antimicrobial • Neurosurgical drainage/decompression • Vaccination
Tumors[7,8]	• Neurosurgical resection • Radiation • Chemotherapy
Autoimmune[9-11]	• Steroids • IV immunoglobulin • Plasmapheresis • Immunosuppressant drugs (e.g., methotrexate, cyclophosphamide, Plaquenil)

TABLE 53.4	Ischemic Stroke Classification		
Thrombotic	**Embolic**	**Lacunar**
Large cerebral vessel occlusions	Cardioembolic	Smaller, arteriolar vessel occlusion
Gradual onset, progressive symptoms; often preceded by transient ischemic attack	Sudden in onset	Presents suddenly or gradually

TABLE 53.5	Ischemic Stroke Risk Factors	
Modifiable Risk Factors	**Nonmodifiable Risk Factors**
Hypertension	Age
Transient ischemic attack/prior stroke	Sex
	Ethnicity
Diabetes mellitus	Family history
Heart disease	
Hyperlipidemia	
Obesity	
Sleep apnea	
Tobacco abuse	
Alcohol abuse/illicit drug abuse	
Hypercoagulable disorder	
Sickle cell disease	

Infection

- Central nervous system (CNS) infections are not common, and immune suppression (e.g., posttransplant, human immunodeficiency virus) increases risk[4]
- Includes bacterial and viral meningitis, encephalitis, CNS parasites, and brain abscess (see Table 53.5)
- Most result from exposure to infected person, contaminated surface/object, or bite from infected animal or insect (Table 53.6)[4]
- Rapid diagnosis and treatment are essential to prevent mortality and sequelae of CNS infections
- Outcome is variable and depends on timing of diagnosis and treatment and severity of infection/inflammation[4-6] (see Tables 53.2 and 53.3).
- Infectious encephalitis is uncommon; many cases with unknown etiology[6]

Tumors

- Approximately 23,000 new brain cancer diagnoses occur yearly. Incidence is higher in industrialized countries and higher in men than women (see Table 53.1).[7]
- Risk factors include exposure to radiation or toxins or history of immunosuppression.

TABLE 53.6	Etiology of Nontraumatic Brain Injuries	
Pathology	**Etiology**

Bacterial meningitis[4,5]	• Often the result of:
	   • *Haemophilus influenzae* b
	   • *Neisseria meningitides*
	   • *Streptococcus pneumonia*
	 • Untreated, mortality rate is 20%
	 • 30%–50% risk of neurological impairments with meningitis

Viral meningitis[4,5]	• Most common cause of meningitis • Presents similarly to bacterial meningitis but less severe • Nonpolio enteroviruses are the most common cause
Encephalitis[5,6]	• Most are viral, but etiology goes undiagnosed in most • Herpes virus is the most common cause of encephalitis in the United States; other viral causes include West Nile virus (arboviruses) • Lyme disease is a common bacterial cause; rabies is a rare bacterial cause • Predilection for frontal and temporal lobes
Parasites[4]	• Typically from consuming contaminated food • Toxoplasmosis causes cystic brain lesions; infections are often subclinical/asymptomatic in immunocompetent people; predilection for the basal ganglia • Cysticercosis is another more common cystic lesion–forming parasite infection and usually results from undercooked pork; complications include seizure and hydrocephalus
Brain abscess[4]	• Etiology: spread from adjacent structure, hematogenous spread, or trauma • Affects the frontal lobes followed by temporal, parietal, cerebellar, and occipital respectively • Common organisms include *Streptococcus, Staphylococcus,* or *Enterococcus,* spp. or anaerobic bacteria

- Glial tumors (e.g., astrocytomas, glioblastomas, and oligodendrogliomas) are the most common primary brain tumor followed by meningiomas.[7]
- Metastatic lesions are more common than primary brain tumors.[8]
- Metastasis affects the cerebral hemispheres more than cerebellum and brainstem.[8]
- Prognosis is determined by tumor type and grade. Glioblastomas are the most aggressive primary brain tumor.[7,8]

TABLE 53.7 Epidemiology of Nontraumatic Brain Injuries

Disorder	Epidemiology	Pathophysiology
Cerebral vasculitis[9]	• Rare cause of stroke, headache, encephalitis, and seizure • Associated with personal or family history of inflammatory disorders • Age of occurrence: 40–60 years • Affects men more than women	• Due to immune complex deposits, direct antibody insult, or cytotoxic T lymphocyte attack on the cerebral vessels.
Multiple sclerosis[10]	• Worldwide prevalence of 2–3 million with a US prevalence of approximately 400,000 • Etiology appears to be multifactorial with hereditary and environmental factors (e.g., exposure to sun and vitamin D levels) playing a role • Epstein-Barr virus identified as a possible risk factor • Significant impairments in 30% of patients within 20–25 years disease onset • Worse prognosis occurs in men with primary progressive variant	• Demyelinating disorder of white matter • Episodic attacks occurring months to years apart and affecting different anatomical areas • Relapsing-remitting (most common) or progressive
Autoimmune encephalitis[11]	• Paraneoplastic or nonparaneoplastic association. • Small cell lung cancer is the most common associated cancer • N-methyl-D-aspartate (NMDA) receptor encephalitis is the most common nonparaneoplastic version • More common in children and younger women • Prognosis is better if nonneoplastic	• Antibody mediated attack on neural tissue commonly affecting the temporal lobes and limbic system

Autoimmune Brain Disorders

- Etiology of autoimmune brain disorders is unknown, and clinical presentation is variable (see Tables 53.1 and 53.7)
- Included in this category: cerebral vasculitis, multiple sclerosis, autoimmune encephalitis (see Table 53.6)
- Imaging studies can be negative initially, especially in autoimmune encephalitis.[9,11]
- Cerebrospinal fluid studies show pleocytosis, increased protein, oligoclonal bands; in multiple sclerosis specifically, gamma globulin may be present.
- Most have poor prognosis, but treatment can improve outcomes and delay progression.

Review Questions

1. What is the most common modifiable risk factor of ischemic stroke?
   a. Hyperlipidemia
   b. Tobacco abuse
   c. Age
   d. Hypertension
2. A 60-year-old man with history of hypertension has witnessed acute onset right-sided hemiplegia and aphasia and is taken emergently to a nearby hospital for evaluation. Systolic blood pressure upon arrival is 175 mm Hg. He is quickly taken for computed tomography (CT) head scan, and no hemorrhage is noted. Which is the next best option for management?
   a. Treatment with intravenous (IV) tissue plasminogen activator
   b. Stat brain magnetic resonance imaging (MRI)
   c. Laboratory work to assess for coagulopathies
   d. Aggressive blood pressure management
3. An otherwise healthy college student presents to urgent care with head and neck pain, fever, light sensitivity, stupor. What is the next best step in management?
   a. CT imaging
   b. MRI
   c. Lumbar puncture
   d. Intravenous antibiotics

Answers on page 401.
Access the full list of questions and answers online.
Available on ExpertConsult.com

References

1. Benjamin EJ, Blaha MJ, Chiuve SE, et al. on behalf of the American Heart Association Statistics Committee and Stroke Statistics Subcommittee. Heart disease and stroke statistics—2017 update: a report from the American Heart Association. *Circulation.* 2017; 135:e229-e445

2. Powers WJ, Rabinstein AA, Ackerson T, et al. 2018 Guidelines for the early management of patients with acute ischemic stroke: a guideline for healthcare professionals from the American Heart Association/American Stroke Association. *Stroke.* 2018;49(3): e46-e99.

3. Kernan WN, Ovbiagele B, Black HR, et al. Guidelines for the prevention of stroke in patients with stroke and transient ischemic attack: a guideline for healthcare professionals from the American Heart Association/American Stroke Association. *Stroke.* 2014; 45(7):2160-2236.

4. Sarrazin JL, Bonneville F, Martin-Blondel G. Brain infections. *Diagn Interv Imaging.* 2012;93:473-490.

5. National Institute of Neurological Disorders and Stroke. *Meningitis and Encephalitis Fact Sheet.* 2018. Available at: https://www.ninds.nih.gov/Disorders/Patient-Caregiver-Education/Fact-Sheets/Meningitis-and-Encephalitis-Fact-Sheet. Accessed January 15, 2019.

6. Tunkel AR, Glaser CA, Bloch KC, et al. The management of encephalitis: Clinical practice guidelines by the Infectious Diseases Society of America. *Clin Infect Dis.* 2009;47(3):303-327.

7. National Cancer Institute at the National Institutes of Health. *Adult Central Nervous System Tumors Treatment (PDQ®)–Health Professional Version.* 2018. Available at: https://www.cancer.gov/types/brain/hp/adult-brain-treatment-pdq. Accessed January 19, 2019.

8. Butowski NA. Epidemiology and diagnosis of brain tumors. *Continuum.* 2015;21(2, Neuro-oncology):301-313. doi:10.1212/01.CON.0000464171.50638.fa.

9. Berlit P. Diagnosis and treatment of cerebral vasculitis. *Ther Adv Neurol Disord.* 2010;3(1):29-42.

10. National Multiple Sclerosis Society. *MS Prevalence.* 2018. Available at: https://www.nationalmssociety.org/About-the-Society/MS-Prevalence. Accessed January 19, 2019.

11. Lancaster E. The diagnosis and treatment of autoimmune encephalitis. *J Clin Neurol.* 2016;12(1):1-13.

12. Colantonio A, Gerber G, Bayley M, Deber R, Yin J, Kim H. Differential profiles for patients with traumatic and non-traumatic brain injury. *J Rehabil Med.* 2011;43(4):311-315.

13. Winstein CJ, Stein J, Arena R, et al. Guidelines for adult stroke rehabilitation and recovery: a guideline for healthcare professionals from the American Heart Association/American Stroke Association. *Stroke.* 2016;47(6):e98-e169.

54

Dual Diagnosis of Traumatic Brain Injury and Spinal Cord Injury

GEMAYARET ALVAREZ, MD, AND KEVIN DALAL, MD

The dual diagnosis of traumatic spinal cord injury (SCI) and traumatic brain injury (TBI) has clinical and diagnostic features of both conditions typically stemming from a single traumatic event. These events are typically blunt traumas, in the case of assaults and falls, and rapid acceleration/deceleration injuries as would be seen in motor vehicle accidents (MVAs). These injuries and the advanced interventions required can make it challenging to identify a TBI, especially a mild one, in the early stages of functional recovery. The associated issues stemming from a dual diagnosis of SCI and TBI together present a unique challenge to the practicing physiatrist, regardless of their subfield of expertise.

Epidemiology

Risk factors for dual diagnosis include male gender and involvement of alcohol intoxication at the onset of injury. The risk of sustaining a TBI along with an SCI is also correlated with level of completeness of the SCI and a more caudal injury, with cervical SCI being more commonly associated with concomitant TBI.

Depending on the risk factors, the incidence of a dual diagnosis may approach 60% according to the SCI Model Systems. The criteria for claiming a TBI include:
- Posttraumatic amnesia
- Initial abnormal Glasgow Coma Scale (GCS) score
- Abnormal brain imaging

Although the overall rate of trauma related to MVAs has declined, the aging population and associated risk of falls has led to an overall increase in TBI-related emergency department (ED) visits. There has been increased vigilance in identifying sports-related concussions in young athletes.

The breakdown of incidence of the dual diagnosis patient are as follows:
- Mild TBI (GCS 13–15) represents 64% to 73% of dual diagnosis patients
- Moderate TBI (GCS 9–12) represents 10% to 23%
- Severe (GCS 3–8) makes up 17% to 23% of cases

This roughly mirrors the prevalence of these subsets of TBI without SCI.

Evaluation and Diagnosis

To assess and evaluate a dual diagnosis injury properly, a detailed screening of the medical records at the time of initial assessment should be performed. Of particular importance are:
- Confirmation of loss of consciousness (LOC)
- GCS
- Duration of posttraumatic amnesia (PTA)
- Behavioral issues
- Initial imaging

Comorbid factors that complicate the SCI presentation and may mask or mimic TBI include:
- Altered mental status caused by orthostasis
- Urinary tract infection stemming from neurogenic bladder
- Intensive care unit psychosis
- Psychoactive medications to treat pain, spasticity, and/or depression[1]

Confounding clinical neurological indices of TBI such as hypoxia, intoxication (alcohol/other), and intubation, all occur with some frequency with SCI and can alter LOC and GCS scores.

Negative brain imaging on initial imaging can frequently mask the presence of mild or even moderate TBI, and positive findings, especially contusions, may be missed in up to 67% of cases.[7] For up to 2 to 3 months after TBI, findings consistent with axonal shear, hemorrhages, or small contusions may be present.[7] Diffusion tensor MRI may show brain motor pathway lesions that contribute to weakness in TBI in patients with SCI.[7]

Possible symptoms of mild and moderate TBI include:
- Headaches
- Dizziness
- Insomnia
- Emotional irritability/lability
- Impaired memory
- Focal weakness
- Visual impairments
- Impaired communication

Rehabilitation

There are no current guidelines regarding the admission process for dual diagnosis patients. Historically, patients would be assigned to either an SCI or TBI unit based on which diagnosis is contributing most to the patient's functional impairment and barriers to recovery.[2] Patients with dual diagnosis are more likely to manifest behavioral issues,

exhibit psychopathology, and have more severe neuropsychological impairment than patients with SCI alone.[3] Concomitant TBI may delay one's ability to tolerate 3 hours of therapy per day and demonstrate the potential to benefit from rehabilitation interventions, thereby delaying rehabilitation admission.

The moderate to severe TBI patient can present additional challenges, including:
- Neuroendocrine dysfunction
- Salt balance
- Obstructive hydrocephalus
- Paroxysmal sympathetic hyperactivity
- Spasticity
- Heterotopic ossification
- Agitation
- Seizures
- Dysphagia
- Depression and anxiety

The management of certain comorbidities may compromise improvement in other areas, such as treating spasticity with agents that may weaken muscular strengthening.

Data from Somner and Witkiewcz on suggested strategies for the management of moderate to severe TBI and SCI are summarized in Table 54.1.[8]

Outcomes

Dual diagnosis patients have more complex factors adversely affecting the functional improvement measures (FIMs). The improvement in scores at discharge relative to

TABLE 54.1 Management of the Confused Patient

Confused/Agitated	Confused/Nonagitated Inappropriate	Confused Appropriate to Automatic Appropriate
Rancho 4	Rancho 5	Rancho 6–7
Provide private room	Therapy sessions still best in quiet area of the gym	Therapy may now focus more on spinal cord injury (SCI) rehabilitation interventions
Restraints only when necessary	Patient responds well to structure and redirection for task completion	Therapy may occur in open gym
Covering brace and feeding tube with shirt/abdominal binder	Now able to follow one- and two-step commands consistently	Orientation group, memory logbook, and signs in room helpful
Full attendant care when possible	Rest breaks and avoidance of overstimulation	Checklist and environmental cues useful in planning/initiating necessary SCI activities such as pressure relief and catheterizations
Minimize overstimulation	Full-time supervision by staff or caregivers still important	Patient should be able to verbalize why braces and treatments are necessary
Regular nursing care, including catheterizations		Paraparetic should learn to don/doff brace, dress in bed, wheelchair mobility
Maintain sleep–wake cycles		Family education
Tilt-in-space wheelchair for pressure relief		Including patient and family in support group
Minimize agitation		
Frequent reorientation by staff		
Cotreatment with one therapist		
Patient instruction should be short one-step commands		
Rest breaks		
Therapy in a quiet gym		
Aggressive and inappropriate behavior to be dealt with firmly/instantly		
Involve psychology for patient family support and therapy		

Adapted from Somner JL, Witkiewicz PM. The therapeutic challenges of dual diagnosis: TBI/SCI. *Brain Inj*. 2004;18(12):1297-1308.

admission (FIM gain) and FIM efficiency (change/unit time) are likely to be lower relative to an SCI patient without TBI, and the length of stay (LOS) may be longer because of the barriers to discharge to home.[7]

In addition, functional cognition and neuropsychological test performance was negatively affected in cases of moderate to severe TBI (Macciocci). Patients with dual diagnosis have poorer memory and problem-solving skills than those without TBI.[8]

In paraplegia, severe TBI has contributed to:
- Lower admission and discharge FIM motor scores
- Longer rehabilitation length of stay
- Lower functional comprehension
- Problem solving, memory, and speed of information processing.

Pain

The prevalence of pain after SCI ranges anywhere from 26% to 96% (Dijkers et al 2009). Studies indicate that pain is consistently denoted as one of the biggest challenges associated with both TBI and SCI. As the patient transitions from the acute inpatient course to outpatient, chronic pain issues can impede the patient's functional independence and ability to participate in rehabilitative programs.

Both the TBI and the SCI may be overlapping etiologies of central or neuropathic pain. Neuropathic pain is typically classified relative to the level of injury, specifically, above level, at level, or below level. The dermatomal level of injury is frequently a transition area where significant neuropathic pain is first noticed and frequently radiates caudally from there down the extremities.

Nociceptive pain may also be present in the forms of either musculoskeletal or visceral pain. Musculoskeletal pain typically affects the supportive connective tissue associated with the spinal column without any native damage to the associated nerves. This pain can be exacerbated by overuse and disproportionate use postinjury. Visceral pain can be linked to numerous organ-based pathologies secondary to SCI, such as renal/bladder calculi, rectal impaction, and abdominal cramping. Visceral pain can be difficult to ascertain as they are typically below level and vague in nature.

The dual diagnosis of TBI superimposes the added risk of headaches to these underlying SCI-derived pain generators. Headaches are present in 59% of brain injury patients, irrespective of the trauma severity (Nampiaparampil, 2008). These headaches resemble typical headache variants such as migraine, tension, or cluster, and may last between 1 and 4 weeks and resolve within 3 months.[13] Beyond 3 months, the pain may be considered chronic and resembles other central pain syndromes. One differentiating outcome is that posttraumatic headache patients manifest movement allodynia, which is not as prevalent in SCI. Complex regional pain syndrome (CRPS) can occur after severe TBI with a frequency comparable to poststroke CRPS (Irvine K and Clark J 2018).

Heterotopic Ossification

One of the distinctive chronic outcomes of both TBI and SCI is the development of heterotopic ossification (HO). HO develops after trauma to the CNS and leads to osteogenesis in the fascial planes. The process is considered inflammatory initially, and then bony matrix is laid down over time. In the SCI patient, the typical pattern of development is adjacent to the hip joint, whereas the TBI patient has a predilection to develop osteogenesis in the elbows followed by the hips and knees.

Typically, the patient presents with increased swelling, spasms, or pain in one or both of the affected extremities. If the process is still in the early inflammatory phase, the diagnosis can be confirmed with triple-phase bone scan. The early determination of serum creatine phosphokinase may help predict the onset and severity of HO (Banovac 2004).

The gold standard of management if the developing masses are identified during the inflammatory period is to manage with weight-adjusted antiinflammatory medications. Banovac described the dosing protocol as 20 mg/kg for the first 2 weeks followed by 10 mg/kg for the following 10 weeks.

If the HO is not identified during the inflammatory window and is evident only on x-ray, then the masses have already ossified, and antiinflammatory medication will not be effective. The patient should be followed to see how they are progressing symptomatically. If there is ankyloses of the joints or intractable pain, then surgical excision may be considered as a final option but comes with the risk of recurrence and significant bleeding perioperatively. The use of radiation therapy has a therapeutic role in preventing postoperative recurrence of HO.

Autonomic Dysfunction

Autonomic dysfunction is common after TBI and SCI and on occasion may be difficult to distinguish symptomatically. Table 54.2 describes the etiology, pathophysiology, symptoms, and management in paroxysmal sympathetic hyperactivity after TBI and autonomics dysreflexia after SCI.

Summary

The traumatic nature of spinal cord injuries can frequently mask a missed diagnosis of TBI. TBI occurring in tandem with SCI is typically mild in intensity and likelier to be associated with a cervical SCI. TBI can add physiological and cognitive barriers to self-care and care direction that impede the patient's functional progress and independence. Certain downstream outcomes are frequently seen in both the TBI and SCI patient, namely HO and chronic pain issues. A proper treatment strategy, beginning with early recognition of TBI and attention to its associated challenges, can optimize the patient's functional recovery from a traumatic injury to the nervous system.

TABLE 54.2	Autonomic Dysreflexia Versus Paroxysmal Sympathetic Hyperactivity	

Autonomic Dysreflexia	Paroxysmal Sympathetic Hyperactivity
Etiology: Spinal cord injury (SCI) at the thoracic level T6 and above	**Etiology:** Traumatic brain injury (TBI), hypoxic/anoxic injury, subarachnoid hemorrhage, stroke, encephalitis, thalamic lesion, vasculitis, postpartum vasoconstriction, cerebral fat embolism
Pathophysiology: Results from noxious stimuli, which in turn trigger sympathetic hyperactivity	**Pathophysiology (theory):** Absence of central inhibitory pathway mechanism on regulation of afferent information, which causes increased stimulation of the sympathetic nervous system
Symptoms: Sudden increase in blood pressure Bradycardia along with tachycardia (caused by opposed vagal stimulation) Pounding headaches Flushing of the skin above the level of the SCI Piloerection Nasal congestion Blurred vision Sweating above the level of SCI	**Symptoms:** Tachycardia Elevated blood pressure Respiratory rate Elevated temperature Posturing
Treatment: Sit patient up Remove noxious stimuli (fecal impaction, bladder distention) Treat hypertension (e.g., nitrates, hydralazine)	**Treatment (challenging to manage):** Environmental management: (e.g., remove indwelling catheters, suctioning, constipation, remove C collars when possible) **Medications (anecdotal):** Bromocriptine - fever dystonia Propranolol - decreases hypertension and heart rate, decrease catecholamines Gabapentin - control autonomic symptoms Intrathecal baclofen: effective but invasive

Review Questions

1. Brain computed tomography (CT) for closed head injury will demonstrate
   a. positive axonal injury.
   b. CT of the brain is the only diagnostic tool for traumatic brain injury (TBI).
   c. CT of the brain can be negative for injury.
   d. magnetic resonance imaging (MRI) will reveal abnormalities only in the first week of injury.

2. What common risk factor has been involved in TBI and spinal cord injury (SCI) at initial injury?
   a. Smoking
   b. Hypertension
   c. Alcohol intoxication
   d. Marijuana use

3. In mild TBI, the strongest diagnostic tool is
   a. conventional CT.
   b. neuropsychological assessment.
   c. MRI.
   d. clinical neurological indices (Glasgow Coma Scale [GCS], posttraumatic amnesia [PTA], loss of consciousness [LOC]).

Answers on page 402.

Access the full list of questions and answers online.
Available on ExpertConsult.com

References

1. Budisin B, Bradbury CC, Sharma B, et al. Traumatic brain injury in spinal cord injury: frequency and risk factors. *J Head Trauma Rehabil.* 2016;31(4):E33-E42

2. Inoue T, Lin A, Ma X, et al. Combined SCI and TBI: recovery of forelimb function after unilateral cervical spinal cord injury (SCI) is retarded by contralateral traumatic brain injury (TBI), and ipsilateral TBI balances the effects of SCI on paw placement. *Exp Neurol.* 2013;248:136-147.

3. Bradbury CL, Wodchis WP, Mikulis DJ, et al. Traumatic brain injury in patients with traumatic spinal cord injury: clinical and economic consequences. *Arch Phys Med Rehabil.* 2008;89: S77-S84.

4. Macciocci S, Seel RT, Thompson N, Byams R, Bowman B. Spinal cord injury and co-occuring traumatic brain injury: assessment and incidence. *Arch Phys Med Rehabil.* 2008;89:1350-1357.

5. Hagen EM, Eide GE, Rekand T, Gilhus NE, Gronning M. Traumatic spinal cord injury and concomitant brain injury: a cohort study. *Acta Neurol Scand Suppl.* 2010;122 (Suppl. 190): 51–57.

6. Bombardier CH, Lee DC, Tan DL, Barber JK, Hoffman JM. HYPERLINK "https://www.ncbi.nlm.nih.gov/pubmed/27084266"

Comorbid Traumatic Brain Injury and Spinal Cord Injury: Screening Validity and Effect on Outcomes.Arch Phys Med Rehabil. 2016 Oct;97(10):1628-34. doi: 10.1016/j.apmr.2016.03.008. Epub 2016 Apr 12.

7. Kushner DS, Alvarez G. Dual diagnosis: traumatic brain injury with spinal cord injury. *Phys Med Rehabil Clin North Am.* 2014; 25(3):681-696, ix-x. doi:10.1016/j.pmr.2014.04.005.

8. Jacqueline L. Sommer & Patti M. Witkiewicz (2004) The therapeutic challenges of dual diagnosis: TBI/SCI, *Brain Injury,* 18:12, 1297-1308

9. Irvine K, Clark J. Chronic pain after tbi: pathophysiology and pain mechanism. *Pain Med.* 2018;19(7):1315-1333

10. Banovac K, Sherman AL, Estores IM, Banovac F. Prevention and treatment of heterotopic ossification after spinal cord injury. *J Spinal Cord Med.* 2004;27(4):376-382.

11. Dijkers M, Bryce T, Zanca J. Prevalence of chronic pain after traumatic spinal cord injury: a systematic review. *J Rehabil Res Dev.* 2009;46:13-29.

12. Nampiaparampil DE. Prevalence of chronic pain after traumatic brain injury. *JAMA.* 2008;300:711-719.

13. Ofek H, Defrin R HYPERLINK "https://www.ncbi.nlm.nih.gov/pubmed/17689190" The characteristics of chronic central pain after traumatic brain injury.Pain. 2007 Oct;131(3):330-40. Epub 2007 Aug 6.

55

Anoxic Brain Injury

MONICA VERDUZCO-GUTIERREZ, MD, AND SIMA A. DESAI, MD

Anoxia is defined by the total absence of oxygen to the tissues or a particular organ such as the brain. The term *anoxic brain injury* (ABI) is frequently used synonymously in the literature with terms *hypoxic-ischemic, anoxic-ischemic, hypoxic,* or *cerebral anoxia.*

One of the earliest documented cases of ABI was in 1945 with eight cases of poisoning from nitrous oxide anesthesia that resulted in persistent deficits in judgment, attention, and memory; loss of insight; apathy; indifference, and restlessness.[1]

Etiology

The etiology of ABI can be related to any event that deprives the brain of sufficient oxygenation. In addition to cardiac arrest and respiratory failure, a variety of disorders such as carbon monoxide poisoning, asphyxiation because of hanging, near drowning, obstructive sleep apnea, complications from anesthesia, metabolic conditions, and pulmonary disease can be attributable causes.[2]

Epidemiology

The majority of data for ABIs are in the setting of cardiac arrest. The majority of cardiac arrest events occur outside of the hospital in a private residence. The incidence of emergency medical services (EMS)-assessed cardiac arrest in the adult population is 347,322 per year, based on the most recent data by the American Heart Association (AHA).[3]

Survival with good functional outcomes was present for a majority of these patients, as defined by independence with activities of daily living (ADLs) with possible residual deficits of hemiplegia, seizures, or memory impairment. There are also large regional variations in survival to hospital discharge and survival with functional recovery.[4] However, as many as 18% of out of hospital cardiac arrest survivors have moderate to severe functional deficits at discharge. But, survival rates to hospital discharge after EMS-treated cardiac arrest increased from 10.2% in 2006 to 12.4% in 2015.[3]

Pathophysiology

There are two primary mechanisms of injury with ABI: primary and secondary. During the primary injury, there is first ischemia and then subsequent reperfusion. During the process of the brain ischemia, there is anoxic depolarization, adenosine triphosphate (ATP) depletion, glutamate release, free radical formation, and nitric oxide production.[5] The primary injury causes considerable neuronal damage, but the successive reperfusion accounts for substantial cerebral ischemia and cell death.[6] Despite the return of spontaneous circulation during cardiac arrest, there is a brief period of hyperemia that is quickly replaced by a longer period of global and multifocal hypoperfusion known as the *no reflow phenomenon.*[5]

Secondary injury occurs immediately after return of spontaneous circulation and is the result of the additive cerebral injury caused by an imbalance of postresuscitation cerebral oxygen delivery.[6] Secondary injury consists of ongoing ischemia, autoregulatory failure, cerebral hypoperfusion, blood-brain barrier breakdown, seizures, oxidative injury, and hyperpyrexia.[7]

There are specific areas of the brain that are more vulnerable to damage than others: the hippocampus (CA1 pyramidal neurons); Purkinje cells of the cerebellum; pyramidal neurons in layers three, five,and six of the neocortex; reticular neurons of the thalamus; neurons of the striatum; and vascular border zone areas.[5]

Examination and Prognosis

Initial evaluations begin with a thorough history regarding the onset of the injury, mechanism, duration of ischemia to reperfusion; medical history; family history; social history including illicit, prescription, and over the counter drug use; prior psychiatric history; functional history; educational history; and social support.

The clinical manifestations of ABIs are varied and complex. Neurologists are often asked to evaluate patients after cardiopulmonary resuscitation and to help provide prognostication. The clinical examination is focused on brainstem reflexes, the presence of generalized myoclonus, and motor responses to noxious stimuli.[8] Additionally, it is important to assess for range of motion, skin breakdown, and muscle tone. In the acute care setting, physicians and families are interested in long term prognostication so that goals of care discussions can be established early.

There are many studies that summarize factors that are associated with poor outcomes. However, each study defines poor outcomes differently (Table 55-1).

In conscious patients, it is important to also assess for cognitive impairments. These cognitive impairments include:

- Attention
- Processing speed
- Memory impairments
- Executive dysfunction
- Language impairments
- Calculation impairments
- Apraxia
- Agnosia
- Visuospatial impairments
- Balint syndrome: simultagnosia, optic ataxia, ocular apraxia
- Anton syndrome: anosognosia for visual impairment
- Alterations in personality and behavior
- Affective dysregulation

Additionally, one should also assess for neurological impairments such as motor deficits, parkinsonism, dystonia, chorea, tremor, tics, athetosis, seizures, and myoclonic syndromes.[9]

Clinical sequelae also include:

- Man-in-a-barrel syndrome: bilateral proximal upper limb paresis with preservation of lower limb function caused by injury between the anterior cerebral artery and middle cerebral artery watershed zone
- Paraparesis and quadriparesis in the upper and lower thoracic and lumbar regions of the spinal cord
- Cortical blindness and Balint syndrome are examples of disorders of sensory function
- Akinetic-rigid syndrome
- Amnestic syndrome caused by hippocampal damage
- Lance-Adams syndrome: significant action myoclonus associated with ataxia[8,9]

Further evaluation by electroencephalogram (EEG) and somatosensory evoked potentials (SSEP) can also help with prognostication. Biochemical markers are also being used for prognosticating outcomes such as serum neuron-specific enolase (NSE) and serum S100.[10,11]

Treatment

The acute period of ischemia is treated with high-quality cardiopulmonary resuscitation (CPR) with the goal of return of spontaneous circulation (ROSC). However, once ROSC has been achieved, it is imperative for postcardiac arrest care to help mitigate the subsequent ischemia-reperfusion injury to multiple organ systems.

The 2015 updated guidelines on postcardiac arrest care by the AHA identify and note several points:

- Identify acute ST elevation, and if present perform urgent coronary angiography with prompt recanalization of any infarct-related artery.
- Avoid and immediately correct hypotension (systolic blood pressure less than 90 mm Hg, mean arterial pressure less than 65 mm Hg).
- Targeted temperature management (TTM) for comatose adults is between 32° and 36°C for at least 24 hours.
- Actively prevent fever in comatose patient after TTM.
- EEG for diagnosis of seizure should monitored frequently or continuously in a comatose patient after ROSC.
- Maintain normocarbia levels and avoiding hypoxia.
- The target range for glucose control remains uncertain.[13]

However, the 2017 guidelines from the American Academy of Neurology (AAN) found level A evidence for the use of TTM for patients with either pulseless ventricular tachycardia or ventricular fibrillation after an out-of-hospital cardiac arrest, to be 32° to 34°C for 24 hours.[14]

Rehabilitation-Specific Treatment

Traumatic brain injury (TBI) and ABI rehabilitation outcomes in a retrospective study found similar functional independent measurement (FIM) scores on discharge between the two groups.[15] However, older studies have shown the ABI group to have a higher discharge rate than skilled nursing facilities compared with TBI and slower recoveries.[16-18]

Physiatrists are an essential part of the post-ABI team and are frequently consulted in the intensive care unit setting to determine the medical and physical readiness for inpatient rehabilitation.

Patients can present with disorders of consciousness (DOC), but other presentations can include cognitive deficits, behavioral changes, affective changes, visual difficulties, movement disorders, spasticity, and alterations in gait. Physiatrists can help differentiate DOC patients with metrics such as the JFK Coma Recovery Scale-Revised (CRS-R) and Individual Quantitative Behavioral Assessment (IQBA) with the help of an interdisciplinary team. Initially, pharmacologic interventions are focused on arousal and increasing participation.[19] However, as the patient progresses, the pharmacological interventions also include treatment for agitation, attention, processing speed, memory deficits, sleep disturbances, depression, headaches, and spasticity.

Spasticity is defined as velocity-dependent increases in muscle tone resulting in resistance to muscle stretch. It is a part of the upper motor neuron syndrome. Determining

TABLE 55.1	Factors Associated with Poor Outcome	
Symptom	**Time Frame**
Anoxia duration	>8–10 min
Duration of cardiopulmonary resuscitation	>30 min
Myoclonic status epilepticus	Day 1
Absent pupillary or corneal reflexes	Days 1–3
Serum neuron-specific enolase (NSE) >33 µg/L	Days 1–3 for nontherapeutic hypothermia patients
Absent N20 responses on somatosensory evoked potentials (SSEP) bilaterally	Days 1–3
Motor response extensor or none	Day 3 for nontherapeutic hypothermia patients; possibly longer for therapeutic hypothermia patients
Electroencephalogram (EEG) with nonreactive background	
EEG with burst suppression and generalized epileptiform activity	
Loss of gray-white matter differentiation on head computed tomography	
Widespread cortical restricted diffusion on brain magnetic resonance imaging	

Data from Fugate, JE, Wijdicks, EFM. Anoxic-Ischemic Encephalopathy. In: Flemming KD, Jones LK, eds *Mayo Clinic Neurology Board Review: Clinical Neurology for Initial Certification and MOC*. New York: Oxford University Press; 2015. p. 35–8; Wijdicks EFM, Hijdra A, Young GB, Bassetti CL, Wiebe S. Practice Parameter: Prediction of outcome in comatose survivors after cardiopulmonary resuscitation (an evidence-based review): Report of the Quality Standards Subcommittee of the American Academy of Neurology. *Neurology*. 2006 Jul 25;67(2):203–10; Bouwes A, Binnekade JM, Kuiper MA, Bosch FH, Zandstra DF, Toornvliet AC, et al. Prognosis of coma after therapeutic hypothermia: A prospective cohort study. *Ann Neurol*. 2012 Feb;71(2):206–12.

when to treat spasticity requires knowledge of not only the advantages and disadvantages of treatment options but also defining and integrating goals of care from the patient, family members, and caretakers.

The treatment of spasticity helps with ambulation, transfers, muscle bulk maintenance, deep vein thrombosis prevention, improved range of motion, improved hygiene, and osteoporosis prevention.[20]

There are conventional oral agents such as baclofen, tizanidine, dantrolene, diazepam, and clonazepam. However, there is limited evidence as to the effect they have on ABI patients. Additionally, the side effects of sedation frequently limit patients from reaching a therapeutic dose. Focal treatment can include the use of injectable intramuscular chemodenervation agents such as botulinum toxin, phenol, and alcohol. Injectable therapies are unique in that specific muscles can be targeted to help with function; whereas others can be left alone if the patient is using their spasticity functionally.[21] However, when more diffuse spasticity is present, intrathecal baclofen pump therapy should be considered. Careful consideration of patient selection must be done as patients require regular medication refills and pump maintenance. Two small studies have been shown to be effective in decreasing spasticity objectively in the severe TBI population.[22,23]

Review Questions

1. Which of these indicates a poor prognostic outcome for anoxic brain injury (ABI) patients?
   a. Anoxic duration is greater than 5 minutes
   b. Cardiopulmonary resuscitation (CPR) duration is greater than 20 minutes
   c. Myoclonic status epilepticus
   d. Electroencephalogram (EEG) with spindle pattern
2. Which pattern on an EEG indicates a better prognostic outcome for ABI patients?
   a. Burst suppression
   b. Nonreactive background
   c. Low amplitude delta activity
   d. Spindle activity

3. What type of lesion results in bilateral upper extremity paresis with preserved lower extremity function?
   a. Infarction between the anterior cerebral artery (ACA) and middle cerebral artery (MCA)
   b. Infarction between the ACA and internal carotid artery
   c. Infarction between the MCA and posterior cerebral artery (PCA)
   d. Infarction between PCA and basilar artery

Answers on page 402.
Access the full list of questions and answers online.
Available on ExpertConsult.com

References

1. Fletcher DE. Personality disintegration incident to anoxia: observations with nitrous oxide anesthesia. *J Nerv Ment Dis.* 1945;102(4):392-403.

2. Hopkins RO, Haaland KY. Neuropsychological and neuropathological effects of anoxic or ischemic induced brain injury. *J Int Neuropsychol Soc.* 2004;10(7):957-961.

3. Benjamin EJ, Virani SS, Chair CV, et al. A report from the American Heart Association. *Circulation.* 2018;137(12):e67-e492.

4. 2017 Cardiac Arrest Registry to Enhance Survival (CARES). Center for Disease Control and Prevention. Available at: https://mycares.net/sitepages/uploads/2018/2017flipbook/index.html?page=26.

5. Busl KM, Greer DM. Hypoxic-ischemic brain injury: Pathophysiology, neuropathology and mechanisms. *Neurorehabilitation.* 2010;26(1):5-13.

6. Sekhon MS, Ainslie PN, Griesdale DE. Clinical pathophysiology of hypoxic ischemic brain injury after cardiac arrest: a "two-hit" model. *Crit Care.* 2017 Dec [cited 2018 Nov 11];21(1). Available at: http://ccforum.biomedcentral.com/articles/10.1186/s13054-017-1670-9.

7. Elmer J, Callaway C. The brain after cardiac arrest. *Semin Neurol.* 2017;37(1):19-24.

8. Fugate, JE, Wijdicks, EFM. Anoxic-Ischemic Encephalopathy. In: Flemming KD, Jones LK, eds. *Mayo Clinic Neurology Board Review: Clinical Neurology for Initial Certification and MOC.* New York: Oxford University Press; 2015:35-38.

9. Anderson CA, Arciniegas DB. Cognitive sequelae of hypoxic-ischemic brain injury: A review. *Neurorehabilitation.* 2010;26:47-63.

10. Wijdicks EFM, Hijdra A, Young GB, Bassetti CL, Wiebe S. Practice parameter: prediction of outcome in comatose survivors after cardiopulmonary resuscitation (an evidence-based review): Report of the Quality Standards Subcommittee of the American Academy of Neurology. *Neurology.* 2006;67(2):203-210.

11. Zandbergen EG, de Haan RJ, Stoutenbeek CP, Koelman JH, Hijdra A. Systematic review of early prediction of poor outcome in anoxic-ischaemic coma. *Lancet.* 1998;352(9143):1808-1812.

12. Bouwes A, Binnekade JM, Kuiper MA, et al. Prognosis of coma after therapeutic hypothermia: A prospective cohort study. *Ann Neurol.* 2012;71(2):206-212.

13. Callaway CW, Donnino MW, Fink EL, et al. Part 8: Post–cardiac arrest care: 2015 American Heart Association Guidelines Update for cardiopulmonary resuscitation and emergency cardiovascular care. *Circulation.* 2015;132(18 suppl 2):S465-S482.

14. Geocadin RG, Wijdicks E, Armstrong MJ, et al. Practice guideline summary: reducing brain injury following cardiopulmonary resuscitation: report of the guideline development, dissemination, and implementation subcommittee of the American Academy of Neurology. *Neurology.* 2017;88(22):2141-2149.

15. Adigüzel E, Yaşar E, Kesikburun S, et al. Are rehabilitation outcomes after severe anoxic brain injury different from severe traumatic brain injury? A matched case-control study. *Int J Rehabil Res.* 2018;41(1):47-51.

16. Shah MK, Al-Adawi S, Dorvlo ASS, Burke DT. Functional outcomes following anoxic brain injury: a comparison with traumatic brain injury. *Brain Inj.* 2004;18(2):111-117.

17. FitzGerald A, Aditya H, Prior A, McNeill E, Pentland B. Anoxic brain injury: clinical patterns and functional outcomes. A study of 93 cases. *Brain Inj.* 2010;24(11):1311-1323.

18. Cullen NK, Crescini C, Bayley MT. Rehabilitation outcomes after anoxic brain injury: a case-controlled comparison with traumatic brain injury. *PM&R.* 2009;1(12):1069-1076.

19. Sawyer KN, Callaway CW, Wagner AK. Life after death: surviving cardiac arrest—an overview of epidemiology, best acute care practices, and considerations for rehabilitation care. *Curr Phys Med Rehabil Rep.* 2017;5(1):30-39.

20. Schultz BA, Bellamkonda E. Management of medical complications during the rehabilitation of moderate-severe traumatic brain injury. *Phys Med Rehabil Clin North Am.* 2017;28(2):259-270.

21. Bhatnagar S, Iaccarino MA, Zafonte R. Pharmacotherapy in rehabilitation of post-acute traumatic brain injury. *Brain Res.* 2016;1640:164-179.

22. Francisco GE, Hu MM, Boake C, Ivanhoe CB. Efficacy of early use of intrathecal baclofen therapy for treating spastic hypertonia due to acquired brain injury. *Brain Inj.* 2005;19(5):359-364.

23. Al-Khodairy AT, Wicky G, Nicolo D, Vuadens P. Influence of intrathecal baclofen on the level of consciousness and mental functions after extremely severe traumatic brain injury: brief report. *Brain Inj.* 2015;29(4):527-532.

56

Disorders of Consciousness

MATTHEW LIN, MD, AND SUNIL KOTHARI, MD

OUTLINE

Nomenclature and Taxonomy

- The three main disorders of consciousness (DoC) are *coma*, the *vegetative state* (VS), and the *minimally conscious state* (MCS).
- It is important to distinguish between arousal and awareness. *Arousal* refers only to the overall level of wakefulness. By itself, wakefulness is not sufficient for consciousness.
- For someone to be conscious, awareness must be present. For clinical purposes, consciousness is defined as the state of awareness of oneself and/or the environment.
- Differing degrees of arousal and awareness distinguish the three DoC from each other (Table 56.1).

TABLE 56.1 Arousal and Awareness in Disorders of Consciousness[3]

	Arousal	Awareness
Coma	-	-
Vegetative state	+/++	-
MCS	+/++	+
Emerged from MCS	++	++

MCS, Minimally conscious state.

- The clinical features of the three disorders of consciousness (coma, VS, MCS) are summarized in Box 56.1.
- Coma is a self-limited state that rarely lasts more than 4 weeks, after which patients will have either died or progressed into at least the VS. The end of coma is heralded by eye opening and the return of sleep-wake cycles.
- Both VS and MCS can last indefinitely. However, the use of temporal adjectives such as *persistent* or *permanent* is now discouraged; instead, the term *chronic* has been recommended as an alternative.[1] In addition, the length of time that a patient has remained in a particular state should be specified (e.g., "in a VS for 10 months").
- Because of the negative connotations of the term *vegetative state,* alternatives have been proposed. Of these alternatives, the most widely used is *unresponsive wakefulness syndrome* (UWS).[1]
- Emergence from MCS occurs when the patient demonstrates evidence of functional communication and/or functional object use. Functional communication is demonstrated when the patient can provide accurate yes/no responses to basic questions. Functional object use is demonstrated when the patient can demonstrate knowledge of the appropriate use of common objects.

> ### • BOX 56.1 Disorders of Consciousness[3]
>
> **Unconscious Conditions**
>
> **Coma**: Complete loss of spontaneous and stimulus-induced arousal; lack of eye opening
> **Vegetative state (VS)**: Return of basic arousal; state of wakeful unawareness
>
> **Conscious Conditions**
>
> **Minimally conscious state (MCS)**: Return of awareness; but awareness may be minimal in degree and inconsistent in manifestation
> **MCS minus**: Presence of nonlinguistically mediated behavior only (e.g., nonreflexive movement, visual pursuit, etc.)
> **MCS plus**: Presence of linguistically mediated behavior (e.g., command following, verbalization, communication)
> **Emerged from MCS**: Return of functional object use and/or functional communication

Epidemiology

- There are an estimated 35,000 people in the United States in the VS and 280,000 in the MCS,[2] but it is likely that these figures underestimate the true prevalence of DoC.[3]

Neural Substrate of Consciousness

- Consciousness is not localized to any single area of the brain but seems to be subserved by large-scale, integrated corticothalamic networks. Patients with higher levels of consciousness demonstrate more widespread activation and a greater degree of integration of these networks.[4]
- One proposed hypothetical model of the consciousness network is the "mesocircuit model."[5]

Approach to Diagnosis

- The general approach to determining a patient's level of consciousness is to use behavioral (and, in the future, nonbehavioral) assessments to detect the presence of awareness of self and/or environment.
- Behaviors that can indicate the presence of consciousness are summarized in Table 56.2.
- Because behaviors that indicate consciousness can be subtle and inconsistent, they can often be missed.
- Numerous studies have documented widespread underestimation of consciousness in these patients. One study found that over 40% of patients diagnosed as being in a VS based on qualitative bedside evaluations were actually conscious when assessed with a standardized behavioral measure. In addition, 10% of patients diagnosed as MCS in this study had actually emerged.[6]

- Factors contributing to misdiagnosis of DoC include the lack of use of standardized assessment tools to supplement bedside examinations, performing a limited number of evaluations (which may miss subtle and inconsistent evidence of awareness), and lack of knowledge about DoC among clinicians. Other factors contributing to misdiagnosis include motor, sensory, or cognitive impairments that confound assessment and reversible factors that impair consciousness, such as sedating medications or concurrent medical problems.
- Before initiating and/or interpreting the results of clinical assessments, the clinician should screen for conditions that can mimic or overlap with a DoC. These include locked-in syndrome, akinetic mutism, and catatonia. In each of these conditions, patients may appear to have a DoC when, in fact, their awareness is likely intact.
- In addition, there should be an evaluation of deficits that can confound the assessment of consciousness[1] (Box 56.2). The presence of these deficits can result in an underestimation of the level (or even presence) of consciousness.
- Finally, reversible causes of impaired consciousness should be identified and addressed before proceeding with and/or interpreting the results of behavioral assessments of consciousness[1] (Box 56.3).

Clinical Assessment

- The current gold standard for evaluation of DoC patients is behavioral assessment, which should include both qualitative assessments (e.g., bedside evaluations)

TABLE 56.2	Behaviors that Distinguish the Vegetative from Minimally Conscious States[3]	
	VS	MCS
Response to pain	Posturing	Localization
Movement	Reflexive/ patterned/ involuntary	Nonreflexive
Visual	Startle	Fixation/pursuit
Affective	Random	Contingent
Vocal	Noncontingent vocalization	Intelligible verbalization
Response to commands	–	Inconsistent
Communication	–	Unreliable yes/no[a]
Object use	–	Object manipulation[a]

[a]Functional communication and/or functional object use indicate emergence from the minimally conscious state.
MCS, Minimally conscious state; VS, vegetative state
Adapted from Eapen, Rehabilitation After Traumatic Brain Injury, 1e. Elsevier; 2019. Table 14.2, p. 193.

• BOX 56.2 Deficits that can Confound the Assessment of Consciousness[3]

- Widespread paresis or paralysis (e.g., critical illness polyneuropathy/myopathy)
- Bilateral cranial nerve III palsies
- Profound primary sensory deficits (e.g., blindness, deafness)
- Higher-order sensory, motor, or cognitive deficits (e.g., aphasia, apraxia, etc.)

• BOX 56.3 Potentially Reversible Causes of Impaired Consciousness[3]

- Understimulation/undermobilization
- Disrupted sleep-wake cycles
- Sedating medications
- Concurrent medical conditions (e.g., infection, hypoxemia, metabolic abnormalities)
- Neuroendocrine abnormalities
- Intracranial abnormalities (e.g., hydrocephalus, large subdural hygromas)
- Seizures (e.g., nonconvulsive status epilepticus)

and more structured assessments, such as standardized scales.

- Because behavioral evidence of consciousness is subtle and inconsistent, the approach to assessment should involve:
  - Multiple evaluations over time[1]
  - Different modes of assessment
  - Assessment by multiple examiners
  - Optimal environmental conditions (including optimal patient arousal)[1]
  - Assessment at various times of day
- For ambiguous or subtle behaviors observed during the bedside qualitative assessment, the likelihood that the behavior suggests consciousness is directly related to the complexity and frequency of the behavior, especially if the behaviors are appropriately related to environmental stimuli.
- Qualitative bedside assessments should be supplemented by standardized rating scales.[1] The Coma Recovery Scale-Revised (CRS-R)[7] is currently the most widely used scale in the United States. It is a 23-item scale composed of six subscales assessing auditory, visual, motor, oromotor/verbal, communication, and arousal functions. The total score can range from 0 to 23.
- Each subscale has a threshold score that implies consciousness. The patient only needs to score as "conscious" on one subscale to be considered conscious based on CRS-R.
- The criteria for emergence from MCS—that is, functional object use and functional communication—are also operationalized by the CRS-R.
- The use of the CRS-R may be supplemented by an individualized quantitative behavioral assessment (IQBA).[8] The IQBA uses a single-subject experimental design to assist in answering specific questions about residual cognitive or behavioral capacities. It is especially useful if the behavioral responses are infrequent or ambiguous.
- The assessment process should also include observations from family members. They are often able to provide observations about behaviors that occur when the clinical team is not present. Additionally, DoC patients have been found to react more frequently to the voice of a family member than to a treating clinician,[9] and CRS-R scores are often higher when family members actively participate in the administration of the measure.[10] Although there is a concern that family members may overinterpret the patient's behaviors, there is evidence that families' beliefs about the patient's level of consciousness matched the diagnostic assessment of the clinical team 76% of the time.[11]

Ancillary Diagnostic Modalities

- Although the behavioral assessments described in the previous section currently form the foundation for the assessment of consciousness, new technologies are likely to play an increasing role in the evaluation of these patients. In particular, the use of both electrophysiological measures (e.g., event-related potentials, specialized electroencephalogram measures) and functional neuroimaging (e.g., functional magnetic resonance imaging [fMRI]) have been recommended in select circumstances.[1]
- The rationale behind the use of these modalities is the growing recognition that even the most comprehensive behavioral assessment may underestimate (or completely miss) the presence of consciousness in a subset of patients.[12] Patients whose awareness can only be detected through electrophysiological measures or functional neuroimaging have been characterized as possessing *covert consciousness.*
- One metaanalysis estimated that at least 15% of patients thought to be in a VS after behavioral assessments are in fact able to follow commands by modifying their brain activity.[13]

Treatment

- The medical and neurological issues faced by patients with DoC overlap with those faced by other patients with significant traumatic brain injury but are often more severe in their manifestations. Patients with a DoC in rehabilitation settings have been found to have a high burden of medical complications and higher rates of transfers to the acute care setting.[14] Common complications include infections, paroxysmal sympathetic hyperactivity, hydrocephalus, metabolic disturbances, and seizures. The rate of new complications seems to diminish as a function of time in an inpatient rehabilitation program and not as a function of time since injury, suggesting that the close monitoring and management in rehabilitation units can reduce the rate of these complications.[1,14]
- Particular attention should be paid to medical and neurological conditions that can impair consciousness (Box 56.3).
- Neuromuscular issues such as weakness, spasticity, and contractures are also more severe in the DoC population. In the DoC patient, these issues have the added significance of limiting motor output, potentially confounding the assessment of the level of consciousness. Frequent use of nerve blocks, chemodenervation, intrathecal baclofen, and orthopedic tendon lengthening is warranted. Clinicians should also routinely screen patients for other neuromusculoskeletal conditions such as occult fractures, heterotopic ossification, peripheral nerve injuries, and the presence of critical illness polyneuropathy/myopathy.
- It is especially important to monitor for and address pain in these patients.[1] Patients with a DoC are at high risk for painful conditions from neuromusculoskeletal issues, skin breakdown, constipation, instrumentation, etc. Functional neuroimaging studies show that patients in MCS are capable of feeling pain.[15] It is currently not thought that patients in a VS are capable of feeling pain, but the high rate of misdiagnosis of VS and the phenomenon of covert awareness would suggest

that adequate analgesic control be the goal for all patients, regardless of the presumed level of consciousness.
- Treatments that aim to enhance the level of consciousness include both medical and nonmedical interventions, especially pharmacological agents.
- Likely to be helpful are standard rehabilitation interventions such as environmental enrichment (increased sensory stimulation and more frequent interpersonal interaction) and aggressive mobilization (including standing programs and body weight–supported gait activities).
- Of the medications available, neurostimulants targeting catecholaminergic pathways are most often used. Of these, amantadine has the strongest evidence base supporting its use, primarily because of a clinical trial that found benefit in posttraumatic DoC.[1,16] Other agents in this category (e.g., methylphenidate, amphetamines, modafinil, and bromocriptine) are reasonable options, although evidence for their benefit in DoC is limited and inconsistent.
- In addition to stimulants, GABA agonists have shown efficacy in a subset of patients with a DoC. In particular, zolpidem has been shown in one trial to improve the complexity and consistency of behavioral responses in approximately 5% of patients.[17] Although the response rate seems to be low, it is reasonable to consider a trial of zolpidem for all patients with a DoC (unless contraindicated) given the relatively low risks associated with its use.
- Other medications such as selective serotonin receptor inhibitors (SSRIs), lamotrigine, and donepezil may have a role, but there is not enough evidence to make specific recommendations.
- In addition to medications, there is growing evidence that certain forms of electrical stimulation may be efficacious in this setting, although none of these modalities are currently in routine clinical use. These modalities include deep brain stimulation (DBS), transcranial direct current stimulation (tDCS), and repetitive transcranial magnetic stimulation (rTMS).
- Most of the care described ideally is delivered in programs that specialize in the care of patients with DoC. National practice guidelines state that clinicians *should* refer patients with DoC to such programs.[1] Sample goals of a DoC program are described in Box 56.4.

• BOX 56.4 Goals of a Disorders of Consciousness Rehabilitation Program[3]

- Assess current level of consciousness.
- Address reversible causes of impaired consciousness.
- Initiate interventions to enhance consciousness.
- Establish a system of communication.
- Identify and magnify residual voluntary movement.
- Address restrictions in range of motion.
- Intensive mobilization and environmental enrichment.
- Prevent and manage secondary medical complications.
- Optimize respiration/nutrition/elimination/integument.
- Provide family education/training/support.
- Establish a plan for aftercare.

Prognosis and Outcomes

- Our ability to prognosticate outcomes for DoC in individual cases is still limited. However, several clinical rules of thumb can be helpful[3]:
  - Patients with traumatic DoC have a significantly better prognosis than those with nontraumatic, especially anoxic, DoC.
  - At any given point in time, patients in MCS have a better prognosis than patients in VS.
  - Rate of recovery is positively correlated with outcome.
- With regard to mortality, patients with traumatic DoC admitted to inpatient rehabilitation were seven times more likely to die than matched individuals in the general population, with a reduction in life expectancy of 12 years.[18] Cardiorespiratory issues were the most common cause of death, with pneumonia being the most common diagnosis associated with death. Mortality rates were higher for older patients and for those with more severe DoC.[18] Studies of patients with a chronic DoC have also found high mortality rates.[19,20]
- Most studies of outcome in VS have focused on the rate of recovery of consciousness. Although the most comprehensive review of this topic is now several decades old,[21] the general thrust of the findings is still relevant, even if the actual percentages reported are not likely to reflect current reality (Table 56.3). In summary: Patients with traumatic VS are more likely to recover consciousness than those with nontraumatic VS, and the longer one remains in VS, the less likely one is to recover consciousness.
- Since this study (see Table 56.3), there have been multiple reports of late recovery of consciousness, indicating that, although rare, it is possible.[1] Still, national practice guidelines suggest that the VS can be described as *chronic* 12 months after traumatic injury and 3 months after nontraumatic injury. In these cases, families should be counseled as to the likelihood of permanent severe disability.[1]
- The prognosis for MCS is much better than that of VS. One study found that for patients in a posttraumatic MCS, the likelihood of a favorable outcome was 38% compared with 2% for those in a posttraumatic VS.[22] In particular, MCS diagnosed within 5 months of onset of traumatic injury is associated with better outcomes.[1]
- Several studies have examined the outcomes of patients admitted to inpatient rehabilitation with posttraumatic

TABLE 56.3 Percentage of Patients in Vegetative State Recovering Consciousness at 1 Year

	VS at 1 Month	VS at 3 Months	VS at 6 Months
Traumatic injury	52%	35%	16%
Nontraumatic injury	15%	7%	0%

VS, Vegetative state.
Adapted from data presented in Reference 21.

DoC (including both VS and MCS) within approximately 30 days after injury.[23-25] One found that, at 1 year, almost 50% had achieved daytime independence in the home and 22% had returned to work or school.[23] Other studies have replicated these findings.[24,25] Most of the patients in these studies had emerged from a DoC during their stay in inpatient rehabilitation. However, one study investigated 2-year outcomes in patients who remained in a DoC at the time of discharge from inpatient rehabilitation and found that close to 20% performed independently on basic motor and cognitive subscales of the Functional Independence Measure (FIM).[25] Together, these studies confirm that outcomes after posttraumatic DoC are much better than had been assumed previously.

- The same behavioral instruments used to assess patients with a DoC (e.g. CRS-R, Disability Rating Scale [DRS]) can also be useful in tracking recovery and aiding in prognostication.[1] Moreover, technologies such as MRI, fMRI, single-photon emission computed tomography (SPECT), and electrophysiological studies (somatosensory evoked potentials [SEPs], event-related potentials [ERPs]) may also play a role in prognostication.[1]

Ethical Issues

- A number of ethical issues arise in the care of patients with DoC, including the ethical implications of diagnostic and prognostic uncertainty, the conduct of research with this population, and the use of novel diagnostic or therapeutic interventions.
- Challenging issues especially surround limiting or withdrawing medical treatment in this population (see the section on Withdrawal of Treatment in the chapter on ethics). Clinicians should be aware that there is both legal and ethical consensus that it is permissible to withdraw treatment for someone in a chronic VS (if there is sufficient evidence of their wishes to that effect),[26] whereas there is no such consensus should a similar request arise in the context of a patient in an MCS.[27] An ethics consultation or the involvement of an ethics committee should be sought in these situations.
- Clinicians should periodically engage in discussions with family members regarding goals of care.[1,28] In addition, clinicians should be familiar with the unique issues that family members of patients with DoC face, including potentially high levels of burden and distress.[3]

Review Questions

1. Which choice describes a patient in minimally conscious state (MCS) plus?
   a. Patient has a sleep-wake cycle and is awake sometimes. Patient demonstrates nonreflexive movements and visual pursuit. Patient does not demonstrate any behavior mediated by language.
   b. Patient has a sleep-wake cycle and is awake sometimes. Patient can consistently demonstrate the appropriate use of a pen to write on paper.
   c. Patient has a sleep-wake cycle and is awake sometimes. Patient is able to consistently follow commands to move his right hand. Patient can verbally answer "yes" or "no" questions but is not consistently correct.
   d. Patient has a sleep-wake cycle and is awake sometimes. Patient does not demonstrate evidence of awareness of self or environment.
   e. Patient does not have any periods of arousal. Patient does not demonstrate evidence of awareness of self or environment.

2. All of these conditions can last indefinitely except
   a. coma.
   b. vegetative state (VS).
   c. MCS
   d. severe disability on the Glasgow Outcome Scale.

3. Studies have shown that the rate of misdiagnosis of the vegetative state (in patients who are actually conscious) is approximately
   a. 10%.
   b. 15%.
   c. 25%.
   d. 35%.

Answers on page 402.
Access the full list of questions and answers online.
Available on ExpertConsult.com

References

1. Giacino JT, Katz DI, Schiff ND, et al. Practice guideline update recommendations summary: disorders of consciousness: report of the guideline development, dissemination, and implementation subcommittee of the American Academy of Neurology; the American Congress of Rehabilitation Medicine; and the National Institute on Disability, Independent Living, and Rehabilitation Research. *Arch Phys Med Rehabil.* 2018;99(9):1699-1709.
2. Berube J, Fins J, Giacino J, et al. *The Mohonk Report: A Report to Congress on Disorders of Consciousness: Assessment,*

Treatment, and Research Needs. Charlottesville, VA: National Brain Injury Research, Treatment, and Training Foundation; 2006.
3. Kothari S, Gilbert-Baffoe E, O'Brien K. Disorders of consciousness. In: Eapen BC, Cifu DX, eds. *Rehabilitation After Traumatic Brain Injury.* St. Louis, MO: Elsevier; 2018;191-214
4. Rodriguez Moreno D, Schiff ND, Giacino J, Kalmar K, Hirsch J. A network approach to assessing cognition in disorders of consciousness. *Neurology.* 2010;75(21):1871-1878.

5. Schiff ND. Recovery of consciousness after brain injury: a mesocircuit hypothesis. *Trends Neurosci*. 2010;33(1):1-9.

6. Schnakers C, Vanhaudenhuyse A, Giacino J, et al. Diagnostic accuracy of the vegetative and minimally conscious state: clinical consensus versus standardized neurobehavioral assessment. *BMC Neurol*. 2009;9:35.

7. Giacino J, Kalmar K. *Coma Recovery Scale-Revised*. The Center for Outcome Measurement in Brain Injury; 2006. Available at: http://www.tbims.org/combi/crs/.

8. Whyte J, DiPasquale MC. Assessment of vision and visual attention in minimally responsive brain injured patients. *Arch Phys Med Rehabil*. 1995;76(9):804-810.

9. Bekinschtein T, Leiguarda R, Armony J, et al. Emotion processing in the minimally conscious state. *J Neurol Neurosurg Psychiatry*. 2004;75(5):788.

10. Sattin D, Giovannetti AM, Ciaraffa F, et al. Assessment of patients with disorder of consciousness: do different Coma Recovery Scale scoring correlate with different settings? *J Neurol*. 2014;261(12):2378-2386.

11. Jox RJ, Kuehlmeyer K, Klein A-M, et al. Diagnosis and decision making for patients with disorders of consciousness: a survey among family members. *Arch Phys Med Rehabil*. 2015;96(2):323-330.

12. Monti MM, Vanhaudenhuyse A, Coleman MR, et al. Willful modulation of brain activity in disorders of consciousness. *N Engl J Med*. 2010;362(7):579-589.

13. Kondziella D, Friberg CK, Frokjaer VG, Fabricius M, Møller K. Preserved consciousness in vegetative and minimal conscious states: systematic review and meta-analysis. *J Neurol Neurosurg Psychiatry*. 2016;87(5):485-492.

14. Whyte J, Nordenbo AM, Kalmar K, et al. Medical complications during inpatient rehabilitation among patients with traumatic disorders of consciousness. *Arch Phys Med Rehabil*. 2013;94(10):1877-1883.

15. Schnakers C, Zasler N. Assessment and management of pain in patients with disorders of consciousness. *PM R*. 2015;7(11 suppl):S270-S277.

16 Giacino JT, Whyte J, Bagiella E, et al. Placebo-controlled trial of amantadine for severe traumatic brain injury. *N Engl J Med*. 2012;366(9):819-826.

17. Whyte J, Rajan R, Rosenbaum A, et al. Zolpidem and restoration of consciousness. *Am J Phys Med Rehabil*. 2014;93(2):101-113.

18. Greenwald BD, Hammond FM, Harrison-Felix C, Nakase-Richardson R, Howe LLS, Kreider S. Mortality following traumatic brain injury among individuals unable to follow commands at the time of rehabilitation admission: a national institute on disability and rehabilitation research traumatic brain injury model systems study. *J Neurotrauma*. 2015;32(23):1883-1892.

19. Estraneo A, Moretta P, Loreto V, Lanzillo B, Santoro L, Trojano L. Late recovery after traumatic, anoxic, or hemorrhagic long-lasting vegetative state. *Neurology*. 2010;75(3):239-245.

20. Luauté J, Maucort-Boulch D, Tell L, et al. Long-term outcomes of chronic minimally conscious and vegetative states. *Neurology*. 2010;75(3):246-252.

21. Multi-Society Task Force on PVS. Medical aspects of the persistent vegetative state (1). *N Engl J Med*. 1994;330(21):1499-1508.

22. Giacino JT, Kalmar K. The vegetative and minimally conscious states: a comparison of clinical features and functional outcome. *J Head Trauma Rehabil*. 1997;12(4).

23. Katz DI, Polyak M, Coughlan D, Nichols M, Roche A. Natural history of recovery from brain injury after prolonged disorders of consciousness: outcome of patients admitted to inpatient rehabilitation with 1-4 year follow-up. *Prog Brain Res*. 2009;177:73-88.

24. Nakase-Richardson R, Whyte J, Giacino JT, et al. Longitudinal outcome of patients with disordered consciousness in the NIDRR TBI Model Systems Programs. *J Neurotrauma*. 2012;29(1):59-65.

25. Whyte J, Nakase-Richardson R, Hammond FM, et al. Functional outcomes in traumatic disorders of consciousness: 5-year outcomes from the National Institute on Disability and Rehabilitation Research Traumatic Brain Injury Model Systems. *Arch Phys Med Rehabil*. 2013;94(10):1855-1860.

26. Shepherd LL. *If That Ever Happens to Me: Making Life and Death Decisions after Terri Schiavo*. Chapel Hill, NC: University of North Carolina Press; 2009:222.

27. Huxtable R. "In a twilight world"? Judging the value of life for the minimally conscious patient. *J Med Ethics*. 2013;39(9):565-569.

28. Kothari S. Chronic disorders of consciousness, In: Creutzfeldt C, Kluger B, Holloway R, eds. *Neuropalliative Care: A Guide to Improving the Lives of Patients and Families Affected by Neurologic Disease*. Springer Publishers; 2019.

57

Complementary and Alternative Medicine

DMITRY ESTEROV, DO, AND BILLIE SCHULTZ, MD

OUTLINE

Given the high complexity and lack of a definitive treatment to overcome the range of sequelae of traumatic brain injury (TBI), patients and families often turn to complementary therapies to assist in recovery from TBI. Complementary alternative medicine (CAM) can offer patients treatment options to assist in a variety of these sequelae, which include overall functional recovery, mental health issues (including anxiety and depression), fatigue, pain relief, and cognitive deficits. CAM therapies also offer a preventive approach in improving health and quality of life overall after a TBI.

Definitions

- CAM: According to the World Health Organization (WHO), it is defined as set of healthcare practices that are not part of that country's own tradition or conventional medicine and are not fully integrated into the dominant healthcare system.

- Integrative medicine combines conventional and CAM treatments for which there is evidence of safety and effectiveness.
- Evidence-based medicine (EBM) is a systematic approach to clinical problem solving with three core principles:
  1. Awareness of best clinical evidence
  2. Individual expertise
  3. Patient values and expectation
- Given the high use of CAM among the general population, it is essential for the clinician to be aware of various CAM approaches and to use EBM to evaluate potential benefit or risk of CAM practices for persons with brain injury.
- The clinician must weigh the possible benefit versus any harms or risks associated with treatment and the overall cost. As a whole, large randomized control trials are lacking for CAM, so the clinician must use best EBM approaches in decision making.

Epidemiology

- As of 2007, 35.5% of adults are using some form of CAM.[1]
- Natural products are the most commonly used CAM modality (Fig. 57.1).
- CAM use is highest in American Indian/Alaska Native populations (Fig. 57.2).
- CAM use among adults is greater among women and those with higher levels of education and higher incomes, and use of CAM has been generally increasing over the past decade (from 2002 - 2012).[1]
- Musculoskeletal complaints are the most common reason for use of CAM.[2]
- In a national health survey in 2012, an estimated 59 million persons ages 4 years and older had at least one expenditure for some type of complementary health approach, resulting in total out-of-pocket expenditures of $30.2 billion.[3]

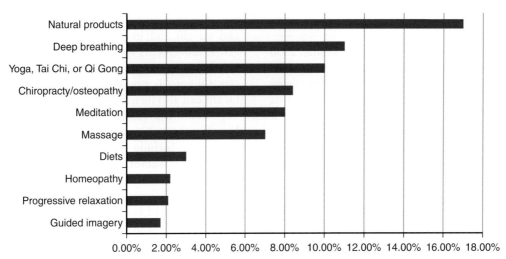

• **Fig. 57.1** Centers for Disease Control and Prevention data of the most commonly used complementary and alternative medicine modalities in 2012. (Adapted from Barnes PM, Bloom B, Nahin R. Complementary and alternative medicine use among adults and children: United States, 2007. *Natl Health Stat Report.* 2008;12:1-23.)

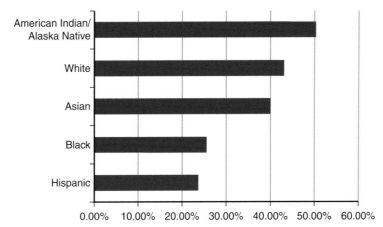

• **Fig. 57.2** Complementary and alternative medicine use by race/ethnicity from 2002 to 2012, per National Health Statistics Reports. (Adapted from Clarke TC, Black LI, Stussman BJ, et al. Trends in the use of complementary health approaches among adults: United States, 2002 - 2012. *Natl Health Stat Report.* 2015;79:1-16.)

Natural Products

According to the Dietary Supplement Health and Education Act (DSHEA), dietary supplements are defined as a category of food, which puts them under different regulations than US Food and Drug Administration (FDA)–approved drugs. Examples include a wide variety of herbs, vitamins, minerals, and probiotics. They are considered safe until proven otherwise.

• The most commonly used natural product is fish oil.[1]
• Manufacturers are not required to test new ingredients or supplements in clinical trials. There is no controlled system for reporting adverse reactions because natural products are usually self-prescribed. Moreover, products such as herbs can often be contaminated or contain a substance other than what is written on the label. In this way, herbal medicines can thus cause adverse effects; may

not be safe during pregnancy, in children, or in the elderly; and may damage specific organ systems.[4]
• There is limited evidence for use of omega-3 fatty acids, zinc, magnesium, creatine, and vitamins D, E, and B3 in TBI.
  • Increased production of free radicals leading to oxidative stress can play a role in the pathogenesis of TBI, and treatment with antioxidants such as vitamin E can theoretically prevent tissue damage and improve outcome.[5]
  • Antiinflammatory supplements such as curcumin resveratrol and lipoic acid have been shown to reduce inflammation in animal models but not studied in clinical trials.[5]
  • Animal models have shown omega-3 fatty acids reduce reactive oxygen species after TBI and reduce TBI-related injuries in areas such as mitochondrial malfunction, excitotoxicity, and oxidative stress.[5]

Acupuncture

The use of acupuncture can be traced back more than 2000 years in China and includes stimulation of anatomical points on the body by a variety of techniques, involving penetrating the skin with thin, solid, metallic needles that are manipulated by the hands or by electrical stimulation. It is based on the principles of traditional Chinese medicine in terms of a vital energy called *qi* that circulates between organ channels called *meridians*.

- The mechanism may involve triggering endogenous opioids or stress-related hormones.[6]
- A Cochrane review of 30 Chinese studies found a high risk of bias and very low methodological quality, although studies suggested that results were efficacious in improving overall function after TBI.[6]
- It is generally well tolerated and safe.
- Acupressure is another form of traditional Chinese medicine that involves the application of pressure to specific points using hands, fingers, or thumbs instead of needles.
  - Although limited evidence exists of use in patients with TBI, acupressure treatment has been associated with lowering stress and anxiety and improving sleep measures in other patient populations.[7]

Hyperbaric Oxygen Therapy

Hyperbaric oxygen therapy (HBOT) is the therapeutic administration of 100% oxygen at environmental pressures greater than 1 atmosphere absolute (ATA). It involves placing the patient in an airtight vessel, increasing the pressure within that vessel, and administering oxygen for respiration. The goal with HBOT is to improve oxygen supply to the injured brain and reduce the swelling associated with low oxygen levels, thus reducing death and disability after TBI.[8]

- In a Cochrane review of seven studies with 71 people, routine use of HBOT in brain-injured patients could not be justified by the findings of this review, although limited evidence was found for use after acute brain injury.[8]
  - Although HBOT may reduce the risk of death and improve the final Glasgow Coma Scale (GCS) score based on some studies, there was no evidence of survivors having a good outcome.
- Side effects include otic trauma, risk of seizures, and pulmonary injury.
- A double-blind, randomized control trial with sham treatment of 60 military members with a combat-related mild TBI found no evidence for efficacy of HBOT.[9]
- Overall, there is insufficient evidence to support use of HBOT in brain injury.
- It is not currently covered by insurance.

Mind-Body Medicine

Mind-body practice uses the power of thoughts and emotions to influence physical health and vice versa. Mindful-based stress reduction is a method that identi-fies thoughts without passing judgment to thoughts, and tai chi and qi gong involve certain postures and gentle movements with mental focus, breathing and relaxation. They are both considered a safe form of exercise. Qi gong is a moving mindfulness practice, whereas tai chi can also be used as a form of martial arts combat. Yoga combines gentle movement and stretching with breathing exercises and meditation. Other relaxation techniques include guided imagery and *humor therapy* (therapeutic humor), which refers to finding ways to increase smiles and laughter to reduce anxiety and possibly boost the immune system.

- Mindful-based stress reduction may regulate autonomic function by regulating parasympathetic tone.[7]
- Tai chi may help after a cerebrovascular accident (CVA) to improve balance and controlled movement in a community-based setting.[7]
- Yoga can potentially help in improving overall function and decreasing anxiety, although evidence is limited.
- Evidence is lacking overall, but mind-body medicine is thought to be safe and may be of benefit in improving quality of life and symptomatology in those with brain injuries.

Music Interventions

Music interventions can be categorized into music therapy and music medicine interventions. Music therapy requires implementation by a trained music therapist, whereas music medicine intervention is defined as listening to prerecorded music.

- Music interventions use after stroke:
  - Studies have been done for those with acquired brain injuries, including a Cochrane review with rhythmic auditory stimulation (RAS) showing a benefit in improving gait parameters after stroke, including gait velocity, stride length, and cadence.[10]
  - Music therapy was found to reduce agitation and improve orientation level in stroke patients.[10]
- Music interventions use in TBI:
  - In patients with disorders of consciousness, music therapy has been studied in recovery, although with poor methodological quality.
  - A study investigating Familiar Auditory Stimulus Training showed it to have some benefit with changes in functional magnetic resonance imaging (fMRI).[11]
  - Overall studies with music interventions have shown a high rate of bias for those with TBI, and more studies are needed to demonstrate efficacy.

Biofeedback

Biofeedback involves sensors that allow the wearer to detect and learn to control functions that are normally autonomous, including heart rate, blood pressure, and muscle tension.

- Systematic reviews indicate biofeedback may help lessen anxiety but is not effective treatment for posttraumatic stress disorder, which may be a concomitant condition after TBI. It is also used to treat tension-type headaches, but studies with posttraumatic headaches specifically are limited.

- There are very few studies in TBI and very small sample sizes, so there is insufficient evidence to justify support, although biofeedback is safe and not associated with any side effects.

Manual Therapies

Massage therapy includes various forms of light touch to deep touch modalities to improve pain and reduce anxiety. It can also be an adjunct to other therapeutic interventions. Craniosacral osteopathy was developed by William Sutherland, DO, as osteopathy in the cranial field in the 1930s, which is taught as part of osteopathic medical school curriculum. Craniosacral therapy was later adapted by John Upledger, DO, who expanded teachings to nonphysician practitioners. The overall general principle is that there is physiological motion in the cranial bones, and practitioners can assess for structural dysfunctions in the physiological motion of those bones and return the structures to normal balance, inducing overall healing.

- Studies are limited, but there is potential use for craniosacral therapy for pain syndromes after TBI and for posttraumatic headaches.
- Given the traumatic nature of brain injury and theoretical alteration in the motion of the cranial bones, craniosacral therapy has potential in restoring proper motion resulting in improved function after TBI.
  - Research has included case reports and small randomized controlled trials, but the methodology of all studies is poor.

Naturopathy

Naturopathy is a healthcare profession emphasizing health and prevention and treatment through methods that encourage a person's inherent self-healing. Naturopathic doctors (NDs) are trained at accredited, 4-year postgraduate naturopathic medical programs. Principles include an inherent power in self-healing process, identifying and removing the cause of illness, emphasizing prevention, and minimizing harm. Treatments include nutrition, homeopathy, natural products, acupuncture, massage, and Traditional Chinese Medicine.

- Most treatments are safe, but natural products may carry risk because they are not Food and Drug Administration regulated or may cause drug interactions.
- Modalities could theoretically improve function after brain injury, given significant overlap with multiple other CAM modalities.
- Medical physicians should be cognizant of types of treatment offered by naturopathic physicians.

Homeopathy

Homeopathy is a form of natural medicine developed by Samuel Hahnemann at end of the 18th century that stimulates the body's self-healing mechanisms to treat illness. The cornerstone principle is *similia similibus curantur,* which means "let likes cure likes." Other principles include the single remedy, in which only one homeopathic remedy is given at one time and the minimum dose principle, in which a tiny dose of medicine is given after a dilute extract is made.

- Theoretical uses after brain injury are to improve overall function, pain, anxiety, and depression and to increase overall health.

Review Questions

1. Which of these is correct regarding complementary and alternative medicine (CAM)?
   a. It is more commonly used in males compared with females,
   b. Its use increased from 2002 - 2012
   c. It is more common in those with lower incomes,
   d. It is more common in those with a lower level of education.
2. What is the most common CAM therapy used among adults?
   a. Meditation
   b. Yoga/tai chi
   c. Massage
   d. Natural products

3. What is the most common ethnicity in the United States to use complementary and alternative medicine?
   a. White
   b. Asian
   c. Black
   d. American Indian/Alaska Native

Answers on page 403.
Access the full list of questions and answers online. Available on ExpertConsult.com

References

1. Clarke TC, Black LI, Stussman BJ, Barnes PM, Nahin RL. *Trends in the Use of Complementary Health Approaches Among Adults: United States, 2002 - 2012.* National health statistics reports; no 79. Hyattsville, MD: National Center for Health Statistics; 2015.

2. Barnes PM, Bloom B, Nahin R. CDC National Health Statistics Report #12. *Complementary and Alternative Medicine use Amongst Adults and Children: United States, 2007.*

3. Nahin RL, Barnes PM, Stussman BJ. Expenditures on complementary health approaches: United States, 2012. National health statistics reports; no 95. Hyattsville, MD: National Center for Health Statistics; 2016.

4. Ernst E. Treatments used in complementary and alternative medicine. *Side Effects of Drugs Annual.* 2005;28:573-586.

5. Drake DF, Hudak AM, Robbins, W. Integrative medicine in traumatic brain injury. *Phys Med Rehabil Clin North Am.* 2017;28: 363-378. doi:10.1016/j.pmr.2016.12.011.

6. Wong V, Cheuk DKL, Lee S, Chu V. Acupuncture for acute management and rehabilitation of traumatic brain injury. *Cochrane Database Syst Rev.* 2013(3):CD007700. doi:10.1002/14651858. CD007700.pub3.

7. Hernández TD, Brenner LA, Walter KH, Bormann JE, Johansson B. Complementary and alternative medicine (CAM) following traumatic brain injury (TBI): opportunities and challenges. *Brain Res.* 2016;1640:139-151. doi:10.1016/j.brainres.2016.01.025.

8. Bennett MH, Trytko B, Jonker B. Hyperbaric oxygen therapy for the adjunctive treatment of traumatic brain injury. *Cochrane Database Syst Rev.* 2012(12):CD004609. doi:10.1002/14651858. CD004609.pub3.

9. Cifu DX, Hart BB, West SL, Walker W, Carne W. The effect of hyperbaric oxygen on persistent postconcussion symptoms. *J Head Trauma Rehabil.* 2014;29(1):11-20.

10. Magee WL, Clark I, Tamplin J, Bradt J. Music interventions for acquired brain injury. *Cochrane Database Syst Rev.* 2017(1): CD006787. doi:10.1002/14651858.CD006787.pub3.

11. Schnakers C, Magee WL, Harris B. Sensory stimulation and music therapy programs for treating disorders of consciousness. *Frontiers in Psychology.* 2016;7:297. doi:10.3389/fpsyg.2016.00297.

58

Neuromodulation and Neuroprosthetics

MIRIAM SEGAL, MD

Neuromodulation

The North American Neuromodulation Society (NANS), founded in 1994, roughly defines neuromodulation as encompassing a number of treatment modalities that exert their effect on the nervous system, typically using implantable techniques and including the stimulation of nerves in the central, peripheral or autonomic nervous systems or through the use of implanted drug delivery systems.[1] The International Modulation Society (INS), founded in 1989, defines neuromodulation as the alteration of nerve activity through targeted delivery of a stimulus, such as electrical stimulation or chemical agents, to specific neurological sites in the body.[2] These definitions, conspicuous in their ambiguity, are a reflection of an emerging and rapidly evolving field with an ever-expanding list of treatments and indications.[3]

Techniques Involving Implanted Devices

Deep Brain Stimulation

Deep brain stimulation (DBS) is used for the treatment of movement disorders and is the most invasive neuromodulation strategy (see Chapter 29).
- **1997:** DBS granted US Food and Drug Administration (FDA) approval for essential tremor.
- **2002:** DBS granted FDA approval for Parkinson's disease (PD) and is quickly adopted as a popular and effective treatment for PD and essential tremor.[4]
- **2003:** FDA provided humanitarian device exemption for DBS treatment of dystonia.[5]
- **2009:** FDA provided humanitarian device exemption for DBS treatment of obsessive-compulsive disorder.[5]

- In the subsequent decade, investigational and off-label uses of DBS were reported in the treatment of various conditions, including pain, major depression, Tourette syndrome and other tic disorders and dyskinesias, obesity, anorexia, addiction, pathological aggression, dementia, and epilepsy[5]
- **2016:** A systematic review examined 78 individual cases in 19 articles discussing the use of DBS for treatment of disorders of consciousness (DoCs) and concluded that no clear evidence exists to support DBS for restoration of consciousness in DoC patients and that in cases where benefit was reported, spontaneous recovery was too confounding[6]
- **2018:** DBS granted FDA approval for treatment resistant epilepsy[7] after the Stimulation of the Anterior Nucleus of the Thalamus for Epilepsy (SANTE) trial and other trials demonstrated sustained efficacy and safety in a treatment-resistant population[8]

Motor Cortex Stimulation

Motor cortex stimulation (MCS) is a neuromodulation technique that is one degree less invasive than DBS and uses implanted *cortical* electrodes.
- Used for various neuropathic pain syndromes
- Greatest efficacy observed in the treatment of deafferentation pain caused by either peripheral (trigeminal nerve injury, phantom limb) or central (post stroke) lesions[9]
- An emerging technique in MCS patient selection has been the use of repetitive transcranial magnetic stimulation (rTMS), which is noninvasive, to predict a positive response to MCS.[10]

Noninvasive Techniques

Developments in noninvasive brain stimulation are rapid as increases in both the technology and the understanding of the brain continue.

Transcranial Electrical Stimulation

Transcranial electrical stimulation (TES) involves stimulation through the use of scalp electrodes.
- **1980:** Merton and Morton first published on this technique.[11]

- High-voltage TES stimulates the cortex underlying the anode, activating corticospinal tract neurons and generating a motor evoked potential (MEP).[12]
- TES is credited as the first technique to allow for the noninvasive study of excitability and propagation along CNS fibers in living, cooperative human beings.[12]
- TES is uncomfortable.

Transcranial Magnetic Stimulation

Transcranial magnetic stimulation (TMS) uses electromagnetic induction as a painless way to induce a current in the brain.[12]

- **1985:** TMS is developed, and because it is painless, it becomes preferred over TES.[12,13]
- TMS of the motor cortex can be used to provide information regarding disease-related changes of corticospinal output in conditions such as multiple sclerosis, stroke, cervical myelopathy, and amyotrophic lateral sclerosis through analysis of MEPs.[12]
- TMS has been used to map brain function; initially it was used to map the motor homunculus through use of the MEP, a convenient output measure.[12]
- The combination of TMS and EEG creates vast possibilities; TMS-evoked cortical activity can be measured and used to study cortical excitability, connectivity, and plasticity.[12]
- These developments have been part of the neuroscience revolution that has shaped the neurorehabilitation approach to incorporate principles of neuroplasticity and motor learning.[14]
- Many therapeutic applications of TMS have surfaced:
  - TMS is approved by the FDA as a preoperative navigational tool.[12]
  - Several TMS devices have now been FDA approved for treating depression.[15]
  - 2014 European expert panel published evidence-based guidelines for therapeutic use of, TMS and ascribed:
    1. Level A evidence (definite efficacy) to the antidepressant effect of high-frequency repetitive TMS (HFrTMS) on the left dorsolateral prefrontal cortex (DLPFC)[16]
    2. Level A evidence for the analgesic efficacy of HFrTMS on the primary motor cortex (M1) of the contralateral hemisphere[16]
    3. Level B evidence (probable efficacy) for low-frequency rTMS (LFrTMS) for depression, HFrTMS on the left DLPFC for the negative symptoms of schizophrenia, and LFrTMS of the contralesional M1 for motor recovery in chronic motor stroke[16]
    4. Several indications reached possible efficacy (Level C) including tinnitus and auditory hallucinations[16]

Peripheral Nerve Stimulation Techniques

Peripheral nerve stimulation techniques are numerous and varied. Some applications of interest to the brain injury specialist include treatments for neurogenic bowel,[17] neurogenic bladder,[18] and chronic pain.[19]

Various neuromodulation strategies exist for treatment of migraine. These include noninvasive vagus nerve stimulation (nVNS), external trigeminal nerve stimulation, occipital and supraorbital transcutaneous nerve stimulation, transcranial direct current stimulation, and alternating current stimulation in addition to TMS.[20] The nVNS device is the only device that is FDA approved for acute and preventive use in cluster headache and that has strong evidence to suggest efficacy in acute and preventive treatment of migraine.[20] Left cervical vagus nerve stimulation is an approved therapy for epilepsy and treatment-resistant depression, but its treatment efficacy for depression has been called into question .[21]

In terms of neuromodulation strategies that use drug delivery systems, most brain injury medicine specialists are familiar with intrathecal pumps. Agents approved by the FDA for intrathecal therapy include morphine and ziconotide for pain and baclofen for spasticity, although several other agents are used off label for the treatment of pain.[2] Intrathecal baclofen (ITB) has also been suggested to be of benefit in patients with paroxysmal sympathetic hyperactivity (PSH) caused by severe TBI.[22]

Neuroprosthetics and Brain Computer Interface

In parallel to the field of neuromodulation, neuroprosthetics is a domain that also involves devices that interface with the nervous system to restore function—the most successful and well known being the cochlear implant.[23] At the heart of neuroprosthetics is the *brain computer interface* (BCI), which is defined as "a system that measures central nervous system activity and converts it into artificial output that replaces, restores, enhances, supplements or improves natural CNS output and thereby changes the ongoing interactions between the CNS and its external or internal environment."[24]

There are five stages making up a typical BCI[25]:
1. Brain signal acquisition
2. Preprocessing
3. Feature extraction/selection
4. Classification
5. Application interface

To put it another way: Brain signals are recorded, processed by a translational algorithm, and then routed to drive a chosen application. One way to categorize BCIs is in terms of invasiveness of signal recording. As a rule, the more invasive the system, the higher/better the signal resolution.[23]

The most common recording methods in the CNS are:
- Scalp EEG
- Electrocorticography (ECoG) that records from the cortical surface of the brain via an implanted electrode array
- Intracortical and depth electrodes, the most invasive technique[23]
- Other modalities for brain signal acquisition include magnetoencephalography (MEG), functional magnetic resonance imaging (fMRI), and functional near infrared spectroscopy (fNIRS)[26]

- Bidirectional systems, capable of electrical stimulation and recording, are also being explored[23]
  - Initially, BCI systems were used to allow the user to control output for environmental control or communication.[25]
  - This has been explored for augmentative and alternative communication for patients who have severely limited ability to control a communication device such as in amyotrophic lateral sclerosis or locked-in syndrome.[27-29]
  - In 2015, Coyle et al. reported four patients in a minimally conscious state who demonstrated consistent and appropriate brain activation on EEG through visual and auditory feedback, suggesting that patients in MCS may be able to operate a BCI-based communication system.[30]

A newly emerging application of BCI and a new frontier in neurorehabilitation is the use of BCI to enhance of motor learning.[25] As an example, a 2018 study demonstrated that BCI coupled to functional electrical stimulation (FES) elicited a clinically relevant and lasting motor recovery in chronic stroke survivors compared with sham FES.[31] In addition, these authors were also able to demonstrate through EEG mapping increased functional connectivity between motor areas of the affected hemisphere in the treatment group, suggesting that BCI–FES therapy can drive functional recovery through "purposeful plasticity."[31]

Review Questions

1. Which of these statements regarding deep brain stimulation (DBS) are true?
   a. The US Food and Drug Administration (FDA) has approved DBS as treatment for dystonia and other movement disorders.
   b. The Stimulation of the Anterior Nucleus of the Thalamus for Epilepsy (SANTE) trial demonstrated that DBS was safe and effective treatment for treatment-resistant epilepsy, leading to the FDA approval for this indication in 2018.
   c. DBS has been shown to improve communication in patients with disorders of consciousness (DoC), but it has not been adopted as a popular treatment because decreased access to treatment.
   d. All of the above
   e. None of the above
2. Which of these treatments are FDA approved for the treatment of depression?
   a. Transcranial magnetic stimulation (TMS)
   b. Left cervical vagus stimulation
   c. Noninvasive vagus nerve stimulation (nVNS)
   d. A and B
   e. A and C
3. Which of these treatments are incorrectly paired with the approved indication?
   a. DBS/Parkinson's tremor, essential tremor, epilepsy
   b. TMS/preoperative navigation, depression
   c. Intrathecal baclofen (ITB)/paroxysmal sympathetic hyperactivity (PSH)
   d. Noninvasive vagus nerve stimulation (nVNS)/cluster headache
   e. Left cervical vagus nerve stimulation/epilepsy, depression

Answers on page 403.
Access the full list of questions and answers online. Available on ExpertConsult.com

References

1. North American Neuromodulation Society. *What is Neuromodulation. About NANS.* Neuromodulation.org [Internet]. Available at: https://neuromodulation.org/Default.aspx?TabID=442.
2. International Neuromodulation Society. *About the INS.* Available at: https://www.neuromodulation.com/about-ins.
3. Levy RM. The evolving definition of neuromodulation. *Neuromodulation Technol Neural Interface.* 2014;17(3):207-210.
4. Gardner J. A history of deep brain stimulation: Technological innovation and the role of clinical assessment tools. *Soc Stud Sci.* 2013;43(5):707-728.
5. Youngerman BE, Chan AK, Mikell CB, McKhann GM, Sheth SA. A decade of emerging indications: deep brain stimulation in the United States. *J Neurosurg.* 2016;125(2):461-471.
6. Vanhoecke J, Hariz M. Deep brain stimulation for disorders of consciousness: Systematic review of cases and ethics. *Brain Stimul.* 2017;10(6):1013-1023.
7. US Food & Drug Administration. *Medtronic DBS System for Epilepsy—P960009/S219.* FDA. Available at: https://www.fda.gov/medical-devices/recently-approved-devices/medtronic-dbs-system-epilepsy-p960009s219.
8. Salanova V, Witt T, Worth R, et al. Long-term efficacy and safety of thalamic stimulation for drug-resistant partial epilepsy. *Neurology.* 2015;84(10):1017-1025.
9. Honey CM, Tronnier VM, Honey CR. Deep brain stimulation versus motor cortex stimulation for neuropathic pain: a minireview of the literature and proposal for future research. *Comput Struct Biotechnol J.* 2016;14:234-237.
10. Lefaucheur JP, Ménard-Lefaucheur I, Goujon C, Keravel Y, Nguyen JP. Predictive value of rTMS in the identification of responders to epidural motor cortex stimulation therapy for pain. *J Pain.* 2011;12(10):1102-1111.
11. Merton PA, Morton HB. Stimulation of the cerebral cortex in the intact human subject. *Nature.* 1980;285(5762):227.
12. Rossini PM, Burke D, Chen R, et al. Non-invasive electrical and magnetic stimulation of the brain, spinal cord, roots and peripheral nerves: basic principles and procedures for routine clinical and research application. An updated report from an I.F.C.N. Committee. *Clin Neurophysiol.* 2015;126(6):1071-1107.
13. Barker AT, Jalinous R, Freeston IL. Non-invasive magnetic stimulation of human motor cortex. *Lancet.* 1985;1(8437):1106-1107.

14. Winstein C, Lewthwaite R, Blanton SR, Wolf LB, Wishart L. Infusing motor learning research into neurorehabilitation practice: a historical perspective with case exemplar from the accelerated skill acquisition program. *J Neurol Phys Ther*. 2014; 38(3):190-200.

15. TMS Devices. *Clinical TMS Society* [Internet]. Available at: https://www.clinicaltmssociety.org/tms/devices.

16. Lefaucheur JP, André-Obadia N, Antal A, et al. Evidence-based guidelines on the therapeutic use of repetitive transcranial magnetic stimulation (rTMS). *Clin Neurophysiol*. 2014;125(11): 2150-2206.

17. Worsøe J, Rasmussen M, Christensen P, Krogh K. Neurostimulation for neurogenic bowel dysfunction. *Gastroenterol Res Pract*. 2013;2013:563294.

18. Sanford MT, Suskind AM. Neuromodulation in neurogenic bladder. *Transl Androl Urol*. 2016;5(1):117-126.

19. Chakravarthy K, Nava A, Christo PJ, Williams K. Review of recent advances in peripheral nerve stimulation (PNS). *Curr Pain Headache Rep*. 2016;20(11):60.

20. Reuter U, McClure C, Liebler E, Pozo-Rosich P. Non-invasive neuromodulation for migraine and cluster headache: a systematic review of clinical trials. *J Neurol Neurosurg Psychiatry*. 2019;jnnp-2018-320113.

21. Howland RH. Vagus nerve stimulation. *Curr Behav Neurosci Rep*. 2014;1(2):64-73.

22. Pucks-Faes E, Hitzenberger G, Matzak H, Verrienti G, Schauer R, Saltuari L. Intrathecal baclofen in paroxysmal sympathetic hyperactivity: impact on oral treatment. *Brain Behav*. 2018;8(11):e01124.

23. Adewole DO, Serruya MD, Harris JP, et al. The evolution of neuroprosthetic interfaces. *Crit Rev Biomed Eng*. 2016;44(1-2):123-152.

24. Wolpaw J, Wolpaw E. *Brain-Computer Interfaces: Principles and Practice*. New York, NY: Oxford University Press; 2012

25. Daly JJ, Huggins JE. Brain-computer interface: current and emerging rehabilitation applications. *Arch Phys Med Rehabil*. 2015;96(3 suppl):S1-S7.

26. Naseer N, Hong KS. fNIRS-based brain-computer interfaces: a review. *Front Hum Neurosci*. 2015;9:3

27. Hill K, Kovacs T, Shin S. Critical issues using brain-computer interfaces for augmentative and alternative communication. *Arch Phys Med Rehabil*. 2015;96(3 suppl):S8-S15.

28. Holz EM, Botrel L, Kaufmann T, Kübler A. Long-term independent brain-computer interface home use improves quality of life of a patient in the locked-in state: a case study. *Arch Phys Med Rehabil*. 2015;96(3):S16-S26.

29. Schettini F, Riccio A, Simione L, et al. Assistive device with conventional, alternative, and brain-computer interface inputs to enhance interaction with the environment for people with amyotrophic lateral sclerosis: a feasibility and usability study. *Arch Phys Med Rehabil*. 2015;96(3):S46-S53.

30. Coyle D, Stow J, McCreadie K, McElligott J, Carroll Á. Sensorimotor modulation assessment and brain-computer interface training in disorders of consciousness. *Arch Phys Med Rehabil*. 2015;96(3):S62-S70.

31. Biasiucci A, Leeb R, Iturrate I, et al. Brain-actuated functional electrical stimulation elicits lasting arm motor recovery after stroke. *Nat Commun*. 2018;9(1):2421.

59

Neuropharmacology

CRAIG DITOMMASO, MD, SUSAN LOUGHLIN, PharmD, BCPS, AND CHRISTOPHER M. FALCO, MD

OUTLINE

Neuropharmacology is a small piece of the overall management of the person with a brain injury. This chapter touches on a few elements of brain injury pharmacology but should not overshadow the necessary work of obtaining an adequate history, performing a thorough examination, discussing the goals of treatment, and applying the correct therapies and interventions. Furthermore, administration of any medication should occur only by brain injury physicians who have had adequate training and who understand the potential benefits, risks, and potential interactions of said medication.

In addition, the authors of this book highly recommend consultation with a clinical pharmacist when appropriate.

Analgesics

Issues of pain are common after a traumatic brain injury (TBI).[1] (Dobscha) This chapter is not the appropriate place to explore complementary or alternative options to pain management, but they should not be ignored by the brain injury physician.

Modalities

The authors of this chapter recommend nonpharmacological treatment of pain whenever possible in the TBI population. Table 59.1 has some of the possible modalities.

Nonopioid Analgesics

Acetaminophen

Mechanism of action (MOA)[2] (Micromedex),[3] (Lexicomp Online): Proposed analgesia through the activation of descending serotonergic inhibitory pathways in the central nervous system (CNS); inhibits the cyclooxygenase (COX) isoenzyme, particularly the COX-2 isoform, by acting as a reducing cosubstrate at the peroxidase site
Side effects (SEs)[3]: Minimal; monitor Liver Function Test with long-term use
Comments: used alone to treat mild pain and in combination with opioid to treat mild and moderate to severe pain
- Advantage: pain relief with little cognitive effect
- Advantage: first line for posttraumatic headache[4] (Watanabe)

Nonsteroidal Antiinflammatory Drugs

MOA: block prostaglandin synthesis resulting in analgesic, antipyretic, and antiinflammatory properties

TABLE 59.1	Modalities
Modality	**Type of Pain Typically Treated**
Heat conduction	Subacute and chronic pain
Convection heat	Subacute pain, limited neuropathic pain
Conversion heat	Subacute muscular pain
Deep heat	Deep muscle pain, chronic muscle pain
Cold	Acute pain and inflammation-related pain
Electrical stimulation/ TENS	Subacute pain, limited neuropathic pain
Traction	Acute joint pain

54. (Akyuz) 55. (Feine) 56. (Gersh)
TENS, transcutaneous electrical nerve stimulation.

Examples: ibuprofen (COX-1 and 2 inhibitor), meloxicam (COX-1 and 2 inhibitor), celecoxib (COX2 inhibitor)
SEs: peripheral edema, dyspepsia, increased liver enzymes, nephrolithiasis
- Advantage: pain relief with little cognitive effect
- Disadvantage: cardiovascular thrombotic events, serious gastrointestinal (GI) bleeding, ulcerations, and GI perforation possible[4A]

Opioid Analgesics

- Advantage: strong pain relief
- Disadvantage: sedation and risk of addiction
- Opioids are also mentioned later in this chapter under Problematic Medications.

Pure Agonists

MOA: bind to mu opioid receptors in CNS and inhibit ascending pain pathways; opioids alter the perception of and response to pain
Examples: morphine, oxycodone, hydrocodone
SEs: drowsiness, headache, nausea, constipation, respiratory and CNS depression
- Disadvantage: active metabolites of morphine can accumulate in renal impairment.[3]

Partial Agonists

MOA: bind to mu opioid receptors in aLL CNS; partial mu agonist and weak kappa antagonist activity
Example: buprenorphine
SEs: similar to
- Advantage: useful similar to pure agonist in addiction because partial mu agonist properties are such that at high doses behaves as an antagonist[3]

Central Agonists

Tramadol

MOA: bind to mu opiate receptors in the CNS and inhibits ascending pain pathways; inhibit norepinephrine and serotonin reuptake
SEs: dizziness, vertigo, constipation, nausea, dyspepsia, respiratory depression
Comments: risk of seizures when taken alone; increased risk of seizure when taken with other medications known to lower seizure threshold
- Disadvantage: risk of seizure[3]

Tapentadol

MOA: binds to mu opiate receptors in the CNS, inhibiting ascending pain pathways; inhibits norepinephrine

Adjuvants/Alternative Pain Medications

Antiepileptic Medications

- Discussed further in the Anticonvulsants section
- Used off label to assist in pain management
  MOA: medication specific

Examples: gabapentin, pregabalin, carbamazepine, topiramate

SEs: peripheral edema, somnolence, weight gain, fatigue, dizziness, hepatic dysfunction, hyponatremia, thrombocytopenia, rash
- Advantage: Some individual antiepileptics have specific uses in pain. Common examples:
  - Carbamazepine: trigeminal neuralgia[3]
  - Gabapentin: neuropathic pain[6A]
  - Valproic acid: headache[7]

Tricyclic Antidepressants
- Discussed further in the Antidepressants section and Table 59.2
- Used off label for years to treat neuropathic pain

MOA: inhibit serotonin and/or norepinephrine reuptake in CNS

SEs: anticholinergic: constipation, xerostomia, blurred vision, urinary retention
- Advantage: individual medications have specific uses:
  - Nortriptyline: fewer anticholinergic properties than other tricyclic antidepressants (TCAs)[7A]
  - Amitriptyline: posttraumatic headache[8]

Serotonin-Norepinephrine Reuptake Inhibitors
- Discussed further in the Antidepressants

MOA: inhibit reuptake of serotonin and norepinephrine and weak inhibitor of dopamine reuptake

Examples: duloxetine, venlafaxine

SEs: insomnia, dizziness, drowsiness, nausea, headache, fatigue

Local Anesthetics
MOA: medication specific

Examples: lidocaine, capsaicin, diclofenac

SEs: exfoliation of skin, papule formation, skin edema, localized erythema, pruritus, rash, xeroderma, increased serum transaminases, dizziness

Anticonvulsants/Antiepileptic Medications

Prophylaxis Versus Treatment
- Based largely on the work of Dikmen and Temkin, various recommendations have been given for seizure treatment and prophylaxis after moderate to severe TBI without penetrating injury.[9-12]
- Full summary of this topic is not possible within this chapter, but a generalized evidence-based approach is present in the organization of this section.[12A]
- Please see Chapter 28 for more information.

Type of Posttraumatic Seizure
- Consider 7 days of prophylactic medications in all cases[9] (Temkin)
  a. Immediate seizure
     i. Seizure occurs within 24 hours of injury.
     ii. Treat acute seizure as appropriate.
     iii. Recommend 7 days of prophylactic medication only.
  b. Early seizure
     i. Seizure occurs within 24 hours to 7 days post injury.
     ii. Treat acute seizure as appropriate.
     iii. Recommend 3 to 6 months of further medication.
  c. Late
     i. Seizure occurs 1 week or more postinjury.
     ii. Treat acute seizure as appropriate.
     iii. Recommend long-term antiepileptic management.
     iv. Late seizures typically reflect more permanent structural damage and require long-term treatment.

Medication Options
Carbamazepine
MOA: limits influx of sodium ions across cell membrane[13]

SEs: sedation, dizziness, hepatic dysfunction, hyponatremia, thrombocytopenia, rash

Gabapentin
MOA: membrane stabilizer that blocks voltage gated calcium channels. It is structurally similar to the neurotransmitter gamma aminobutyric acid (GABA), but it has no effects on GABA receptors[13]

SEs: Somnolence, sedation, dizziness, peripheral edema
- Advantage: commonly used for neuropathic pain as discussed in section A
- Advantage: may help with paroxysmal sympathetic hyperactivity[14]
- Disadvantage: generally not considered primary antiepileptic[14A]

Lamotrigine
MOA: inhibits the release of glutamate and inhibits voltage-sensitive sodium channels and calcium channels[13] stabilizing neuronal membranes

SEs: nausea, peripheral edema, insomnia, skin rash
- Disadvantage: must be slowly titrated to prevent life-threatening skin rashes

Levetiracetam
MOA: The mechanism of action is unknown but may involve inhibition of calcium channels.

TABLE 59.2	Tricyclic Antidepressants			
Amitriptyline	Amoxapine	Desipramine	Doxepin	Imipramine
Maprotiline	Nortriptyline	Protriptyline	Trimipramine	

SEs: drowsiness, aggression, irritability, anorexia, dizziness
- Advantage: Typically the drug of choice for seizure prophylaxis[15,15A]

Phenobarbital

MOA: long-acting sedative hypnotic; suppresses high-frequency firing in neurons through actions on sodium channels
SEs: bradycardia, hypotension, respiratory depression
- Disadvantage: requires slower administration rate
- Disadvantage: very sedating and typically used as last line as an anticonvulsant because of its slow rate of administration[15B]

Phenytoin

MOA: stabilizes neuronal membranes, decreasing seizure activity through changes in sodium, potassium, and calcium conductance and membrane potentials
SEs: bradycardia, cardiac arrhythmia, nausea, vomiting, nystagmus, tremors, gingival hyperplasia
- Disadvantage: significant cognitive deficits in TBI patients[10]
- Disadvantage: serum levels should be checked frequently

Valproic Acid

MOA: increases availability of GABA to neurons; blocks sodium channels and therefore decreases repetitive neuronal firing
SEs: headache, drowsiness, nausea, thrombocytopenia, diplopia
- Advantage: mood stabilizing; see Anxiolytics/Mood Stabilizers
- Advantage: may have few cognitive side effects[11]

Topiramate

MOA: blocks sodium channels[13] and enhances GABA A activity
SEs: drowsiness, memory impairment, nausea, diarrhea
- Disadvantage: There are some case reports of hyperammonemia when used with valproic acid.[16A]

Antispasticity Agents

Spasticity often follows TBI, especially in the severe TBI population. The use of the medications in this section is an option but is often limited by their side effects.

Gaba Agonists

Baclofen

MOA: acts as GABA agonist, hyperpolarizes afferent fiber terminals, reducing release of excitatory transmitters in brain and spinal cord
SEs: drowsiness, confusion, headache, nausea, vomiting, hypotension, urinary retention, weakness[16B]
- Advantage: oral and intrathecal formulations available
- Disadvantage: abrupt withdrawal of intrathecal baclofen can be fatal

- Symptoms of withdrawal include hyperpyrexia, altered mental status, muscle rigidity, multiple organ failure, death.[16C]

Benzodiazepines

MOA: binds to GABA receptors and enhance the inhibitory effect of GABA; enhances inhibitory effect of GABA through increased neuronal permeability to chloride ions[16D]
Examples: alprazolam, clonazepam, diazepam, lorazepam
SEs: drowsiness, hypotension, dizziness, amnesia, disinhibition, agitation, respiratory depression, dependency/abuse, confusion, hypotension
- Disadvantage: usually avoided in patients with brain injury because of CNS depression, worsening cognitive impairments[16]

Alpha Antagonists

Clonidine

MOA: an alpha-2 adrenergic agonist; it controls symptoms of autonomic dysfunction through decreased sympathetic outflow from CNS
SEs: decrease in peripheral resistance, muscle relaxation, hypotension, bradycardia, and renal vascular resistance
- Disadvantage: less commonly used in spasticity given the side effects

Tizanidine

MOA: a central alpha-2 adrenergic agonist; increases presynaptic inhibition, reducing facilitation of spinal motor neurons
SEs: hypotension, drowsiness, dizziness, xerostomia, bradycardia
- Disadvantage: requires monitoring of liver function, blood pressure, renal function

Calcium Channel

Dantrolene

MOA: interferes with excitation-contraction coupling in the muscle fiber by preventing release of calcium and thereby decreasing catabolic processes and spasticity
SEs: flushing, drowsiness, dysphagia, nausea, vomiting, hepatitis
- Disadvantage: has potential for hepatotoxicity and requires regular liver function tests

Marijuana/Tetrahydrocannabinol

- Animal studies have identified activation of cannabinoid type 1 receptor, resulting in reduction in glutaminergic transmission and thus in reduction of spasticity.
- In humans, the data for use in spasticity is inconsistent and confounded by the multiple cannabinoid products; future studies are required to adequately assess the usefulness in spasticity.[16CC]

Neurotoxins

Botulinum Toxin A

MOA: binds to the c-terminus of the SNAP-25 protein
Examples: onabotulinum toxin A, incobotulinum toxin A, abobotulinum toxin A
SEs: weakness, anaphylaxis[16E]
- Advantage: works locally with few if any systemic side effects
- Disadvantage: effects last 2 to 6 months

Antibiotics

The use of antibiotics in the TBI population requires understanding of a few special principles. Those issues are described here:
- Beta-lactams (e.g., penicillins and cephalosporins) can lower seizure thresholds at high doses that penetrate the CNS or in patients with renal failure. The mechanism is thought to be through interfering with the inhibitory effects of GABA. The overall risk is thought to be low.[17]
- Carbapenems readily penetrate the CNS and have an increased risk of seizure over the other beta-lactams through the same mechanism. In addition, they can significantly decrease valproic acid serum levels; therefore, their concomitant use is not recommended or an additional antiseizure medication should be administered.[17]
- Fluoroquinolones have been implicated in seizure risk in patients with renal dysfunction. Fluoroquinolones have also been known to cause encephalopathies and delirium, which can be difficult to separate from posttraumatic confusion.[17]

Sedatives/Hypnotics

There are a number of possible reasons for the administration of these medications in the TBI population. Specific medications that are commonly used are described here.

Benzodiazepines

MOA: bind to GABA receptors and enhance the inhibitory effect of GABA; enhance inhibitory effect of GABA through increased neuronal permeability to chloride ions[16C]
Examples: lorazepam, diazepam, alprazolam, clonazepam
SEs: drowsiness, hypotension, dizziness, amnesia, disinhibition, agitation, respiratory depression, dependency/abuse, confusion, hypotension
- Disadvantage: relatively contraindicated in brain injury patients because of high risk of delirium, memory impairment,[16] falls, and neurological recovery delay

Beta Blockers

MOA: antagonize beta receptors
Examples: propranolol, carvedilol
SEs: Hypotension, bradycardia, dizziness, fatigue
- Advantage: Propranolol is considered first-line treatment for posttraumatic agitation/aggression; its CNS effects

are a result of its highly lipophilic nature thus allowing it to readily cross the blood-brain barrier; the desired clinical effect for posttraumatic agitation often requires higher doses (200–400 mg/day).[17A,17B]
- Advantage: Propranolol may also improve autonomic dysfunction in patients with severe TBI and paroxysmal sympathetic hyperactivity.[17C]

Doxepin

MOA: tricyclic antidepressant that has potent histamine (H1) antagonist effects at very low doses.
SEs: nausea, xerostomia, dizziness, hypertension, orthostatic hypotension, cardiac arrhythmias, extrapyramidal symptoms

GABA A–Positive Allosteric Modulators or "Z Drugs"

MOA: GABA A receptor agonist (specific sedating effects are induced via the α1 subtype)
Examples: zolpidem, zaleplon, zopiclone, eszopiclone
SEs: nausea, vomiting, drowsiness, anxiety, confusion complex sleep-related behavior, hallucinations, possible amnesia
- Advantage: similar to benzodiazepines, but they bind to GABA A receptors in a different manner; this reduces the risk of tolerance, dependence, and/or withdrawal; potential for complications remains however[18]
- Advantage: Immediate-release formulations have a duration of action of 2 to 4 hours and facilitate sleep initiation more so than sleep maintenance.
- Advantage: The controlled-release formulations' duration of action is 6 to 8 hours and therefore be more effective for sleep maintenance.

Melatonin

MOA: acts on melatonin receptors (MT1 and MT2) in the suprachiasmatic nucleus to induce sleep and facilitate normal circadian rhythms
SEs: usually benign, can cause nightmares, hallucinations, confusion, and vertigo
- Disadvantage: optimal dosing in the brain injury population is unclear; the unregulated and variable dosing of over-the-counter (OTC) formulations further complicates this issue

Prazosin

MOA: alpha-1 blocker; alpha-1 adrenergic receptor antagonist
SEs: Dizziness, headaches, drowsiness, weakness
- Mixed research on benefit for PTSD[18A]

Ramelteon

MOA: melatonin receptor (MT1 and MT2) agonist
SEs: drowsiness, dizziness

Suvorexant

MOA: antagonizes orexin 1 and orexin 2 receptors (dual orexin receptor antagonist), thereby facilitating both sleep initiation and maintenance

SEs: headaches, dizziness, abnormal dreams, diarrhea, xerostomia, cough, upper respiratory infection

Trazodone

MOA: at low doses, it acts as an effective sleep aid through its antagonism of serotonin (5HT2A), histamine (H1), and adrenergic (α1) receptors.[19,20]

SEs: orthostatic hypotension, nausea, vomiting, QT prolongation, priapism

Neurostimulants/Cognitive Enhancers

There remains tremendous optimism in the rehabilitation field for medications to improve cognition or aspects of cognitive function after a TBI. As best described by Wortzel and Arciniegas,[21] pharmacological interventions should be "best regarded as adjunctive to nonpharmacologic interventions." Nonpharmacological cognitive interventions are prioritized given that most of the studies involving pharmacological interventions for cognition are rather small and somewhat underwhelming.[22]

Amantadine

MOA: increases pre- and postsynaptic dopamine, dopamine receptor agonist, and uncompetitive N-methyl-D-aspartate (NMDA) receptor antagonist

SEs: orthostatic hypotension, dizziness, hallucinations, xerostomia, livedo reticularis, congestive heart failure exacerbation, neuroleptic malignant syndrome (with abrupt discontinuation)

- Advantage: often used in the TBI population for hypoarousal, akathisia, parkinsonism, impaired cognition, and posttraumatic agitation.[23,24]
- Advantage: The best evidence lies in the disorders of consciousness population in which a randomized clinical trial found improvements in patients who were vegetative or minimally conscious.[25]
- Disadvantage: A study of TBI patients who did not have a disorder of consciousness found no consistent cognitive improvement with amantadine.[26]
- Disadvantage: must be renally adjusted based on creatinine clearance

Bromocriptine

MOA: D2 receptor agonist

SEs: dizziness, nausea, diarrhea, hypotension, hypoglycemia

- Advantage: Improves executive function in TBI patients[27]
- Advantage: Due to its propensity to lower blood pressure, it is a good neurostimulant option for patients who are experiencing dysautonomia.

- Disadvantage: may result in orthostatic hypotension in some patients

Dextroamphetamine/Amphetamine

MOA: promotes the release and inhibits the reuptake of norepinephrine and dopamine

SEs: hypertension, tachycardia, irritability, insomnia, appetite suppression

- Advantage: similar indications as methylphenidate but with less research

Donepezil

MOA: acetylcholinesterase inhibitors

SEs: nightmares, anorexia, nausea, vomiting

- Advantage: Donepezil may help with attention, working memory, and executive dysfunction, so it is often used in TBI.[28,29]
- Advantage: Donepezil works centrally with minimal peripheral activity and may have fewer side effects than rivastigmine.
- Advantage: It is often given in the morning to improve performance during the day and limit nightmares.

Levodopa/Carbidopa

MOA: Levodopa crosses the blood-brain barrier and serves as a dopamine precursor; carbidopa inhibits the peripheral metabolism of levodopa by inhibiting decarboxylation thereby increasing plasma levodopa levels.

SEs: orthostasis, nausea, hallucinations

- Advantage: can be used as a neurostimulant and/or for parkinsonism following brain injury

Memantine

MOA: strong NMDA receptor antagonist

SEs: tiredness, body aches, joint pain, dizziness, nausea, vomiting, diarrhea, constipation

- Advantage: benefit may have more to do with slowing secondary damage than improving the function in TBI

Methylphenidate

MOA: promotes the release and inhibits the reuptake of norepinephrine and dopamine

SEs: Hypertension, tachycardia, irritability, insomnia, appetite suppression

- Advantage: Studies in TBI population have demonstrated improvement in attention, poor initiation, hypoarousal, aphasia, executive dysfunction, depression, and apathy in TBI samples.[30-34A]
- Advantage: also has antidepressant properties as described in the Antidepressants section
- Advantage: Methylphenidate is not found to increase the risk of seizures in the TBI population.[32]

Modafinil

MOA: exact mechanism not clear; increases dopamine by blocking dopamine transporters
SEs: dizziness, anxiety, insomnia
- Advantage: Food and Drug Administration (FDA)–approved indications are obstructive sleep apnea, narcolepsy, and shift work-related sleep disorder.
- Advantage: commonly used off label for hypoarousal and disorders of consciousness in the brain injury population[35]
- See the Antifatigue Agents section for more information.

Rivastigmine

MOA: an acetylcholinesterase inhibitor
SEs: Anorexia, nausea, vomiting
- Advantage: Rivastigmine is typically tasked with improving attention, working memory, and executive dysfunction in TBI.[36]
- Disadvantage: It may have more side effects than donepezil.

Antidepressants

Selective Serotonin Reuptake Inhibitors

Selective serotonin reuptake inhibitors (SSRIs)are indicated for various neuropsychiatric disorders that may arise following a brain injury, including depression, anxiety, emotional lability, pathological laughing and crying, and posttraumatic agitation.

Among the SSRIs, there is considerable overlap in terms of side effect profiles, all possessing a sizeable risk of dizziness, insomnia, diarrhea, syndrome of inappropriate antidiuretic hormone secretion (SIADH), QT prolongation, and sexual dysfunction. Platelet inhibition and hemorrhage is another known effect, however the clinical implications vis-à-vis intracranial hemorrhage are not clear.

Each individual SSRI is noted to have distinct secondary pharmacological properties that result in additional unique therapeutic and adverse effects.

Citalopram
- Advantage: generally well tolerated
- Disadvantage: It has a high (maybe the highest) risk of QT prolongation of all SSRIs.[37]

Escitalopram
- Advantage: It is considered to have the most favorable SE profile of all SSRIs.
- Disadvantage: likely prolongs the QT interval[37] (Ojero-Senard)

Fluoxetine
- Advantage: the most activating of the SSRIs
- Advantage: It has demonstrated neurorecovery properties in stroke patients.[37A]
- Advantage: low risk of withdrawal symptoms upon abrupt discontinuation because of very long half-life

- Disadvantage: many drug interactions because of CYP450 inhibition

Paroxetine
- Disadvantage: It has limited utility in the brain injury population because of anticholinergic effects.

Sertraline
- Advantage: may be somewhat activating
- Advantage: well studied in TBI population[38,38A] (Fann)
- Advantage: may help with aggression and irritability after TBI[39]
- Disadvantage: lower risk of QT prolongation compared with other SSRIs

Serotonin-Norepinephrine Reuptake Inhibitors

- Serotonin-norepinephrine reuptake inhibitors (SNRIs) are covered also in the Analgesics section.

Duloxetine

MOA: potent serotonin and norepinephrine reuptake inhibition; weak dopamine reuptake inhibition
SEs: nausea, headaches, fatigue
- Advantage: FDA approved for a variety of pain syndromes
- Advantage: less sedating than most other agents used for neuropathic pain

Venlafaxine

MOA: potent serotonin and norepinephrine reuptake inhibition, weak dopamine reuptake inhibition
SEs: nausea, insomnia, dizziness, hypertension
- Advantage: The extended-release formulation is better tolerated than the immediate-release formulation.
- Advantage: Metabolically, venlafaxine is converted into the active metabolite desvenlafaxine (another SNRI).

Tricyclic Antidepressants

Although very effective antidepressants because of their serotonin and norepinephrine reuptake inhibition, tricyclic antidepressants (TCAs) should be used with caution after a TBI because of the anticholinergic, antihistaminic, and alpha-1 adrenergic effects; see Table 59.2 for a list of tricyclic antidepressants.
- TCAs are associated with an increased risk of cardiac arrhythmias and seizures.
- Amitriptyline has been used in TBI-related agitation [40] and for posttraumatic headaches.[8]
- TCAs are also covered in the Analgesics section.

Other Antidepressants
Bupropion

MOA: several proposed mechanisms: norepinephrine-dopamine reuptake inhibitor (NDRI) or dopaminergic and serotonergic agonist[40A]

SEs: insomnia, headache, agitation, dizziness, xerostomia, weight loss, seizures

- Disadvantage: contraindicated in patients with history of seizures, which limits utility in the severe brain injury population

Methylphenidate

MOA: promotes the release and inhibits the reuptake of norepinephrine and dopamine

SEs: hypertension, tachycardia, irritability, insomnia, appetite suppression

- Advantage: Methylphenidate is proven to be an effective antidepressants in the TBI population, especially as an augment to SSRIs.[38]
- Covered in the Neurostimulants/Cognitive Enhancers section.

Mirtazapine

MOA: noradrenergic and specific serotonin antidepressant (NaSSA); blocks presynaptic alpha-2 adrenergic receptors, thereby increasing the release of serotonin and norepinephrine; also blocks serotonin and histamine receptors

SEs: drowsiness, xerostomia, weight gain

- Advantage: can also be used as an effective appetite stimulant at low doses (typically 7.5 mg)[41]

Agents for Pathological Laughing and Crying

Pathological laughing and crying (PLC) or pseudobulbar affective disorder (PSA) are well recognized after TBI. SSRIs should be considered first line for PLC given effectiveness and rapid onset (often within a few days). TCAs, neurostimulants (amantadine, methylphenidate), and dextromethorphan/quinidine are also reasonable options.[41A]

Antipsychotics

Typical (First-Generation) Antipsychotics

- The typical antipsychotics act via widespread blocking of D2 receptors; very effective at controlling the positive symptoms of psychosis
- These drugs are associated with numerous undesirable side effects, including sedation, cognitive impairment, apathy, akathisia, hyperprolactinemia, anticholinergic effects, and movement disorders/extrapyramidal symptoms.
- These drugs may be used in the setting of acute agitation/aggression but are otherwise of very limited utility in the brain injury population.
- Haloperidol is the most commonly used typical antipsychotic.
- The authors of this chapter encourage you to use these medications as little as possible.

Haloperidol

MOA: widespread blocking of D2 receptors

SEs: Sedation, cognitive impairment, apathy, akathisia, hyperprolactinemia, anticholinergic effects, and movement disorders/extrapyramidal symptoms

- Disadvantage: likely prolongs the duration of posttraumatic amnesia (PTA) and may slow recovery[42,42A]

Atypical (Second-Generation) Antipsychotics

- Like the typical antipsychotics, the atypical antipsychotics are effective at managing psychosis by blocking D2 receptors.
- Unlike the typical antipsychotics, however, these drugs also possess serotonin receptor antagonist activity that affords a lower risk of extrapyramidal symptoms and hyperprolactinemia.
- Atypical antipsychotics are more likely than the typical antipsychotics to cause cardiometabolic problems, including weight gain, hypertension, diabetes, elevated lipids, etc.
- Each of the specific agents within this class has unique properties and actions that may be useful for certain neurobehavioral sequelae after brain injury.

Aripiprazole

- Advantage: Unique MOA (partial D2 agonist) may help with depression.[42B]

Clozapine

- Advantage: may improve aggression and psychosis in TBI
- Disadvantage: hematological risk of life-threatening agranulocytosis[43] and sedation

Olanzapine

- Advantage: may improve post-TBI psychosis[44,45]
- Disadvantage: sedating and typically causes weight gain[46]

Quetiapine

- Advantage: may decrease irritability, aggression, and psychosis[47]
- Advantage: Questionable improvement in cognitive function
- Advantage: dose-dependent effect: sedative, antidepressant, antipsychotic
- Disadvantage: sedation and weight gain common[46]

Risperidone

- Disadvantage: high risk of hyperprolactinemia
- Disadvantage: high risk of extrapyramidal syndrome

Ziprasidone

- Advantage: may help with rapid deescalation of aggressive behavior
- Disadvantage: increased risk of QT prolongation[48] (Addiow)[46]

Anxiolytics/Mood Stabilizers

Because anxiety and labile mood are often present after brain injury, neuropharmacological management is often attempted.

This section will mention a few of the more common medications that can be used, but it should be stressed that the first-line approach should be psychological interventions, counseling, environmental strategies, and meditation.

Buspirone

MOA: unknown but likely related to its affinity for serotonin (5-HT1A) receptors
SEs: dizziness, nausea, headache, nervousness, lightheadedness, drowsiness, feeling tired, blurred vision

Divalproex

MOA: increases availability of GABA to neurons, blocks sodium channels and therefore decreases repetitive neuronal firing
SEs: headache, drowsiness, nausea, thrombocytopenia, diplopia
- Advantage: Although also used for seizures and migraine, divalproex and its cousin valproic acid are often used as mood stabilizers in TBI.[49]

Lithium

MOA: unknown, but lithium interacts throughout the CNS and is thought to decrease norepinephrine release and increase serotonin synthesis
SEs: tremor, increased thirst, increased urination, diarrhea, vomiting, weight gain, impaired memory

Valproic Acid

MOA: increases availability of GABA to neurons, blocks sodium channels and therefore decreases repetitive neuronal firing
SEs: headache, drowsiness, nausea, thrombocytopenia, diplopia
- Advantage: Serum levels can be checked to assist in preventing toxicity.
- Advantage: Wroblewski[50] presented a case series that demonstrated improvements in depression and mania in TBI patients
- Advantage: In a study by Dikmen et al,[11] valproate did not result in changes in cognition in a TBI sample; this may make valproic acid a good choice for those working on cognitive improvement
- Advantage: potent antiepileptic as discussed in the Anticonvulsants/Antiepileptic Medications section

Antifatigue Agents

Fatigue is a common complaint after TBI, but there has been little success with pharmacological interventions.

Modafinil

MOA: exact mechanism not clear; increases dopamine by blocking dopamine transporters
SEs: dizziness, anxiety, insomnia

- Disadvantages: often used to assist with somnolence and posttraumatic narcolepsy; research with TBI populations is inconsistent[51] (Castriotta) [52] (Kaiser) [53] (Jha)
- See section L for more information

Zolpidem

MOA: GABA A receptor agonist (specific sedating effects are induced via the alpha-1 subtype)
SEs: nausea, vomiting, drowsiness, anxiety, confusion, complex sleep-related behavior, hallucinations, possible amnesia
- Disadvantage: Despite evidence for improving consciousness in patients with disorders of consciousness,[53A] there is no evidence for improvement in fatigue or other psychological complaints (nonsleep issues) in TBI.[53AA]

Problematic Medications

Histamine-2 Blockers

Histamine-2 blockers, including cimetidine, famotidine, nizatidine, ranitidine, and others, are often used to assist with gastroesophageal reflux disorder, gastritis, and gastrointestinal prophylaxis. There is a risk of worsening delirium and confusion with these medications.

Metoclopramide

Metoclopramide is often used for poor gastric motility. It has been observed to cause cognitive deficits and extrapyramidal side effects.

Opioids

Opioids are available in too numerous in formulation to name. Opioids are covered briefly in the Analgesics section. Although often necessary to control pain, they may cause somnolence, dizziness, and addiction. Recent epidemiological research indicates that TBI may make addiction more likely, thus the need to monitor closely.[53AB]

Tricyclic Antidepressants

Covered in the tend to have anticholinergic properties and should be avoided if possible.

Benzodiazepines

Benzodiazepines are thought to worsen cognitive deficits after TBI and increase somnolence. Please see the Hypnotics section for more information.

Anticholinergic Medications

Anticholinergic medications are covered in various earlier sections. All medications with anticholinergic properties may cause anticholinergic side effects. There are peripheral

TABLE 59.3	Common Anticholinergic Medications		
Amitriptyline	Atropine	Benztropine	Carisoprodol
Chlorpheniramine	Chlorpromazine	Cyclobenzaprine	Cyproheptadine
Dicyclomine	Diphenhydramine	Doxepin	Fluphenazine
Hydroxyzine	Imipramine	Loratadine	Meclizine
Metaxalone	Methocarbamol	Oxybutynin	Perphenazine
Promethazine	Scopolamine	Thioridazine	Tizanidine

anticholinergic effects such as decreased salivation, decreased bronchial secretions, and increased heart rate. There are central effects such as impaired concentration, confusion, attention deficit, and memory impairment. It is the central effects that are often problematic in the TBI population. See Table 59.3 for a list of anticholinergic medications.

In summary, neuropharmacology is a growing and ever-changing field of study. Many reviews have been previously published, and those reviews may serve as a good starting point for further education.[22,53B,53C,53D,54E] The information in this chapter should be taken at face value

and with the understanding that every patient reacts to every medication in a unique way that often changes as the patient changes and their brain heals. This may depend a great deal on who the patient was before the brain injury and the nature and severity of the brain injury itself. Furthermore, those interested in the care of the brain injuries should always respect the dangers of polypharmacy. We recommend regular review of the Beers criteria of the American Geriatric Society[53F] and minimization or avoidance of medications on the Beers criteria without strong reason to administer and/or expert guidance.

Review Questions

1. Which of these medications is known to place a patient at higher risk of seizures?
   a. Hydrocodone
   b. Tramadol
   c. Gabapentin
   d. Methylphenidate

2. A 45-year-old man was involved in a high-speed motor vehicle accident with documented seizure by emergency medical services (EMS) shortly after the wreck. Which option is most appropriate to control his seizures and maximize his cognitive recovery?
   a. 3 to 6 months of phenytoin
   b. Indefinite antiepileptic treatment with valproic acid
   c. No antiepileptic medication
   d. 1 week of levetiracetam

3. A 26-year-old woman with a history of moderate TBI and posttraumatic epilepsy with new-onset trigeminal neuralgia presents to your office. To prevent polypharmacy, which of these medications may be the best option to control her pain?
   a. Carbamazepine
   b. Oxycodone
   c. Levetiracetam
   d. Diazepam

Answers on page 403.
Access the full list of questions and answers online.
Available on ExpertConsult.com

References

1. Dobscha SK, Clark ME, Morasco BJ, Freeman M, Campbell R, Helfand M. Systematic review of the literature on pain in patients with polytrauma including traumatic brain injury. *Pain Med.* 2009;10(7):1200-1217.
2. Micromedex® (electronic version). Greenwood Village, CO: IBM Watson Health. Available at: https://www.micromedexsolutions.com/.
3. Lexicomp Online, Lexi-Drugs, Hudson, Ohio: Wolters Kluwer Clinical Drug Information, Inc.; 2019; February 3, 2019. ** Note: Applies to all mechanism of action and side effect descriptions except where noted**
4. Watanabe TK, Bell KR, Walker WC, Schomer K. Systematic review of interventions for post-traumatic headache. *PM&R.* 2012;4:129-140.

4A. Trelle S, Reichenbach S, Wandel S, et al. Cardiovascular safety of non-steroidal anti-inflammatory drugs: network meta-analysis. *BMJ.* 2011;342:1-11.
6A. Quilici S, Chancellor J, Löthgren M, et al. Meta-analysis of duloxetine vs. pregabalin and gabapentin in the treatment of diabetic peripheral neuropathic pain. *BCM Neurology.* 2009;9(6):1-14.
7. Packard RC. Treatment of chronic daily posttraumatic headache with divalproex sodium. *Headache.* 2000;40:736-739.
7A. Baldessarini RJ. Drug therapy of depression and anxiety disorders. In: Brunton LL, ed. *Goodman & Gilman's The Pharmacological Basis of Therapeutics.* 11th ed. New York, NY: McGraw-Hill Companies; 2006:429-459.
8. Erickson JC, Neely ET, Theeler BJ. Posttraumatic headache. *Continuum.* 2010;16(6):55-78.

9. Temkin NR, Dikmen SS, Winn HR. Posttraumatic Seizures. *Neurosurg Clin North Am.* 1991;2(2):425-435.

10. Dikmen SS, Temkin NR, Miller B, Machamer J, Winn HR. Neurobehavioral effects of phenytoin prophylaxis of post-traumatic seizures. *JAMA.* 1991;265(10):1271-1277.

11. Dikmen SS, Machamer JE, Winn HR, Anderson GD, Temkin NR. Neuropsychological effects of valproate in traumatic brain injury. *Neurology.* 2000;54:895-902.

12. Temkin NR, Dikmen SS, Anderson GD, et al. Valproate therapy for prevention of posttraumatic seizures: a randomized trial. *J Neurosurg.* 1999;91:593-600.

12A. Chang BS, Lowenstein DH. Practice parameter: Antiepileptic drug prophylaxis in severe traumatic brain injury. *Neurology.* 2003;60:10-16.

13. Sills GJ. Mechanisms of action of antiepileptic drugs. In: Sander JW, Walker MC, Smalls JE, eds. *Epilepsy 2011: From Science to Society. A Practical Guide to Epilepsy.* London, UK: ILAE; 2011.

14. Baguley IJ, Heriseanu RE, Gurka JA, Nordenbo A, Cameron ID. Gabapentin in the management of dysautonomia following severe traumatic brain injury: a case series. *J Neurol Neurosurg Psychiatry.* 2007;78:539-541.

14A. Kanner AM, Ashman E, Gloss D, et al. Practice guideline update summary: efficacy and tolerability of the new antiepileptic drugs I: treatment of new-onset epilepsy. *Epilepsy Curr.* 2018;18(4):260-268.

15. Zimmermann LL, Martin RM, Girgis F. Treatment options for posttraumatic epilepsy. *Curr Opin Neurol.* 2017;30(6):580-586.

15A. Zafar SN, Khan AA, Ghauri AA, Shamim MS. Phenytoin versus levetiracetam for seizure prophylaxis after brain injury—a meta analysis. *BCM Neurol.* 2012;12:30-38.

15B. Glauser T, Shinnar S, Gloss D, et al. Evidence-based guideline: Treatment of convulsive status epilepticus in children and adults: Report of the guideline committee of the American Epilepsy Society. *Epilepsy Curr.* 2016;16(1):48-61.

16. Levy M, Berson A, Cook T, et al. Treatment of agitation following traumatic brain injury: a review of the literature. *Neurorehabilitation.* 2005;20:279-306.

16A. Noh Y, Kim DW, Chu K, et al. Topiramate increases the risk of valproic acid-induced encephalopathy. *Epilepsia.* 2013;54(1):e1-e4.

16B. Chou R, Peterson K, Helfand M. Comparative efficacy and safety of skeletal muscle relaxants for spasticity and musculoskeletal conditions: a systematic review. *J Pain Symptom Manage.* 2004;28(2):140-175.

16C. Coffey RJ, Edgar TS, Francisco GE, et al. Abrupt withdrawal from intrathecal baclofen: recognition and management of a potentially life-threatening syndrome. *Arch Phys Med Rehabil.* 2002;83:735-741.

16CC. Nielsen S, Murnion B, Campbell G, Young H, Hall W. Cannabinoids for the treatment of spasticity. Dev Med Child Neurol. 2019;61(6):631-638. doi:10.1111/dmcn.14165.

16D. Costa E, Guidotti A, Mao CC, Suria A. New concepts on the mechanism of action of benzodiazepines. *Life Sci.* 1975;17:167-185.

16E. Anton C. Botulinum toxins: adverse effects. *Adverse Drug Reaction Bulletin.* 2011;267:1027- 1030.

17. Sutter R, Rüegg S, Tschudin-Sutter S. Seizures as adverse events of antibiotic drugs: a systematic review. *Neurology.* 2015;85(15):1332-1341.

17A. Fleminger S, Greenwood RJ, Oliver DL. Pharmacological management for agitation and aggression in people with acquired brain injury. *Cochrane Database Systemic Review.* 2006; 18 (4).

17B. Brooke MM, Patterson DR, Questad KA, Cardenas D, Farrel-Roberts L. The treatment of agitation during initial hospitalization after traumatic brain injury. *Arch Phys Med Rehabil.* 1992;73(10):917-921.

17C. Schroeppel TJ, Sharpe JP, Magnotti LJ, et al. Traumatic brain injury and β-blockers: not all drugs are created equal. *J Trauma Acute Care Surg.* 2014;76(2):504-509.

18. Li Pi Shan RS, Ashworth NL. Comparison of lorazepam and zopiclone for insomnia in patients with stroke and brain injury: a randomized, crossover, double-blinded trial. *Am J Phys Med Rehab.* 2004; 83 (6): 421-427.

18A. Raskin MA, Peskind ER, Chow B, et al. Trial of prazosin for post-traumatic stress disorder in military veterans. *N Engl J Med.* 2018;378:507-517.

19. Stahl SM. Mechanism of action of trazodone: a multifunctional drug. *CNS Spectr.* 2009;14(10):536-546.

20. Stahl, Stephen M. "Mechanism of action of trazodone: a multifunctional drug." Psychopharmacology Educational Updates, vol. 6, no. 3, Mar. 2010. Gale OneFile: Health and Medicine, https://link.gale.com/apps/doc/A238349063/HRCA?u=txshracd2509&sid=HRCA&xid=79d73ce8. Accessed 23 Apr. 2020

21. Wortzel HS, Arciniegas DB. Treatment of post-traumatic cognitive impairments. *Curr Treat Options Neurol.* 2012;14:493-508.

22. Chew E, Zafonte RD. Pharmacological management of neurobehavioral disorders following traumatic brain injury—a state-of-the-art review. *J Rehabil Res Dev.* 2009;46(6):851-878.

23. Al-Adawi S, Hoaglin H, Vesali F, Dorvlo AS, Burke DT. Effect of amantadine on the sleep-wake cycle of an inpatient with brain injury. *Brain Inj.* 2009;23(6):559-565.

24. Meythaler JM, Brunner RC, Johnson A, Novack TA. Amantadine to improve neurorecovery in traumatic brain injury—associated diffuse axonal injury: a pilot double-blind randomized trial. *J Head Trauma Rehabil.* 2002:17(4);300-313.

25. Giacino JT, Whyte J, Bagiella E, et al. Placebo-controlled trial of amantadine for severe traumatic brain injury. *N Engl J Med.* 2012;366(9):819-826.

26. Hammond FM, Sherer M, Malec JF, et al. Amantadine did not positively impact cognition in chronic traumatic brain injury: a multi-site, randomized, controlled trial. *J Neurotrauma.* 2018;35(19):2298-2305.

27. McDowell S, Whyte J, D'Esposito M. Differential effect of a dopaminergic agonist on prefrontal function in traumatic brain injury patients. *Brain.* 1998;121:115-1164.

28. Zhang L, Plotkin RC, Wang G, Sandel ME, Lee S. Cholinergic augmentation with donepezil enhances recovery in short-term memory and sustained attention after traumatic brain injury. *Arch Phys Med Rehabil.* 2004;85:1050-1055.

29. Ballesteros J, Güemes I, Ibarra N, Quemada JI. The effectiveness of donepezil for cognitive rehabilitation after traumatic brain injury: a systematic review. *J Head Trauma Rehabil.* 2008;23(3):171 180.

30. Whyte J, Hart T, Schuster K, Fleming M, Polansky M, Coslett HB. Effects of methylphenidate on attentional function after traumatic brain injury. A randomized, placebo-controlled trial. *Am J Phys Med Rehabil.* 1997;76(6):440-450.

31. Whyte J, Hart T, Vaccaro M, et al. Effects of methylphenidate on attention deficits after traumatic brain injury a multidimensional, randomized, controlled trial. *Am J Phys Med Rehabil.* 2004;83(6):401-420.

32. Willmott C, Ponsford J. Efficacy of methylphenidate in the rehabilitation of attention following traumatic brain injury: a randomized, crossover, double blind, placebo controlled inpatient trial. *J Neurol Neurosurg Psychiatry.* 2009;80(5):552-557.

33. Gualtieri CT, Evans RW. Stimulant treatment for the neurobehavioural sequalae of traumatic brain injury. *Brain Inj.* 1998;2(4):273-290.

34. Kaelin DL, Cifu DX, Matthies B. Methylphenidate effect on attention deficit in the acutely brain-injured adult. *Arch Phys Med Rehabil.* 1996;77:6-9.

34A. Hornstein A, Lennihan L, Seliger G, Lichtman S, Schroeder K. Amphetamine in recovery from brain injury. *Brain Inj.* 1996;10(2):145-148.

35. Teitelman E. Off-label uses of modafinil. *Psychiatry Online.* 2001;158(8):1341. doi:10.1176/ajp.158.8.1341.

36. Silver JM, Koumaras B, Chen M, et al. Effects of rivastigmine on cognitive function in patients with traumatic brain injury. *Neurology.* 2006;67:748-755.

37. Ojero-Senard A, Benevent J, Bondon-Guitton E, et al. A comparative study of QT prolongation with serotonin reuptake inhibitors. *Psychopharmacology.* 2017;234:3075-3081.

37A. Chollet F, Tardy J, Albucher JF, et al. Fluoxetine for motor recovery after acute ischaemic stroke (FLAME): a randomised placebo-controlled trial. *Lancet Neurol.* 2011;10(2):123-130.

38. Lee H, Kim SW, Kim JM, Shin IS, Yang SJ, Yoon JS. Comparing effects of methylphenidate, sertraline, and placebo on neuropsychiatric sequelae in patients with traumatic brain injury. *Hum Psychopharmacol.* 2005;20:97-104.

38A. Fann JR. Uomoto JM, Katon WJ. Sertraline in the treatment of major depression following mild traumatic brain injury. *J Neuropsychiatry Clin Neurosci.* 2000;12(2):226-232.

39. Kant R, Smith-Seemiller L, Zeiler D. Treatment of aggression and irritability after head injury. *Brain Inj.* 1998:12(8):661-666.

40. Mysiw WJ, Jackson RD, Corrigan JD. Amitriptyline for posttraumatic agitation. *Am J Phys Med Rehabil.* 1988;67:29-33.

40A. Eison, AS, Temple DL. Buspirone: Review of its pharmacology and current perspectives on its mechanism of action. *Am J Med.* 1986;80(S3B):1-9.

41. Anttila SA, Leinonen EV. A review of the pharmacological and clinical profile of mirtazapine. *CNS Drug Rev.* 2001;7(3):249-264.

41A. Arciniegas DB, Wortzel HS. Emotional and behavioral dyscontrol after traumatic brain injury. *Psychiatr Clin North Am.* 2014;37(1):31-53.

42. Mysiw WJ, Bogner JA, Corrigan JD, Fugate LP, Clinchot DM, Kadyan V. The impact of acute care medications on rehabilitation outcome after traumatic brain injury. *Brain Inj.* 2006;20(9):905-911.

42A. Rao N, Jellinek HM, Woolston DC. Agitation in closed head injury: haloperidol effects on rehabilitation outcomes. Arch Phys Med Rehabil. 1985;66:30-34.

42B. Berman RM, Fava M, Thase ME, et al. Aripiprazole augmentation in major depressive disorder: a double-blind, placebo-controlled study in patients with inadequate response to antidepressants. *CNS Spectr.* 2009;14(4):197-206.

43. Michals ML, Crismon ML, Roberts S, Childs A. Clozapine response and adverse effects in nine brain-injured patients. *J Clin Psychopharmacol.* 1993;13:198-203.

44. Viana Bde M, Prais HA, Nicolato R, Caramelli P. Posttraumatic brain injury psychosis successfully treated with olanzapine. *Prog Neuropsychopharmacol Biol Psychiatry.* 2010;34:233-235.

45. Umansky R, Geller V. Olanzapine treatment in an organic hallucinosis patient. *Int J Neuropsychopharmacology.* 2000;3(1):81-82.

46. Elovic EP, Jasey NN Jr, Eisenberg ME. The use of atypical antipsychotics after traumatic brain injury. *J Head Trauma Rehabil.* 2008;23(2):132-135.

47. Kim E, Bijlani M. A pilot study of quetiapine treatment of aggression due to traumatic brain injury. *J Neuropsychiatry Clin Neurosci.* 2006;18(4):547-549.

48. Addiow WS, Shamliyan TA. Effects of atypical antipsychotic drugs on QT interval in patients with mental disorders. *Ann Transl Med.* 2018;6(8):147.

49. Chatham Showalter, PE, Netsky Kimmel D. Agitated symptom response to divalproex following acute brain injury. *J Neuropsychiatry Clin Neurosci.* 2000;12(3):395-397

50. Wroblewski BA, Joseph AB, Kupfer J, Kalliel K. Effectiveness of valproic acid on destructive and aggressive behaviours in patients with acquired brain injury. *Brain Inj.* 1997;11(1):36-47.

51. Castriotta RJ, Atanasov S, Wilde MC, Masel BE, Lai JM, Kuna ST. Treatment of sleep disorders after traumatic brain injury. *J Clin Sleep Med.* 2009;5(2):137-144.

52. Kaiser PR, Valko PO, Werth E, et al. Modafinil ameliorates excessive daytime sleepiness after traumatic brain injury. *Neurology.* 2010;75:1780-1785.

53. Jha A, Weintraub A, Allshouse A, et al. A randomized trial of modafinil for the treatment of fatigue and excessive daytime sleepiness in individuals with chronic traumatic brain injury. *J Head Trauma Rehabil.* 2008;23(1):52-63.

53A. Whyte J, Myers R. Incidence of clinically significant responses to zolpidem among patients with disorders of consciousness: A preliminary placebo controlled trial. *Am J Phys Med Rehab.* 2009;88(5):410-418.

53AA. Larson EB, Zollman FS. The effect of sleep medications on cognitive recovery from traumatic brain injury. *J Head Trauma Rehabil.* 2010;25(1):61-67.

53AB. Miller SC, Baktash SH, Webb TS, et al. Risk for addition-related disorders following mild traumatic brain injury in a large cohort of active-duty US airmen. *Am J Psychiatry.* 2013; 170:383-390.

53B. Arciniegas DB, Topkoff J, Silver JM. Neuropsychiatric aspects of traumatic brain injury. *Curr Treat Options Neurol.* 2000; 2:169-186.

53C. Lee HB, Lyketsos CG, Rao V. Pharmacological management of the psychiatric aspects of traumatic brain injury. *Int Rev Psychiatry.* 2003;15:359-370.

53D. Liepert J. Pharmacotherapy in restorative neurology. *Curr Opin Neurol.* 2008;21:639-643.

53E. Writer BW, Schillerstrom JE. Psychopharmacological treatment for cognitive impairment in survivors of traumatic brain injury: A critical review. *J Neuropsychiatry Clin Neurosci.* 2009;21(4):362-370.

53F. American Geriatrics Society. American Geriatrics Society 2015 Updated Beers Criteria for potentially inappropriate medication use in older adults. *J Am Geriatr Soc.* 2015.

54. Akyuz G, Kenis O. Physical therapy modalities and rehabilitation techniques in the management of neuropathic pain. *Am J Phys Med Rehabil.* 2014;93(3):253-259.

55. Feine JS, Lund JP. An assessment of the efficacy of physical therapy and physical modalities for the control of chronic musculoskeletal pain. *Pain.* 1997;71(1):5-23.

56. Gersh MR, Wolf SL. Applications of transcutaneous electrical nerve stimulation in the management of patients with pain. *Phys Ther.* 1985;65:314-336.

60

Neurodegeneration and Dementia

BRETON M. ASKEN, MS, ATC, STEPHEN CORREIA, PHD, ABPP-CN,
AND STEPHEN T. MERNOFF, MD, FAAN

The views expressed in this article are those of the authors and do not necessarily reflect the position or policy of the Department of Veterans Affairs.

Concerns about long-term effects of repetitive head impact exposure date back to the 1920s and 1930s with reports of "punch drunk syndrome" and "dementia pugilistica" in both current and former boxers. The modern incarnation, chronic traumatic encephalopathy (CTE), has sparked renewed interest in the complex links of repetitive head impacts, brain injury, and incident risk for neurodegenerative disease.

TBI History

A comprehensive history of head impact exposure includes consideration of:
- Moderate to severe traumatic brain injury (TBI)
- Single or isolated instances of mild TBI (mTBI), often called *concussion*
- Repetitive subclinical head impact exposure, also known as *subconcussive blows*, which refers to head impacts presumably resulting in physiological disruption that do not manifest symptomatically; such impacts are common in populations playing collision sports (most notably boxing and American football), engaging in certain military activities, and exposed to frequent assaults (e.g., domestic violence)

Confounding Factors

Both methodological and person-specific factors complicate the current understanding of the relationship between brain trauma and neurodegenerative disease or dementia.

Such factors include:
- Differing definitions of outcomes: specific disease states (CTE, Alzheimer disease) versus a clinical syndrome (mild cognitive impairment, dementia)
- Differing methods for defining *brain trauma* or neurological outcomes: severity indicators, subjective report, medical records, etc.
- Age when exposed to brain trauma: e.g., youth, adolescence, or young adulthood versus middle-aged or elderly
- Uncertain contribution of non-brain trauma factors to subsequent development of neurodegenerative disease or dementia, for example, genetic risk, psychiatric disorders, substance use, sociodemographics, and cognitive reserve indicators

Research Controversies

Autopsy findings in patients deceased shortly after severe TBI indicate neuropathologic features that overlap neurodegenerative diseases such Alzheimer disease (Johnson et al., 2010). However, the mechanisms translating acute brain injury to a progressive and neurodegenerative process are poorly characterized. Mild TBI research is notably inconsistent both with findings and methodology. Variable definitions for mTBI history, time since injury, operationalization of outcomes (e.g., specific diseases versus dementia syndromes), and follow-up duration contribute to mixed and contradictory results (Asken & Bauer, 2018). Studies that show increased risk after mTBI typically report relative risk and hazard ratios between 1.5 and 2.0, whereas others have found no such relationship. Importantly, studies have shown that the degree of risk specifically associated with mTBI history typically drops to clinically negligible magnitudes when factoring in non-TBI risk factors for poor later-life neurologic health. These factors also often convey a stronger risk for neurodegenerative disease/dementia than mTBI when compared directly.

Mechanistic Theories

Mechanistic theories about the implications of single TBI events on later neurodegenerative processes may not directly overlap with the hypothesized links between repetitive mild/

subclinical events and later neurodegeneration. The attention paid specifically to CTE stems from case series studying individuals with years of exposure to both multiple mTBIs and repetitive subclinical head impacts (Bieniek et al., 2015, Mez et al., 2017). A recent consensus meeting established general—but not universal—agreement that the pathognomonic CTE lesion is perivascular accumulation of hyperphosphorylated tau in an irregular dotlike pattern affecting neurons, astrocytes, and cell processes preferentially at the depths of cortical sulci (McKee et al., 2016). Like most neurodegenerative diseases, CTE is often a mixed pathology (Mez et al., 2017; Stein et al., 2015). The largest CTE case series to date, including 177 retired professional football players, showed that 61% of cases had diffuse or neuritic $A\beta$ plaques, 48% had TDP-43, and 24% had α-synuclein (Mez et al., 2017).

Summary

Brain trauma, however defined, may increase relative risk for CTE or other neurodegenerative diseases, but accurate quantification of risk remains unclear because of unknown CTE prevalence and incidence rates. There are currently no validated CTE biomarker profiles. The presumed regional specificity of tau deposits in CTE suggests advanced neuroimaging such as positron emission tomography (PET-tau) holds promise, but fluid biomarkers may struggle to adequately differentiate CTE from other neurodegenerative tauopathies like frontotemporal lobar degeneration (FTLD) and Alzheimer disease (Elahi & Miller, 2017).

Further, the clinical manifestation of CTE is complicated by the presence of non–brain trauma factors (see earlier) common among at-risk populations that directly and indirectly affect cognition, behavior, and mood (Asken et al., 2016, Asken et al., 2017). Ongoing longitudinal studies and clinical trials enrolling more diverse cohorts and using advanced assessment methods (e.g., advanced brain imaging, fluid biomarkers, and comprehensive neuropsychological testing) are likely to advance rapidly our understanding of CTE, its symptoms, and individual-level risk factors for poor neurological outcomes of brain trauma exposure.

Review Questions

1. According to the National Institute of Neurological Disorders and Stroke (NINDS) and National Institute of Biomedical Imaging and Bioengineering (NIBIB) provisional diagnostic criteria, what is the pathognomonic neuropathologic sign of chronic traumatic encephalopathy (CTE)?
   a. Intracellular phosphorylated tau in the form of neurofibrillary tangles and neuropil threads deposited in the pre-α layer of transentorhinal cortex; extracellular $A\beta$ plaques in neocortical regions
   b. Perivascular accumulation of hyperphosphorylated tau in an irregular dotlike pattern affecting neurons, astrocytes, and cell processes preferentially at the depths of cortical sulci
   c. α-Synuclein inclusions within neuronal perikarya and neuronal processes along with pigment loss in the substantia nigra
   d. Degeneration of cortical and subcortical structures within frontal and temporal regions typically related to tau and/or TDP-43 pathology
2. CTE is predominantly characterized as a tauopathy but often presents as mixed pathology at autopsy. Which of these most accurately shows the relative frequency of other neurodegenerative proteins, from most to least frequent, within current CTE case series?
   a. $A\beta$ > TDP-43 > α-synuclein
   b. α-synuclein > TDP-43 > $A\beta$
   c. $A\beta$ > α-synuclein > TDP-43
   d. TDP-43 > α-synuclein > $A\beta$
3. The overwhelming majority of CTE cases are individuals with past exposure to head trauma. What is the strongest identified risk factor for developing CTE pathology?
   a. Single or isolated instances of mild traumatic brain injury (mTBI) during childhood and adolescence
   b. A moderate to severe traumatic brain injury (TBI) at any point in the lifespan
   c. Multiple concussions/mTBIs occurring within a "window of vulnerability" (i.e., while still recovering from prior concussion/mTBI)
   d. Extensive exposure to both mTBIs and repetitive subclinical head impacts (i.e., "subconcussive" blows) throughout life

Answers on page 403.
Access the full list of questions and answers online. Available on ExpertConsult.com

61

Basic Statistics and Research Methods

MAURO ZAPPATERRA, MD, PHD, AND DIXIE ARAGAKI, MD

OUTLINE

A basic familiarity with statistical terms and research methodology is helpful when critically assessing literature for practical evidence-based clinical application. Statistics is the study of the collection, analysis, interpretation, presentation, and organization of data. Statistical analysis helps determine the likelihood that an observed result occurred by chance alone or with a relationship to a study variable.

Key Terms and Concepts

Hypothesis

- An assumption or proposed explanation, a belief
- States the expected relationship between variables
- Is testable: can be rejected or not rejected

Null Hypothesis (H$_0$)

- Assumed to be true unless there is evidence to the contrary
- States there is no difference between groups being tested
- If the researcher is interested in whether there exists a relationship exists between two groups or a difference between two treatments, then the null hypothesis is: "There is no relationship between the two groups" or "No difference exists between the two treatments or variables under study."
- Researchers' bias is to try to disprove the null hypothesis

Alternative (Research) Hypothesis (H$_A$)

- There is a relationship or difference between the variables under study.
- Often represents what the researcher is trying to prove

Hypothesis Testing

- State the hypothesis.
- Choose a statistical significance level denoted as alpha (α).
  - Probability of type I error (Table 61.1)
  - The threshold value that p-values are measured against
  - By convention, α is set between 0.01 and 0.10, usually set at 0.05.
- Determine the sample size, the total number of subjects involved in the study, needed to determine statistical significance.

TABLE 61.1	Hypothesis Testing Decisions: H$_0$ = Null Hypothesis	
Decision	H$_0$ is true	H$_0$ is false
Reject H$_0$	Type I error = α	Correct decision
Fail to Reject H$_0$	Correct decision	Type II error = β (1-power)

- Test the hypothesis by applying a statistical test to the collected data to determine how likely the observed results are because of chance.
- A statistical test will generate a calculated p-value
  - P = probability, the probability the observed data occurred by chance
  - P = 0.5 is a 50% probability the observed data occurred by chance
  - P = 0.05 is a 5% probability the observed data occurred by chance
  - Small p-values (0.05, 0.01, 0.001) suggest that the null hypothesis is unlikely or very unlikely to be true
- Statistical significance: compare obtained p-value from statistical test to the significance level (alpha)
- If p-value is less than alpha → reject null hypothesis, the result is statistically significant; observed data is unlikely to occur by chance
- If p-value is greater than alpha → accept the null hypothesis; the result is not statistically significant; observed data are likely to occur by chance

Hypothesis Testing Errors (Table 61.1)

Type I Error = Alpha (α)

- A true null hypothesis is rejected.
- Considered more serious than type II errors
- If α = 0.05, then the null hypothesis is rejected if the sample would only happen 5% of the time if the null hypothesis is true. Therefore, there is a probability of 0.05 that the null hypothesis will be rejected when in fact it is true.

Type II Error = Beta (β) = (1-Power)

- A false null hypothesis is not rejected
- If the null hypothesis is not rejected, it may still be false, because the sample may not be big enough to identify the false null hypothesis.

Statistical Power

- The ability to reject a false null hypothesis
- 1- β, where β = risk of type II error defined earlier
- The higher the power, the greater probability of producing statistically significant results.
- Statistical power is increased by:
  - Larger sample size
  - Larger effect size
  - Larger alpha level
  - Test direction (e.g., one-tailed t-test)
  - Using parametric statistics
  - Decreasing error
- For instance, if alpha is changed from 0.05 to 0.01, the power of the study will decrease, because alpha is changed to a smaller number.

Types of Data or Scales of Measurement

Categorical

- **Nominal data:** nonordered category for classification (e.g., sex, ethnicity, city, political party)
- **Ordinal data:** ordered category, allows one to rank in terms of less or more (e.g., Likert scales, percentile ranks)

Continuous

- **Interval data:** score or numerical data with equal intervals with no absolute zero score (e.g., temperature in degrees Fahrenheit and degrees Celsius)
- **Ratio data:** interval data with absolute zero value (e.g., weight, height, money in bank account, temperature in Kelvins)

Variables

- Things that are measured, controlled, or manipulated in research
- Dependent variable (DV)
  - The variable that depends on another variable (independent variable)
  - Variable that is measured or registered (e.g., pain, body mass index [BMI], Glasgow Coma Scale [GCS])
  - Usually the outcome variable
- Independent variable (IV)
  - The variable that is believed to affect the status of another variable (DV)
  - Variable that is manipulated (e.g., therapy type, drug dose)
  - Usually considered the intervention or treatment
- To determine which variable is the DV and IV, one can use this phrase: What is the effect of the IV on the DV?

Descriptive Statistics

- Used to describe a sample or population characteristics (e.g., diagnoses, height, weight, body mass index, temperature, pain scores, treatment outcomes)

Data Distribution (Fig. 61.1)

When a large enough number of samples are collected or observations made, the data for many variables will follow a normal distribution (a symmetrical, bell-shaped curve with values and data points equally distributed above and below the mean). Data that are not normally distributed are called *skewed* or *kurtotic*. In a positive skew, there is a larger proportion of data points with lower values. In a negative skew, there is a larger proportion of data points of higher values.

Measures of Central Tendency (See Fig. 61.1)

- Used to summarize the collected data with a single number that best describes the central or middle value

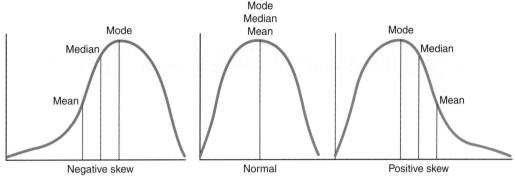

• **Fig. 61.1** Common measures of central tendency as related to normal and skewed distribution.

- When the data are normally distributed, mean = median = mode.
- When the data are skewed, mean ≠ median ≠ mode.
- Mean
  - The arithmetic average of a group, calculated by adding all the values and dividing by the total number of values
  - Used for normally distributed data
- Median
  - The middle value or score that divides the distribution in half
  - The number for which 50% of the scores are larger and 50% of the scores are smaller; the number at the 50th percentile
- Mode
  - The value with greatest frequency

Measures of Variability

- Indicate the amount of dispersion within a distribution of data
- The larger the variance or standard deviation (SD), the greater the dispersion of values around the mean of the data.
- Range
  - The difference between the maximum and minimum value
  - Based only on the two most extreme scores
- Variance
  - The average of the squared difference from the mean
- SD (Fig. 61.2)
  - The average deviation of spread or dispersion from the mean
  - The square root of the variance
  - Expressed in units of measurement of the variable
  - ± 1 SD = 68.3% of data, ± 2 SD = 95.4%, ± 3 SD = 99.7%

Confidence Intervals

When data are collected, they are only from a sample of the "true population." The actual "true" value of the population is not known, because data from the entire population was not collected. The confidence interval is a range, from the sample

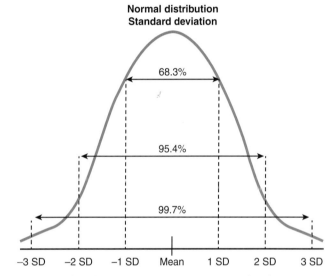

• **Fig. 61.2** Standard deviation measurements as related to normally distributed data.

data, that is likely to contain the true population value. This is a calculated range (interval) in which the researcher can be fairly sure (confident) the true value lies. A 95% confidence interval represents a significance level of 0.05.

Inferential Statistics

- Tests that allow researchers to make inferences or judgments about a larger population based on the data collected from a smaller sample
- Random selection decreases selection bias and sampling error
- Using the proper statistical test, inferences can be made regarding similarities, differences, relationships, and associations
- The **chi-square test** is used to analyze nominal data such as observations of frequency.
- The **student's t-test** and the **analysis of variance (ANOVA)** are the two most common statistical tests for interval and ratio data. The t-test evaluates the hypothesis between two means, and the ANOVA compares two or more means.

TABLE 61.2	Test Accuracy Classification			
		Truth		
		Has Disease	**Does Not Have Disease**	
Test result	Positive	True positives (A)	False positives (B)	PPV = A/(A + B)
	Negative	False negatives (C)	True negatives (D)	NPV = D/(C + D)
		Sensitivity = A/(A + C)	Specificity = D/(B + D)	

NPV, Negative predictive value; *PPV*, positive predictive value.

Accuracy Classification (Table 61.2)

- **Sensitivity:** percentage of people who have the disorder and accurately identified by test
- **Specificity:** percentage of people who do not have the disorder and accurately identified by test
- **Positive predictive value (PPV):** probability that people who test positive have the disorder
- **Negative predictive value (NPV):** probability that people who test negative do not have the disorder

Types of Clinical Research

Experimental Studies

Randomized Control Trials

- Gold standard for clinical trials
- Best if double blinded so the subject and researcher are blinded to the treatment or intervention provided; this decreases selection bias
- Randomization provides comparable groups for most factors (confounders similar in each group) so that differences in outcome can be attributed to intervention; this decreases sample bias.

Observational Studies

Cohort

- Start with an identified group or cohort that shares a characteristic (e.g., exposed to drug X, underwent a medical procedure, admission GCS of 5)
- Follow the group to determine who develops the outcome of interest
- Used to determine incidence and prevalence
- Relative risk (RR) can be calculated; RR = probability of an outcome occurring with an exposure versus the probability of the outcome occurring without the exposure.

- Large cohort studies include Framingham Heart Study and Nurses' Health Study.

Case Control

- Comparing cases (people with a condition/disease) to controls (no condition/disease)
- Start with the outcome/condition and identify a sample of people with the condition
- Identify a similar control group
- Usually look back in time (retrospective) to determine exposure differences
- Calculate risk in the cases and controls using odds ratio (OR); OR = odds of outcome in exposed versus odds of outcome in nonexposed
- Example: tobacco smoking and lung cancer

Case Series

- Descriptive study
- Track patients with known exposure or given treatment
- No control group

Cross-Sectional

- Data are collected from population or subset of population at one point in time
- Cannot make inferences about causality
- Can assess prevalence
- Examples include surveys, census

Potential Bias in Research

- **Selection bias:** difference in selecting groups
- **Measurement bias:** difference in measuring variables
- **Performance bias:** difference in care provided
- **Detection bias:** difference in outcome assessment
- **Attrition bias:** difference in withdrawals from the study

Review Questions

1. Which of these actions will reduce the power of a hypothesis test?
   a. Increasing sample size
   b. Increasing alpha, the significance level
   c. Increasing beta, the probability of a type II error
   d. Increasing effect size
2. Five friends take an intelligence (IQ) test. The scores are 90, 100, 105, 110, and 110. Which of these statements is true?
   a. The mean is 105, and the mode is 110.
   b. The mean is 103, and the median is 105.
   c. The mean is 105, and the median is 110.
   d. The mean is 105, and the mode is 105.

3. If a researcher does not reject a true null hypothesis, the researcher is making a
   a. type I error.
   b. type II error.
   c. type III error.
   d. correct decision.

Answers on page 404.
Access the full list of questions and answers online.
Available on ExpertConsult.com

References

1. Gerstman B. *Basic Biostatistics*. Sudbury, MA: Jones & Bartlett Learning; 2014.
2. Fletcher R, Fletcher S, Fletcher G. *Clinical Epidemiology*: The Essentials. 5th ed. Lippincott Williams & Wilkins; Pennsylvania 2012.
3. McClave J, Sincich T. *Statistics*. 10th ed. Prentice Hall; New Jersey 2006.

62

Ethics and Law

BONNY S. WONG, MD, JEAN E. WOO, MD, AND SUNIL KOTHARI, MD

Decision-Making Capacity

One of the most common ethical issues encountered in brain injury medicine centers on the circumstances in which it is permissible (or even obligatory) to restrict the freedom of patients to make and act on their own decisions. Because decision-making capacity (DMC) is often impaired after brain injury, clinicians are often faced with the challenge of balancing the requirement to respect a patient's autonomy with the obligation to ensure the patient's well-being.

Autonomy

Patient autonomy is the foundational value in Western bioethics and law. It is broadly defined as the patient's right to make decisions regarding his or her healthcare.[1] However, for a patient's decisions to be counted as autonomous and thereby respected, he or she must possess the appropriate capacity to reason and choose. When patients possess the necessary capacities, they are said to have DMC. In that case, their decisions must be respected even if others believe the decisions are not ideal or even contrary to the patient's best interests.[1]

Competency versus Capacity

Although both *competency* and *capacity* refer to the patient's capability to make autonomous decisions, each is determined differently and is used in different contexts.

- *Competency*: a legal term that can only be determined by the court
- Decision-making *capacity:* assessed by a clinician in the healthcare setting

General Principles of Decision-Making Capacity[1]

- DMC is domain specific. A patient can lack DMC in some areas (e.g., financial management) but not others (e.g., healthcare decisions).
- Even within a domain, the DMC required will vary depending on the complexity of the decision to be made. Evaluate the way a patient's abilities match up with the demands of the particular decision to be made.
- Decision making is a process. Assess *how* a decision is made; not *what* is decided.
- Evaluation of DMC should involve direct observation of the patient making the decision in question. Avoid *inferring* from the patient's diagnosis or particular cognitive deficits.

Specific Abilities Required for Decision-Making Capacity

There is a broad consensus in bioethics and the law regarding the abilities that constitute DMC. The most widely used model was first proposed by Paul Applebaum and Thomas Grisso[2] (Box 62.1).

- The patient must be able to *express a choice*, whether verbally or behaviorally.
- For healthcare decision making, the patient must be able to *understand* relevant information including:
  - The nature and rationale of the treatment
  - Its risks and benefits, including their likelihood
  - The risks and benefits (and their likelihoods) of alternative treatments, including the option of no treatment

- The ability to *express a choice*
- The ability to *understand* information relevant to the decision to be made
- The ability to *appreciate* the significance of that information for one's own situation
- The ability to *reason* with the relevant information in a logical manner

• BOX 62.2 Alternate Decision Makers, in Order of Priority

1. Current guardian
2. Designated healthcare power of attorney
3. Surrogate decision maker designated by state statute
4. Court appointed guardian

- The patient should *appreciate* the relevance of this information for their own situation, an ability that is often impaired in patients with diminished insight after brain injury.
- The patients must be able to *reason* with the relevant information in a logical and coherent manner. This would include the ability to recognize how the various options align with their values and to imagine the consequences of the various outcomes. The recommended strategy for assessing a patient's ability to reason in the appropriate manner is to ask the patient to think out loud as they consider the decision at hand.

Additional Considerations in the Assessment of Decision-Making Capacity

- Address factors that might adversely affect a patient's performance, such as distraction, fatigue, and the effects of sedating medications, before the assessment.
- Conduct serial evaluations given the degree to which cognitive capacities can fluctuate after brain injury.
- Obtain collateral information from others, such as family members, about how the patient makes and executes decisions in other contexts.
- Use formal assessment of the patient's specific cognitive deficits and strengths, such as provided by neuropsychological testing. Keep in mind that neuropsychological testing is not a substitute for the direct clinical assessment of DMC.[1]
- Although the method for assessing DMC described earlier is widely accepted, be aware of the limitations of the model when applied to patients with brain injuries.[1]

When a Patient Lacks Decision-Making Capacity

When it is determined that a patient lacks DMC for a specific decision(s), an alternate mechanism for decision-making must be identified. Clinicians should be guided by the law in their jurisdiction on how to proceed in these situations. In most jurisdictions, there is a hierarchy of alternatives (Box 62.2).

- Clinicians should first determine whether a guardian exists.
- If not, then it should be determined whether there exists a properly designated healthcare power of attorney.

- If one does not exist, then most (but not all) states have statutes that identify legally recognized surrogate decision makers. For example, in order of priority, a statute might designate a spouse, followed by adult children, parent(s), siblings, etc.
- If none of these mechanisms identifies an individual who could serve as a surrogate decision maker, then a guardian might need to be appointed by the court.[1]

It is important to keep in mind that there are constraints on the decisions that surrogate decision makers can make.

- Some jurisdictions restrict the types of decisions that certain surrogates can make (for example, surrounding withdrawal of treatment).
- Surrogates are expected to make decisions as they believe the patient would have made them. This is known as *substituted judgment*.
- However, if the patient's wishes are not known or cannot be inferred, the surrogate must then make decisions in the patient's *best interests*.
- It should be emphasized that the surrogate's own desires cannot be the basis of the decision; rather, surrogates must rely on either *substituted judgment* or the patient's *best interests* in making their decisions.
- Patients can and should still be involved in decisions that affect their lives, even if they do not possess DMC. In these situations, the concepts of *assent* and *dissent* may be useful to clinicians.[3]

Withdrawal of Treatment

- Discussions frequently arise regarding withdrawal of treatment in patients with a severe brain injury, especially those with a disorder of consciousness.[1,4]
- Several factors complicate decision making in these situations, especially early after a brain injury:
  - *Prognostic uncertainty*: There is increasing evidence suggesting that our ability to prognosticate in the acute setting is limited.[5]
  - *Prognostic pessimism*: Despite our lack of ability to prognosticate accurately, there is widespread pessimism about the outcomes of these acutely injured patients that is likely unwarranted.[6] National guidelines specifically counsel against uniformly assuming a poor prognosis within the first 28 days after injury.[7]
  - *Diagnostic uncertainty*: There is a high rate of underestimation of consciousness in patients after brain injury, with studies suggesting that over one-third of

patients diagnosed as being in a vegetative state are actually conscious.[8]

- *Underestimation of quality of life*: Clinicians significantly underestimate the quality of life of people with disability,[9] which can significantly affect the information the clinicians provide and the recommendations they make.[10]
- *Minimal legal guidance for the minimally conscious state*: Well-known court cases (for example, those involving Karen Quinlan, Nancy Cruzan, and Terri Schiavo) have all addressed issues surrounding the chronic vegetative state; the legal issues surrounding withdrawal of treatment in minimally conscious patients have not yet been systematically addressed.[4]
- Clinicians should keep in mind all of these factors when engaging in discussions and decisions regarding withdrawal of treatment.[4,11]

Legislation

Americans with Disabilities Act

The Americans with Disabilities Act (ADA) was passed and signed into law in 1990 by President George H.W. Bush and was built on the foundation of the Rehabilitation Act of 1973.[12] It was amended in 2008 and reauthorized in 2010. For protection under the ADA, a *disability* is defined as an impairment that substantially limits one or more major life activities, a record of such an impairment, or being regarded as having such an impairment.[13]

The ADA:
- Protects the civil liberties of individuals with disabilities
- Prohibits discrimination by all public entities
- Specifies equal access to employment, public places, transportation, and telecommunications

Return to Work and Return to School

People with brain injuries have varying degrees of physical, cognitive, emotional, and/or psychosocial impairments that can make return to work and return to school particularly challenging.

The US Equal Employment Opportunity Commission (EEOC) enforces Title 1 of the ADA, which prohibits discrimination on the basis of disability in employment.[12] Under this, employers are responsible for providing reasonable accommodations to employees with disabilities, unless a particular accommodation provides an undue hardship on the business or employer.

Reasonable accommodations may include:
- Job restructuring
- Modifying work schedules
- Acquiring adaptive or assistive equipment or devices
- Reassigning tasks
- Modifying the workplace and office layout to improve accessibility
- Providing support services

Vocational rehabilitation specialists can provide one-to-one individualized assistance with job search and placement

services through tailored interventions and advocacy level services. In addition, they can identify supports needed to help the person succeed at work.[14]

Under the Individuals with Disabilities Education Act (IDEA), school-age children with disabilities are entitled to educational assistance such as Individualized Education Programs (IEPs) and accommodations such as modification of classroom equipment, use of assistive technology devices, modification of testing procedures, and psychosocial behavioral plans in the classroom.[15]

Traumatic Brain Injury Act

The Traumatic Brain Injury Act (TBI) of 1996 was signed by President Bill Clinton and was the first federal legislation that addressed the needs of individuals with TBI.[16] There have been multiple amendments and reauthorizations of the TBI Act, with the most current being the TBI Program Reauthorization Act of 2018.[17]

The purpose of the TBI Act was to:
- Reduce the incidence of TBI through prevention and surveillance projects conducted by the Centers for Disease Control and Prevention
- Conduct TBI research through the National Institutes of Health
- Improve access to rehabilitation healthcare and related services by state grants authorized by the Health Resources & Services Administration, which was later transitioned to the Administration for Community Living

Medicolegal Issues

Independent Medical Examination

Requests for an independent medical examination (IME) generally come from attorneys, insurance companies, government agencies, or employers. During an IME, an examiner assumes a unique role that entails certain expectations:

- Evaluate a patient as an independent examiner, not as a treating physician. Keep in mind that there is no therapeutic relationship, no expectation of ongoing care, and a limited duty of confidentiality.[18]
- Do not provide medical advice or care during or after the interaction[18] and inform the examinee of the unique role of the independent medical examiner and the evaluation.
- Perform the examination using standardized, widely available, and evidence-based methods.
- Be aware that the examinee may be ambivalent or even hostile during the interaction and that the examinee may withhold information or even fabricate or exaggerate symptoms for secondary gain. Inform the examinee that incomplete effort, bias, or withholding of information will be documented.
- Use symptom validity tests to detect evidence of response bias.[19]
- The ideal approach has been summarized as one of "trust but verify."[18]

Review Questions

1. Which of these is not true about decision-making capacity (DMC) after brain injury?
   a. A patient can lack DMC for financial affairs but retain DMC for healthcare decisions.
   b. A patient with expressive aphasia automatically loses DMC.
   c. Patients may have DMC for some healthcare decisions but not others.
   d. If a patient with a brain injury has DMC, their decisions must be honored even if their decisions are not in their best interests.

2. Which of these is not considered a component of DMC?
   a. Understanding the clinical recommendation being made
   b. Appreciating the relevance of the clinical recommendation to one's own situation
   c. Agreement with an evidence-based clinical recommendation
   d. Being able to express a choice about following or not following a recommendation

3. Which of these is true about surrogate decision makers for an incapacitated patient?
   a. The patient's next of kin should always be the surrogate decision maker.
   b. A surrogate decision maker should override a patient's previously expressed wishes if it is in the patient's best interests.
   c. The decisions of a legally recognized surrogate cannot be challenged in court.
   d. There may be limits on the types of decisions a surrogate decision maker is authorized to make.

Answers on page 404.
Access the full list of questions and answers online.
Available on ExpertConsult.com

References

1. Kothari S, Kirschner K. Decision-making capacity after brain injury: clinical assessment and ethical implications. In: Zasler N, Katz D, Zafonte R, eds. *Brain Injury Medicine: Principles and Practice*. 1st ed. New York, NY: Demos Medical Pub.; 2006: 1205-1222.
2. Grisso T, Appelbaum PS. *Assessing Competence to Consent to Treatment: A Guide for Physicians and Other Health Professionals*. New York, NY: Oxford University Press; 1998.
3. Kothari S, Kirschner K. Beyond consent: assent and empowerment in brain injury rehabilitation. *J Head Trauma Rehabilitation*. 2003;18(4):379-382.
4. Kothari S. Chronic disorders of consciousness. In: Creutzfeldt C, Kluger B, Holloway R, eds. *Neuropalliative Care: A Guide to Improving The Lives of Patients and Families Affected by Neurologic Disease*. Berlin, Germany: Springer Publishers; 2019.
5. Lazaridis C. Withdrawal of life-sustaining treatments in perceived devastating brain injury: the key role of uncertainty. *Neurocrit Care*. 2019;30(1):33-41.
6. Turgeon AF, Lauzier F, Simard J-F, et al. Mortality associated with withdrawal of life-sustaining therapy for patients with severe traumatic brain injury: a Canadian multicentre cohort study. *CMAJ*. 2011;183(14):1581-1588.
7. Giacino JT, Katz DI, Schiff ND, et al. Practice guideline update recommendations summary: disorders of consciousness. *Neurology*. 2018;91(10):450-460.
8. Schnakers C, Vanhaudenhuyse A, Giacino J, et al. Diagnostic accuracy of the vegetative and minimally conscious state: clinical consensus versus standardized neurobehavioral assessment. *BMC Neurol*. 2009;9(1).
9. Kothari S. Clinical (mis)judgments of quality of life after disability. *J Clin Ethics*. 2004;15(4):300-307.
10. Kothari S, Kirschner K. Abandoning the golden rule: the problem with "putting ourselves in the patient's place." *Top Stroke Rehabil*. 2006;13(4):68-73.
11. Fins JJ. Affirming the right to care, preserving the right to die: disorders of consciousness and neuroethics after Schiavo. *Palliat Support Care*. 2006;4:169-178.
12. Americans with Disabilities Act of 1990, P.L. No.101-336, Vol 104 Stat. 328. Available at: http://finduslaw.com/americans-disabilities-act-1990-ada-42-us-code-chapter-126. Accessed February 13, 2019.
13. Bodine C. Americans with Disabilities Act and the reauthorization of the Rehabilitation Act. In: *Braddom's Physical Medicine & Rehabilitation*. 5th ed. Philadelphia, PA: Elsevier; 2015:408.
14. West M, Targett P, Crockatt S, Wehman P. Return to work following traumatic brain injury. In: Zasler N, Katz D, Zafonte R, eds. *Brain Injury Medicine: Principles and Practice*. 2nd ed. New York, NY: Demos Medical Pub; 2013:1353-1355.
15. Individuals with Disabilities Education Act (IDEA); 1997. Available at: http://idea.ed.gov/. Accessed February 13, 2019.
16. Traumatic Brain Injury Act of 1996, P.L. No. 104-652 [cited 2019 Feb 12]. Available at: https://www.congress.gov/congressional-report/104th-congress/house-report/652/1.
17. Traumatic Brain Injury Program Reauthorization Act of 2018, P.L No. 115-377 [cited 2019 Feb 12]. Available at: https://www.congress.gov/115/bills/hr6615/BILLS-115hr6615enr.xml.
18. Ameis A, Zasler N, Martelli M, Bush S. Clinicolegal issues. In: Zasler N, Katz D, Zafonte R, eds. *Brain Injury Medicine: Principles and Practice*. 2nd ed. New York, NY: Demos Medical Pub.; 2013:1391-1414.
19. Bush S, Ruff R, Troster A, et al. Symptom validity assessment: practice issues and medical necessity. *Arch Clin Neuropsychol*. 2005;20(4):419-426.

Answer Key

Chapter 1

1.1 Answer: B
Subdural hematomas result from tearing of bridging veins with resulting blood product forming in the meninges in the space below the dura but above the arachnoid. The remaining three intracranial bleeds generally result from arterial tearing and involve blood product accumulating between the skull and dura (epidural hematoma), arachnoid and pia (SAH), or below the pia in the actual brain parenchyma (intraparenchymal hemorrhage).

Reference: Blumenfeld H. *Neuroanatomy Through Clinical Cases.* 2nd ed. Sunderland, MA: Sinauer Associates; 2010.

1.2 Answer: A
Hydrocephalus can occur when there is overproduction, underreabsorption, or blockage of flow. AVMs are the most common cause of a SAH, which would present in an acute manner. A Chiari malformation is more likely congenital and contributory to chronic versus acute hydrocephalus. An arachnoidal tumor would also more likely cause slowly progressive hydrocephalus. Answer D is incorrect because extracommunicating hydrocephalus is not one of the two types.

Reference: Blumenfeld H. *Neuroanatomy Through Clinical Cases.* 2nd ed. Sunderland, MA: Sinauer Associates; 2010 [chapter 5].

1.3 Answer: C
In addition to controlling aspects of eye movement, cranial nerve III (oculomotor) controls pupillary constriction; thus dilated and nonresponsive ("blown") pupils most likely would result from dysfunction of this cranial nerve, which has it nuclei in the midbrain. Although cranial nerve IV (trochlear) and VI (abducens) control downward and lateral eye movements respectively, these cranial nerves do not control pupillary constriction.

Reference: Blumenfeld H. *Neuroanatomy Through Clinical Cases.* 2nd ed. Sunderland, MA: Sinauer Associates; 2010.

Chapter 2

2.1 Answer: C
Apoptosis is programmed cell death that occurs as part of the secondary processes that are set in motion by a primary brain injury. All other choices are potential features of primary brain injury.

2.2 Answer: B
Axonal and neuronal injury leads to influx of calcium ions. Accumulating intracellular calcium then initiates a cascade of issues including mitochondrial calcium uptake, activation of intracellular proteases, and impaired adenosine triphosphate (ATP) production caused by mitochondrial compromise.

2.3 Answer: D
All of the networks except D have been recognized as intrinsic connectivity networks operating in the brain during active cognitive function.

Chapter 3

3.1 Answer: D
In the absence of details, it is hard to determine severity based on loss/alteration of consciousness or posttraumatic amnesia. The patient reports cognitive deficits and neurological symptoms of balance dysfunction. Although a thorough examination is important, in this scenario, advanced imaging would help rule out a moderate or severe injury. CT would be appropriate in the acute setting. Neuropsychological testing should be included as part of the patient's future workup.

3.2 Answer: C
The patient's initial diagnosis was incorrect, and he is suffering an early-onset seizure that is associated with intracranial pathology. Late-onset seizures start 7 days after injury. Concussions and mTBI are not typically prophylactically medicated for seizures.

3.3 Answer: A
Best motor response is the best acute predictor of outcome.[5]

Chapter 4

4.1 Answer: B
Gunshot wounds are the most common cause of penetrating brain injury and are also the leading cause of mortality.[1]

4.2 Answer: C
Projectiles that enter the brain and then exit at a distal site are classified as a perforating wound. This type of wound pattern carries the most severe prognosis.[9]

4.3 Answer: B
Primary injury is the result of direct brain tissue damage caused by a blast wave.[16]

Chapter 5

5.1 Answer: A
Absent bilateral median SSEPs is consistent with breath death. Both reverberating arterial flow and small peaks in early systole are compatible with brain death. Brain perfusion (hollow skull phenomenon) with hexamethylpropyleneamine-oxime (HMPAO) should be absent for brain death.

Reference: Cant BR, Hume AL, Judson JA, Shaw NA. The assessment of severe head injury by short-latency somatosensory and brain-stem auditory evoked potentials. *Electroencephalogr Clin Neurophysiol.* 1986;65(3): 188-195.

5.2 Answer: D
Hypoxemia is a possible confounder, and prerequisite target is Pao_2 ≥200 mg Hg; thus 100 mm Hg does not meet this target. Temperature requisite for hypothermia is > 32°C. Severe endocrine abnormality should be absent, but blood glucose level of 180 mg/dL should not affect neurological examination. Sedative and paralytic drugs need to be stopped for five to seven elimination half-lives; because propofol's elimination half-life is about 30 minutes, it should not be a major confounder 5 hours after cessation.

Reference: Wijdicks EF, Varelas PN, Gronseth GS, Greer DM. Evidence-based guideline update: determining brain death in adults: report of the Quality Standards Subcommittee of the American Academy of Neurology. *Neurology.* 2010;74(23):1911-1918.

5.3 Answer: C
Apnea is confirmed if there is no respiratory movement after approximately 8 minutes on an apnea test, so the testing can continue at 5 minutes.
The apnea test should be aborted and patient should be reconnected to the ventilator if there is evidence of respiratory movement, refractory hypotension (systolic blood pressure [SBP] <90 mm Hg), or worsening hypoxemia (pulse oximetry <85%).

Reference: Rabinstein AA. Coma and brain death. *Continuum (Minneap Minn).* 2018;24(6):1708-1731.

Chapter 6

6.1 Answer: C
Based upon Centers for Disease Control and Prevention (CDC) data reports, falls are the overall leading cause of TBI.[7]

6.2 Answer: B
Based upon CDC surveillance data reports, MVAs are the leading cause of TBI-related deaths in persons ages 15 to 24 years.[7]

6.3 Answer: D
Estimates vary based upon the resource, but it is estimated that 75% to 90% of all TBIs are classified as mild.[2,3,7]

Chapter 7

7.1 Answer: D
Urinary catecholamines and serum cholesterol have not proven useful in diagnosing TBI. APOE genotype can be a useful *prognostic* biomarker but not a diagnostic one.

7.2 Answer: C
Sensitivity is the probability that a true positive case will test positive. 1 − sensitivity = the odds that a test will miss a positive case. When a test is positive, the odds that the patient has the disease (choice A) is called the *positive predictive value* (PPV). When a test is negative, the odds that the patient is disease free (choice B) is the negative predictive value (NPV). Both NPV and PPV require information on the prevalence in a specific population. Choice D refers to specificity, the probability that a true negative case will test negative.

7.3 Answer: B
S100B is also detected in the serum after extracranial injury (e.g., pulmonary contusion). This would give positive results in patients who are true negatives for TBI, therefore decreasing specificity.

Chapter 8

8.1 Answer: C
The GCS is a widely used tool to assess and monitor an individual's level of consciousness. It takes three domains into consideration: eye opening, verbal response, and motor response. The motor response takes into consideration reflexive movements versus being aware of a stimulus and ceasing it or completing a specific motor task at hand. Eye opening and verbal response may help predict prognosis when considered in the total GCS score but not individually. The GCS may be influenced by confounding factors such as sedatives or being intubated. Following commands is part of the motor response of the GCS.

References: Majdan M, Steyerberg EW, Nieboer D, et al. Glasgow coma scale motor score and pupillary reaction to predict six-month mortality in patients with traumatic brain injury: comparison of field and admission assessment. *J Neurotrauma.* 2015;32(2):101-108.
McNett M. A review of the predictive ability of Glasgow Coma Scale scores in head-injured patients. *J Neurosci Nurs.* 2007;39(2):68-75.

8.2 Answer: A
Age plays a significant role in predicting prognosis. An underdeveloped brain or one that does not have the resiliency to recover have a greatest risk for worse outcomes. Those who are less than 4 years of age or older than 65 years of age have the greatest risk for poor outcomes.

Reference: Zasler ND, Katz DI, Zafonte RD. *Brain Injury Medicine: Principles and Practice.* 2nd ed. New York, NY: Demos Medical Pub.; 2013.

8.3 Answer: A
Coma is defined as the absence of eye opening, absence of sleep–wake cycle, and absence of spontaneous/purposeful movements. A patient in a coma has no awareness or interaction with the surrounding environment. Choice C clinically describes vegetative state. Eye opening and sleep–wake cycles are usually occurring together.

References: Cuccurullo, SJ. *Physical Medicine and Rehabilitation Board Review.* 3rd ed. New York, NY: Demos Medical Pub.; 2015.
Zasler ND, Katz DI, Zafonte RD. *Brain Injury Medicine: Principles and Practice.* 2nd ed. New York, NY: Demos Medical Pub.; 2013.

Chapter 9

9.1 Answer: B
Elevation of the patient's head of bed reduces intracranial hypertension by encouraging venous drainage from the brain. Hyperventilation with goal end-tidal carbon dioxide (ETCO$_2$) 30 to 35 mm Hg will lead to cerebral vasoconstriction and lowered cerebral blood flow/volume. Osmotherapy using mannitol or hypertonic saline can treat cerebral herniation by promoting the osmotic shift of fluid from the intracellular to the interstitial and intravascular space, whereas hypotonic fluids would lead to osmotic shift of fluid into the intracellular space causing increased intracranial pressure and worsening of cerebral herniation. Propofol decreases the cerebral metabolic rate and cerebral blood flow to treat elevated intracranial pressure.

9.2 Answer: E
Initial evaluation of all patients with suspected TBI is based on the Advanced Trauma Life Support (ATLS) guidelines. The ABCDE mnemonic defines the primary survey, which includes **a**irway and cervical spine stabilization, **b**reathing and ventilation, **c**irculation, **d**isability/neurological status, and **e**xposure/environment. Obtaining information on a patient's medical history is part of the secondary survey that occurs once the patient is stabilized.

9.3 Answer: D
The GCS is a measurement of the severity of neurological impairment based on assessment of eye opening, verbal responses, and motor responses. The GCS has a possible score range of 3 to 15. Categories of TBI severity using the GCS are defined as 13 to 15 for mild injuries, 9 to 12 for moderate injuries, and 3 to 8 for severe injuries.

Chapter 10

10.1 Answer: A
Autoregulation refers to the ability of the cerebral vasculature to maintain CBF at a constant level even in the face of very high or very low arterial pressures. The other terms listed are not generally used to describe this aspect of cerebral metabolism or are not applicable to this situation.

Reference: Rangel-Castilla L, Gasco J, Nauta HJW, et al. Cerebral pressure autoregulation in traumatic brain injury. *Neurosurg Focus.* 2008;(4);E7.

10.2 Answer: D
A secondary insult is any deviation from normal physiological conditions which, in a TBI patient, can exacerbate the damage caused by the primary insult. The other choices are incorrect.

Reference: Whitaker-Lea WA, Valadka AB. Acute management of moderate-severe traumatic brain injury. *Phys Med Rehabil Clin N Am.* 2017;28(2):227-43.

10.3 Answer: A
So far, all treatments instituted as prophylaxis against elevated intracranial pressure (ICP) and/or poor outcome from severe TBI have failed to demonstrate benefit. Hypothermia is one such treatment. Clinical trials have documented no significant differences between normothermic and hypothermic groups in rates of infections or hemorrhagic complications. Target temperature can be reached within several hours of initiation of hypothermia.

References: Clifton GL, Miller ER, Choi SC, et al. Lack of effect of induction of hypothermia after acute brain injury. *N Engl J Med.* 2001;344(8):556-563.
Clifton GL, Coffey CS, Fourwinds S, et al. Early induction of hypothermia for evacuated intracranial hematomas: a post hoc analysis of two clinical trials: Clinical article. *J Neurosurg.* 2012;117(4):714-720.

Chapter 11

11.1 Answer: C
Current recommendation for glucose control in the ICU is targeting glucose between 140 and 180 mg/dL. Tight glucose control in older studies showed possible mortality benefit but in more recent studies has not shown any benefit in reducing mortality and improving neurological outcomes. Instead, it can increase potential harm by increasing the risk of hypoglycemia. Overt hypoglycemia and hyperglycemia should be avoided to mitigate the effects of secondary toxicity to the brain.

11.2 Answer: C
The Brain Trauma Foundation's fourth guideline recommends targeting CPP at 60 to 70 mm Hg for best

outcomes based on current available evidence. Low CPP can lead to further ischemic insults, whereas high CPP can induce detrimental cerebral hyperemia. High CPP has also been associated with higher incidence of acute respiratory distress syndrome, likely caused by greater vasopressor use.

11.3 Answer: A

In a patient with a TBI who is comatose or unable to give a reliable neurological examination (e.g., GCS <8, intubated and sedated), it is recommended to monitor intracerebral pressure to rule out intracranial hypertension. It is most commonly performed with insertion of an external ventricular drain. TBI patients who are intubated do have higher risk of pneumonia, but prophylactic antibiotics have not been shown to reduce its incidence. Currently prophylactic antibiotics are only recommended for patients with depressed skull fractures. Induced hypertension to increase CPP has not led to improved neurological recovery and is not currently advised.

Chapter 12

12.1 Answer: C

All the other options are therapy strategies used to decrease intracranial pressure (ICP) after a traumatic brain injury (TBI). However, the midline shift and uncal herniation shown in this patient's head computed tomography (CT) suggest a rapidly expanding hematoma that is displacing the cerebral structures into adjacent compartments, which, if unreversed, may lead to brainstem compression with after cardiorespiratory arrest. To prevent this fatal outcome, a STAT decompressive craniectomy is performed in order to give the cerebrum room for expansion, without furtherly increasing the ICP and compromising the brainstem.

12.2. Answer: D

Brain herniation is one of the most common complications after cerebral surgery and TBI with increased ICP. This patient presenting with fixed and dilated pupils and decerebrate posturing, is showing signs of rapid central transtentorial herniation (CTH). Fixed and dilated pupils and possibly, decorticate posturing, might be the only signs of CTH because the patient is already sedated and mechanically ventilated, preventing the clinician from recognizing Cheyne-Stokes breathing or the development of coma. As herniation progresses and the brainstem is pushed further down, Duret's hemorrhages will appear, which are hemorrhagic areas seen in the brainstem caused by the stretching and rupturing of the perforating arteries branching off the basilar artery.

12.3 Answer: A

The patient in this question developed rapid transtentorial herniation, most likely as a result of

second-impact syndrome (SIS). SIS occurs in patients who suffer a second concussion before symptoms of a first one fully resolve, leading to a specific form of brain swelling that is sometimes impossible to control, and can result in rapid brain herniation and subsequent death. Concussions in football players are fairly common, and early return to play (RTP) is as well. The patient in this question stem most likely suffered a previous concussion recently, and postconcussive symptoms had not fully resolved by the time he suffered this second blow to the head.

Chapter 13

13.1 Answer: D

Temporal bone fractures increase risk of delayed CN VII palsies. Lyme disease may also cause a Bell's palsy, but this is less likely given the clinical history. A central CN VII palsy has nasolabial fold flattening and no involvement of the frontalis.

Reference: Guerrissi J. Facial nerve paralysis after intratemporal and extratemporal blunt trauma. *J Craniofac Surg.* 1997;8(5):431-437.

13.2 Answer B

See Modified Ashworth Scale table.

Reference: Braddom R. *Physical Medicine and Rehabilitation.* 4th ed. Philadelphia, PA: Elsevier Saunders; 2011:1148.

13.3 Answer A

Stereognosis is the inability to identify objects placed in the hand. Tactile extinction is the inability to perceive multiple stimuli simultaneously, but being able to recognize the same stimuli independently. Proprioception is the awareness of the position of one's body.

Reference: Russell S, Triola M. *The Precise Neurological Exam.* New York, NY: NYU School of Medicine; 1995-2006. Available from https://informatics.med.nyu.edu/modules/pub/neurosurgery/sensory.html. Accessed May 27, 2019.

Chapter 14

14.1 Answer: D

IL-8 was found to be correlated with increased ICP and cerebral hypoperfusion, which can result in poor prognosis after severe TBI. Compared with other markers of neuroinflammation, increased IL-8 levels were specifically correlated with increased times spent with ICP >20 mm Hg and CPP <60 mm Hg. Therefore IL-8 may be predictive of impending secondary injury after severe TBI and has the potential to be detected before clinical manifestation of secondary injury becomes apparent.[4]

14.2 Answer: B

Low CSF glucose:lactate ratio was observed in those who did not survive their TBI. This study also found that high CSF lactate was independently associated with poor outcomes after TBI.[6] Elevated CSF lactate has also been correlated with worse neurological outcomes. Increased lactate concentration is believed to be related to altered cerebral metabolism after injury resulting in lactate overproduction and decreased lactate clearance from the brain parenchyma.[6]

14.3 Answer: B

S100B is an astroglial protein that is sensitive to brain injury but not specific to TBI and therefore can be elevated with any cerebral injury such as from a cerebrovascular accident. It has been shown that normal serum S100B levels correlate with negative intracranial findings on CTH and therefore may have prognostic value in deciding which patients will require a CTH.[11]

Chapter 15

15.1 Answer: C

CT is the imaging modality of choice in acute head trauma because it is widely available, it is fast, it is the most sensitive modality for the detection of intra- and extraaxial hemorrhage, and it is superior in the detection of bony details, including fractures of the skull and/or face.

15.2 Answer: C

It is an axial slice of noncontrast-enhanced head CT with bilateral subdural hematomas. Notice the crescentic shape of the hematomas that spreads diffusely across cranial convexities. Also notice how the hematomas can extend across cranial sutures but not dural attachments.

15.3 Answer: A

Chapter 16

16.1 Answer: D

The ABS can be used to serially track symptoms of agitation, including disinhibition, aggression, and emotional lability. It can be scored by multiple members of the treatment team and correlated with a patient's medication regimen. Total scores of the ABS commonly are used as thresholds to guide the administration of agitation medications on an as-needed basis. The Orientation Log is a measure of cognitive recovery. The PART-O-17 and CHIEF are both measures social participation.

16.2 Answer: C

The Rancho LCFS VII level describes an individual with brain injury who presents cognitively and behaviorally as automatic and appropriate, requiring minimal assistance with activities of daily living (but with ongoing deficits of judgment and insight).

16.3 Answer: B

A comprehensive neuropsychological assessment would be the most appropriate next step among the choices provided. This patient presents with multiple cognitive complaints that could be characterized better with a comprehensive neuropsychological evaluation. Such testing also has the benefit of including baseline intellectual function for interpreting the results. Although the MoCA may be somewhat more robust than the MMSE, the comprehensive neuropsychological evaluation will provide more detailed diagnostic information that can inform work accommodations and other interventions. Although brain imaging and EEG might reveal abnormalities in neurological functioning, they would not be able to characterize how any abnormality is expressed in terms of functional ability.

Chapter 17

17.1 Answer: A

Medicare requires that patients admitted to IRFs need medical supervision by a rehabilitation physician. Medicare requires ongoing therapeutic intervention of multiple therapy disciplines, and one therapy discipline would not satisfy that requirement. Medicare requires rehabilitation nursing support, multiple therapy disciplines, ability to tolerate 3 hours of therapy per day at least 5 days a week, medical stability to benefit from rehabilitation services, and an expectation to make measurable and significant improvement within a reasonable timeframe.

Reference: Medicare Learning Network. *Inpatient Rehabilitation Therapy Services: Complying With Documentation Requirements.* Center for Medicare & Medicaid Services. Available from https://www.cms.gov/Outreach-and-Education/Medicare-Learning-Network-MLN/MLNProducts/Downloads/Inpatient_Rehab_Fact_Sheet ICN905643.pdf

17.2 Answer: B

A 3-day intensive care unit length of stay at the acute hospital immediately preceding the LTACH admission or 96 hours of mechanical ventilation services during the LTACH admission are the Medicare requirements for admission.

Reference: Medicare Learning Network. *Long-Term Care Hospital Prospective Payment System.* Chicago, IL: American Hospital Association; 2018. Available from https://www.cms.gov/Outreach-and-Education/Medicare-Learning-Network-MLN/MLNProducts/Downloads/Long-Term-Care-Hospital-PPS-Fact-Sheet-ICN006956.pdf

17.3 Answer: D

There is no Medicare requirement for the amount of rehabilitation therapy at LTACHs. Inpatient rehabilitation facilities (IRFs) are required by Medicare to provide 3 hours of therapy 5 days a week.

Reference: Medicare Learning Network. *Long-Term Care Hospital Prospective Payment System.* Chicago, IL: American Hospital Association; 2018. Available from https://www.cms.gov/Outreach-and-Education/Medicare-Learning-Network-MLN/MLNProducts/Downloads/Long-Term-Care-Hospital-PPS-Fact-Sheet-ICN006956.pdf

Chapter 18

18.1   Answer: B
Reference: Biso S, Wongrakpanich S, Agrawal A, et al. A review of neurogenic stunned myocardium. *Cardiovasc Psychiatry Neurol.* 2017;2017:5842182. doi: 10.1155/2017/5842182.

TCM and NSM may both be seen acutely after traumatic brain injury. TCM is distinguished by involvement of segments of the left ventricle wall, whereas imaging in NSM reveals global left ventricle involvement. Mild elevations in troponin and up to 10 days of persistent elevated sympathetic tone may be observed in both conditions.

18.2   Answer: A
Reference: Scantlebury DC, Prasad A. Diagnosis of takotsubo cardiomyopathy. *Circ J.* 2014;78(9):2129-39.

Per Mayo criteria for the diagnosis of takotsubo cardiomyopathy, there is a segmental left ventricle wall abnormality in the absence of corresponding ischemic ECG changes, also in the absence of obstructive coronary disease. Mildly elevated troponin levels may be present. Restrictive cardiomyopathy syndromes are not associated with TBI.

18.3   Answer: D
Reference: Gregory T, Smith M. Cardiovascular complications of brain injury. *Continuing Education in Anaesthesia Critical Care & Pain.* 2012;12(2):67-71. doi:10.1093/bjaceaccp/mkr058.

Torsades de pointes is a dangerous arrhythmia associated with prolonged QTc that may lead to ventricular fibrillation and fatality. Sinus tachycardia and premature atrial tachycardias may be seen commonly after TBI related to elevated sympathetic tone, not to a prolonged QTc.

Chapter 19

19.1   Answer: B
Patient is exhibiting signs and symptoms of gastro-esophageal reflux disease (GERD) with symptoms of burning sternal pain and cough secondary to the reflux of tube feedings. Studies show that lower esophageal sphincter dysfunction accompanies acute head injury, increases risk of regurgitation, and contributes to risk of aspiration after early gastric feeding. Nutrition in patients with low GCS scores should be parenteral or via the jejunum if they are unable to tolerate feedings.

Reference: Saxe JM, Ledgerwood AM, Lucas CE, et al. Lower esophageal sphincter dysfunction precludes safe gastric feeding after head injury. *J Trauma.* 1994;37(4):581-586.

19.2   Answer: C
Patient is exhibiting signs and symptoms of delayed gastric emptying, which is associated with TBI. This is suspected with feeding intolerance associated with high residuals. This can be manifested by vomiting, abdominal distention, and increased gastric residual volumes. Studies have shown that the combination of erythromycin and metoclopramide therapy exhibited greater benefits than erythromycin or metoclopramide alone and demonstrated less associated tachyphylaxis.

References: Dickerson RN, Mitchell JN, Morgan LM, et al. Disparate response to metoclopramide therapy for gastric feeding intolerance in trauma patients with and without traumatic brain injury. *J Parenter Enteral Nutr.* 2009;33(6):646-655.
Nguyen NQ, Chapman M, Fraser RJ, et al. Prokinetic therapy for feed intolerance in critical illness: one drug or two? *Crit Care Med.* 2007;35(11):2561-2567.

19.3   Answer: C
Intensive insulin therapy in maintaining blood glucose levels 80 to 100 mg/dL may result in cerebrospinal fluid (CSF) glucose values below the normal threshold and increase the risk of hypoglycemia. Blood glucose levels >200 mg/dL are a poor predictor of outcome and are associated with increased risk of morbidity and mortality. Maintaining blood glucose concentrations at 100 to 180 mg/dL should result in improved CSF glucose values and reduce the risk of hypoglycemia.

References: McClave SA, Martindale RG, Vanek VW, et al. Guidelines for the provision and assessment of nutrition support therapy in the adult critically ill trauma patient: Society of Critical Care Medicine (SCCM) and American Society for Parenteral and Enteral Nutrition (ASPEN). *J Parenter Enteral Nutr.* 2009;33(3):277-316.
Vespa P, Boonyaputthikul R, McArthur DL, et al. Intensive insulin therapy reduces microdialysis glucose values without altering glucose utilization or improving the lactate/pyruvate ratio after traumatic brain injury. *Crit Care Med.* 2006;34:850-856.
Young B, Ott L, Dempsey R, et al. Relationship between admission hyperglycemia and neurologic

outcome of severely brain-injured patients. *Ann Surg.* 1989;210(4):466-472.

Chapter 20

20.1 Answer: C
The most common bladder abnormality after brain injury is urinary incontinence. Urinary dysfunction in this population will often involve detrusor hyperreflexia because of an uninhibited and intact reflex pathway and is, therefore, characterized by varying degrees of urge incontinence. It is best to avoid using indwelling Foley catheters for treatment because of risk for infection and development of small, poorly compliant bladder.

References: Chua K, Chuo A, Kong KH. Urinary incontinence after traumatic brain injury: incidence, outcomes and correlates. *Brain Inj.* 2003;17(6):469-478.
Schneider H, Stein A. Genitourinary system. In: Christian A, ed. *Medical Management of Adults with Neurologic Disabilities.* New York, NY: Demos Medical Publishing; 2009.
Weld KJ, Wall BM, Mangold TA, et al. Influences on renal function in chronic spinal cord injured patients. *J Urol.* 2000;164(5):1490-1493.

20.2 Answer: D
When spontaneous voiding returns, PVRs should be measured to verity adequate bladder emptying. PVRs should be less than 100 cc. Elevated PVRs indicate urinary retention and concern for spastic bladder and spastic external sphincter (detrusor sphincter dyssynergia). Urodynamic testing should be performed for diagnostic purposes to determine cause and/or mechanism of neurogenic bladder. BUN and Cr can be measured when there is concern for kidney insufficiency or damage. Urinalysis and urine culture should be performed when there is concern for infection.

Reference: Schneider H, Stein A. Genitourinary system. In: Christian A, ed. *Medical Management of Adults with Neurologic Disabilities.* New York, NY: Demos Medical Publishing; 2009.

20.3 Answer: B
Timed voiding, also known as *bladder training*, refers to scheduled urination for people with a overactive bladder. In timed voiding, individuals adopt a schedule of regular bladder emptying (e.g., every 3–4 hours). Timed voiding also may help with behavioral training in cognitively impaired patients. Intermittent catheterization is used for patients with urinary retention. Indwelling Foley catheters should be avoided because of multiple associated complications such as urinary tract infections (UTIs), urethral strictures, and development of a small, poorly compliant bladder. Antispasmodic medications are used with caution in TBI patients given the potential negative side effects on cognition and known sedation, and they should not be used for initial management.

References: Schneider H, Stein A. Genitourinary System. In: Christian A, ed. *Medical Management of Adults with Neurologic Disabilities.* New York, NY: Demos Medical Publishing; 2009.
Weld KJ, Wall BM, Mangold TA, et al. Influences on renal function in chronic spinal cord injured patients. *J Urol.* 2000;164(5):1490-1493.

Chapter 21

21.1 Answer: B
Prolonged coma duration has been associated with an increased risk for the development of HO.
History of seizure disorder and gender have not been shown to be associated with development of HO. Long bone and extremity fractures, not facial fractures, may also be a risk factor. Other risks may include use of mechanical ventilation and presence of spasticity.

Reference: van Kampen P, Martina J, Vos P, et al. Potential risk factors for developing heterotopic ossification in patients with severe traumatic brain injury. *J Head Trauma Rehabil.* 2011;26(5):384-391.

21.2 Answer: C
The hips are the most common location for the development of HO in TBI patients.
The elbows are the next most common location. HO of the shoulders and knees is also seen, but to a lesser extent.

Reference: Sullivan M, Torres S, Mehta S, et al. Heterotopic ossification after central nervous system trauma. *Bone Joint Res.* 2013;2(3):51-57.

21.3 Answer: B
Plain x-ray can be an effective tool to evaluate for maturity of HO. Bone scan can be a sensitive method for early detection. DEXA does not appear to correlate with HO development. Alkaline phosphatase levels may aid in initial diagnosis but are not correlated with maturation.

Reference: Sullivan M, Torres S, Mehta S, et al. Heterotopic ossification after central nervous system trauma. *Bone Joint Res.* 2013;2(3):51-57.

Chapter 22

22.1 Answer: D
The most common physical symptom experienced after TBI is headache.[1]

22.2. Answer: B
Individuals with preexisting headache and women are more likely to report posttraumatic headache. The

severity of TBI was not related to the incidence of posttraumatic headache.[5]

22.3   Answer: A
Migraine-type headaches account for approximately 35% of posttraumatic headaches with probable migraine-type headaches accounting for another 25%. Tension-type headaches account for approximately 20% of posttraumatic headaches, and cervicogenic headaches account for approximately 10%. Patients may experience multiple types of headache.[7]

Chapter 23

23.1   Answer: A
Hyponatremia commonly occurs after brain injury. Although differentiating CSW and SIADH at times can be difficult, it is very important to distinguish because they are managed differently. Laboratory values for both can be very similar, which is why establishing fluid status is important. CSW usually occurs with high urine output and is a hypovolemic state and would be treated with fluid and sodium replacement, whereas SIADH would require fluid restriction.

Reference: Zasler ND, Katz DI, Zafonte RD. *Brain Injury Medicine: Principles and Practice*. 2nd ed. New York, NY: Demos Medical Pub.; 2013. Chapter 53.

23.2   Answer: C
Thyroid screening tests usually involve TSH and free T4 if deficient replacement is given in the form of T4 hormone. Thyroid hormone abnormalities have been associated with cognitive issues in TBI.

23.3   Answer: D
Although hyponatremia is one of the most common electrolyte abnormalities after neurological injury, it is not a hormone. Growth hormone deficiency has been identified as the most common hormonal abnormality after TBI.

Reference: Zasler ND, Katz DI, Zafonte RD. *Brain Injury Medicine: Principles and Practice*. 2nd ed. New York, NY: Demos Medical Pub.; 2013. Chapter 53.

Chapter 24

24.1   Answer: B
Reference: Baguley IJ, Nicholls JL, Felmingham KL, et al. Dysautonomia after traumatic brain injury: a forgotten syndrome? *J Neurol Neurosurg Psychiatry*. 1999;67(1):39-43.

PSH is associated with longer coma, lower Functional Independence Measure (FIM) score at discharge, longer hospital stay, greater healthcare costs, and increased morbidity and mortality rates, compared with other

severe traumatic brain injury (TBI) patients. Although FIM scores have been shown to be lower than for non-PSH patients, patients with PSH do show functional improvement during rehabilitation.

24.2   Answer: C
Reference: Baguley IJ, Perkes IE, Fernandez-Ortega JF, et al. Paroxysmal sympathetic hyperactivity after acquired brain injury: consensus on conceptual definition, nomenclature, and diagnostic criteria. *J Neurotrauma*. 2014;31(17):1515-1520.

Common clinical features during episodes of PSH include tachycardia, tachypnea, hypertension, hyperthermia, diaphoresis, and posturing.

24.3   Answer: D
References: Perkes I, Baguley IJ, Nott MT, et al. A review of paroxysmal sympathetic hyperactivity after acquired brain injury. *Ann Neurol*. 2010;68(2):126-135. Pertab JL, Merkley TL, Cramond AJ, et al. Concussion and the autonomic nervous system: an introduction to the field and the results of a systematic review. *NeuroRehabilitation*. 2018;42(4):397-427.

Autonomic dysfunction such as heart rate variability, abnormal tilt testing, baroreflex dysfunction, syncope, and postural orthostatic tachycardia syndrome (POTS) have been noted in patients with mild TBI. PSH is seen in moderate and severe TBI patients and those with hypoxic brain injury or stroke.

Chapter 25

25.1   Answer: C
Phenol is less costly, more technically difficult to administer, and carries a higher risk of dysesthesia compared with botulinum toxin. Phenol requires less frequent administration than botulinum toxin because its effect can last from months to years.[5,6]

25.2   Answer: B
Both MAS 1 and 1+ are associated with a "catch" during ROM, but MAS 1 is a catch followed by a release, whereas MAS 1+ exhibits a catch followed by slight resistance in the remainder of ROM.[1]

25.3   Answer: C
MAS 2 indicates a marked increase in muscle tone throughout ROM, but the joint is easily moved. MAS 3 would indicate a considerable increase in tone; passive movement is difficult.[1]

Chapter 26

26.1   Answer: C
The presentation of hydrocephalus can be subtle and different than the classic triad of ataxia, incontinence and change in mental status. Arrest in progression,

which is seen with the decline in progress in therapy with this presentation, increased spasticity, and vomiting are all clinical signs of possible hydrocephalus. At this time imaging of the head is warranted. Labs were normal therefore there is less concern for systemic infection. Posttraumatic seizures can be a possibility, but less likely based on clinical picture. Neurostimulants can be used in the management of traumatic brain injury, but first further work up is needed.

Reference: Ivanhoe CB, Durand-Sanchez A, Spier ET. Acute rehabilitation. In: Zasler ND, Katz DI, Zafonte RD, eds. *Brain Injury Medicine Principles and Practice.* 2nd ed. New York, NY: Demos Medical Publishing; 2013.

26.2   Answer: C
The patient is presenting with shunt failure. The most common cause of shunt dysfunction is proximal occlusion of the ventricular catheter (this occurs in at least 30% of shunt dysfunction cases). Overdrainage of the shunt may make proximal occlusion more likely as the catheter tip abuts the ventricular wall. Distal shunt obstruction may occur from loculation of peritoneal content around the distal catheter tip. Disconnection of shunt components accounts for 15% of shunt revisions.

Reference: Long DF. Diagnosis and management of late intracranial complications of traumatic brain injury. In: Zasler ND, Katz DI, Zafonte RD, eds. *Brain Injury Medicine Principles and Practice.* 2nd ed. New York, NY: Demos Medical Publishing; 2013:726-747.

26.3   Answer: C.
The presence of subarachnoid and intraventricular hemorrhage place him at higher risk for development of posttraumatic hydrocephalus. Older age, lower GCS score, and decompressive craniectomy are other risk factors that can lead to the development of hydrocephalus.

Reference: Chen H, Yuan F, Chen SW, et al. Predicting posttraumatic hydrocephalus: derivation and validation of a risk scoring system based on clinical characteristics. *Metab Brain Dis.* 2017;32(5):1427-1435.

Chapter 27

27.1   Answer: A
Olfactory nerve injury should be considered in the differential diagnosis for bland-tasting food, weight loss, and anorexia in a patient with mild TBI.

Injury to the olfactory nerve is the only CN injury commonly associated with mild TBI, which makes CN XII, IX, and X injury less likely. CN IX does provide taste sensation to the posterior one-third of the tongue but is not a commonly injured CN and is not associated with mild TBI. Even a conscious patient with a mild injury may be unaware of anosmia; more often, the patient complains of altered taste sensation that may lead to anorexia.

References: Costanzo R, Zasler N. Epidemiology and pathophysiology of olfactory and gustatory dysfunction in head trauma. *J Head Trauma Rehabil.* 1992;7(1):15-24.
Welge-Lüssen A, Hilgenfeld A, Meusel T, et al. Long-term follow-up of posttraumatic olfactory disorders. *Rhinology.* 2012;50(1):67-72.

27.2   Answer: D
The CN most susceptible to injury in the setting of TBI is the olfactory nerve (CN I).

Higher incidences of olfactory injury are correlated with increased severity of TBI, with anosmia in 25% to 30% of patients with severe head injury, in 15% to 19% of those with moderate head injury, and in 0% to 16% of those with mild injuries. CN VIII is the third most commonly injured CN in TBI. The trigeminal (CN V) and lower CNs (CN IX–XII) are rarely injured. CN I injury is the only CN injury commonly associated with mild TBI.

References: Costanzo R, Zasler N. Epidemiology and pathophysiology of olfactory and gustatory dysfunction in head trauma. *J Head Trauma Rehabil.* 1992;7(1):15-24.
Welge-Lüssen A, Hilgenfeld A, Meusel T, et al. Long-term follow-up of posttraumatic olfactory disorders. *Rhinology.* 2012;50(1):67-72.

27.3   Answer: C
INO is a disorder of conjugate lateral gaze in which the affected eye shows impairment of adduction. When an attempt is made to gaze contralaterally (relative to the affected eye), the affected eye adducts minimally, if at all. The contralateral eye abducts with nystagmus. In INO, the divergence of the eyes leads to horizontal diplopia. If the right eye is affected, the patient will see double when looking to the left. Convergence is generally preserved. INO is caused by disruption in the medial longitudinal fasciculus.

Horner syndrome is characterized by miosis, ptosis, and anhidrosis and does not include the symptoms reported by the patient. Oculomotor nerve injury would result in a down-and-out position, ptosis, and a dilated pupil on the affected side. Abducens nerve injury will cause diplopia caused by the unopposed muscle tone of the medial rectus muscle, and the affected eye is pulled to look toward the midline.

References: Beck RW, Meckler RJ. Internuclear ophthalmoplegia after head trauma. *Ann Ophthalmol.* 1981;13(6):671-675.
Cerovski B, Vidovifá T, Papa J, et al. Minor head trauma and isolated unilateral internuclear ophthalmoplegia. *J Emerg Med.* 2006;31(2):165-167.

Chon J, Kim M. Bilateral internuclear ophthalmoplegia following head trauma. *Indian J Ophthalmol.* 2017;65(3):246-247.

Chapter 28

28.1 Answer: C
PTS is classified temporally as immediate (within 24 hours), early (between 1 and 7 days), and late (after 1 week).[1,2,4]

28.2 Answer: B
Based on the description of generalized tonic–clonic movements, patient possibly had a generalized seizure. Because it occurred within 24 hours after his head injury, the seizure is classified as immediate. Current guidelines are to treat TBI patients with an AED for 1 week for seizure prophylaxis. If an early or late PTS occurs, long-term treatment is indicated. Long-term seizure prophylaxis is not recommended for immediate PTS.[1,4,13-16]

28.3 Answer: D
Most PTS are the partial seizures. Left untreated, seizures can lead to increased intracranial pressure, neurometabolic demand, and further secondary brain injury. In this patient case, EEG and serum prolactin are not recommended because of limited diagnostic sensitivity and the inability of this patient to tolerate EEG. Empiric AED treatment with close monitoring of patient response is reasonable after excluding other acute causes for this patient's behavior.[1,2,4,9-12]

Chapter 29

29.1 Answer: D
Motor learning is a cognitive process to acquire, retain, and retrieve motor plans to execute actions with speed, accuracy, coordination, and consistency to achieve task goals. Whereas motor disorders (resulting from pyramidal tract injury) or a movement disorder may hinder motor learning somewhat by making practice more challenging, motor learning is a cognitive process.

29.2 Answer: C
The FLAME trial was published in 2011 and included 118 patients with ischemic stroke from nine centers in France who were randomized to fluoxetine versus placebo. Results suggested that fluoxetine did enhance motor recovery at 3 months. FOCUS, however, a randomized, double-blind RCT, included 3127 patients with ischemic and hemorrhagic stroke across 103 hospitals in the United Kingdom. The results of FOCUS were published in 2018 and did not demonstrate any benefit of fluoxetine on functional outcome at 6 months. The treatment group did have an increase rate of fractures.

29.3 Answer: C
A high-amplitude, postural, and kinetic tremor is the most common movement disorder after severe TBI, followed by hemidystonia. The true incidence of parkinsonism resulting from brain injury is unclear because the epidemiological relationship between parkinsonism and brain injury in terms of cause versus effect remains unknown. Spasticity is a feature of upper motor neuron syndrome, which is a motor disorder and not a movement disorder.

Chapter 30

30.1 Answer: B
Patients are at risk of developing a pressure injury if they have reduced mobility, complex medical conditions and hospitalizations, cognitive impairments such as brain injury or dementia, and motor and sensory impairments such as stroke or spinal cord injury. Although, eczema affects the skin and vitamin D, which is produced by the skin, it is a known risk factor for pressure injuries.

Reference: Bergstrom N, Braden B, Kemp M, et al. Multi-site study of incidence of pressure ulcers and the relationship between risk level, demographic characteristics, diagnoses, and the prescription of preventive interventions. *J Am Geriatr Soc.* 1996;44(1):22-30.

30.2 Answer: D
Although psychosocial factors and lifestyle are extrinsic risk factors for the development of pressure ulcers, race on its own is not an independent risk factor. Issues that may be indirectly related to socioeconomic status, such as familial support, access to specialized healthcare, and independence of community mobility, affect social integration and thus may contribute to a lifestyle that inherently increases the risk for developing pressure ulcers. Incontinence is an intrinsic risk factor. Moisture from incontinence, immobility, and the inability to consciously perform postural maneuvers, sensory impairment, and impaired nutritional status may lead to impaired response to healing (see Table 30.1).

Reference: Bergstrom N, Braden B, Kemp M, Champagne M, Ruby E. Multi-site study of incidence of pressure ulcers and the relationship between risk level, demographic characteristics, diagnoses, and the prescription of preventive interventions. *J Am Geriatr Soc.* 1996;44(1):22-30.

30.3 Answer: C
In any position, the iliac crest is not a pressure-loaded area or an area at risk of sheer injury.

Reference: Kruger EA, Pires M, Ngann Y, et al. Comprehensive management of pressure ulcers in spinal cord injury: current concepts and future trends. *J Spinal Cord Med.* 2013;36(6):572-585.

Chapter 31

31.1   Answer: B
Patients with TBI admitted to the intensive care unit (ICU) are at high risk of pneumonia, with the incidence as high as 93% among those with severe TBI because of problems with eating and drinking. The incidence correlates with injury severity, and these factors indicate more severe injury: decrease level of alertness, lower tone in the lower esophageal sphincter, or relaxation of the muscles in the larynx leading to reduced airway closure.

Reference: Hansen TS, Larsen K, Enberg AW. The association of functional oral intake and pneumonia in patients with severe traumatic brain injury. *Arch Phys Med Rehabil.* 2008;89(11):2114-2120.

31.2   Answer: C
Swallowing characteristics of dysphagic patients after TBI were comparable to those of dysphagic stroke patients. Some studies suggest the problem results from pharyngeal phase dysfunction, whereas others suggest oral phase dysfunction. Common to both are finding among these studies on videofluoroscopic swallowing studies (VFSS) are aspiration/penetration, decreased laryngeal elevation, and reduced epiglottis inversion.

Reference: Lee WK, Yeom J, Lee WH, et al. Characteristics of dysphagia in severe traumatic brain injury patients: a comparison with stroke patients. *Ann Rehabil Med.* 2016;40(3):432-439.

31.3   Answer: C.
The Four Phases Model describes drinking and swallowing liquid, whereas the Process Model describes eating and swallowing of solid food. The Four Phase Model is subdivided into the oral preparatory stage, the oral propulsive stage, the pharyngeal stage, and the esophageal stage.

Risk of aspiration is greatest in the pharyngeal phase, as successful passage of food requires a coordinated inhibition of breathing to prevent aspiration.

Reference: Matsuo K, Palmer JB. Anatomy and physiology of feeding and swallowing: normal and abnormal. *Phys Med Rehabil Clin N Am.* 2008; 19(4):691-707.

Chapter 32

32.1   Answer: B.
Aphasia is a disorder of language that occurs after injury to one or more of the brain areas responsible for language, which is usually located in the left hemisphere. Aphasia can occur suddenly (after a head injury or stroke) or gradually as a result of a brain tumor or a progressive neurological disease.

Reference: NIH National Institute on Deafness and Other Communication Disorders. Aphasia. 2017. Available from https://www.nidcd.nih.gov/health/aphasia

32.2   Answer: A
Broca's aphasia occurs after injury/damage usually to the left frontal lobe of the brain in the area posterior/inferior to the postcentral gyrus. Because the frontal lobe is important to motor movements, this often results in right-sided weakness/paralysis involving the arm/leg.

Reference: Ardila A, Bernal B, Rosselli M. How localized are language brain areas? A review of Brodmann areas involvement in oral language. *Arch Clin Neuropsychol.* 2016;31(1):112-122.

32.3   Answer: D
Wernicke's aphasia occurs after damage to the posterior third of the superior gyrus in the temporal lobe. Also known as *fluent aphasia*, patients speak in long complete sentences that have no meaning, with made-up words, unaware of their mistakes; have difficulty understanding speech; and have difficulty with repeating phrases.

Reference: Fager SK HM, Brady S, Barlow SM, et al. In Cifu D, ed. *Braddom's Physical Medicine and Rehabilitation.* Philadelphia, PA: Elsevier Health Sciences; 2015:54.

Chapter 33

33.1   Answer: C
Studies have shown that individuals engaged in lawsuits or pursuing disability perform worse on cognitive testing. Individuals with mild TBI often experience complete recovery after TBI, whereas many individuals with severe TBI have residual impairments. Gender is not associated with differential outcomes, although younger age at time of injury is associated with better outcomes. Often described as a *cognitive reserve*, individuals with higher preinjury intelligence have better cognitive outcomes than those with low preinjury functioning.

33.2   Answer: D
Preexisting amnesia is not a term used in TBI. *Anterograde amnesia* refers to memory loss for events immediately after a TBI. PTA is synonymous with anterograde amnesia. Retrograde amnesia is loss of events preceding a TBI and occurs in some cases of severe TBI.

33.3   Answer: D
PTA can be assessed prospectively at bedside/inpatient at regular intervals. Standardized measures are very helpful to obtain objective assessment of PTA. On clinical interview, the interviewer can ask the patient

what was the first memory they had after their injury to assess PTA retrospectively. Computerized batteries can assess cognitive abilities but not duration of PTA.

Chapter 34

34.1   Answer: C
This veteran is presenting with a constellation of symptoms of posttraumatic Meniere's. Audiogram shows sensorineural hearing loss at both high and low frequencies.

Reference: Smouha E. Inner ear disorders. *NeuroRehabilitation*. 2013;32(3):455-462.

34.2   Answer: C
Brainstem contusion is a central cause of vertigo. Vertical gaze nystagmus is found in central lesions. Saccadic pursuit is also seen in central disorders. Dynamic visual acuity test is positive in peripheral disorders. All other choices are peripheral sources of dizziness.

Reference: Chandrasekhar SS. The assessment of balance and dizziness in the TBI patient. *NeuroRehabilitation*. 2013;32(3):445-454.

34.3   Answer: A
The symptoms of diplopia, difficulty reading, headache, and dizziness are seen in vergence deficits. The testing is consistent with a convergence insufficiency. Convergence insufficiency is the most common oculomotor deficit after TBI. Oculomotor therapy, prisms, and patching are treatments. Oculomotor is recommended as primary treatment of convergence insufficiency, prisms secondary, and patching sparingly. Sumatriptan will not help the visual disorder.

Reference: Fox SM, Koons P, Dang SH. Vision rehabilitation after traumatic brain injury. *Phys Med Rehabil Clin N Am*. 2019;30(1):171-188.

Chapter 35

35.1   Answer: A
An appropriate first-line treatment for apathy after traumatic brain injury is a psychostimulant such as methylphenidate or amphetamine. Bupropion may be beneficial, but this patient's history of epilepsy is a relative contraindication to bupropion pharmacotherapy.

References: Reekum R, Reekum E. Apathy. In: Arciniegas DB, Nasler ND, Vanderploeg RD, et al., eds. *Management of Adults with Traumatic Brain Injury*. Washington, DC: American Psychiatric Publishing; 2013:283-302.

Starkstein SE, Pahissa J. Apathy following traumatic brain injury. *Psychiatr Clin North Am*. 2014;37(1):103-112.

35.2   Answer: C
The presence of a premorbid personality disorder must be given strong consideration when evaluating individuals with emotional dyscontrol after TBI. This patient's superficial conversation, exaggerated expressions, exclusion of her boyfriend from providing history, and increased emotionality across all topics and emotional states are most consistent with histrionic personality disorder.

Reference: Arciniegas DB, Wortzel HS. Emotional and behavioral dyscontrol after traumatic brain injury. *Psychiatr Clin North Am*. 2014;37(1):31-53.

35.3   Answer: B
Only dextromethorphan/quinidine is FDA approved for the treatment of pseudobulbar affect (pathological laughter and crying), but selective serotonin reuptake inhibitors (SSRIs) remain appropriate first-line pharmacotherapy.

Reference: Yang LP, Deeks ED. Dextromethorphan/quinidine: a review of its use in adults with pseudobulbar affect. *CNS Drugs*. 2015;75(1):83-90.

Chapter 36

36.1   Answer: B
The ABS is the only validated measure of agitation in the TBI population. The OAS was originally developed for the mental health population. The GOAT is a reliable and validated indicator of PTA in the TBI population but does not measure agitation. RLAS represents the typical progression of recovery in TBI. A component of stage IV describes a confused agitated patient but does not measure agitation.

Reference: Castaño Monsalve B, Laxe S, Bernabeu Guitart M, et al. Behavioral scales used in severe and moderate traumatic brain injury. *NeuroRehabilitation*. 2014;35(1):67-76.

36.2   Answer: D
First-line management of agitated behavior should include environmental modification, including limiting the number of visitors. Bilateral wrist restraints may worsen agitation. Medication management can be considered if agitation persists despite environmental and behavioral modification. A beta blocker may be appropriate, but nonselective lipophilic beta blockers such as propranolol are preferred over selective, moderately lipophilic choices such as metoprolol. Although haloperidol can be effective to manage a patient during an acute agitation crisis, it should not be used first line.

Reference: Bhatnagar S, Iaccarino MA, Zafonte R. Pharmacotherapy in rehabilitation of postacute traumatic brain injury. *Brain Res*. 2016;1640:164-179.

36.3   Answer: B

In this case it may be appropriate to initiate treatment with an antipsychotic given the paranoia and delusions. Atypical antipsychotics are preferred over typical antipsychotics because of more favorable side effect profile and deleterious effect on recovery with typical antipsychotics.

Reference: Kalra I, Watanabe T. Mood stabilizers for traumatic brain injury-related agitation. *J Head Trauma Rehabil.* 2017;32(6):E61-E64.

Chapter 37

37.1   Answer: B

K-complexes and sleep spindles are part of N2 (stage 2) sleep, which indicate a transition into deeper sleep, where heart rate and blood pressure drop.

Reference: Patel AK, Araujo JF. Physiology, sleep stages. [Updated 2018 Oct 27]. In: *StatPearls* [Internet]. Treasure Island, FL: StatPearls Publishing; 2018.

37.2   Answer: B

The BNI Fatigue Scale was created to adequately assess fatigue during early stages after a brain injury, it is designed particularly for acute inpatient rehabilitation setting.

Reference: Borgaro S, Gierok S, Caples H, et al. Fatigue after brain injury: initial reliability study of the BNI Fatigue Scale. *Brain Inj.* 2004;18(7):685-690.

37.3   Answer: A

All these medications act as stimulants, but out of these options, research for treatment of fatigue after TBI has only found moderate evidence for use of methylphenidate.

Reference: Johansson B, Wentzel AP, Andrell P, et al. Evaluation of dosage, safety and effects of methylphenidate on posttraumatic brain injury symptoms with a focus on mental fatigue and pain. *Brain Inj.* 2014;28(3):304-310.

Chapter 38

38.1   Answer: C

Preinjury psychiatric history, in particular preinjury anxiety, depression, and substance abuse, remains the most robust risk factor for postinjury depression and anxiety. There is little evidence indicating that injury severity affects risk for depression or anxiety. Although some studies have shown increased risk of depression and anxiety associated with age and education level; others have not shown this association.

References: Fann J, Burington B, Leonetti A, et al. Psychiatric illness following traumatic brain injury in an adult health maintenance organization population. *Arch Gen Psychiatry.* 2004;61:53-61.

Gould K, Ponsford J, Johnston L, et al. The nature, frequency and course of psychiatric disorders in the first year after traumatic brain injury: a prospective study. *Psychol Med.* 2011;41:2099-2109.

Scholten A, Haagsma J, Cnossen M, et al. Prevalence of and risk factors for anxiety and depressive disorders after traumatic brain injury: a systematic review. *J Neurotrauma.* 2016;33:1969-1994.

38.2   Answer: D

There are numerous mechanisms through which depression and anxiety can develop after TBI. These include both biological mechanisms and psychosocial, adjustment-related mechanisms. Depression and anxiety can arise as a person struggles to adjust to temporary or lasting disability, losses, or role changes within the family and society. With respect to biological mechanisms, focal and diffuse injuries to prefrontal and limbic regions may result in disruption of neural circuits, which may contribute to affective disturbance, increasing risk for depression and anxiety. Although age at injury could be a risk factor for depression and anxiety, it is not mechanistically linked (i.e., does not play a causal role) in the development of postinjury depression or anxiety.

References: Hoofien D, Gilboa A, Vaki E. Traumatic brain injury (TBI) 10-20 years later: a comprehensive outcome study of psychiatric symptomatology, cognitive abilities and psychosocial functioning. *Brain Inj.* 2001;15(3):189-209.

Jorge RE, Arciniegas DB. Mood disorders after TBI. *Psychiatr Clin North Am.* 2014;37(1):13-29.

Jorge RE, Robinson RG, Arndt SV, et al. Comparison between acute- and delayed-onset depression following traumatic brain injury. *J Neuropsychiatry Clin Neurosci.* 1993;5(1):43-49.

38.3   Answer: B

For a diagnosis of major depression, the individual must be experiencing five or more symptoms during the same 2-week period and at least one of the symptoms should be either depressed mood or loss of interest or pleasure. Other ancillary symptoms include significant weight change or change in appetite, sleep disturbance, psychomotor agitation or retardation, fatigue, feelings of worthlessness, difficulty concentrating, and recurrent thoughts of death or suicidal ideation.

Reference: *Diagnostic and Statistical Manual of Mental Disorders: DSM-5.* Arlington, VA: American Psychiatric Association; 2013.

Chapter 39

39.1   Answer: C

39.2   Answer: D

Choice A is incorrect because education has not been identified as a risk factor. Choice B is incorrect because age during the trauma has not been identified as a risk factor. Choice C is incorrect because age during the trauma is not an identified risk factor for PTSD.

39.3   Answer: B
PTSD is found in 11% to 39% of bipolar patients. Major depressive disorder occurs in half of patients with PTSD. Generalized anxiety disorder is found in 40% of patients with PTSD and 20% of those with PTSD also have a substance use disorder.

Chapter 40

40.1   Answer: B
Cultural factors may significantly influence one's baseline behavior in relation to social norms. For example, personal space and physical contact during casual conversation can vary widely across cultures. Variations in these types of behaviors could be misconstrued as disinhibition if cultural norms are not appropriately considered. Age, blood type, and specific injury characteristics such as length of posttraumatic amnesia are not likely to significantly bias one's assessment and diagnosis of posttraumatic disinhibition.

Reference: Wortzel HS, Silver JS. Behavioral dyscontrol. In: Silver JM, McAllister TW, Arcinegas DB, eds. *Textbook of Traumatic Brain Injury.* 3rd ed. Washington, DC: American Psychiatric Association Publishing; 2019:395-411.

40.2   Answer: A
Positive reinforcement, such as rewarding either appropriate behavior or avoiding undesired behavior is a common element in typical behavior modification plans. All members of the treatment team, rather than one individual, should participate in the implementation of behavior modification plan. Removing the opportunity to rest would be a maladaptive form of punishment that is not likely going to improve the patient's ability to control behavior. Benzodiazepines are not an indicated treatment for disinhibition, and administering medication in response to disinhibition is not a behavioral modification strategy.

Reference: Arcinegas DB, Wortzel HS. Emotional and behavioral dyscontrol after TBI. *Psychiatr Clin N Am.* 2014;37:31-53.

40.3   Answer: D
Pharmacotherapy for posttraumatic disinhibition includes serotonin reuptake inhibitors (SSRIs) as first-line treatment. Atypical antipsychotics warrant consideration when patients do not respond to other approaches.

Reference: Wortzel HS, Silver JS. Behavioral dyscontrol. In: Silver JM, McAllister TW, Arcinegas DB,

eds. *Textbook of Traumatic Brain Injury.* 3rd ed. Washington, DC: American Psychiatric Association Publishing; 2019:395-411.

Chapter 41

41.1   Answer: A
Reference: Zasler ND, Katz DI, Zafonte RD. *Brain Injury Medicine: Principles and Practice.* 2nd ed. New York, NY: Demos Medical Pub.; 2013.

41.2   Answer: B
Alcohol use peaks 2 years postinjury and stabilizes afterward.

Reference: Merkel SF, Cannella LA, Razmpour R, et al. Factors affecting increased risk for substance use disorders following traumatic brain injury: What we can learn from animal models. *Neurosci Biobehav Rev.* 2017;77:209-218.

41.3   Answer: C
Liver function tests should be monitored on patients taking naltrexone because of risk of hepatotoxicity.

Reference: Zasler ND, Katz DI, Zafonte RD. *Brain Injury Medicine: Principles and Practice.* 2nd ed. New York, NY: Demos Medical Pub.; 2013.

Chapter 42

42.1   Answer: B
Kluver-Bucy syndrome is caused by damage to the bilateral anterior temporal lobes and can present with symptoms such as hypersexuality, hyperorality, and exploratory behaviors.[3] Frontal lobe injuries can also lead to hypersexual responses because of disinhibition[2] and apathy, attention deficits, and initiation impairments.[5,6]

42.2   Answer: B
Cognitive deficits such as attention and concentration difficulties can interfere with patient's ability to maintain an erection or focus on sexual activities.[4] Spasticity is a functional deficit that can cause difficulty with body positioning, movement, and pain.[7] Fatigue is also a physical factor that can contribute to decreased desire and frequency of sexual activity.[9] Depression is an emotional factor that can lead to decreased sexual desire and arousal.[5,7]

42.3   Answer: A
The reticular activating system is in the midbrain/pons and is involved with consciousness. Damage to this structure can cause decreased levels of arousal and alertness, which can lead to decreased sexual function. The brainstem also makes connections to other areas of the brain such as the limbic and

paralimbic structures, which include the hippocampus, amygdala, and hypothalamus. These areas are also involved in sexual function and behavior.[6]

Chapter 43

43.1 Answer: A
Based on assessment of range of motion (ROM), spasticity, and strength not only providing therapy but a device to maximize function and safety needs to be considered.

Reference: Rogozinski BM, Schwab SE, Kesar TM. Effects of an articulated ankle foot orthosis on gait biomechanics in adolescents with traumatic brain injury: a case-series report. *Phys Med Rehabil Int.* 2018;5(2)pii: 1144.

43.2 Answer: B
Because of the severity of his impairments early in his recovery, his prognosis for full recovery is diminished.

Reference: Hylin MJ, Kerr AL, Holden R. Understanding the mechanisms of recovery and/or compensation following injury. *Neural Plast.* 2017;2017: 7125057.

43.3 Answer: B
The presentation of "wild, wet, and wobbly" is new for this patient. Periodic examinations and transdisciplinary approach can assist with ruling in or out secondary complications.

Reference: Whyte J, Nordenbo AM, Kalmar K, et al. Medical complications during inpatient rehabilitation among patients with traumatic disorders of consciousness. *Arch Phys Med Rehabil.* 2013; 94(10):1877 1883.

Chapter 44

44.1 Answer: C
AT means any item, piece of equipment or product system, whether acquired commercially off the shelf, modified, or customized, that is used to increase, maintain, or improve the functional capabilities of children with disabilities. (Federal Register, August 19, 1991, p. 41272).

44.2 Answer: D
The federal regulations went on to state that an array of services is included when considering applications of AT. Such services include activities such as evaluation of a person's needs for AT devices, purchasing or leasing AT devices for people, designing and fabricating devices, coordinating services offered by those who provide AT services, providing training or technical assistance to a person who uses AT, and training and technical assistance to those who work with people who use AT devices, such as teachers or employers.

44.3 Answer: B
The Individuals With Disabilities Education Act (IDEA), passed in 1997, Public Law 105-17 guarantees the right of all children with disabilities to a free and appropriate public education in the least restrictive environment. Most important is the development of an Individualized Education Program (IEP) for every student who is enrolled in special education, which are now extended to preschool programs for students who are entitled to an Individualized Family Services Plan (IFSP) and to those who are eligible for rehabilitation services through the development of an Individualized Written Rehabilitation Plan (IWRP).

Chapter 45

45.1 Answer: C
After 8 weeks in a coma, your chance of having a good outcome is approaching zero. TTFC correlates with emergence from coma. There are many jobs where aphasia is not a significant barrier to RTW. Anosognosia becomes a larger issue over time and is a bigger barrier to RTW long term. Psychiatric illness is treatable even if associated with TBI.

45.2 Answer: C
Retirement goals are not considered DVR. Likewise, CMS is not interested in DVR goals because CMS recipients are over the age of 65 or on disability. Most IRFs do not support these services because they are primarily under CMS guidelines.

45.3 Answer: C
Intellectual quotient, medical comorbidities, and time since injury correlate very little, if at all, with RTW.

Chapter 46

46.1 Answer: C
The relationship is bidirectional, because patient functioning can affect caregiver functioning, and caregiver functioning can affect patient outcome. A and B are each only partially correct, because they only account for one direction. D is incorrect because research demonstrates a bidirectional relationship.

46.2 Answer: B
Family caregivers most often rate the need for information as most important. Choices A, C, and D list other important needs, but these are not consistently identified as most important by caregivers themselves in research.

46.3 Answer: C
During acute inpatient rehabilitation, family members may be experiencing an emotional roller coaster ranging from fear of possible death to joy of the patient's survival. They will be receiving communications from multiple members of the trauma team and may have difficulty processing and recalling all the information. A is incorrect, because this applies most to the inpatient rehabilitation setting, where gains in functioning tend to be rapid and family members may expect the same pace of gains and a full recovery. B is incorrect because it applies most to the postacute rehabilitation phase, when patients are at home and family members are learning to navigate their daily lives. D is incorrect because family members may process grief and distress throughout all phases of recovery, making this factor not as salient as choice C.

Chapter 47

47.1 Answer: B
Current guidelines for mild traumatic brain injury (mTBI, formerly "concussion") advise against imaging studies unless there is suspicion for more severe injury. Severe injury can include vomiting, loss of consciousness, worsening headache, suspicion of skull fracture and Glasgow Coma Score less than 15. Head CT is the preferred imaging in severe cases. In mTBI, clinical counseling for families to monitor for signs of evolving injury can guide care. Current protocols have not set standardized timelines for graded return to learn/play.

Reference: Lumba-Brown A, Yeates KO, Sarmiento K, et al. Centers for Disease Control and Prevention guideline on the diagnosis and management of mild traumatic brain injury among children. *JAMA Pediatr.* 2018;172(11):e182853.

47.2 Answer: A
Whereas growth hormone deficiency is the most common endocrine dysfunction in adults with TBI, precocious puberty was found to be the most common endocrine deficiency in children. Precocious puberty is a unique feature of pediatric TBI, requiring GnRH agonist therapy to slow the progression of puberty.

Reference: Kaulfers AM, Backeljauw PF, Reifschneider K, et al. Endocrine dysfunction following traumatic brain injury in children. *J Pediatr.* 2010; 157(6):894-899.

47.3 Answer: C
Studies have documented premorbid ADHD in 10% to 22% of children, whereas other studies theorize a link between TBI and subsequent ADHD. Awareness of this can guide clinicians in appropriate classroom

settings and available resources. None of the other choices describe this behavior pattern.

References: Adeyemo BO, Biederman J, Zafonte R, et al. Mild traumatic brain injury and ADHD: a systematic review of the literature and meta-analysis. *J Atten Disord.* 2014;18(7):576-584.
Max JE, Lansing AE, Koele SL, et al. Attention deficit hyperactivity disorder in children and adolescents following traumatic brain injury. *Dev Neuropsychol.* 2004;25(1-2):159-177.

Chapter 48

48.1 Answer: B
Statistically, unintentional falls represent the leading cause of TBI in the elderly population. Transportation-related accidents such as motor vehicle collisions represent the second leading cause of TBI in the elderly.

48.2 Answer: D
The aging CNS demonstrates a decline in its ability to handle stress. Choices A through C all represents potential reasons for poor outcomes after TBI.

48.3 Answer: B
Patients who are recovering from a brain injury benefit from a low-stimulus environment. Loud noises, busy rooms, and a large number of visitors may all be causes of overstimulation in a patient, leading to behavioral dysregulation. Other causes of behavioral dysregulation include pain and constipation, thus treating both is a reasonable treatment approach for dysregulated behavior.

Chapter 49

49.1 Answer: C
Medics and corpsmen are the first responders in military medicine.

49.2 Answer: B
The MACE (Military Acute Concussion Examination) is the initial assessment tool used to screen service Members with suspected acute traumatic brain injury.

49.3 Answer: C
Tertiary blast injures are those that result from being thrown by the blast wind.

Chapter 50

50.1 Answer: D
In the setting of the child demonstrating improvement in her overall symptoms, lingering headaches can persist and can be managed with as-needed pain

medications such as acetaminophen or ibuprofen. Normalization of school should be continued and modifications provided if needed, such as rest breaks to go to the nurse's office or extension on assignments/tests. Removal from school should not be recommended if the child is improving in her symptoms. Providing reassurance of recovery and reaffirming that reintegration is beneficial for recovery are crucial.

50.2 Answer: C
Worsened symptoms after concussion symptoms have been improving is most likely related to factors other than the injury sustained. Children and parents should be counseled on this, and investigating why the child has worsened symptoms should be further pursued. Often, it can be related to psychosocial stressors at home or at school, such as tests or even bullies. Identifying the source of the increase in symptoms can lead to the most appropriate management options.

50.3 Answer: A
Sleep should always be managed first, because poor sleep can lead to other symptoms of headache, mood changes, and cognitive inefficiencies. When identified, sleep disorders should always be prioritized.

Chapter 51

51.1 Answer: A
Neck strength was a significant predictor of concussion among high school athletes. Increased neck strength decreases head acceleration, rapid changes in velocity, and displacement after collision, which way reduce the risk of sports-related concussion.[21-23]

51.2 Answer: D
Men have over twice the rate of TBI-related deaths and TBI related hospitalizations compared with women, suggesting men may be at higher risk of suffering a more severe brain injury.[3]

51.3 Answer: C
Progesterone administration in patients with TBI has shown conflicting results in clinical studies. Although limited studies have shown some benefits, others have shown progesterone had no effect on disability outcomes as scored by the Glasgow Outcome Scale.[7-9]

Chapter 52

52.1 Answer: D
There is no universally accepted definition of PCS. It is loosely described as a constellation of symptoms occurring in individuals with mild traumatic brain injury (mTBI). The onset and duration of symptoms remain vague, but the DSM-IV states symptom duration of at least 3 months.

Reference: Castillo RJ, Carlat DJ, Millon T, et al. *Diagnostic and Statistical Manual of Mental Disorders.* 4th ed. Washington, DC: American Psychiatric Association Press; 2007.

52.2 Answer: D
Limitations when using diagnostic criteria exist, and strict adherence to these guidelines is not recommended. The most obvious limitation seen is the emphasis of subjective symptoms over objective findings (e.g., neuropsychological tests).

Reference: Smith-Seemiller L, Fow NR, Kant R, et al. Presence of post-concussion syndrome symptoms in patients with chronic pain vs mild traumatic brain injury. *Brain Inj.* 2003;17(3):199-206.

52.3 Answer: B
Prolongation of symptoms however, such as those seen in patients with PCS, are thought to be perpetuated by early psychological distress, preexisting mental health disorders, and mental health sequalae. Several studies have suggested early psychological factors also play an important etiological role in PCS.

References: Silverberg ND, Iverson GL. Etiology of the post-concussion syndrome: physiogenesis and psychogenesis revisited. *NeuroRehabilitation.* 2011; 29(4):317-329.
Stein MB, Jain S, Giacino JT, et al. Risk of posttraumatic stress disorder and major depression in civilian patients after mild traumatic brain injury: a TRACK-TBI study. *JAMA Psychiatry.* 2019;76(3):249-258.

Chapter 53

53.1 Answer: D
Ischemic stroke is the leading cause of long-term disability in the United States. As such, addressing risk factors is important in preventing new and recurrent strokes. Affecting more than 70% of patients, hypertension is the most common modifiable risk factor for stroke. Other treatable factors that are targets for stroke prevention include hyperlipidemia, diabetes, tobacco abuse, and hypercoagulable disorders. Age is a nonmodifiable risk factor.

Reference: Kernan WN, Ovbiagele B, Black HR, et al. Guidelines for the prevention of stroke in patients with stroke and transient ischemic attack: a guideline for healthcare professionals from the American Heart Association/American Stroke Association. *Stroke.* 2014;45(7):2160-2236.

53.2 Answer: A
Acute stroke management guidelines recommend early use of tissue plasminogen activator (tPA) to help with early reperfusion of ischemic brain. MRI is helpful in diagnosing subtle, early stroke not seen

on CT imaging, but imaging should not delay administration of tPA. Aside from glucose testing, laboratory testing is not prioritized over tPA administration, and it is assumed that most individuals do not have bleeding tendencies. Although pressure management is part of acute stroke management, treatment with thrombolytics are prioritized if systolic pressures are less than 185 and diastolic pressures are less than 110.

Reference: Powers WJ, Rabinstein AA, Ackerson T, et al. 2018 Guidelines for the Early management of patients with acute ischemic stroke: a guideline for healthcare professionals from the American Heart Association/American Stroke Association. *Stroke.* 2018;49(3):e46-e99.

53.3   Answer: C
Common presenting symptoms of meningitis are fever, headache, light sensitivity, and stiff neck. Because of the risk of mortality, early diagnosis is essential and urgent lumbar puncture with cerebrospinal fluid analysis and culture is indicated for diagnosis of suspected meningitis. IV antibiotics should be initiated after lumbar puncture. CT and MRI are indicated if clinical presentation suggests contraindication to lumbar puncture, if focal neurological deficits, seizures.

Reference: National Institute of Neurological Disorders and Stroke. Meningitis and Encephalitis Fact Sheet. 2018. Available at: https://www.ninds.nih.gov/Disorders/Patient-Caregiver-Education/Fact-Sheets/Meningitis-and-Encephalitis-Fact-Sheet. Accessed January 15, 2019.

Chapter 54

54.1   Answer: C
Radiological findings consistent with mild and moderate TBIs, in particular findings of contusions, may be missed in up to 67% of scans, especially when the scans are read by inexperienced radiologists.[13] (Kushner Alvarez). MRI scans may reveal abnormalities for up to 2 to 3 months after brain trauma. Included findings are consistent with areas of axonal shear injury and/or small contusions or hemorrhages.

54.2   Answer: C
The combination of SCI and concomitant TBI is associated with alcohol consumption.

54.3   Answer: D
The strongest diagnostic information comes from clinical neurological indices (GCS score,[41] PTA,[42] LOC[43]) taken at the scene of the accident and at the emergency department.

Chapter 55

55.1   Answer: C
Myoclonic status epilepticus is a reflection of severe brain injury rather than a treatable entity. It indicates a very poor prognosis.

Anoxic duration of greater than 8 to 10 minutes and CPR duration of greater than 30 minutes are indicators of poor prognosis. EEG with a nonreactive background, burst suppression, and generalized epileptiform activity also indicate poor prognostic outcome.

Reference: Fugate, JE, Wijdicks, EFM. Anoxic-ischemic encephalopathy. In: Flemming KD, Jones LK, eds. *Mayo Clinic Neurology Board Review: Clinical Neurology for Initial Certification and MOC.* Oxford University Press; 2015:35-38.

55.2   Answer: D
Favorable EEG patterns after a traumatic brain injury (TBI) include normal activity, rhythmic theta activity, frontal rhythmic delta activity, and spindle pattern.

On the other hand, nonreactive background, low-amplitude delta activity, nonreactive, and burst suppression patterns are associated with poor prognosis.

Reference: Lew HL, Lee RD, Pan SSL, et al. Electrophysiologic assessment techniques: evoked potentials and electroencephalography. In: Zasler, ND, Katz DI, Zafonte RD, eds. *Brain Injury Medicine: Principles and Practice.* New York, NY: Demos; 2007:159.

55.3   Answer: A
Man-in-a-barrel syndrome is a result of an infarction between the ACA and MCA that results in bilateral upper extremity paresis with preserved lower extremity function.

Balint syndrome is infarction between the MCA and PCA with asimultagnosia, optic ataxia, and ocular apraxia. There is no syndrome that results between the ACA and ICA or PCA and basilar artery.

Reference: Fugate, JE, Wijdicks, EFM. Anoxic-ischemic encephalopathy. In: Flemming KD, Jones LK, eds. *Mayo Clinic Neurology Board Review: Clinical Neurology for Initial Certification and MOC.* Oxford University Press; 2015:35-38.

Chapter 56

56.1   Answer: C
Choice C reflects a patient in MCS (as evidenced by the presence of arousal and awareness). The patient is in MCS *plus* because he demonstrates language-mediated abilities. He displays receptive language ability to understand a command to move his right hand and expressive language ability to verbalize "yes" or "no" when questioned. There is no evidence that the patient has emerged from MCS because he is not able to correctly

answer simple "yes" or "no" questions consistently. Choice A describes a patient in MCS minus; choice B, a patient who has emerged from MCS; choice D, a patient in VS; and choice E, a comatose patient.[3]

56.2 Answer: A
Coma is a self-limited state that rarely lasts beyond 4 weeks. Choices B, C, and D describe states that can persist indefinitely.[3]

56.3 Answer: D
Numerous studies have documented that at least one-third of patients diagnosed as being in a vegetative state are in fact conscious.[6]

Chapter 57

57.1 Answer: B
Explanation: CAM use among adults is greater among women and those with higher levels of education and higher incomes, and use of CAM has been generally increasing over the past decade.

Reference: Clarke TC, Barnes PM, Black LI, et al. Use of yoga, meditation, and chiropractors among U.S. adults aged 18 and over. *NCHS Data Brief.* 2018;325:1-8.

57.2 Answer: D
Based on data from 2012, natural products including nonvitamin and nonmineral supplements were the most commonly used form of CAM.

Reference: Clarke TC, Black LI, Stussman BJ, et al. Trends in the use of complementary health approaches among adults: United States, 2002 - 2012. *Natl Health Stat Report.* 2015;79:1-16.

57.3 Answer: D
American Indian/Alaska Native population has the highest use of CAM modalities.

Reference: Barnes PM, Bloom B, Nahin R. Complementary and alternative medicine use among adults and children: United States, 2007. *Natl Health Stat Report.* 2008;12:1-23.

Chapter 58

58.1 Answer: B
DBS is not FDA approved for dystonia, but it does have humanitarian device exemption for dystonia and OCD, which is not the same status as FDA device approval but does make it easier to access for off-label and investigational use. DBS is FDA approved for parkinsonian tremor and essential tremor and has been used in other movement disorders as investigational or off label. In terms DoC, a systematic review looking at 78 cases in 19 articles concluded that no clear evidence exists to support DBS for restoration of consciousness or communication in DoC patients and that in cases where benefit was reported, spontaneous recovery was too confounding

58.2 Answer: D
Several TMS devices are FDA approved for treating depression. A 2014 European expert panel published evidence-based guidelines ascribing level A evidence (definite efficacy) to the antidepressant effect of high frequency, repetitive TMS (HFrTMS) on the left dorsolateral prefrontal cortex (DLPFC). Left cervical vagus nerve stimulation is an approved therapy for epilepsy and treatment-resistant depression, but its treatment efficacy for depression has been called into question. The nVNS device is the only device that is FDA approved for acute and preventive use in cluster headache and that has strong evidence to suggest efficacy in acute and preventive treatment of migraine. It is not being used for depression.

58.3 Answer: C
Although some reports have suggested that ITB is helpful in PSH, this is not an approved indication.

Chapter 59

59.1 Answer: B
Hydrocodone has no known effect on seizures. Gabapentin is an antiepileptic. Methylphenidate has not demonstrated an increased risk of seizures in the studies that have been conducted on traumatic brain injury (TBI) patients.

59.2 Answer: D
Immediate seizures do not require more than 1 week of prophylactic medication, and levetiracetam and valproic acid are less cognitively limiting than phenytoin.

59.3 Answer: A
Carbamazepine may be effective for both her epilepsy and her trigeminal neuralgia.

Chapter 60

60.1 Answer: B
A 2015 NINDS/NIBIB consensus meeting produced general agreement that irregular tau deposition in the perivascular spaces within sulcal depths was specific to CTE and differentiated the disease from other tauopathies.

The incorrect responses are more characteristic of other neurodegenerative diseases: choice A of Alzheimer's disease, C of Lewy body/Parkinson's disease, and D of frontotemporal lobar degeneration.

Reference: McKee AC, Cairns NJ, Dickson DW, et al. The first NINDS/NIBIB consensus meeting to define neuropathological criteria for the diagnosis of chronic traumatic encephalopathy. *Acta Neuropathol.* 2016;131(1):75-86.

60.2   Answer: A

The largest CTE case series to date, including 177 retired professional football players, showed that 61% of cases had either diffuse or neuritic Aβ plaques, 48% had TDP-43, and 24% had α-synuclein. Mixed pathology frequency increased with age and CTE severity. Overall, 98 of the 177 cases (55%) were considered "pure CTE."

References: Mez J, Daneshvar DH, Kiernan PT, et al. Clinicopathological evaluation of chronic traumatic encephalopathy in players of American football. *JAMA.* 2017;318(4):360-370.
Stein TD, Montenigro PH, Alvarez VE, et al. Beta-amyloid deposition in chronic traumatic encephalopathy. *Acta Neuropathol.* 2015;130(1):21-34.

60.3   Answer: D

There is a consistent (though not yet causal) link between cumulative exposure to *both* repeated concussion and persistent subclinical head impacts, such as those routinely occurring in certain collision sports and military activities. Individual tolerability differences and a dose-response understanding remain elusive. Ongoing research may ultimately suggest that answers A–C also confer some increased relative risk for neurodegenerative pathology. However, findings from selected—albeit biased—case series to date indicate that choice D is the strongest relative risk factor for CTE pathology.

References: Bieniek KF, Ross OA, Cormier KA, et al. Chronic traumatic encephalopathy pathology in a neurodegenerative disorders brain bank. *Acta Neuropathol.* 2015;130(6):877-889.
Johnson VE, Stewart W, Smith DH, et al. Traumatic brain injury and amyloid-β pathology: a link to Alzheimer's disease? *Nat Rev Neurosci.* 2010;11(5):361-370.

Chapter 61

61.1   Answer: C

Power is the ability to reject a false null hypothesis. Power is (1-beta) where beta is the risk of a type II error. By increasing beta, power is decreased. Increasing sample size, increasing significance level (alpha), and increasing effect size are all ways of increasing power.

61.2   Answer: B

The mean is the mathematic average of the numbers (90 + 100 + 105 + 110 + 110)/5 = 103. The median is the middle value = 105. The mode is the most frequent value = 110.

61.3   Answer: D

Not rejecting a true null hypothesis is making the correct decision. A type I error is when a true null hypothesis is rejected (i.e., when the experimental hypothesis is said to be correct when in fact it is not). A type II error is when a false null hypothesis is not rejected (i.e., when the experimental hypothesis is correct, but the difference or association was not found with the data used). A type III error does not exist.

Chapter 62

62.1   Answer: B

Expressive aphasia by itself does not preclude DMC; patients likely can still comprehend information, reason, and express a choice nonverbally. DMC is domain-specific and patients can retain DMC in some domains but not others. Likewise, DMC can be decision specific, and patients retain DMC for some decisions but not others. The healthcare choices of a person with DMC should always be honored, regardless of their diagnosis.

Reference: Kothari S, Kirschner K. Decision-making capacity after brain injury: clinical assessment and ethical implications. In: Zasler N, Katz D, Zafonte R, eds. *Brain Injury Medicine: Principles and Practice.* 1st ed. New York, NY: Demos Medical Pub.; 2006:1205-1222.

62.2   Answer: C

Agreement or disagreement with a clinical recommendation is not directly relevant to the assessment of DMC. DMC is about *how* a patient makes decisions, not *what* they decide.

Reference: Grisso T, Appelbaum PS. *Assessing Competence to Consent to Treatment: a Guide for Physicians and Other Health Professionals.* New York, NY: Oxford University Press; 1998.

62.3   Answer: D

Many jurisdictions limit the scope of decisions that a surrogate decision maker is authorized to make. If the patient has a guardian or had executed a durable power of attorney for healthcare, those individuals supersede next of kin. Surrogates are expected to make decisions as the patient would have wanted them to be made (substituted judgment). Any disagreement surrounding who should serve as a surrogate or the decisions that are made can be brought to the courts.

Reference: Kothari S, Kirschner K. Decision-making capacity after brain injury: clinical assessment and ethical implications. In: Zasler N, Katz D, Zafonte R, eds. *Brain Injury Medicine: Principles and Practice.* 1st ed. New York, NY: Demos Medical Pub.; 2006:1205-1222.

Index

Note: Page numbers followed by "b," "f," and "t" indicate boxes, figures, and tables respectively.